外 泌 体
临床纲要

Exosomes
A Clinical Compendium

主编
Lawrence R. Edelstein
John R. Smythies
Peter J. Quesenberry
Denis Noble

主译
郭尚春　陶诗聪

上海科学技术出版社

图书在版编目（CIP）数据

外泌体：临床纲要 /（美）劳伦斯 R.埃德尔斯坦等主编；郭尚春，陶诗聪主译. -- 上海：上海科学技术出版社，2025.3
书名原文：Exosomes: A Clinical Compendium
ISBN 978-7-5478-6162-2

Ⅰ.①外… Ⅱ.①劳… ②郭… ③陶… Ⅲ.①临床医学－医学检验 Ⅳ.①R446.1

中国国家版本馆CIP数据核字（2023）第070408号

This edition of Exosomes: A Clinical Compendium by Lawrence Edelstein, John Smythies, Peter Quesenberry and Denis Noble is published by arrangement with Elsevier Inc. Suite 800, 230 Park Avenue, New York, NY 10169, USA.
上海市版权局著作权合同登记号　图字：09-2020-505号

外泌体：临床纲要
主编　Lawrence R. Edelstein　John R. Smythies
　　　Peter J. Quesenberry　Denis Noble
主译　郭尚春　陶诗聪

上海世纪出版（集团）有限公司
上海科学技术出版社　出版、发行
（上海市闵行区号景路159弄A座9F-10F）
邮政编码 201101　www.sstp.cn
江阴金马印刷有限公司印刷
开本 787×1092　1/16　印张 23.25
字数 480千字
2025年3月第1版　2025年3月第1次印刷
ISBN 978-7-5478-6162-2/R·2752
定价：198.00元

本书如有缺页、错装或坏损等严重质量问题，请向印刷厂联系调换

Exosomes: A Clinical Compendium, First Edition
Lawrence R. Edelstein, John R. Smythies, Peter J. Quesenberry, Denis Noble
ISBN: 978-0-12-816053-4
Copyright © 2020 Elsevier Inc. All rights reserved.
Authorized Chinese translation published by Shanghai Scientific & Technical Publishers.

《外泌体：临床纲要》（郭尚春、陶诗聪　主译）
ISBN: 978-7-5478-6162-2

Copyright © Elsevier Inc. and Shanghai Scientific & Technical Publishers. All rights reserved.
No part of this publication may be reproduced or transmitted in any form or by any means, electronic or mechanical, including photocopying, recording, or any information storage and retrieval system, without permission in writing from Elsevier Inc. Details on how to seek permission, further information about the Elsevier's permissions policies and arrangements with organizations such as the Copyright Clearance Center and the Copyright Licensing Agency, can be found at our website: www.elsevier.com/permissions.
This book and the individual contributions contained in it are protected under copyright by Elsevier Inc. and Shanghai Scientific & Technical Publishers (other than as may be noted herein).

This edition of Exosomes: A Clinical Compendium is published by Shanghai Scientific & Technical Publishers under arrangement with ELSEVIER INC.
This edition is authorized for sale in China only, excluding Hong Kong, Macao and Taiwan Region. Unauthorized export of this edition is a violation of the Copyright Act. Violation of this Law is subject to Civil and Criminal Penalties.

本版由 ELSEVIER INC. 授权上海科学技术出版社有限公司在中国大陆地区（不包括香港、澳门以及台湾地区）出版发行。
本版仅限在中国大陆地区（不包括香港、澳门以及台湾地区）出版及标价销售。未经许可之出口，视为违反著作权法，将受民事及刑事法律之制裁。
本书封底贴有 Elsevier 防伪标签，无标签者不得销售。

注　意

本书涉及领域的知识和实践标准在不断变化。新的研究和经验拓展我们的理解，因此须对研究方法、专业实践或医疗方法作出调整。从业者和研究人员必须始终依靠自身经验和知识来评估和使用本书中提到的所有信息、方法、化合物或本书中描述的实验。在使用这些信息或方法时，他们应注意自身和他人的安全，包括注意他们负有专业责任的当事人的安全。在法律允许的最大范围内，爱思唯尔、译文的原文作者、原文编辑及原文内容提供者均不对因产品责任、疏忽或其他人身或财产伤害及/或损失承担责任，亦不对由于使用或操作文中提到的方法、产品、说明或思想而导致的人身或财产伤害及/或损失承担责任。

内容提要

外泌体是细胞外囊泡的一种,参与调控重要的细胞生理活动,在免疫应答、炎症反应、血管生成、凋亡、凝血和废物处理等生理过程中发挥了关键作用,是基础与临床研究的热点之一。本书对外泌体的最新研究做了全面的综述,包括外泌体的基础研究、实验室新进展、临床新发现,以及在血液、免疫、泌尿、神经、呼吸、心血管、内分泌等系统疾病诊治中的应用。

本书内容前沿,对外泌体研究相关人员、生物医药基础研究人员、临床研究人员,以及其他对外泌体领域感兴趣的读者都非常有参考价值。

译者名单

主　译　郭尚春　陶诗聪

译　者（按姓氏拼音排序）
　　　　　白翔宇　重庆医科大学附属第一医院
　　　　　曹建平　中国疾病预防控制中心寄生虫病预防控制所
　　　　　陈金梅　上海交通大学医学院附属第六人民医院
　　　　　陈书瑶　上海交通大学医学院
　　　　　陈小华　上海交通大学医学院附属第六人民医院
　　　　　崔国红　上海交通大学医学院附属第九人民医院
　　　　　邓　辉　上海交通大学医学院附属第六人民医院
　　　　　邓青松　上海交通大学医学院附属第六人民医院
　　　　　董江涛　河北医科大学第三医院
　　　　　高　远　上海交通大学医学院附属第六人民医院
　　　　　高晨珊　上海交通大学医学院附属松江医院
　　　　　关洁莹　广州中医药大学基础医学院
　　　　　郭尚春　上海交通大学医学院附属第六人民医院
　　　　　国海东　上海中医药大学
　　　　　何姝航　上海交通大学医学院附属第六人民医院
　　　　　何耀华　上海交通大学医学院附属第六人民医院
　　　　　侯　磊　上海交通大学医学院附属松江医院
　　　　　胡长平　中南大学湘雅药学院
　　　　　黄　宁　郑州大学第一附属医院
　　　　　黄　扬　上海电力医院
　　　　　黄晶焕　上海交通大学医学院附属第六人民医院
　　　　　李　琦　上海交通大学医学院附属第一人民医院
　　　　　李文哲　太原康明眼科医院
　　　　　李晓林　上海交通大学医学院附属第六人民医院

李旭冉	上海交通大学医学院附属第六人民医院
刘珀霖	上海交通大学医学院附属第六人民医院
陆　健	上海市第八人民医院
覃　丽	湖南中医药大学
沈玉娟	中国疾病预防控制中心寄生虫病预防控制所
沈志翰	上海交通大学医学院附属第六人民医院
宋　伟	上海交通大学医学院附属第六人民医院
陶诗聪	上海交通大学医学院附属第六人民医院
田彬功	上海交通大学医学院附属第一人民医院
田思嫚	河北医科大学第三医院
王　昂	上海交通大学医学院
王　锋	上海交通大学医学院附属第一人民医院
吴家琛	上海交通大学医学院附属第六人民医院
吴若愚	上海交通大学医学院附属仁济医院
吴文灿	温州医科大学
徐泽全	上海交通大学医学院附属第六人民医院
姚　驰	东南大学附属中大医院
余　奇	上海泰和诚肿瘤医院
张　任	江西中医药大学第二附属医院
张光远	东南大学附属中大医院
张文梅	上海交通大学医学院附属第六人民医院
张雅楠	上海交通大学医学院附属松江医院
郑军华	上海交通大学医学院附属仁济医院
周静怡	上海交通大学医学院附属第一人民医院
周晓辉	上海交通大学医学院附属第六人民医院
朱颖婷	中山大学中山眼科中心
庄昊俊	上海交通大学医学院附属第六人民医院

主译简介

郭尚春

医学博士,上海交通大学医学院附属第六人民医院研究员,博士研究生导师。曾于2018年作为访问学者在英国牛津布鲁克斯大学工作一年。主持了4项国家自然科学基金项目,并于2019年入选上海市浦江人才计划,2022年入选上海交通大学医学院"双百人"计划。研究领域主要包括运动系统组织再生与康复治疗新方法。近年来发表21篇SCI期刊论文,获得5项国家发明专利授权,其中1项外泌体相关专利已成功实现了成果转化,此外还参与编写专著1部。担任多个项目评审专家,包括国家自然科学基金、上海市科学技术委员会和上海市体育局项目,同时也是上海市生物医学工程学会生物材料专业委员会、上海市口腔医学会口腔材料专业委员会、国际胞外囊泡协会(ISEV)通讯委员会和国际骨关节炎研究学会(OARSI)通讯委员会的委员。

陶诗聪

医学博士,上海交通大学医学院附属第六人民医院骨科主治医师,上海交通大学医学院青年教师。曾于2019年赴瑞士参加AO Davos Courses进修学习。主持国家自然科学基金青年项目和面上项目各1项,入选2020级上海市"医苑新星"青年医学人才培养资助计划。致力于运动系统疾病的早期诊断和治疗研究。发表SCI期刊论文24篇,并申请了相关专利,目前已获授权12项,其中4项为国家发明专利。担任中国康复医学会康复辅具应用专业委员会副秘书长和青年工作委员会常务委员,同时担任《中华创伤杂志》、*Biomaterials Translational*、*BMEF*以及*Burns & Trauma*等期刊的青年编委。曾先后担任国际骨关节炎研究学会(OARSI)出版委员会(Publication Committee)委员。

主编简介

Lawrence R. Edelstein

美国加州德尔马市 Medimark Corporation 总裁兼创始人。

Lawrence R. Edelstein 博士是一位神经科学家,同时也是制药行业的资深顾问。他的研究领域涵盖多感官融合与整合(屏状核)及细胞间通信(如外泌体和间质细胞)。Edelstein 博士对外泌体的兴趣源自他与 John Smythies 和 Denis Noble 合作编辑的专题期刊 *Epigenetic Information-Processing Mechanisms in the Brain*。这一研究促成了多篇同行评审的论文,Edelstein 博士及其团队在这些论文中深入探讨并理论化了外泌体这一看似无处不在、跨界系的细胞组分所发挥的多样化功能。此外,Edelstein 博士还与 John Smythies 及 Vilayanur S. Ramachandran 合作编著了 *The Claustrum — Structural,Functional and Clinical Neuroscience* 一书[①]。

John Raymond Smythies

John Raymond Smythies,M.B.B. Chir.,M.D.,F.R.C.P.,F.R.C. Psych.(1922—2019),曾任美国加州大学圣地亚哥分校心理学系综合神经科学项目主任,是一位杰出的神经精神病学家和神经科学家,并且在这两个领域均有卓越贡献。他与 Humphry Osmond 共同提出了首个关于精神分裂症的生化理论——甲基转移假说。近年来,随着研究发现精神分裂症中 DNA 甲基化的异常变化,该假说重新引起了科学界的关注。Smythies 教授的研究领域广泛,包括致幻类药物的神经药理学、突触功能的神经解剖学(特别是突触可塑性、内吞作用及氧化还原因素的作用)、儿茶酚胺代谢产物在大脑中的作用,以及大脑与意识关系的理论。Smythies 教授在晚年进一步发展了与外泌体、间质细胞和屏状核功能相关的基础性假设和理论,以及大脑中的表观遗传信息处理机制。Smythies 教授曾担任国际精神神经内分泌学会主席(1970—1974)、世界卫生组织顾问(1963—1968),并长期担任 *International Review of Neurobiology* 编辑(1958—1991)。他于 1968 年当选为雅典娜俱乐部会员。在职业生涯中,他曾任阿拉巴马大学伯明翰分校医学院荣誉教授和 Charles Byron Ireland 精神病学教授,还曾任加州大学圣地亚哥分校大脑与认知中心的访问学者,以及伦敦大学学院神经学研究所的高级研究员。他发表了超过 240 篇科学论文,并著有 16 本专著[②]。

Peter J. Quesenberry

美国罗得岛州人,医学博士,布朗大学沃伦·阿尔伯特医学院 Paul Calabresi 肿瘤学教授。

他在弗吉尼亚大学取得医学学位，随后在大学医院和波士顿市医院完成住院医师培训，并在圣伊丽莎白医院深造，完成了血液/肿瘤学研究员项目。

Quesenberry教授是干细胞生物学和细胞外囊泡研究领域的权威学者。他曾担任国际血液学会主席，并在1990—1998年间担任 Experimental Hematology 期刊主编，以及 Year Book of Hematology 白细胞板块编辑（1987—1998年）。近年来，他还担任 Journal of Extracellular Vesicles 的联合主编，对推动该领域的前沿研究做出了重要贡献。

Denis Noble

英国牛津人，牛津大学生理学、解剖学和遗传学系心血管生理学名誉教授。

Denis Noble，C.B.E.，Ph.D.，F.R.S.是英国著名生理学家和生物学家，曾于1984—2004年担任牛津大学心血管生理学 Burdon Sanderson 教席，现为名誉教授，并兼任计算生理学的联合主任。他是系统生物学领域的开创者之一。

Noble教授在1960年基于与导师 Otto Hutter 的研究，发现了心脏的两种主要钾离子通道，并开发了首个可行的心脏数学模型。这些开创性研究成果分别发表在 Nature（1960年）和 The Journal of Physiology（1962年）上。之后，在与 Dick Tsien、Dario DiFrancesco 和 Don Hilgemann 等人的合作下，这一模型演变成为如今100多种心脏细胞模型的基础。

他于2009年在日本京都举行的国际生理科学联合会（IUPS）大会上当选学会主席，并在2013年于英国伯明翰的大会上连任。作为系统生物学的科普先驱，Noble教授撰写了第一本相关领域的科普书 The Music of Life，近期的演讲主要集中探讨系统生物学对进化生物学的影响。

Noble教授在学术领域建树颇丰，发表了超过500篇论文，并著有11本专著[3]。

---

[1] www.elsevier.com/books/the-claustrum/smythies/978-0-12-404566-8
[2] https://en.wikipedia.org/wiki/John_Raymond_Smythies
[3] https://en.wikipedia.org/wiki/Denis_Noble

编者名单

主编

Lawrence R. Edelstein，John R. Smythies，Peter J. Quesenberry，Denis Noble

编者 括号中的数字为编者编写内容的起始页

Divya Aickara（165），Department of Dermatology and Cutaneous Surgery，University of Miami，Miami，FL，United States

Riccardo Alessandro（1，57），Department of Biomedicine，Neuroscience and Advanced Diagnostics，University of Palermo，Palermo，Italy

Shamila D. Alipoor（261），Molecular Medicine Department，Institute of Medical Biotechnology，National Institute of Genetic Engineering and Biotechnology（NIGEB），Tehran，Iran

Ramaroson Andriantsitohaina（235），SOPAM，U1063，INSERM，UNIV ANGERS，SFR ICAT，Bat IRIS-IBS；Angers University Hospital，Angers，France

Jun Araya（211），Division of Respiratory Diseases，Department of Internal Medicine，The Jikei University School of Medicine，Tokyo，Japan

Koji Asano（71），Department of Urology，Jikei University School of Medicine，Tokyo，Japan

Evangelos Badiavas（165），Department of Dermatology and Cutaneous Surgery，University of Miami，Miami，FL，United States

Matthew A. Bailey（177），University/BHF Centre for Cardiovascular Science，Queen's Medical Research Institute，University of Edinburgh，Edinburgh，United Kingdom

Scott Bonner（196），University of Oxford，Department of Paediatrics，Oxford，United Kingdom

Han Chen（16），Microscopy Imaging Facility，Penn State Hershey Medical Center，Hershey，PA，United States

Yong Cheng（86），Department of Biological Sciences，Eck Institute for Global Health，Center for Rare and Neglected Diseases，University of Notre Dame，Notre Dame，IN，United States

Raul Coimbra（223），Division of Trauma，Surgical Critical Care，Burns and Acute Care Surgery，Department of Surgery，University of California San Diego，San Diego，CA，United States

Alice Conigliaro（1），Department of Biomedicine，Neuroscience and Advanced Diagnostics，University of Palermo，Palermo，Italy

Denis Corbeil（28），Biotechnology Center and Center for Molecular and Cellular Bioengineering，Technische Universität Dresden，Dresden，Germany

Chiara Corrado（1），Department of Biomedicine，Neuroscience and Advanced Diagnostics，University of

Palermo, Palermo, Italy

Todd W. Costantini (223), Division of Trauma, Surgical Critical Care, Burns and Acute Care Surgery, Department of Surgery, University of California San Diego, San Diego, CA, United States

Dragos Cretoiu (138), Department of Cell and Molecular Biology and Histology, Carol Davila University of Medicine and Pharmacy; Alessandrescu-Rusescu National Institute of Mother and Child Health, Fetal Medicine Excellence Research Center, Bucharest, Romania

Sanda Maria Cretoiu (138), Department of Cell and Molecular Biology and Histology, Carol Davila University of Medicine and Pharmacy, Bucharest, Romania

André Cronemberger-Andrade (124), Laboratory of Cellular Immunology and Biochemistry of Fungi and Protozoa, Department of Pharmaceutical Sciences, Federal University of São Paulo (UNIFESP), Diadema, SP, Brazil

James W. Dear (177), University/BHF Centre for Cardiovascular Science, Queen's Medical Research Institute, University of Edinburgh, Edinburgh, United Kingdom

Alexandru Florian Deftu (138), Department of Anatomy, Animal Physiology and Biophysics, Faculty of Biology, University of Bucharest; Life, Environmental and Earth Sciences Division, Research Institute of the University of Bucharest (ICUB), Bucharest, Romania

Antonia Teona Deftu (138), Department of Anatomy, Animal Physiology and Biophysics, Faculty of Biology, University of Bucharest; Life, Environmental and Earth Sciences Division, Research Institute of the University of Bucharest (ICUB), Bucharest, Romania

Shin Egawa (71), Department of Urology, Jikei University School of Medicine, Tokyo, Japan

Brian P. Eliceiri (223), Division of Trauma, Surgical Critical Care, Burns and Acute Care Surgery, Department of Surgery, University of California San Diego, San Diego, CA, United States

Simona Fontana (1), Department of Biomedicine, Neuroscience and Advanced Diagnostics, University of Palermo, Palermo, Italy

Yu Fujita (211), Division of Molecular and Cellular Medicine, National Cancer Center Research Institute; Division of Respiratory Diseases, Department of Internal Medicine, The Jikei University School of Medicine, Tokyo, Japan

Andrew F. Hill (196), La Trobe University, La Trobe Institute for Molecular Science, Melbourne, VIC, Australia

Robert W. Hunter (177), University/BHF Centre for Cardiovascular Science, Queen's Medical Research Institute, University of Edinburgh, Edinburgh, United Kingdom

Tsukasa Kadota (211), Division of Molecular and Cellular Medicine, National Cancer Center Research Institute; Division of Respiratory Diseases, Department of Internal Medicine, The Jikei University School of Medicine, Tokyo, Japan

Ju-Seop Kang (317), Department of Pharmacology & Clinical Pharmacology Lab, College of Medicine, Hanyang University, Seoul, Republic of Korea

Nobuyoshi Kosaka (71, 211, 295), Division of Molecular and Cellular Medicine, National Cancer Center Research Institute; Department of Molecular and Cellular Medicine, Institute of Medical Science;

Department of Translational Research for Extracellular Vesicles, Institute of Medical Science, Tokyo Medical University, Tokyo, Japan

Kazuyoshi Kuwano (211), Division of Respiratory Diseases, Department of Internal Medicine, The Jikei University School of Medicine, Tokyo, Japan

Soazig Le Lay (235), SOPAM, U1063, INSERM, UNIV ANGERS, SFR ICAT, Bat IRIS-IBS, Angers, France

Aurelio Lorico (28), College of Medicine, Touro University Nevada, Henderson, NV, United States; Mediterranean Institute of Oncology, Viagrande, Italy

Imre Mäger (196), University of Oxford, Department of Paediatrics, Oxford, United Kingdom

M. Carmen Martinez (235), SOPAM, U1063, INSERM, UNIV ANGERS, SFR ICAT, Bat IRIS-IBS; Angers University Hospital, Angers, France

Jeffrey D. McBride (165), Department of Dermatology and Cutaneous Surgery, University of Miami, Miami, FL, United States

Esmaeil Mortaz (261), Clinical Tuberculosis and Epidemiology Research Center, National Research Institute of Tuberculosis and Lung Diseases (NRITLD); Department of Immunology, Faculty of Medicine, Shahid Beheshti University of Medical Sciences, Tehran, Iran

Soumyalekshmi Nair (245), Exosome Biology Laboratory, Centre for Clinical Diagnostics, UQ centre for Clinical Research, Royal Brisbane and Women's Hospital, The University of Queensland, St Lucia, QLD, Australia

Denis Noble (329), Department of Physiology, Anatomy & Genetics, University of Oxford, Oxford, United Kingdom

Takahiro Ochiya (71, 211, 295), Division of Molecular and Cellular Medicine, National Cancer Center Research Institute; Department of Molecular and Cellular Medicine, Institute of Medical Science, Tokyo Medical University, Tokyo, Japan

Siew-Wai Pang (103), Department of Medical Sciences, School of Healthcare and Medical Sciences, Sunway University, Petaling Jaya, Malaysia

Beatrice Mihaela Radu (138), Department of Anatomy, Animal Physiology and Biophysics, Faculty of Biology, University of Bucharest; Life, Environmental and Earth Sciences Division, Research Institute of the University of Bucharest (ICUB), Bucharest, Romania

Stefania Raimondo (57), Department of Biomedicine, Neuroscience and Advanced Diagnostics, University of Palermo, Palermo, Italy

Laura Saieva (57), Department of Biomedicine, Neuroscience and Advanced Diagnostics, University of Palermo, Palermo, Italy

Carlos Salomon (245), Exosome Biology Laboratory, Centre for Clinical Diagnostics, UQ centre for Clinical Research, Royal Brisbane and Women's Hospital, The University of Queensland, St Lucia, QLD, Australia; Department of Clinical Biochemistry and Immunology, University of Concepción, Concepción, Chile; Department of Obstetrics and Gynecology, Ochsner Baptist Hospital, New Orleans, LA, United States

Jeffery S. Schorey (86), Department of Biological Sciences, Eck Institute for Global Health, Center for Rare and Neglected Diseases, University of Notre Dame, Notre Dame, IN, United States

Jeffrey M. Sundstrom (16, 283), Department of Ophthalmology, Penn State College of Medicine; Department of Ophthalmology, Penn State Hershey Medical Center, Hershey, PA, United States

Sin-Yeang Teow (103), Department of Medical Sciences, School of Healthcare and Medical Sciences, Sunway University, Petaling Jaya, Malaysia

Ana Claudia Torrecilhas (124), Laboratory of Cellular Immunology and Biochemistry of Fungi and Protozoa, Department of Pharmaceutical Sciences, Federal University of São Paulo (UNIFESP), Diadema, SP, Brazil

Fumihiko Urabe (71), Division of Molecular and Cellular Medicine, National Cancer Center Research Institute; Department of Urology, Jikei University School of Medicine, Tokyo, Japan

Sarah R. Weber (16, 283), Department of Ophthalmology, Penn State College of Medicine; Department of Ophthalmology, Penn State Hershey Medical Center, Hershey, PA, United States

Eduard Willms (196), University of Oxford, Department of Paediatrics, Oxford, United Kingdom

Matthew J. A. Wood (196), University of Oxford, Department of Paediatrics, Oxford, United Kingdom

Patricia Xander (124), Laboratory of Cellular Immunology and Biochemistry of Fungi and Protozoa, Department of Pharmaceutical Sciences, Federal University of São Paulo (UNIFESP), Diadema, SP, Brazil

Junjie Xiao (138), Department of Cardiology, The First Affiliated Hospital of Nanjing Medical University, Nanjing; Cardiac Regeneration and Ageing Lab, Experimental Center of Life Sciences, School of Life Science, Shanghai University, Shanghai, China

Zhongdang Xiao (295), State Key Laboratory of Bioelectronics, School of Biological Science and Medical Engineering, Southeast University, Nanjing, China

Yuanjun Zhao (16, 283), Department of Ophthalmology, Penn State College of Medicine; Department of Ophthalmology, Penn State Hershey Medical Center, Hershey, PA, United States

Mi Zhou (23, 283), Department of Ophthalmology, Penn State College of Medicine; Department of Ophthalmology, Penn State Hershey Medical Center, Hershey, PA, United States

Yueyuan Zhou (295), Division of Molecular and Cellular Medicine, National Cancer Center Research Institute, Tokyo, Japan; State Key Laboratory of Bioelectronics, School of Biological Science and Medical Engineering, Southeast University, Nanjing, China

中文版前言

科学的探索是一场无尽的旅程，每一个发现都有可能引发一场认知的革新，深刻改变我们对世界的理解。在这个旅程中，生物医学研究者们一直在探索新的领域和新的可能性。近年来，一种被称为外泌体的细胞外囊泡，已经逐步成为研究的前沿和热点。这些微小而复杂的外泌体不仅揭示了一种全新的细胞间通信机制，也为我们提供了一种全新的视角去理解生命的运作。更为重要的是，外泌体的研究为疾病的诊断和治疗提供了新的可能性。它们可以携带和传递各种生物分子，包括蛋白质、脂质和RNA，这使得它们在疾病的发生、发展和治疗中扮演了重要的角色。例如，外泌体可以作为生物标志物用于疾病的早期诊断，也可以作为药物的载体用于疾病的治疗。这些都是外泌体研究的重要方向，也是我们未来需要深入探索的领域。

《外泌体：临床纲要》这本书，是对外泌体研究的一次全面梳理，它集结了全球范围内的专家和研究者的智慧，共同探讨外泌体在健康和疾病状态下的作用，以及它们在临床诊断和治疗中的应用。这本书的内容涵盖了外泌体的生物学基础、生物生成和分泌机制、生物功能及在疾病中的作用等多个方面，为读者提供了一个全面的相关知识的汇总，帮助读者更好地理解、研究和应用外泌体。

这本书的中文版由一群专业的译者倾力翻译，他们准确、生动地传达了原文的精髓，使得这本书能够更好地服务于国内同道。他们的辛勤工作，使得这本书的中文版在保持原著精神的同时，也具有了独特的魅力。

科学研究是一场无止境的探索，每一次发现都会带来新的问题和挑战，推动我们不断前行。外泌体的研究，同样充满了未知和可能，它们如同生命的信使，携带着丰富的信息，等待我们去解读。期待随着研究的深入，外泌体能在更多的领域发挥其独特的作用，为人类的健康和福祉做出更大的贡献。这是我们对科学进步的一次重要期待，也是我们对未来的一次重要展望。

最后，我要向每一位读者表示最深的感谢。是你们的热情关注和坚定支持，让我们有动力去完成这本书的翻译工作，将这个重要的科学领域的知识带给更多的人。你们的每一次阅读，每一次分享，都是对我们工作的肯定和鼓励。希望这本书能为你们的学习和研究带来帮助，能够启发你们的思考，激发你们的灵感。期待你们能够在科研的道路上取得更大的成就，无论是在外泌体的研究领域，还是在其他的科学领域，你们的每一次进步，都是对人类知识的丰富和拓展。

让我们一起探索外泌体的奥秘，揭示生命的秘密。

主　译

英文版前言

短时间内快速增多的期刊文章数量及其引用次数最能清楚地说明某项重大临床和科学发现的预期价值,紧随其后的是在该发现基础上迅速成立生物制药初创企业,并争相用内部开发和引进授权的化合物来补充各自的产品线。一个典型的例子就是外泌体,这是一种看似无处不在、不分门别类的细胞外囊泡,来源于核内体,在细胞间通信的背景下迅速成为焦点,其有效载体包括现成的 miRNA、mRNA、lncRNA 和转录因子。可以说,外泌体最引人注目的方面及存在的原因是其在跨代表观遗传中的作用,这也是我们最后一章的主题。

我关注外泌体的起因是我曾作为客座编辑和我的同事 John Smythies 及 Denis Noble 参与了期刊 *Epigenetic information-processing mechanisms in the brain* 的工作。在该期刊中,我和同事从理论上解释了外泌体在大多数活生物体中发挥了多重功能作用的原因,引发了一系列同行评议文章的发表。经过两年多的努力,我们非常高兴看到这项工作取得的成果。

作为一名神经科学家、作者、编辑和科学类期刊的创始主编,我有一些出版经验,我很快注意到现有外泌体领域资料中还缺少一个多学科组成部分。而目前时机已经成熟,可以出版一本有关外泌体的专著,但实现该目标相当艰巨,我邀请了全球被同行认可的专家医生和众多医学领域的研究人员投稿,每个人在探讨中都有平等的发言权。《外泌体:临床纲要》旨在为读者全面、及时地提供有关外泌体在健康和疾病状态下的信息。在第 21 章,诸位作者总结了最新的实验室和临床发现,阐明了前瞻性研究工作的前进方向。

对于初步接触外泌体的学者,我想说,我认为外泌体是临床诊断、治疗研究的最新方向,欢迎各位尽情探索!对于推进了该领域发展的研究者,外泌体已经并将继续在其临床和研究工作中发挥不可或缺的作用,感谢你们坚持不懈的努力,因为没有你们,这本书就不能完成。

Lawrence Edelstein,Ph.D.

致　谢

在编写这本书的早期,细胞外囊泡的研究,特别是外泌体的研究,一直以惊人的速度加速发展,趋势非常明显。这一点在其对整个医学学科的临床意义上表现得最为显著。首先,我们十分感谢诸位作者,他们都是各自领域公认的专家。我们还要感谢爱思唯尔的编辑不断地提供指导和帮助,特别是 Mica Haley、Tracy Tufaga、Swapna Praveen、Mohana Natarajan、Jyotsna Gopichandran、AndréWolff 和 Jaclyn Truesdell。最后,感谢已故的编者 John Smythies,其在神经编码、修复和同源机制方面发表了一系列文章,提出了有关外泌体和特络细胞存在理由的理论/假说,可以说,如果没有他,这本书不会问世。

特别鸣谢

以此纪念一位绅士般的科学家和最高级别的学者——John Raymond Smythies，M. B. B. Chir. , M. D. , F. R. C. Psych. , F. R. C. P.[①]。

引用 John 于 1946—1949 年间在英国皇家海军志愿预备队担任外科中尉时经常使用的一个英国早期海事短语："一切井然有序，整装待发！"任务圆满完成。

[①] https：// en.wikipedia.org/wiki/John_Raymond_Smythies

常用术语缩略词

ACD	allergic contact dermatitis	变应性接触性皮炎
AF4	asymmetric flow field-flow fractionation	非对称场流分离技术
AFM	atomic force microscopy	原子力显微镜
AIDS	acquired immunodeficiency syndrome	获得性免疫缺陷综合征
AKI	acute kidney injury	急性肾损伤
ALL	acute lymphoblastic leukemia	急性淋巴细胞白血病
ALP	alkaline phosphatase	碱性磷酸酶
ALS	amyotrophic lateral sclerosis	肌萎缩侧索硬化
AMD	age-related macular degeneration	年龄相关性黄斑变性
AMI	acute myocardial infarction	急性心肌梗死
AML	acute myeloid leukemia	急性髓细胞性白血病
Ang	angiopoietin	血管生成素
APC	antigen presenting cell	抗原提呈细胞
APD	action potential duration	动作电位时程
APOBEC3G	apolipoprotein B mRNA-editing enzyme-catalytic polypeptide-like 3G	载脂蛋白 B mRNA 编辑酶催化多肽样 3G
APP	amyloid precursor protein	淀粉样前体蛋白
ARE	antioxidant response element	抗氧化响应元件
AREG	amphiregulin	双调蛋白
ARMM	ARRDC1-mediated microvesicle	含 arrestin 结构域的蛋白 1 介导的微泡
ARRDC1	arrestin domain-containing protein 1	含 arrestin 结构域的蛋白 1
ART	antiretroviral therapy	抗反转录病毒治疗
ASC	adipose derived multipotent stem cell	脂肪来源多能干细胞
ASMC	airway smooth muscle cell	气道平滑肌细胞
BALF	bronchoalveolar lavage fluid	支气管肺泡灌洗液
BBB	blood-brain barrier	血脑屏障
BEC	bronchial epithelial cell	支气管上皮细胞
BM	bone marrow	骨髓
BMDC	bone marrow-derived dendritic cell	骨髓源性树突状细胞
BMMC	bone marrow-derived mast cell	骨髓源性肥大细胞
BPD	bronchopulmonary dys plasia	支气管肺发育不良

BPH	benign hyperplasia	前列腺良性增生
Bro1/Alix	BCK1-like resistance to osmotic shock protein-1/apoptosis linked gene 2 interacting protein X	BCK1样抗渗透压休克蛋白-1/凋亡相关基因-2相互作用蛋白 X
CA19-9	carbohydrate antigen 19-9	糖类抗原19-9
CCL2	C-C motif chemokine ligand 2	C-C基序趋化因子配体2
CDS	cytosolic DNA sensors	胞质 DNA 传感器
CEA	carcinoembryonic antigen	癌胚抗原
CFH	complement factor H	补体因子 H
CFP	culture filtrate protein	培养滤液蛋白
CFTR	cystic fibrosis transmembrane conductance regulator	囊性纤维化跨膜传导调节蛋白
circRNA	circular RNA	环状 RNA
CKD	chronic kidney disease	慢性肾脏疾病
CLL	chronic lymphocytic leukemia	慢性淋巴细胞白血病
CLR	C-type lectin receptor	C 型凝集素受体
CML	chronic myeloid leukemia	慢性髓细胞性白血病
CNS	central nervous system	中枢神经系统
CRPC	castration-resistant prostate cancer	去势抵抗型前列腺癌
Cryo-EM	cryogenic electron microscopy	冷冻电子显微镜
CSF	cerebrospinal fluid	脑脊液
CTSK	cathepsin K	组织蛋白酶 K
DC	dendritic cell	树突状细胞
DGK α	diacylglycerol kinase α	二酰甘油激酶 α
DNA	deoxyribonucleic acid	脱氧核糖核酸
DR	diabetic retinopathy	糖尿病视网膜病变
DRE	digital rectal examination	直肠指检
dsDNA	double-stranded DNA	双链 DNA
EAE	experimental autoimmune encephalomyelitis	实验性自身免疫性脑脊髓炎
ECM	extracellular matrix	细胞外基质
ECP	eosinophil cationic protein	嗜酸性粒细胞阳离子蛋白
EDE	erythrocytes-derived exosomes	红细胞衍生外泌体
EDN	eosinophil-derived neurotoxin	嗜酸性粒细胞衍生神经毒素
EE	early endosomes	早期内体
EGFR	epidermal growth factor receptor	表皮生长因子受体
ELISA	enzyme-linked immunosorbent assay	酶联免疫吸附试验
EMTU	epithelial mesenchymal trophic unit	上皮-间充质营养单位
EPC	endothelial progenitor cell	内皮祖细胞
EPO	eosinophil peroxidase	嗜酸性粒细胞过氧化物酶

EPX	eosinophil peroxidase	嗜酸性粒细胞过氧化物酶
ESCRT	endosomal sorting complex request for transport	内吞体分选转运复合体
EV	extracellular vesicle	胞外囊泡
FGF	fibroblast growth factor	成纤维细胞生长因子
GA	geographic atrophy	地图状萎缩
GBM	glioblastoma multiforme	胶质母细胞瘤
GFAP	glial fibrillar acidic protein	胶质纤维酸性蛋白
GFP	green fluorescent protein	绿色荧光蛋白
GMP	good manufacturing practices	良好操作规范
GPX1	glutathione peroxidase 1	谷胱甘肽过氧化物酶1
GvHD	graft-versus-host disease	移植物抗宿主病
HF	heart failure	心力衰竭
HGF	hepatocyte growth factor	肝细胞生长因子
HIF	hypoxia-inducible factor	缺氧诱导因子
hnRNPA2B1	heterogeneous nuclear ribonucleoprotein A2B1	异质核糖核蛋白A2B1
hnRNP	heterogeneous nuclear ribonucleoprotein	异质核糖核蛋白
HRS	hepatocyte growth factor regulated tyrosine kinase substrate	肝细胞生长因子调节的酪氨酸激酶底物
HSC	hematopoietic stem cell	造血干细胞
HSP	heat shock protein	热休克蛋白
IBD	inflammatory bowel disease	炎症性肠病
IFN	interferon	干扰素
IGF-IR	insulin-like growth factor 1 receptor	胰岛素样生长因子1受体
IL	interleukin	白细胞介素
ILV	intraluminal vesicle	管腔内囊泡
IMTP	ischemic myocardium-targeting peptide	缺血心肌靶向肽
INM	inner nuclear membranes	核内膜
IPF	idiopathic pulmonary fibrosis	特发性肺纤维化
IRD	inherited retinal degenerations	遗传性视网膜变性
IUGR	intrauterine growth restriction	宫内生长受限
LAMP2A	lysosome associated membrane protein 2A	溶酶体相关膜蛋白2A
LFIA	lateral flow immunoassay	侧流免疫层析法
lncRNA	long non-coding RNA	长链非编码RNA
LPG	lipophosphoglycan	磷酸酯多糖
LPS	lipopolysaccharide	脂多糖
LTR	long-tandem repeats	长串联重复序列
M/XDR-TB	multidrug-resistant and extensively drug-resistant TB	耐多药和广泛耐药结核病

MAGE	melanoma-associated antigen	黑色素瘤相关抗原
MAPK	mitogen-activated protein kinase	丝裂原活化蛋白激酶
MBP	major basic protein	主要碱性蛋白
MCP-1	monocyte chemotactic protein-1	单核细胞趋化蛋白-1
MDSC	myeloid-derived suppressor cell	髓源性抑制细胞
MDS	myelodysplastic syndromes	骨髓增生异常综合征
MenSC	menstrual blood-derived stem cell	经血来源的干细胞
MHC	major histocompatibility complex	主要组织相容性复合物
miRNA	micro RNA	微小 RNA
ML	mesenteric lymph	肠系膜淋巴
MLN	mesenteric lymph node	肠系膜淋巴结
MM	multiple myeloma	多发性骨髓瘤
MMP	matrix metalloproteinase	基质金属蛋白酶
MR	mannose receptor	甘露糖受体
mRNA	messenger RNA	信使 RNA
MRP1	multidrug resistance-associated protein 1	多药耐药相关蛋白 1
MS	mass spectrometry	质谱分析技术
MS	multiple sclerosis	多发性硬化
MSC	mesenchymal stem cell	间充质干细胞
mtDNA	mitochondrial DNA	线粒体 DNA
MVB	multivesicular bodies	多囊体
MyD88	myeloid differentiation primary response protein 88	髓系分化主要反应蛋白 88
NAE	envelope-associated endosome	核膜相关早期内体
N-ALE	nuclear envelope invagination-associated late endosome	核膜内陷相关晚期内体
NCG	non-caseating granuloma	非干酪样肉芽肿
NDE	neuron-derived exosome	神经源性外泌体
NGF	nerve growth factor	神经生长因子
NK	natural killer	自然杀伤
NPS	natriuretic peptide system	利尿钠肽系统
Nrf2	nuclear factor erythroid 2-related factor 2	核因子 2 相关因子 2
NTA	nanoparticle tracking analysis	纳米颗粒跟踪分析技术
NV	neovascularization	新生血管
OB	osteoblast	成骨细胞
OC	osteoclast	破骨细胞
OMC	oncosuppressor-mutated cell	肿瘤抑制突变细胞
ONM	outer nuclear membranes	核外膜
PAMP	pathogen-associated molecular pattern	病原体相关分子模式

PA	phosphatidic acid	磷脂酸
PBMC	peripheral blood mononuclear cell	外周血单个核细胞
PCA	principle component analysis	主成分分析
PD-1	programmed death 1	程序性死亡 1
PDCD4	programmed cell death 4	程序性细胞死亡 4
PDGF	platelet-derived growth factor	血小板衍生生长因子
PD-L1	programmed death-ligand 1	程序性死亡配体-1
PDR	proliferative diabetic retinopathy	增生型糖尿病视网膜病变
PEDF	pigment epithelium-derived factor	色素上皮衍生因子
PGE2	prostaglandin E2	前列腺素 E2
PI3P	phosphatidyl inositol monophosphate	磷脂酰肌醇一磷酸
piRNA	p-element-induced wimpy testis-interacting RNA	PIWI 相互作用 RNA
PLD2	phospholipase D2	磷脂酶 D2
PMN	pre-metastatic niche	转移前生态位
PMV	platelet-derived exosome	血小板衍生外泌体
PPCM	peripartum cardiomyopathy	围生期心肌病
PRR	pattern recognition receptor	模式识别受体
PSA	prostate-specific antigen	前列腺特异性抗原
PSCA	prostate stem cell antigen	前列腺干细胞抗原
PTEN	phosphatase and tensin homolog	磷酸酶张力蛋白同源物
qRT-PCR	quantitative reverse transcription polymerase chain reaction	定量逆转录聚合酶链反应
RAAS	renin-angiotensin-aldosterone system	肾素-血管紧张素-醛固酮系统
RARβ	retinoic acid receptor β	视黄酸受体 β
RDEB	recessive dystrophic epidermolysis bullosa	隐性营养不良型大疱性表皮松解症
RGC	retinal ganglion cell	视网膜神经节细胞
RIG1	retinoic acid-inducible gene 1 protein	维 A 酸诱导基因 1 蛋白
RISC	RNA-induced silencing complex	RNA 诱导沉默复合体
Rlc	RISC-loading complex	RISC 负载复合物
RNAi	RNA interference	RNA 干扰
ROS	reactive oxygen species	活性氧
RPE	retinal pigment epithelium	视网膜色素上皮
rRNA	ribosomal RNA	核糖体 RNA
S1P	sphingosine 1-phosphate	一磷酸鞘氨醇
SASP	senescence associated secretory phenotype	衰老相关分泌表型
SDF-1	stromal-derived growth factor-1	基质衍生生长因子-1
SEC	sinusoidal endothelial cell	肝窦内皮细胞
SEM	scanning electron microscopy	扫描电子显微镜
SERS	surface-enhanced Raman spectroscopy	表面增强拉曼光谱

Smases	neutral sphingomyelinases	中性鞘磷脂酶
snoRNA	small nucleolar RNA	小核仁 RNA
snRNA	small nuclear RNA	小核 RNA
SOCS	suppressor of cytokine signaling	细胞因子信号传送阻抑物
SOD1	superoxide dismutase 1	超氧化物歧化酶 1
SRA	serum resistance-associated protein	血清耐药相关蛋白
SRP	signal recognition particle	信号识别颗粒
ssDNA	single-stranded DNA	单链 DNA
STAM1/2	signal transducing adaptor molecule 1/2	信号转导调节分子 1/2
STAR	signaling transduction and activation of RNA	RNA 信号转导和激活蛋白
SUMO-1	small ubiquitin-like modifier type 1	小泛素样修饰物 1
TAM	tumor-associated macrophage	肿瘤相关巨噬细胞
TBI	traumatic brain injury	颅脑损伤
TDE	tumor-derived exosome	肿瘤源性外泌体
TEM	transmission electron microscopy techniques	透射电子显微技术
TERF1	telomeric repeat-binding factor 1	端粒重复结合因子 1
TGF-β	transforming growth factor beta	转化生长因子 β
TIMP	tissue inhibitor of metalloproteinase	组织金属蛋白酶抑制物
TLR	Toll-like receptor	Toll 样受体
TMPRSS2	type 2 transmembrane serine protease	2 型跨膜丝氨酸蛋白酶
TNF	tumor necrosis factor	肿瘤坏死因子
TRAIL	TNF-related apoptosis-inducing ligand	肿瘤坏死因子相关凋亡诱导配体
TRAP	tartrate-resistant acid phosphatase	抗酒石酸酸性磷酸酶
Treg	regulatory T cell	调节性 T 细胞
TSA	trichostatin A	曲古抑菌素 A
Tsg101	tumor susceptibility gene 101	肿瘤易感基因 101
UHG	uniquely human gene	独特人类基因
UPR	unfolded protein response	未折叠蛋白反应
VAMP7	vesicle associated membrane protein 7	囊泡有关的膜蛋白 7
VEGF	vascular endothelial growth factor	血管内皮生长因子
VSMC	vascular smooth muscle cell	血管平滑肌细胞
VSP	variable surface protein	可变表面蛋白
YBX1	Y-box protein Ⅰ	Y-框蛋白 Ⅰ

目 录

第1章 外泌体的基本机制
  Exosome basic mechanisms ·········· 1
 一、外泌体的生物合成及释放 ·········· 1
 二、ESCRT及其在外泌体生物合成中的作用 ·········· 1
 三、ESCRT非依赖的外泌体生物合成机制 ·········· 3
 四、MVB向质膜转运并释放外泌体 ·········· 4
 五、基础成分和货物 ·········· 6
 六、作用机制 ·········· 9

第2章 外泌体分离方法及表征
  Methods for exosome isolation and characterization ·········· 16
 一、概述 ·········· 16
 二、外泌体分离方法 ·········· 17
 三、外泌体表征方法 ·········· 20
 四、外泌体货物 ·········· 23
 五、总结 ·········· 25

第3章 实体瘤中的外泌体、微泡及其伴侣
  Exosomes, microvesicles, and their friends in solid tumors ·········· 28
 一、概述 ·········· 28
 二、(肿瘤)细胞来源胞外囊泡的细胞摄取 ·········· 29
 三、胞外囊泡和肿瘤微环境 ·········· 33
 四、抗肿瘤药物的环境分类和致癌性——对胞外囊泡的影响 ·········· 39
 五、胞外囊泡的临床应用 ·········· 40
 六、基于胞外囊泡的临床肿瘤治疗研究 ·········· 47
 七、总结与展望 ·········· 47
 致谢 ·········· 48

第4章 血液系统恶性肿瘤：外泌体在肿瘤进展中的作用
　　　　Hematologic malignancies: The exosome contribution in tumor progression ········ 57
　一、血液系统恶性肿瘤与肿瘤微环境 ·· 57
　二、胞外囊泡对造血的生理调节和病理改变 ·· 57
　三、胞外囊泡介导的内皮重构 ·· 59
　四、胞外囊泡对骨髓基质细胞的重编程 ·· 60
　五、胞外囊泡改变骨稳态 ·· 61
　六、胞外囊泡调节免疫细胞的功能 ·· 62
　七、胞外囊泡介导耐药性 ·· 66
　八、外泌体在疾病诊断和药物治疗监测中的临床意义 ·································· 66
　九、总结 ·· 67
　致谢 ·· 67
　利益冲突 ·· 67

第5章 前列腺小体的生理和病理功能：从基础研究到临床应用
　　　　Physiological and pathological functions of prostasomes: From basic
　　　　research to clinical application ·· 71
　一、概述 ·· 71
　二、前列腺上皮细胞：前列腺小体的起源 ·· 72
　三、前列腺小体的生理功能 ·· 73
　四、前列腺肿瘤来源的前列腺小体 ·· 76
　五、前列腺小体的病理学功能 ·· 77
　六、前列腺小体的临床应用：前列腺癌的生物治疗 ···································· 78
　七、总结 ·· 82
　致谢 ·· 82
　利益冲突 ·· 82

第6章 外泌体在细菌感染中的作用和治疗应用
　　　　The function and therapeutic use of exosomes in bacterial infections ··········· 86
　一、概述 ·· 86
　二、胞外囊泡 ·· 86
　三、外泌体合成 ·· 88
　四、胞外囊泡、病原体和感染性疾病 ·· 89
　五、外泌体和胞外囊泡在分枝杆菌感染中的组成和功能 ······························ 90
　六、外泌体和胞外囊泡在其他细菌感染中的组成和功能 ······························ 93
　七、胞外囊泡作为预防细菌感染的疫苗 ·· 95
　八、胞外囊泡作为药物传递系统 ·· 96

九、外泌体作为传染病诊断的生物标志物 ································· 97
十、总结 ··· 98

第 7 章 外泌体在 HIV-1 感染中的新兴治疗作用
Emerging therapeutic roles of exosomes in HIV-1 infection ················· 103
一、概述 ··· 103
二、外泌体与 HIV-1：鸡还是蛋？ ······································ 103
三、外泌体对 HIV-1 的双刃剑作用 ······································ 104
四、外泌体与自噬 ··· 106
五、外泌体作为 HIV-1 的生物标志物 ···································· 107
六、靶向外泌体的治疗潜力 ··· 109
七、经验教训 ·· 113
八、总结 ··· 117

第 8 章 寄生虫病胞外囊泡
Extracelluar vesicels in parasitic disease ································· 124
一、胞外囊泡和寄生虫 ··· 124
二、利什曼原虫 ·· 124
三、克氏锥虫 ·· 127
四、布氏锥虫 ·· 129
五、疟原虫 ··· 130
六、刚地弓形虫 ·· 131
七、十二指肠贾第虫 ··· 132
八、总结 ··· 132

第 9 章 外泌体作为心脑血管疾病的细胞间通信信使
Exosomes as intercellular communication messengers for cardiovascular and cerebrovascular diseases ································· 138
一、概述 ··· 138
二、外泌体的产生和释放 ·· 139
三、外泌体表征及研究和分析方法 ······································ 142
四、外泌体与冠状动脉疾病 ··· 144
五、心肌缺血和梗死中的外泌体 ·· 145
六、心力衰竭中的外泌体 ·· 147
七、外泌体在心肌肥厚中的作用 ·· 151
八、外泌体在心律失常中的作用 ·· 151
九、外泌体在脑血管疾病中的作用 ······································ 152

十、总结 ··· 155

第 10 章　皮肤生物学和皮肤病中的外泌体
Exosomes in cutaneous biology and dermatologic disease ············· 165

一、角质形成细胞是上层皮肤的主要细胞，分泌外泌体调节黑素细胞产生的
色素 ··· 165

二、角质形成细胞和免疫系统外泌体调节修饰细胞外基质蛋白质的成纤维细胞
表达 ··· 167

三、角质形成细胞外泌体可调控免疫系统 ·· 168

四、真皮成纤维细胞，特别是真皮乳头细胞，分泌外泌体刺激毛囊生长的阶段称为
生长期 ··· 169

五、纤维化疾病使成纤维细胞外泌体表达失调 ·· 169

六、含有磷脂酶活性的肥大细胞刺激朗格汉斯细胞将脂质抗原提呈给 T 细胞 ······ 170

七、大疱性类天疱疮患者体液中的外泌体增强病原性炎症 ······························ 171

八、皮肤修复 ··· 171

九、与外泌体相关的细胞间黏附分子如恶性细胞分泌的桥粒黏蛋白能调节细胞外
环境促进肿瘤进展 ··· 173

十、外泌体对恶性黑色素瘤的发病机制起重要作用 ·································· 173

十一、外泌体的循环信号存在于转移性鳞状细胞癌，特别是在隐性营养不良型大疱性
表皮松解症患者中 ··· 174

十二、黑色素瘤患者血液循环中的外泌体标志转移和预后恶化 ························· 175

十三、总结 ··· 175

第 11 章　泌尿系统中的外泌体
Exosomes in nephrology ·· 177

一、概述 ··· 177

二、尿液外泌体 ··· 178

三、外泌体用作生物标志物 ·· 181

四、外泌体在肾脏与尿路中的生物学作用 ·· 184

五、外泌体疗法的潜在应用 ·· 188

六、总结 ··· 189

第 12 章　神经退行性疾病中的胞外囊泡
Extracellular vesicles in neurodegenerative disorders ····················· 196

一、概述 ··· 196

二、胞外囊泡介导健康的中枢神经系统维护 ·· 198

三、神经退行性疾病中的胞外囊泡 ·· 199

四、总结 ·· 205

第 13 章　纤维化疾病中的胞外囊泡：纤维化诊断和治疗的新应用
　　Extracellular vesicles in fibrotic diseases: New applications for fibrosis
　　diagnosis and treatment ··· 211
　　一、概述 ·· 211
　　二、纤维化机制 ·· 212
　　三、胞外囊泡在器官纤维化发病机制中的作用 ··· 212
　　四、胞外囊泡在纤维性疾病诊断中的作用 ·· 215
　　五、胞外囊泡作为纤维化治疗的新应用 ··· 217
　　六、总结和展望 ·· 219
　　致谢 ··· 219

第 14 章　炎症疾病中外泌体介导的免疫细胞信号交流机制
　　Mechanisms of exosome-mediated immune cell crosstalk in inflammation
　　and disease ··· 223
　　一、在免疫细胞相互作用过程中外泌体的转运参与炎症反应 ····································· 223
　　二、外泌体生物发生和分泌途径与健康和疾病的相关性 ·· 224
　　三、疾病中体内释放外泌体的机制 ·· 225
　　四、肿瘤学中的外泌体和免疫检查点抑制 ·· 225
　　五、外泌体在创伤与缺血/再灌注损伤中的作用 ··· 226
　　六、外泌体与炎症性肠病 ·· 227
　　七、外泌体与伤口愈合 ··· 227
　　八、外泌体与糖尿病 ·· 228
　　九、外泌体释放的物种特异性机制的潜力 ·· 228
　　十、外泌体和技术驱动的进步 ·· 229
　　十一、总结 ··· 229

第 15 章　代谢综合征中的外泌体
　　Exosomes in metabolic syndrome ··· 235
　　一、概述 ·· 235
　　二、MetS 的不同组分 ·· 235
　　三、胞外囊泡：MetS 成分的生物标志物 ·· 237
　　四、胞外囊泡：MetS 的生物学效应 ··· 239
　　五、外泌体作为宿主与微生物群之间新的交流方式 ·· 242
　　六、总结 ·· 242

致谢 ··· 242

第 16 章　外泌体在妊娠与生殖医学中的作用潜力
　　　　　　Potential role of exosomes in reproductive medicine and pregnancy ········ 245
　　一、概述 ··· 245
　　二、胞外囊泡的多样性、生成和分泌 ·· 245
　　三、妊娠期外泌体的来源和功能 ·· 247
　　四、外泌体与妊娠并发症 ·· 253
　　五、总结 ··· 255
　　致谢 ··· 255

第 17 章　外泌体在呼吸系统疾病中的作用
　　　　　　Exosomes in respiratory disease ·· 261
　　一、外泌体在肺部微环境和肺部疾病发病中的作用 ·· 262
　　二、肺部微环境中效应免疫细胞和结构细胞衍生外泌体的作用 ·································· 264
　　三、外泌体在肺疾病中的作用 ·· 266
　　四、外泌体在呼吸系统疾病中的临床应用：临床试验和未来展望 ································ 275

第 18 章　外泌体在视网膜疾病中的作用
　　　　　　Exosomes in retinal diseases ·· 283
　　一、概述 ··· 283
　　二、一般发病机制 ·· 284
　　三、基于外泌体的治疗方法 ··· 290
　　四、总结 ··· 290

第 19 章　MSC 外泌体在再生医学中的应用
　　　　　　MSC-exosomes in regenerative medicine ·· 295
　　一、概述 ··· 295
　　二、来源于间充质基质细胞的外泌体 ·· 296
　　三、MSC-EV 在再生医学中的应用 ··· 297
　　四、再生医学中的外泌体修饰 ·· 302
　　五、MSC-外泌体在再生医学中的临床应用 ·· 307
　　六、局限与挑战 ··· 307
　　七、总结和展望 ··· 310
　　利益冲突 ·· 310

第 20 章　外泌体作为药物在各种临床情况下的可能性
The potential of exosomes as theragnostics in various clinical situations ············ 317
一、外泌体作为疾病的生物标志物和感染的治疗或疫苗候选物 ················ 317
二、胞外囊泡作为药物传递系统 ·· 320

第 21 章　外泌体、芽球、泛生和达尔文
Exosomes, gemmules, pangenesis and Darwin ································· 329
一、概述 ··· 329
二、达尔文主义观点 ·· 329
三、新达尔文主义（现代综合）观点 ··································· 333
四、新趋势观点 ··· 336
五、外泌体和 miRNA 跨代作用的现代研究 ··························· 338
致谢 ··· 338

第 1 章

外泌体的基本机制
Exosome basic mechanisms

Alice Conigliaro, Chiara Corrado, Simona Fontana, Riccardo Alessandro

Department of Biomedicine, Neuroscience and Advanced Diagnostics, University of Palermo, Palermo, Italy

一、外泌体的生物合成及释放

外泌体的生物合成与管腔内囊泡(intraluminal vesicle,ILV)的形成有关,始于质膜的第一次内陷,而后形成早期内体这一非常靠近内膜表面的低密度囊泡。

内吞作用和受体介导的内吞作用可以使不同的物质内化,而早期内体负责分选它们。配体与受体在细胞表面相互作用后,即与其受体分离,而后位于早期内体中,并通过内体运输囊泡转移至晚期内体。相反,受体则可在细胞膜表面循环利用或通过晚期内体-溶酶体途径部分降解,从而关闭信号,降低细胞表面的受体数量。

在细胞内经由微管介导的途径,早期内体会经过各种不同的修饰。它们可以相互融合或与含有酸性水解酶的囊泡融合,从而形成被称为多囊体(multivesicular bodies,MVB)的中间结构,而 MVB 中含有 ILV。ILV 的形成是第二次膜内陷,由内体膜参与。

MVB 由两种不同的机制产生:第一种,由内体分选转运复合体(endosomal sorting complex request for transport,ESCRT)负责 MVB 的形成;另一种,MVB 起源于膜上含有特定结构域(即脂筏)的内体(图 1-1)。

在这一点上,包含 ILV 的 MVB 可以遵循两种不同的命运。首先,MVB 可以与其他 MVB 或与晚期内体融合,并接收源自反面高尔基体的含溶酶体酶的囊泡。在此情况下,MVB 在成熟过程中酸性越来越强,从而激活酸性水解酶,以消化 MVB 内的各种分子,并实现这些分子在真核细胞溶酶体中的转化。这条途径可以实现跨膜蛋白和脂质快速而稳定的周转。此外,MVB 向质膜迁移并与其融合,将 ILV 作为外泌体释放到细胞外。因此,外泌体是源自内膜的,唯一一种内体性溶酶体来源的分泌囊泡。

二、ESCRT 及其在外泌体生物合成中的作用

来自不同细胞类型或体液的外泌体中发现了大量的 ESCRT 蛋白,证明了外泌体生物合成中 ESCRT 的作用。因此,许多成分被学界公认为是外泌体的标记物。

到目前为止,ESCRT 途径很好地解释了 ILV 和 MVB 形成的机制。ESCRT 由 5 个多聚体胞浆复合物组成:ESCRT 0、Ⅰ、Ⅱ、Ⅲ和 Vps4[1](图 1-1)。

包含在早期内体内的特定泛素化蛋白,它们的泛素化位点被 ESCRT-0 识别,并被其置于富含磷脂酰肌醇一磷酸(phosphatidyl inositol monophosphate,PI3P)的特殊内体区域。

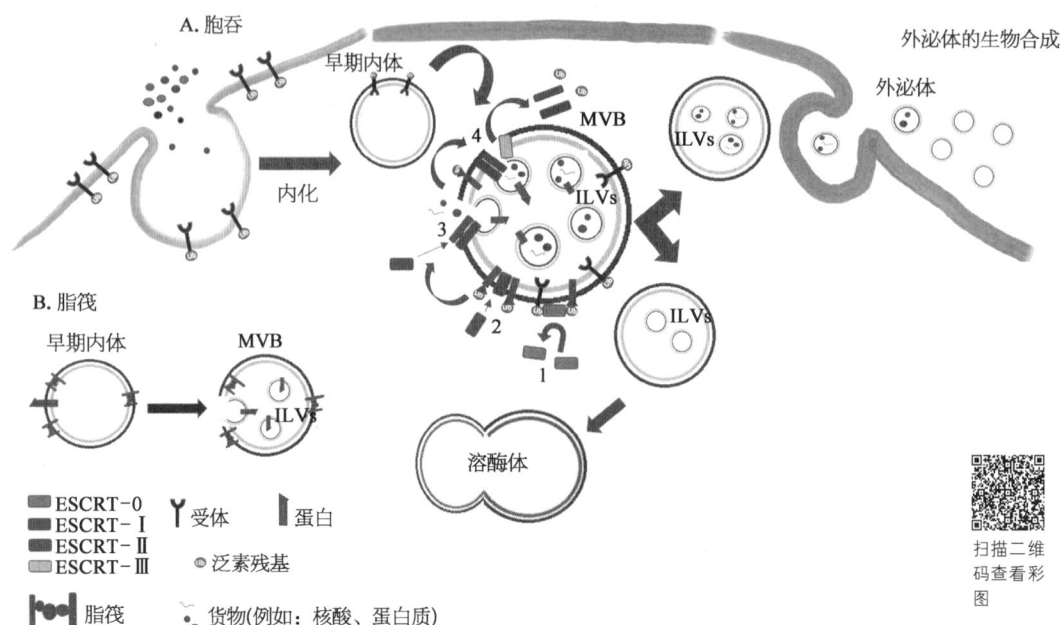

图 1-1 外泌体的生物合成。外泌体的生物合成可以通过不同的机制发生。A. 胞吞：受体-配体在细胞表面相互作用后，配体与其受体分离并进入早期内体中。而受体可以在膜表面上再循环或通过晚期内体-溶酶体途径部分降解。早期内体随后形成包含 ILV 的 MVB。ESCRT 负责 MVB 的形成。(1) ESCRT0 结合泛素残基，从而募集 ESCRT Ⅰ，最终破坏了 ESCRT0 (2)。(3) ESCRT Ⅱ 启动内体膜的内陷并结合 ESCRT Ⅲ (4)，后者使蛋白质上的泛素残基脱离并使膜完全内陷（膜出芽），从而产生 ILV。MVB 向质膜迁移并与质膜融合，ILV 作为外泌体释放。或者，MVB 可以与其他 MVB 或晚期内体融合，从反面高尔基体接收一组包含溶酶体酶的囊泡，这些酶可以实现溶酶体内的转化。B. 脂筏：MVB 也可以源自膜上包含特定结构域（即脂筏）的内体

ESCRT-0 由两个亚基组成，称为肝细胞生长因子调节的酪氨酸激酶底物（hepatocyte growth factor regulated tyrosine kinase substrate，HRS）和信号转导调节分子 1/2（signal transducing adaptor molecule 1/2，STAM 1/2），它们彼此结合并能够识别泛素蛋白和 PI3P 富集区。这能够募集 ESCRT-Ⅰ，一种由肿瘤易感基因 101（tumor susceptibility gene 101，TSG101）、Vps28、Vps37 和多囊体 12（multi-vesicular body 12，Mvb12）组成的异构体复合体。

ESCRT-Ⅰ 替换 ESCRT-0，并募集了 ESCRT-Ⅱ，它由四个亚基组成：Vps22-EAP30、Vps36-EAP45 和 Vps25-EAP20 的两个亚基。ESCRTI-Ⅱ 可以启动内体膜的内陷，从而内化不同的分子/货物，如核酸或蛋白质。

ESCRT-Ⅲ 是另一个异四聚体复合物（Vps20-CHMP6；Snf7-CHMP4；Vps24-CHMP3；Vps2-CHMP2），ESCRT-Ⅲ 的激活及其随后被募集至内体是由 ESCRT-Ⅱ 的亚基 Vps25 与 Vps20 的结合介导。ESCRT-Ⅲ 的作用是将泛素残基从蛋白质中分离出来，并使膜完全内陷（膜出芽），从而产生 ILV。货物的去泛素化也经由 ESCRT-Ⅲ 招募的辅助亚基介导，如 BCK1 样抗渗透压休克蛋白-1/调亡相关基因-2 相互作用蛋白 X（BCK1-like resistance to osmotic shock protein-1/apoptosis linked gene 2 interacting protein X, Bro1/Alix),在与 Snf7 结合后,招募 Doa4 酶(降解 α4),以完成货物的去泛素化[2]。最后,其他衔接蛋白帮助 Vps4-ESCRT Ⅲ 相互作用,并活化 Vps4 ATP 酶,这是最终膜出芽和切断、ESCRT 亚基去除、回收和货物递送所必需的。

综上所述,ESCRT 复合体控制着从 ILV 萌芽到货物选择、膜重塑和 ILV 并入 MVB 的整个过程。一项关于 ESCRT 复合体 23 种组分 RNAi 的有趣研究阐明了他们中只有少数几个是外泌体生物合成中必不可少的。实际上,在这些亚基中,Hrs、Tsg101 和 STAM1 同时沉默(ESCRT0/Ⅰ复合物)能够减少外泌体的分泌。相反,抑制 CHMP4C、VPS4B、VTA1 和 Alix(ESCRTⅢ复合物)会增加外泌体的分泌[3]。最近的研究表明,与刚才提到的 VPS4 作用相反,抑制 VPS4 减少了外泌体的释放[4]。此外,Alix 通过与几种 ESCRT 蛋白(如 Tsg101 或 CHMP4)相互作用,参与了蛋白组分/货物装载、ILV 出芽及其并入 MVB 中的过程。

从内体出芽到 ILV 形成,在外泌体生物合成的所有步骤中,有多种蛋白质与 ESCRT 复合体协同作用。

多配体聚糖结合蛋白是一种可溶性蛋白,通过其 PDZ 结构域充当细胞内衔接蛋白,招募多配体蛋白聚糖[携带硫酸乙酰肝素链(heparan sulfate chains, HS)的膜蛋白]。多配体蛋白聚糖通过 HS 结合许多配体,如黏附分子和生长因子,从而允许它们与其受体相互作用,并协助胞吞过程。最近的证据表明,Alix 与多配体聚糖结合蛋白的 N 端结合,并将多配体蛋白聚糖与 ESCRT 装置连接起来。因此,这种异三聚体复合物不仅参与外泌体的分选和装货(稍后讨论),还参与内体的出芽和外泌体的生物合成[5,6]。

一种 GTP 结合蛋白:ADP-核糖化因子 6(ADP-ribosylation factor 6,ARF6)与晚期内体转运和多配体聚糖结合蛋白-外泌体的产生有关。ARF6 能够激活磷脂酰肌醇(4)-磷酸 5-激酶[phosphatidyl-inositol (4)-phosphate 5-kinase, PIPK],参与 PIP2 的合成。PIP2 的合成支持多配体聚糖结合蛋白-多配体蛋白聚糖从核周区室向质膜的募集[7]。

ARF6 上游的另一种激酶:癌蛋白 Src 负责调节多配体聚糖结合蛋白/多配体蛋白聚糖的活性。Src 通过对多配体聚糖结合蛋白/多配体蛋白聚糖的酪氨酸残基进行磷酸化,作用于内体转运,从而刺激内体出芽和特异性多配体聚糖结合蛋白依赖性的外泌体生物合成[8]。

热休克蛋白(heat shock protein,HSP)是广泛参与蛋白质聚集和折叠的伴侣蛋白。人们最初研究这些蛋白在细胞内通路中的作用,随后的观察表明它们也存在于细胞外。而现在众所周知,HSP 是一种由非经典途径分泌的蛋白质,其中大部分是由外泌体分泌的。有趣的是,HSP 还通过与 ESCRT 蛋白的协作和相互作用参与外泌体的生物合成[9]。

三、ESCRT 非依赖的外泌体生物合成机制

通过同时去除关键 ESCRT 蛋白发现,MVB 的生物合成和 ILV 的形成也可以通过 ESCRT 非依赖的机制来保证,表明这一过程的调控比预期的要复杂得多。由于 ESCRT 复合体的缺乏,尽管保持了早期和晚期内体的分化,实际上也导致了使 MVB 增大这种深层的形态改变。

这说明了虽然ILV在这种情况下数量和大小有所不同,因它们的形成可能是通过一种ESCRT非依赖的胞吞分选机制,并提出了这一假设:即在高等真核生物中,外泌体生物合成的两种机制可以共存并一起发挥作用。细胞类型和细胞内稳态可能是通过这两种生物合成机制之一,来调控不同亚群外泌体。

ESCRT突变的细胞仍然能够形成ILV,这也是由它们膜的脂质成分所致。众所周知,单层膜脂质的生物物理特性,如头部基团的大小、酰基链的长度和饱和度是影响膜曲率的基础。

脂筏是向内弯曲的、具有富含胆固醇和鞘脂的内体的特殊区域,并可能通过跨膜的pH梯度决定MVB的形成。在这种没有ESCRT辅助的情况下,内体的膜内陷是由于磷脂酶介导的从鞘磷脂转变而来的神经酰胺的合成。由于神经酰胺的锥形形态,它们独自或与胆固醇结合产生有利于膜变形和ILV出芽的特定结构域。

此外,神经酰胺通过转化为一磷酸鞘氨醇(sphingosine 1 - phosphate,S1P),并在MVB膜上结合其受体[10],从而诱导外泌体生物合成。

中性鞘磷脂酶(neutral sphingomyelinases,SMases)是神经酰胺中参与鞘磷脂转化的酶,它优先定位于高尔基体-内质网,但也存在于质膜上,从而参与外泌体的生物合成。在特定的细胞类型中抑制SMases可以降低外泌体释放的某些蛋白质,证明神经酰胺对于产生有利于膜出芽的微区是必不可少的[11]。

其他脂质修饰酶,磷脂酶D2(phospholipase D2,PLD2)和二酰甘油激酶α(diacylglycerol kinase α,DGKα),通过产生有利于膜内陷的磷脂酸(phosphatidic acid,PA)和神经酰胺,参与外泌体的生物合成。

另一方面,鞘磷脂对膜上的胆固醇有很高的亲和力,它的水解增加了胆固醇从质膜向细胞内膜的迁移,从而提高膜的流动性。事实上,众所周知,胆固醇分子聚集在脂质区域,从而影响质膜脂质的有序排列和最终的囊泡脱落。

许多蛋白质介导ESCRT非依赖的外泌体生物合成机制,如CD9、CD63和CD81等四次跨膜蛋白,它们是最初在B淋巴细胞中鉴定出的跨膜蛋白,通常参与细胞融合、迁移和细胞黏附[13]。此外,四次跨膜蛋白在外泌体中含量丰富,因此,通常被认为是外泌体的标记。特别是四次跨膜蛋白具有四个穿膜域,在这些穿膜域上它们与许多其他的蛋白质、胆固醇和神经节苷脂相互作用,从而生成TEM域(富含四次跨膜蛋白的结构域)。TEM域最终会影响膜弯曲和肌动蛋白聚合。此外,四次跨膜蛋白介导货物分选和ILV形成,如CD9参与质膜融合;而CD63与多配体蛋白聚糖类似,与多配体聚糖结合蛋白的PDZ结构域相互作用[14]。

四、MVB向质膜转运并释放外泌体

MVB决定不与溶酶体融合,而是移向质膜以释放外泌体的机制,目前尚不清楚。

然而,很显然,外泌体释放到细胞外进入细胞外微环境中,是由于MVB与质膜融合过程中特定的蛋白质-蛋白质和蛋白质-脂质的相互作用引起的。

参与这一膜融合事件的蛋白质当然是SNARE蛋白、拴系因子以及许多小的GTP酶。

SNARE 蛋白通常参与囊泡与靶膜的融合,这种融合是通过 1 个囊泡中的 R‑SNARE 与靶膜中 2～3 个 Q‑SNARE 形成 3～4 个亚基的复合物来实现。R‑SNARE 囊泡相关膜蛋白 7(vesicle associated membrane protein 7,VAMP7)的过表达导致细胞周围形成扩大的 MVB,从而减少外泌体的释放[15]。与此一致,敲除另一种 R‑SNARE YKT6 可降低外泌体分泌的 Tsg101 水平[16]。

微管和细胞骨架蛋白(如肌动蛋白及其结合蛋白)介导 MVB 转运至胞膜。肌动蛋白的结合蛋白即皮层蛋白在 MVB 转运中的作用已通过敲除或过表达实验得以证实,实验验证了皮层蛋白的敲除/过表达分别减少/增加了外泌体的释放[17]。

小 GTP 酶中的 RAB 家族主要参与内体的运输,最近还发现其参与了膜运输,即沿细胞骨架的囊泡运输、MVB 与质膜的对接和外泌体释放。许多研究已经证明了 RAB27 和 RAB35 在 MVB 与质膜的对接中发挥主要作用[18-20]。有趣的是,参与晚期内体运输的 RAB7 下调,以及导致大内体形成的 RAB5 过表达,会抑制接触 SDC/多配体聚糖结合蛋白的外泌体释放[5,21]。其他小 GTP 酶类也参与外泌体释放,如 Rho/Rac/cdc42 家族[22]。

前文中提到的四次跨膜蛋白也参与了 ESCRT 非依赖的外泌体释放,并在外泌体生物合成中发挥作用。四次跨膜蛋白可以在质膜的 TEM 域中找到,但它们也能够通过其他蛋白质与细胞骨架的相互作用,影响它们通过外泌体的释放。

我们提到膜脂对于膜弯曲很重要,并可以因此调节 MVB 的形成。此外,脂质也在 MVB 与质膜融合中起到关键作用,从而增加了外泌体的分泌。

添加一种能增加细胞脂质的醚脂前体,能够增加外泌体的释放[23,24]。与这一实验观察一致,添加胆固醇会增加典型的外泌体蛋白,如 Alix 或 CD63[23,24]。相反,在另一个细胞模型中,抑制胆固醇的合成代谢却增加了几种外泌体蛋白的分泌[25]。

外泌体的释放还受到钙等其他成分或各种不同机制的影响。钙能够影响调节质膜的对称性的酶,例如转位酶或磷脂促翻转酶。转位酶能够将磷脂酰丝氨酸和磷脂酰乙醇胺从质膜外层向内层转位,促进脂质跨膜移动,影响外泌体的释放。

用钙离子载体处理可增加细胞内钙水平,增加外泌体分泌[26]。此外,突触结合蛋白这一钙敏感性蛋白一般与囊泡运输相关,也能够调节外泌体的分泌[27]。

最近的证据表明,ISG 化是一种新型的泛素化修饰,能够通过促进蛋白质聚集和通过自噬体-溶酶体室促进 MVB 降解来控制外泌体的释放。特别是 TSG101 的 ISG 化,它的降解足以影响外泌体分泌[28]。

细胞应激,如辐射、化疗氧化应激或缺氧,都是增加外泌体释放的信号。有趣的是,最新的证据表明,应激条件下 MVB 命运中可识别出一种新因素作为假定"分界点",决定进入外泌体或溶酶体途径。细胞外小热休克蛋白 αB-晶状体蛋白(αB‑crystallin,αBC)就是其中一个例子。在氧化应激条件下释放的外泌体富含 αBC。有趣的是,Gangalum 及其合作者证明,αBC 抑制会导致溶酶体标记物 LAMP1 和晚期内体标记物 RAB7 的表达增加,表明了内体-溶酶体途径的激活[29]。这些数据使我们能够推测 αBC 在外泌体释放中起到关键作用。

五、基础成分和货物

在过去十年中进行的大量组学研究清楚地表明,外泌体包含并运输多种类型的生物大分子,这些大分子在递送至靶细胞后仍能维持其全部活性。这种生物活性物质,包括核酸(DNA 和所有类型的 RNA)、脂质,以及可溶性或膜结合蛋白,都与生产细胞的类型和功能状态严格相关,尽管它不是其内容的同一子集。近年来,越来越多的证据清楚地表明,将大分子内化到外泌体中不是一个随机过程,但是驱动该过程的生物学和分子机制仍远未得到充分地阐述[30]。外泌体作为细胞间通信介质的功能特性及其调控靶细胞行为的能力都与它们所载货物特别相关,因此研究外泌体分子组分的深层表征以及转导内化过程通路的研究是目前外泌体研究领域的关键[31]。此外,由于外泌体的货物和生物分子内化机制与疾病状态特别相关,外泌体被广泛认为是新型生物标记物的潜在来源。

在以下各节中,我们将详细介绍外泌体的分子组成,并描述这些分子进入囊泡的已知机制。

蛋白质:外泌体包含一组来自亲代细胞的复杂蛋白质(胞浆蛋白、核蛋白、线粒体蛋白、核糖体蛋白和膜结合蛋白)。来自多种蛋白质组学研究的数据清楚地表明,在这些外泌体蛋白中,有些蛋白存在于所有细胞来源的外泌体中,因此可被视为"外泌体标记";而另一些蛋白则决定了与来源细胞特定相关的独特的外泌体特征,决定了外泌体的性质和活性。

具体而言,在通常用作标记物的囊泡特异性蛋白中,有各种胞质蛋白,如 14-3-3 蛋白和特定的 HSP,以及与外泌体生物合成过程相关的几种蛋白,如四次跨膜蛋白(CD9、CD63、CD81)、凝集素、GTP 酶、主要组织相容性复合体(major histocompatibility complex,MHC)分子和 ESCRT 复合体的蛋白质(Alix 和 TSG101)[32,33]。

除了包含这些稳定存在的蛋白质,外泌体还包含许多与起始细胞表型特异相关的离散蛋白质亚群,外泌体可通过这些蛋白质分别对近端和远端受体细胞的特性重新编程。越来越多对肿瘤来源外泌体(tumor-derived exosome,TDE)的研究表明,由于其蛋白质含量的不同,这些纳米囊泡在调节细胞存活、肿瘤进展、转移和化疗药物耐药性方面具有独特的作用[31]。Lyden 团队的一个著名研究表明,整合素组成的变化会差异性地影响 TDE 的组织特异性定植,从而诱导器官特异性转移前微环境的形成[34]。

基于 SWATH 的定量蛋白组学分析强调,与那些侵袭性较低的肿瘤细胞释放的外泌体相比,转移性结肠肿瘤细胞释放的外泌体显著富集了几种细胞骨架相关蛋白和 RhoA/ROCK 信号相关蛋白,如 RacGAP1 和凝血酶。人们已经证明转移性肿瘤细胞来源的外泌体能够在肿瘤微环境中传播恶性特性,同时影响肿瘤细胞的可塑性和内皮细胞的行为,并且这种能力与它们的蛋白质特征特别相关。RacGAP1 和凝血酶已被确定为转移性肿瘤来源的外泌体在靶细胞中起诱导作用的关键介质[35]。

许多研究证明,用抗肿瘤化合物治疗肿瘤细胞可以改变 TDE 的基础蛋白组成,从而改变它们的促肿瘤作用。Taverna 等的报道称,姜黄素是一种因其抗肿瘤作用而知名的植物来源化合物,用其治疗后,慢性髓细胞性白血病细胞释放的外泌体(姜黄素/CML-外泌体)中的蛋白质货物得到了显著改变。特别是,与未经处理的 CML 细胞释放的外泌体相比,姜黄素/CML外泌体的促血管生成蛋白减少，同时抗血管生成活性的蛋白增加。这些变化导致CML外泌体的一些能力丧失，包括促进血管生成和改变内皮组织屏障的能力[36]。

尽管越来越多的研究已经提供了许多有关外泌体蛋白质组成的细节，清楚地表明它们是细胞类型相关的，并且可能受到不同细胞条件或治疗的影响，但蛋白质装载的机制尚未完全明了。与外泌体蛋白分选有关的描述与表征最多的系统是由ESCRT家族成员介导的，但是越来越多的证据表明，外泌体蛋白分选系统也有几种非依赖ESCRT的途径[37]。此外，外泌体中特定蛋白质子集的富集表明它们的分选可以由特定机制驱动。外泌体中检测到的许多蛋白质都会经历翻译后修饰（post-translational modification，PTM），如糖基化、磷酸化、泛素化或类泛素化修饰。该观察结果表明，PTM可以赋予蛋白质特定的性质，这些特性在调节蛋白质被分选后进入外泌体的过程中起着至关重要的作用[38]。此外，在蛋白质装载到外泌体的ESCRT非依赖机制中，研究者们还描述了由脂筏和神经酰胺介导的机制。有趣的是，据报道，某些蛋白在脂筏被破坏后（趋化因子、αB-晶状体蛋白、干细胞表面标志物）或神经酰胺代谢通路被阻断后失去了外泌体的定位（CD63）[37]。

核酸：外泌体包含了不同类型的核酸，如单链DNA（single-stranded DNA，ssDNA）和双链DNA（double-stranded DNA，dsDNA）、线粒体DNA（mitochondrial DNA，mtDNA）、信使RNA（messenger RNA，mRNA）、微小RNA（micro RNA，miRNA）和长链非编码RNA（long non-coding RNA，lncRNA）[31]。

DNA：外泌体中存在DNA分子（exoDNA）已被广泛报道[39]。无论是从细胞培养上清液分离的外泌体，还是人和小鼠体液中的外泌体都发现了线粒体和基因组的DNA，经DNA酶处理表明ds-DNA（不同于ssDNA和RNA）主要存在于外泌体的内部而不是外部[40-42]。有证据表明，在正常人类嗜中性粒细胞的外泌体DNA中检测到了来自K562细胞的*BCR/ABL*杂合基因的exoDNA，证实了外泌体具有介导DNA水平转移的能力[43]。即使外泌体介导DNA转移的生理学意义尚未完全清楚，但有证据表明，在受体细胞中外泌体DNA可以集中到胞核[44]。此外，最近有人提出，外泌体分泌的基因组DNA片段可以通过避免DNA在细胞质中的积累而在维持细胞内平衡方面发挥重要作用，调控细胞衰老或凋亡[45]。外泌体中存在一些基因组DNA，可以反映亲代肿瘤细胞中如*P53*、*KRAS*和*EGFR*等基因的突变状态，这一事实有力地支持了外泌体DNA的诊断价值及其临床潜力[40,42,46]。尽管DNA在外泌体中的存在得到了充分的证明，并且其特征已得到了广泛描述，但是对DNA装载到外泌体的机制仍然存在许多疑问。据报道，基于其来源的细胞外泌体可以包含不同类型的DNA（如在星形胶质细胞和胶质母细胞瘤来源的外泌体中发现了mtDNA，但在其他细胞来源外泌体中没有发现）[42,47]。因此有研究者假设，不同细胞类型有不同的特异机制对外泌体装载DNA进行动态调节。另一方面，在外泌体中，DNA片段均匀地分布在整个基因组中，而不偏向于特定区域，这表明外泌体中的DNA分选是一个随机过程[40,42]。

RNA：所有细胞类型释放的外泌体都同时富含编码mRNA和非编码RNA，其中非编码RNA如miRNA、lncRNA、核糖体RNA（ribosomal RNA，rRNA）和环状RNA（circular RNA，circRNA）[37,48]。在过去几年里出现了很多关于外泌体内RNA分子选择性装载的有趣数据[48-50]。由于人们对miRNA作为能够驱动细胞表型基因表达的关键调控因子的兴趣与日俱增,这些小 RNA 的分选机制更是受到了特别关注。有证据表明,原始细胞的 miRNA 谱与其所分泌外泌体的 miRNA 谱有所不同,这有力地表明了这些细胞的外泌体分选不可能是随机发生的[51,52]。

迄今为止的报道称有多种途径和分子参与外泌体 miRNA 的分选,但是这个复杂系统的许多方面仍有待进一步探索。

当前研究的数据表明,miRNA 进入外泌体可以通过某些 miRNA 中存在的特定序列以及它们与某些酶或其他蛋白质的相互作用来引导[31,53]。RNA 结合蛋白是调节外泌体 miRNA 含量的主要蛋白之一。Y-框蛋白Ⅰ(Y-box proteinⅠ,YBX1)似乎是外泌体中特定 miRNA 分选,以及 miRNA EXO 基序(GGAG)或蛋白 SYNCRIP 结合异质核糖核蛋白 A2B1(heterogeneous nuclear ribonucleoprotein A2B1,hnRNPA2B1)所必需的,后者是肝细胞内外泌体 miRNA 分选机制的重要组成部分[31,37,54,55]。

据报道,除了 RNA 结合蛋白,其他蛋白在调节外泌体中 miRNA 的装载中也起着关键作用。敲除 Argonaute 2(Ago2)、Alix 和中性鞘磷脂酶 2(neutral sphingomyelinase 2,nSMase 2)等蛋白质的实验表明,它们直接参与了外泌体 miRNA 水平的调节[29]。转录后修饰也被认为可驱动 miRNA 分选进入外泌体。Koppers-Lalic 等证明了非模板核苷酸的添加与 EV 中 miRNA 的富集(3'-尿嘧啶化)或在原代细胞内的保留(3'-腺苷酸化)有关[56]。此外,据报道,当其目标转录本转录表达水平较高时,miRNA 会保留在细胞质中,表明 mRNA-miRNA 的相互作用可调节进入外泌体的过程[57]。同时也有人提出了将 MVB 的筏样区域作为 miRNA 靶标[58]。最后,Melo 等报道了与乳腺癌相关的外泌体包含了与 RISC-Loading Complex 相关的前体 miRNA,显示出此细胞具有不依赖细胞将前体 miRNA 加工为成熟 miRNA 的能力[59]。

将 miRNA 包装到外泌体中,可以在物理上保护它们免受酶的降解,从而确保将其有效地水平转移到其他细胞中,从而诱导不同生理和病理过程的激活。在过去十年中进行的许多研究都集中在外泌体 miRNA 对调节肿瘤微环境中的作用。多种外泌体 miRNA,如 miR-9、miR-105 或 miR-21,因其在调节肿瘤增殖、血管生成、免疫系统活性、转移和其他支持肿瘤进展的生物学特性中的重要作用而被广泛报道[31,53]。

除了转运 miRNA,外泌体还携带多种 lncRNA,已知这些 lncRNA 可通过翻译抑制或竞争性内源性 RNA 调节基因表达[31]。

lncRNA 与其他生物分子一样,可能是选择性分选进入外泌体中的,因为一些 lncRNA 在外泌体中富集,而另一些则几乎不存在。同样,决定外泌体 lncRNA 种类的机制也不是很清楚。特定的蛋白质似乎作为 lncRNA 载体,推动其内化到外泌体,但目前还没有明确的数据[53]。人们已经证明外泌体衍生的长链非编码 RNA 参与了肿瘤进展多个环节的调控[53]。

最后,一个值得考虑的有趣方面是,外泌体在所有患者体内的血液、尿液和其他体液中具有极高的稳定性,为检测作为疾病生物标记物的 miRNA 和 lncRNA 提供了稳定的来源。许多研究报告了一些令人关注的数据,这些数据涉及疾病患者和健康个体之间外泌体 miRNA 和 lncRNA 数量和组成的不同,这表明循环外泌体 miRNA 和 lncRNA 可以用于液体活检和无创生物标记物、早期检测、诊断和对患者进行临床干预[48,53-55]。

脂质：目前尚无一个完整的外泌体脂质数据集，但很清楚的是，外泌体脂质双分子层具有区别于亲代细胞的独特脂质组成。其特征是选择性地富集了鞘磷脂、胆固醇、磷脂酰丝氨酸、磷脂酰胆碱、磷脂酰乙醇胺和神经节苷脂 GM3[31]。外泌体脂质不对称地分布在双分子层的两侧，并形成脂质筏状结构域，可能在外泌体结构和形成中具有特定的作用[31,60]。

来自肝肿瘤细胞（Huh7）和间充质干细胞（mesenchymal stem cell，MSC）的外泌体富含心磷脂，而恶性胶质细胞瘤细胞（U87）的外泌体富含鞘磷脂，表明外泌体脂质组成可能取决于其来源的细胞类型[61]。外泌体中也富含神经酰胺，参与外泌体向多囊体腔内出芽，并且有报道称，抑制中性鞘磷脂这一神经酰胺前体的合成可显著降低外泌体的释放。囊泡状脂质对于外泌体的生物发生、释放和与靶细胞的相互作用并非必不可少，但是人们认为它能够调节病理生理通路的生物活性成分。早在 2002 年 Kim 等就发现，肿瘤细胞的细胞外膜囊泡可通过自身转运的鞘磷脂促进血管生成[62]。因此，外泌体也被称为携带 GTP 激活的磷脂酶和前列腺素的细胞间信号传导小体，从活化细胞到静息细胞[63]。

最近，对从前列腺癌患者和健康志愿者收集的尿液外泌体进行了脂质组学研究，其提供了初步但有意义的结果，支持了将外泌体脂质作为生物标志物[60]。

外泌体成分和货物分选的进一步表征将有助于更好地了解这些天然纳米载体的生物学相关性，并将为开发创新的诊断和治疗策略提供新的知识。

六、作用机制

最初，外泌体被认为是用作处理细胞垃圾，但随后，大量的文章发现它们具有通过水平传递信息来调节生理和病理状态的关键作用。包装在这些磷脂球内部的大分子和生物活性化合物，从外泌体产生的细胞转移到体内的接收细胞，这些接收细胞分布在近端或远端。外泌体作为细胞间相互交流的方式之一，在维持体内稳态方面有着显著作用，因此对他们的研究也被定义为"新内分泌学"[63]。此外，在包括精液、血液、尿液、脑脊液和乳汁在内的不同体液中对这些囊泡的鉴定也印证了这一定义。

当前，越来越多的研究小组正在对外泌体的世界进行更深入的研究，以了解这种递送系统的交流策略，并加以利用。

不幸的是，由于许多因素会影响细胞/外泌体的相互作用，外泌体在与受体细胞相互作用后的最终效应是难以预测的。

首先，外泌体是选择性的信使，它们优先与特定细胞类型结合。一项旨在研究外泌体与肿瘤转移之间关系的有趣研究表明，在组织驻留基质细胞中，只有极少数会摄取肿瘤细胞外泌体，且这种能力依赖于外泌体整合素[33]。人们采用蛋白质组学方法表征从肿瘤细胞释放的外泌体尽管在组织学来源上有所不同，但却有共同的转移优先部位。由于这项研究，Hoshino 等证明了 TDE 受其整合素（integrins，ITG）的驱动，选择靶向特定器官的转移位点及组织内的基质细胞。实际上，含有 ITGα6β4 和 ITGα6β1 的外泌体会被 S100A4 阳性细胞内化，而 ITGαvβ5 的表达则允许外泌体被 F4/80$^+$ 巨噬细胞摄取[33]。

外泌体一旦到达正确的位置并被作为受体的细胞类型识别，就可以采用不同的策略改造受体细胞，具体取决于细胞-外泌体接触的分子相互作用。外泌体传递信息的分子机制包括受体细胞的激活和下游信号通路、膜融合、外泌体内化和核转位。

从外部开始，外泌体-受体细胞相互作用的第一步可能是配体/受体结合。

暴露于外泌体表面的配体与受体细胞上的特定膜受体结合，并激活它们，从而激活信号转导通路。

研究最深入的例子是外泌体介导的细胞死亡，是多种肿瘤细胞用于增强免疫耐受性的策略。肿瘤细胞来源的外泌体，通过在表面表达死亡信号，如程序性死亡配体-1（programmed death-ligand 1，PD-L1）或 Fas 配体，通过诱导 T 细胞和 NK 细胞的凋亡来系统性抑制免疫系统[64,65]。在生理条件下，作为免疫调节信号的介质，外泌体也与抗原提呈细胞（antigen presenting cell，APC）协同作用。一篇有趣的文献指出，免疫小鼠的树突状细胞（dendritic cell，DC）可在血浆中释放 MHC Ⅱ$^+$/FasL$^+$ 外泌体，这种外泌体能够通过 Fas 激活 Ag 特异性的免疫抑制反应[66]。根据收集到的数据，人们现在提出了使用表达 TRAIL 的工程化外泌体向肿瘤细胞传递促凋亡信号的策略[67]。

在细胞膜配体和受体的修饰下，外泌体可参与通常由细胞-细胞接触方式介导的过程，如发育、器官形成和组织稳态[68]。例如，内皮细胞产生暴露 Notch 配体 Dll4 的外泌体，一旦暴露于受体细胞表面，就会促进 Notch 的裂解和激活，最终导致体外培养细胞的血管分支和密度增加。由于囊泡持续与活化的受体连接，在内化阶段，这些囊泡会与受体一起转运到细胞内[69]。此外，也发现 Hedgehog 和 WNT 家族的分泌蛋白均能够促进形态发生信号的传递，这一过程可通过将其直接装载于外泌体双分子层或作为外泌体相关蛋白这两种方式实现。而带有膜相关 TGF-$β_1$ 的外泌体能够激活接受细胞 TGF-β 受体[70,71]。

肿瘤来源外泌体中存在其他可激活信号转导的外泌体，如表达双调蛋白（AREG）的外泌体，这些外泌体可从多种肿瘤细胞中分离出来，通过激活接收细胞中的 EGFR 影响骨髓微环境[72]或促进肿瘤骨转移[73]。

尽管外泌体能够从外部启动细胞内通路，但在大多数情况下，与蛋白的相互作用会驱动囊泡在接受细胞中内化。对小鼠外泌体预处理的人肥大细胞内小鼠蛋白进行鉴定，可以明确地证明此内化过程。同样重要的是，在 Montecalvo 等设计的实验[74]中发现，用负载荧光素的外泌体处理表达荧光素酶的细胞能够诱导其发光。

迄今为止，人们已经描述了多种参与驱动外泌体内化的机制[75,76]，还有可能发现其他多种机制（图 1-2）。

通过蛋白水解处理或使用特异性阻断外泌体内化的抗体，可鉴定某些内吞途径激活相关的蛋白质-蛋白质相互作用。

如前所述，受体介导的内吞作用是参与外部物质内化从而产生早期内体的机制之一，也是外泌体生物发生的第一步。另一方面，受体介导的内吞作用需要外泌体表面配体与其在质膜上的特定配体结合。这种结合是通过网格蛋白介导的胞吞途径进行的[77]，通过促进包被蛋白在细胞膜内表面上的组装，形成网格蛋白包被的囊泡，而后通过一种大型的 GTP 酶

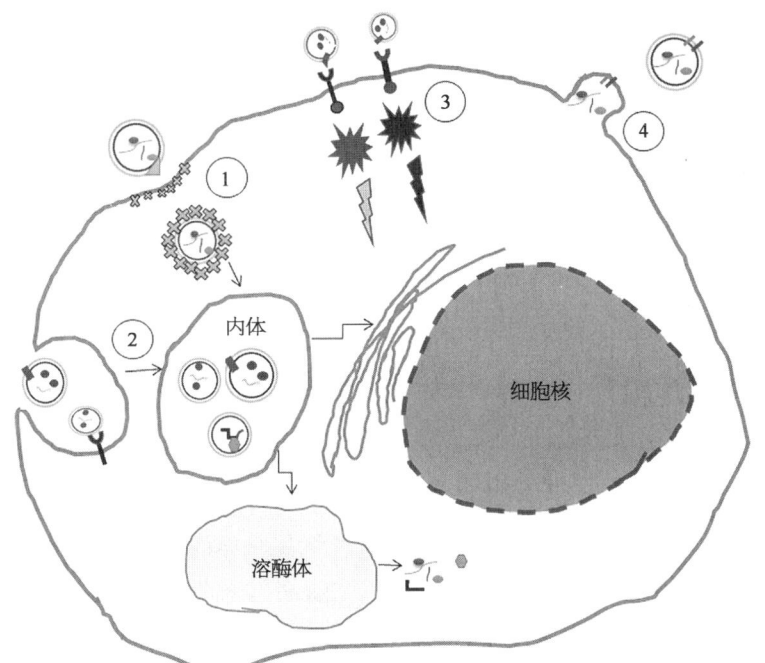

图 1-2 作用机制。内化作用(1~2):1. 依赖网格蛋白的,或 2. 非依赖内吞途径的囊泡,其聚合到内体,而后转到溶酶体或细胞核。3. 细胞内通路的激活:配体/受体相互作用激活信号转导。4. 融合:膜融合后释放生物活性分子

扫描二维码查看彩图

发动蛋白螺旋领环,从细胞膜上脱离。Tian 等掌握了依赖网格蛋白的内吞作用可吸收外泌体的正式证据,这表明,用阳离子两亲药物处理细胞而引起的网格蛋白减少,可显著抑制外泌体的内化[78]。

另外,外泌体可以通过非经典的内吞途径进入细胞,该途径是由质膜中的脂筏、胆固醇和富含鞘磷脂的微域介导的。如上所述,脂筏通过小窝或非小窝途径在膜上移动并实现平顺的内陷。有趣的是,用膜胆固醇消耗实验或抑制胆固醇生物合成实验表明,HUVEC 的外泌体摄取呈剂量依赖性降低,最高可达 60%[79]。

外泌体的吞噬作用发生在吞噬细胞和其他免疫细胞(即巨噬细胞、DC 和 γδT 细胞)中,它依赖于肌动蛋白细胞骨架、磷脂酰肌醇 3-激酶(phosphatidylinositol 3-kinase,PI3K)和发动蛋白 2。此外,EV 的一个共同特征是在外膜上暴露出磷脂酰丝氨酸,这一特征可介导外泌体的内化,也可被许多参与凋亡小体吞噬的质膜受体所识别。

在这一点上,有趣的是在生理上,胞吞作用和吞噬作用都将内化的货物驱动到内体-溶酶体的降解途径中。然而大量的证据表明,外泌体货物在接收细胞中仍具有生物活性。

内化外泌体如何逃避溶酶体降解的问题目前仍在研究中。最近,Lorico 研究小组提出了一种可能的策略,他们在间充质基质细胞和乳腺肿瘤细胞中发现一种中间隔室,用于将内吞的 EV 或其中一部分(如 CD9/CD133 蛋白复合物)直接递送至接受细胞的核中。特别的是,他们确定了一个名为 VOR 的三联体复合物,它由 ER 蛋白 VAP-A 和晚期内体蛋白

ORP1L 和 Rab7 组成，后者将晚期内体驱动到核孔附近，并从那里运至核质[80]。

但是，不同的内化机制可能会提高货物的递送效率。

接受细胞表面上外泌体蛋白质的表征证明了外泌体货物递送机制中的膜融合。例如，四跨膜蛋白超家族自身的相互作用及其与一系列分子的相互作用，这些分子包括蛋白质、脂质和碳水化合物，其同时还形成了 TEM 结构域，如前所述，此结构域可参与包括膜融合在内的多种生物学功能。迄今为止，尽管只有很少的证据支持该假说，但这在很大程度上解释了 TEM 在外泌体内化中的作用[31]。另外，整合素也参与了膜融合和特异性抗体掩蔽，如 CD61、CD51 和 CD54，证明了它们在 DC 摄取外泌体方面的关键作用。

如上所述，外泌体是收集和运送生物活性化合物的容器。外泌体能够通过向邻近和远处组织输送不同的分子货物改造受体细胞，调节特定组织和（或）全身的代谢，磷脂结构可以保护货物免受降解，并保持其生物活性。

因此，外泌体影响受体细胞的多种机制与所载货物有着密切联系。例如，如前所述，外泌体既可以通过激活细胞外膜上受体，也可以通过将其介导的某种活化受体递送入细胞内的方式来激活细胞内信号传导。Song 等证明了肿瘤细胞来源的外泌体富含磷酸化的受体酪氨酸激酶，如磷酸化表皮生长因子受体（epidermal growth factor receptor，EGFR）和人表皮生长因子受体 2（human epidermal growth factor receptor 2，HER-2），一旦进入肿瘤相关的单核细胞，就会激活 MAPK 通路，从而提高其存活率[81]。此外，肿瘤细胞来源的外泌体含有与 miRNA 相关的 RISC 负载复合物（RISC-loading complex，Rlc），包括 Dicer、TRBP 和 AGO2，它们可将 miRNA 前体加工为成熟的 miRNA，并在靶细胞中诱导 Dicer 依赖的 mRNA 降解[58]。

内分泌学家对外泌体进行了大量研究，以了解其增强激素信号传导的能力。例如，如果子宫内膜细胞载入了滋养层细胞内化的外泌体蛋白，则会影响黏附、迁移、侵袭和细胞外基质重塑等功能，从而促进着床与妊娠[82]。Crewe 等的最新数据[83]证实了外泌体在代谢信号中的作用。这些学者用一种新型的小鼠模型取得了进展，该模型能够追踪外泌体在体内的运动，证明了内皮细胞向脂肪组织传递了系统能量平衡"实时更新"的信号。他们特别说明了，来自脂肪组织的内皮细胞捕获了来自血液的信号分子，即可溶性或白蛋白结合的营养素和激素，将其包装在外泌体中，并将这些外泌体优先发送至邻近的脂肪细胞。

另外，外泌体还参与了组织动态平衡的维持。特别是间充质干细胞（mesenchymal stem cell，MSC）来源的外泌体。这些囊泡携带的酶，能够修复再灌注心肌中糖酵解缺陷、ATP 的生产以及修复与组织修复十分相关的生长因子（即血小板衍生生长因子、表皮生长因子、成纤维细胞生长因子）和具有抗炎作用的生物活性分子。有趣的是，数据表明，在组织损伤模型的多种器官再生过程中，MSC 来源的外泌体与亲代干细胞一样有效，因此我们建议将 MSC 分泌的外泌体作为一种新型的非细胞治疗手段[84]。

尽管外泌体递送的大量生物活性大分子能够调节接受细胞，但大多数实验证据都涉及外泌体携带的 RNA，尤其是非编码 RNA 所诱导的效应。对于外泌体改变受体细胞行为的机制，人们研究最深入的肯定是 miRNA 递送。目前，我们知道不同细胞和组织来源外泌体中 miRNA 的选择性分选涉及了多种通路和分子[30]。Pegtel 等[85]首先证明了，得益于外泌体的负载,成熟的 miRNA 可以在体内运输而免受 RNA 酶的降解。有趣的是,人们对外泌体中的核酸进行了更深入的分析,发现有大量的 RNA 片段,大小分布在 25～700 个核苷酸之间,其中 miRNA 只占小部分,然而 tRNA 片段和 Y - RNA 似乎是其中最丰富的,不过它们在受体细胞中的作用仍需探索[86]。另外,越来越多的证据表明外泌体递送的 lncRNA 在靶细胞表型的调节中起到作用。它们是长于 200 个核苷酸的单链 RNA 片段,尽管在外泌体中的数量少于小 RNA,但在控制基因表达方面保留了多种功能。例如,缺氧膀胱肿瘤细胞释放的外泌体富含致癌的 lncRNA - UCA1,能够诱导肿瘤微环境重塑以促进肿瘤生长[60]。同样,神经胶质瘤细胞和肝癌干细胞分别通过释放包含 lncRNA POU3F3 和 lncRNA H19[61, 62]的外泌体来促进血管生成。LncRNA 通过招募和驱动多蛋白复合物到特定的基因位点参与表观遗传调节,控制选择性剪接和蛋白质翻译,最终通过互补区域吸附多种 miRNA 从而重塑它们的细胞质模式。迄今为止的所有数据都验证了我们对外泌体作用的了解只是冰山一角,而它们正在从"细胞垃圾"变为"细胞宝藏"。

(高远 邓青松 刘珀霖 何姝航 沈志翰 王昂 译,郭尚春 审校)

参考文献

[1] Henne WM, Buchkovich NJ, Emr SD. The ESCRT pathway. Dev Cell 2011; 21(1): 77 - 91.
[2] Luhtala N, Odorizzi G. Bro1 coordinates deubiquitination in the multivesicular body pathway by recruiting Doa4 to endosomes. J Cell Biol 2004; 166(5): 717 - 29.
[3] Colombo M, et al. Analysis of ESCRT functions in exosome biogenesis, composition and secretion highlights the heterogeneity of extracellular vesicles. J Cell Sci 2013; 126(Pt 24): 5553 - 65.
[4] Jackson CE, et al. Effects of inhibiting VPS4 support a general role for ESCRTs in extracellular vesicle biogenesis. Biophys J 2017; 113(6): 1342 - 52.
[5] Baietti MF, et al. Syndecan-syntenin-ALIX regulates the biogenesis of exosomes. Nat Cell Biol 2012; 14(7): 677 - 85.
[6] Friand V, David G, Zimmermann P. Syntenin and syndecan in the biogenesis of exosomes. Biol Cell 2015; 107(10): 331 - 41.
[7] Ghossoub R, et al. Syntenin-ALIX exosome biogenesis and budding into multivesicular bodies are controlled by ARF6 and PLD2. Nat Commun 2014; 5: 3477.
[8] Imjeti NS, et al. Syntenin mediates SRC function in exosomal cell-to-cell communication. Proc Natl Acad Sci U S A 2017; 114(47): 12495 - 500.
[9] Reddy VS, et al. Extracellular small heat shock proteins: exosomal biogenesis and function. Cell Stress Chaperones 2018; 23(3): 441 - 54.
[10] Kajimoto T, et al. Ongoing activation of sphingosine 1-phosphate receptors mediates maturation of exosomal multivesicular endosomes. Nat Commun 2013; 4: 2712.
[11] Trajkovic K, et al. Ceramide triggers budding of exosome vesicles into multivesicular endosomes. Science 2008; 319 (5867): 1244 - 7.
[12] Alonso R, et al. Diacylglycerol kinase alpha regulates the secretion of lethal exosomes bearing Fas ligand during activation-induced cell death of T lymphocytes. J Biol Chem 2005; 280(31): 28439 - 50.
[13] Charrin S, et al. Tetraspanins at a glance. J Cell Sci 2014; 127(Pt 17): 3641 - 8.
[14] Latysheva N, et al. Syntenin-1 is a new component of tetraspanin-enriched microdomains: mechanisms and consequences of the interaction of syntenin-1 with CD63. Mol Cell Biol 2006; 26(20): 7707 - 18.
[15] Fader CM, et al. TI-VAMP/VAMP7 and VAMP3/cellubrevin: two v-SNARE proteins involved in specific steps of the autophagy/multivesicular body pathways. Biochim Biophys Acta 2009; 1793(12): 1901 - 16.
[16] Ruiz-Martinez M, et al. YKT6 expression, exosome release, and survival in non-small cell lung cancer. Oncotarget 2016; 7(32): 51515 - 24.
[17] Sinha S, et al. Cortactin promotes exosome secretion by controlling branched actin dynamics. J Cell Biol 2016; 214(2): 197 - 213.
[18] Ostrowski M, et al. Rab27a and Rab27b control different steps of the exosome secretion pathway. Nat Cell Biol 2010; 12 (1): 19 - 30; sup. pp 1 - 13.
[19] Bobrie A, et al. Rab27a supports exosome-dependent and -independent mechanisms that modify the tumor microenvironment and can promote tumor progression. Cancer Res 2012; 72(19): 4920 - 30.
[20] Hsu C, et al. Regulation of exosome secretion by Rab35 and its GTPase-activating proteins TBC1D10A-C. J Cell Biol 2010; 189(2): 223 - 32.
[21] Wegner CS, et al. Ultrastructural characterization of giant endosomes induced by GTPase-deficient Rab5. Histochem Cell Biol 2010; 133(1): 41 - 55.
[22] Loomis RJ, et al. Citron kinase, a RhoA effector, enhances HIV-1 virion production by modulating exocytosis. Traffic

2006; 7(12): 1643 - 53.
[23] Phuyal S, et al. The ether lipid precursor hexadecylglycerol stimulates the release and changes the composition of exosomes derived from PC-3 cells. J Biol Chem 2015; 290(7): 4225 - 37.
[24] Strauss K, et al. Exosome secretion ameliorates lysosomal storage of cholesterol in Niemann-Pick type C disease. J Biol Chem 2010; 285(34): 26279 - 88.
[25] Llorente A, van Deurs B, Sandvig K. Cholesterol regulates prostasome release from secretory lysosomes in PC-3 human prostate cancer cells. Eur J Cell Biol 2007; 86(7): 405 - 15.
[26] Savina A, et al. Exosome release is regulated by a calcium-dependent mechanism in K562 cells. J Biol Chem 2003; 278(22): 20083 - 90.
[27] Hoshino D, et al. Exosome secretion is enhanced by invadopodia and drives invasive behavior. Cell Rep 2013; 5(5): 1159 - 68.
[28] Villarroya-Beltri C, et al. ISGylation controls exosome secretion by promoting lysosomal degradation of MVB proteins. Nat Commun 2016; 7: 13588.
[29] Gangalum RK, et al. Inhibition of the expression of the small heat shock protein alphaB-crystallin inhibits exosome secretion in human retinal pigment epithelial cells in culture. J Biol Chem 2016; 291(25): 12930 - 42.
[30] Conigliaro A, et al. Exosomes: nanocarriers of biological messages. Adv Exp Med Biol 2017; 998: 23 - 43.
[31] Andreu Z, Yanez-Mo M. Tetraspanins in extracellular vesicle formation and function. Front Immunol 2014; 5: 442.
[32] Hurley JH, Odorizzi G. Get on the exosome bus with ALIX. Nat Cell Biol 2012; 14(7): 654 - 5.
[33] Hoshino A, et al. Tumour exosome integrins determine organotropic metastasis. Nature 2015; 527(7578): 329 - 35.
[34] Schillaci O, et al. Exosomes from metastatic cancer cells transfer amoeboid phenotype to non-metastatic cells and increase endothelial permeability: their emerging role in tumor heterogeneity. Sci Rep 2017; 7(1): 4711.
[35] Taverna S, et al. Curcumin modulates chronic myelogenous leukemia exosomes composition and affects angiogenic phenotype via exosomal miR-21. Oncotarget 2016; 7(21): 30420 - 39.
[36] Li SP, et al. Exosomal cargo-koading and synthetic exosome-mimics as potential therapeutic tools. Acta Pharmacol Sin 2018; 39(4): 542 - 51.
[37] Moreno-Gonzalo O, Fernandez-Delgado I, Sanchez-Madrid F. Post-translational add-ons mark the path in exosomal protein sorting. Cell Mol Life Sci 2018; 75(1): 1 - 19.
[38] Kalluri R, LeBleu VS. Discovery of double-stranded genomic DNA in circulating exosomes. Cold Spring Harb Symp Quant Biol 2016; 81: 275 - 80.
[39] Kahlert C, et al. Identification of double-stranded genomic DNA spanning all chromosomes with mutated KRAS and p53 DNA in the serum exosomes of patients with pancreatic cancer. J Biol Chem 2014; 289(7): 3869 - 75.
[40] Lazaro-Ibanez E, et al. Different gDNA content in the subpopulations of prostate cancer extracellular vesicles: apoptotic bodies, microvesicles, and exosomes. Prostate 2014; 74(14): 1379 - 90.
[41] Thakur BK, et al. Double-stranded DNA in exosomes: a novel biomarker in cancer detection. Cell Res 2014; 24(6): 766 - 9.
[42] Cai J, et al. Functional transferred DNA within extracellular vesicles. Exp Cell Res 2016; 349(1): 179 - 83.
[43] Cai J, et al. Extracellular vesicle-mediated transfer of donor genomic DNA to recipient cells is a novel mechanism for genetic influence between cells. J Mol Cell Biol 2013; 5(4): 227 - 38.
[44] Takahashi A, et al. Exosomes maintain cellular homeostasis by excreting harmful DNA from cells. Nat Commun 2017; 8: 15287.
[45] Wan JCM, et al. Liquid biopsies come of age: towards implementation of circulating tumour DNA. Nat Rev Cancer 2017; 17(4): 223 - 38.
[46] Guescini M, et al. Astrocytes and glioblastoma cells release exosomes carrying mtDNA. J Neural Transm (Vienna) 2010; 117(1): 1 - 4.
[47] Sun Z, et al. Emerging role of exosome-derived long non-coding RNAs in tumor microenvironment. Mol Cancer 2018; 17(1): 82.
[48] Bolukbasi MF, et al. miR-1289 and "zipcode"-kike sequence enrich mRNAs in microvesicles. Mol Ther Nucleic Acids 2012; 1: e10.
[49] Gao T, Shu J, Cui J. A systematic approach to RNA-associated motif discovery. BMC Genomics 2018; 19(1): 146.
[50] Baglio SR, et al. Human bone marrow- and adipose-mesenchymal stem cells secrete exosomes enriched in distinctive miRNA and tRNA species. Stem Cell Res Ther 2015; 6: 127.
[51] Hessvik NP, et al. Profiling of microRNAs in exosomes released from PC-3 prostate cancer cells. Biochim Biophys Acta 2012; 1819(11 - 12): 1154 - 63.
[52] Sun Z, et al. Effect of exosomal miRNA on cancer biology and clinical applications. Mol Cancer 2018; 17(1): 147.
[53] Momen-Heravi F, Getting SJ, Moschos SA. Extracellular vesicles and their nucleic acids for biomarker discovery. Pharmacol Ther 2018; 192: 170 - 87.
[54] Garcia-Romero N, et al. Extracellular vesicles compartment in liquid biopsies: clinical application. Mol Aspects Med 2018; 60: 27 - 37.
[55] Koppers-Lalic D, et al. Nontemplated nucleotide additions distinguish the small RNA composition in cells from exosomes. Cell Rep 2014; 8(6): 1649 - 58.
[56] Squadrito ML, et al. Endogenous RNAs modulate microRNA sorting to exosomes and transfer to acceptor cells. Cell Rep 2014; 8(5): 1432 - 46.
[57] Janas T, Janas MM, Sapon K. Mechanisms of RNA loading into exosomes. FEBS Lett 2015; 589(13): 1391 - 8.
[58] Melo SA, et al. Cancer exosomes perform cell-independent microRNA biogenesis and promote tumorigenesis. Cancer Cell 2014; 26(5): 707 - 21.
[59] Skotland T, Sandvig K, Llorente A. Lipids in exosomes: current knowledge and the way forward. Prog Lipid Res 2017; 66: 30 - 41.

[60] Haraszti RA, et al. High-resolution proteomic and lipidomic analysis of exosomes and microvesicles from different cell sources. J Extracell Vesicles 2016; 5: 32570.
[61] Yi X, et al. The feasibility of using mutation detection in ctDNA to assess tumor dynamics. Int J Cancer 2017; 140(12): 2642-7.
[62] Subra C, et al. Exosomes account for vesicle-mediated transcellular transport of activatable phospholipases and prostaglandins. J Lipid Res 2010; 51(8): 2105-20.
[63] Guay C, Regazzi R. Exosomes as new players in metabolic organ cross-talk. Diabetes Obes Metab 2017; 19(Suppl 1): 137-46.
[64] Chen G, et al. Exosomal PD-L1 contributes to immunosuppression and is associated with anti-PD-1 response. Nature 2018; 560(7718): 382-6.
[65] Lugini L, et al. Immune surveillance properties of human NK cell-derived exosomes. J Immunol 2012; 189(6): 2833-42.
[66] Kim SH, et al. MHC class II+ exosomes in plasma suppress inflammation in an antigen-specific and Fas ligand/Fas-dependent manner. J Immunol 2007; 179(4): 2235-41.
[67] Rivoltini L, et al. TNF-related apoptosis-inducing ligand (TRAIL)-armed exosomes deliver proapoptotic signals to tumor site. Clin Cancer Res 2016; 22(14): 3499-512.
[68] McGough IJ, Vincent JP. Exosomes in developmental signalling. Development 2016; 143(14): 2482-93.
[69] Sheldon H, et al. New mechanism for Notch signaling to endothelium at a distance by Deltalike 4 incorporation into exosomes. Blood 2010; 116(13): 2385-94.
[70] Raimondo S, et al. Chronic myeloid leukemia-derived exosomes promote tumor growth through an autocrine mechanism. Cell Commun Signal 2015; 13: 8.
[71] Yu L, et al. Exosomes with membrane-associated TGF-beta1 from gene-modified dendritic cells inhibit murine EAE independently of MHC restriction. Eur J Immunol 2013; 43(9): 2461-72.
[72] Corrado C, et al. Chronic myelogenous leukaemia exosomes modulate bone marrow microenvironment through activation of epidermal growth factor receptor. J Cell Mol Med 2016; 20(10): 1829-39.
[73] Taverna S, et al. Amphiregulin contained in NSCLC-exosomes induces osteoclast differentiation through the activation of EGFR pathway. Sci Rep 2017; 7(1): 3170.
[74] Montecalvo A, et al. Mechanism of transfer of functional microRNAs between mouse dendritic cells via exosomes. Blood 2012; 119(3): 756-66.
[75] Mulcahy LA, Pink RC, Carter DR. Routes and mechanisms of extracellular vesicle uptake. J Extracell Vesicles 2014; 3: 24641, 1-14.
[76] McKelvey KJ, et al. Exosomes: mechanisms of uptake. J Circ Biomark 2015; 4: 7.
[77] Kaksonen M, Roux A. Mechanisms of clathrin-mediated endocytosis. Nat Rev Mol Cell Biol 2018; 19(5): 313-26.
[78] Tian T, et al. Exosome uptake through clathrin-mediated endocytosis and macropinocytosis and mediating miR-21 delivery. J Biol Chem 2014; 289(32): 22258-67.
[79] Svensson KJ, et al. Exosome uptake depends on ERK1/2-heat shock protein 27 signaling and lipid raft-mediated endocytosis negatively regulated by caveolin-1. J Biol Chem 2013; 288(24): 17713-24.
[80] Santos MF, et al. VAMP-associated protein-A and oxysterol-binding protein-related protein 3 promote the entry of late endosomes into the nucleoplasmic reticulum. J Biol Chem 2018; 293(36): 13834-48.
[81] Song X, et al. Cancer cell-derived exosomes induce mitogen-activated protein kinase-dependent monocyte survival by transport of functional receptor tyrosine kinases. J Biol Chem 2016; 291(16): 8453-64.
[82] Greening DW, et al. Human endometrial exosomes contain hormone-specific cargo modulating trophoblast adhesive capacity: insights into endometrial-embryo interactions. Biol Reprod 2016; 94(2): 38.
[83] Crewe C, et al. An endothelial-to-adipocyte extracellular vesicle axis governed by metabolic state. Cell 2018; 175(3): 695-708.e13.
[84] Lou G, et al. Mesenchymal stem cell-derived exosomes as a new therapeutic strategy for liver diseases. Exp Mol Med 2017; 49(6): e346.
[85] Pegtel DM, et al. Functional delivery of viral miRNAs via exosomes. Proc Natl Acad Sci U S A 2010; 107(14): 6328-33.
[86] Tosar JP, et al. Assessment of small RNA sorting into different extracellular fractions revealed by high-throughput sequencing of breast cell lines. Nucleic Acids Res 2015; 43(11): 5601-16.

延伸阅读

[87] Yanez-Mo M, et al. Biological properties of extracellular vesicles and their physiological functions. J Extracell Vesicles 2015; 4: 27066.

第 2 章

外泌体分离方法及表征
Methods for exosome isolation and characterization

Mi Zhou[a], Sarah R. Weber[a], Yuanjun Zhao[a], Han Chen[b], Jeffrey M. Sundstrom[a]

[a]Department of Ophthalmology, Penn State Hershey Medical Center, Hershey, PA, United States,
[b]Microscopy Imaging Facility, Penn State Hershey Medical Center, Hershey, PA, United States

一、概述

不论是在生理还是病理条件下，几乎所有类型的细胞均可释放 EV[1]。外泌体是一类直径为 30～150 nm 的 EV，在 MVB 内作为腔内囊泡产生。外泌体也存在于多种体液，包括血液、尿液、脑脊液（cerebrospinal fluid，CSF）、玻璃体、腹水和母乳[2-7]之中。外泌体形成的机制尚有争议。目前一种常见的理论认为，外泌体通过一个 ESCRT 依赖的通路形成[8]。另一种关于多囊体形成和外泌体来源的观点是神经酰胺依赖通路理论[9]。神经酰胺是一种脂质，被认为有助于 MVB 膜内陷。Rab27 是小 GTP 酶中 Rab 家族的成员，已被证明可以控制外泌体分泌通路，特别是在 MVB 对接质膜时起到作用[10,11]。由于其异质性，选择一种适当的方法来分离和检测这些小囊泡至关重要。

大量证据表明，外泌体在细胞间交流中起着关键作用，因为这些囊泡以生物分子的形式封装了来自其亲代细胞的"信息"，包括蛋白质、脂质和核酸。这些信息会在不同的生理病理条件下特异性表达。例如，产生于 DC 和 T 细胞的外泌体已被证明携带细胞因子到它们的受体细胞[12]。产生于肿瘤细胞的外泌体参与了肿瘤细胞发生和转移的多个步骤，包括肿瘤细胞增殖、肿瘤细胞转移、免疫逃逸和血管生成[13]。另外，一些研究已经证实外泌体通过传播神经毒性物质参与神经退行性疾病的发展，如阿尔茨海默病和帕金森病[14,15]。

除了在细胞间交流的作用，外泌体可能也有一些有效的临床应用。外泌体越来越多地被作为诊断用生物指标和治疗用靶向药物运送载体[16,17]。一家名为 Exosome Diagnostics 的生物科技公司已经开发出几个突破性的基于外泌体的肺癌和前列腺癌诊断工具。Kamerkar 等发现外泌体有助于胰腺癌中原癌基因 KRAS 的靶向治疗。相对于脂质体，工程化外泌体可以通过向特定靶点递送 RNA 干扰（RNA interference，RNAi）提高肿瘤抑制的效率[18]。

为了同时在基础科学和临床环境中推进外泌体的研究，适当的制备和表征技术尤为重要。本文回顾了目前外泌体分离和表征技术，并突出其实验局限性。这里讨论的分离技术包括差速离心分离、超滤、密度梯度离心分离、沉淀和基于免疫俘获的分离方法。关于外泌体的表征,我们讨论了一些外泌体可视化的常用方法,主要运用透射电子显微技术(electron microscopy techniques,TEM)。我们同样讨论了许多外泌体的定量方法,包括纳米颗粒跟踪分析技术(nanoparticle tracking analysis,NTA)、非对称场流分离技术(asymmetric flow field-flow fractionation,AF4)、抗脉冲传感技术(resistance pulse sensing,RPS)。我们描述了流式细胞仪和 ExoView(NanoView Biosciences,Boston,MA)平台作为探测外泌体表面标记和亚型表征的工具。最后,我们讨论了追踪外泌体和界定外泌体货物的方法,包括蛋白质组学和微 RNA 测序技术。

二、外泌体分离方法

(一) 差速离心

最早开发差速离心是为了将外泌体从网织红细胞中分离出来,是目前最常用的外泌体分离方法[19]。这种方法的原理是通过连续的离心步骤将细胞、细胞碎片和大囊泡分离出来。简而言之,实验样品会分别在 300、2 000 和 10 000×g 的离心条件下分离出细胞、死细胞和细胞碎片。外泌体在 100 000×g 离心下获得。由于在这个过程中会丢失一大部分的囊泡,这种方法更适用于包含大体积初始样本的实验。根据 Kowal 等的研究,通过这种方法得到的外泌体 70% 由直径 50~150 nm 的囊泡组成,其余囊泡直径>150 nm(20%)或直径<50 nm(10%)[20]。

(二) 过滤和超速离心

过滤是另一种分离外泌体的常见方法。这种方法的原则是根据分子量和分子大小,利用膜过滤器将外泌体从其他样本成分中分离出来。

这种方法有两个主要步骤:① 利用孔径在 0.1~0.22 μm 的膜过滤器将外泌体从较大的微粒,如细胞、细胞碎片、细胞微粒中分离出来。② 利用分子量在 3~100 kDa 的过滤器将外泌体从较小的颗粒,如可溶性蛋白质、蛋白聚集物中分离出来。已经研发出许多商用膜过滤器,如有着 500 mL 容量和 0.22 μm 孔径的康宁一次性 Bottle-Top 过滤器,以及用于 3~100 kDa 蛋白质的 Amicon 离心过滤器 Ultra。如果需要进一步缩减体积,可以将含有外泌体的样品在 100 000~200 000×g 下离心至外泌体团块。

(三) 密度梯度离心

密度梯度离心是利用囊泡大小和质量密度的差异,制造密度梯度来分离外泌体。在离心分离步骤中,粒子穿过各梯度,直到到达其密度与周围溶液相匹配的点。蔗糖和碘克沙醇是两种常见的密度梯度制造介质。相对于蔗糖,碘克沙醇更稳定、黏性更低[21]。样品装载有两种方式:顶部装载和底部装载。底部装载相对于顶部装载更有优势,因为可溶性蛋白质会在超速离心时留在底部,但如果是顶部装载,可溶性蛋白质会沉淀在此梯度。

Greening 等从 OptiPrep(MilliporeSigma,US)(密理博西格玛,美国)报道了一种基于密度的利用碘克沙醇分离的方法[22]。实验样品首先在 100 000×g 下超速离心 2 小时。粗制的外泌体颗粒将在磷酸盐缓冲液（phosphate-buffered saline，PBS）中重悬，并且经顶部装载进入碘克沙醇梯度缓冲液中。在100 000×g下超速离心18小时后，管中会存在12个分层，而外泌体会在从上到下的第7个部分，而后收集这12个部分对其进行下游分析（图2-1A）。

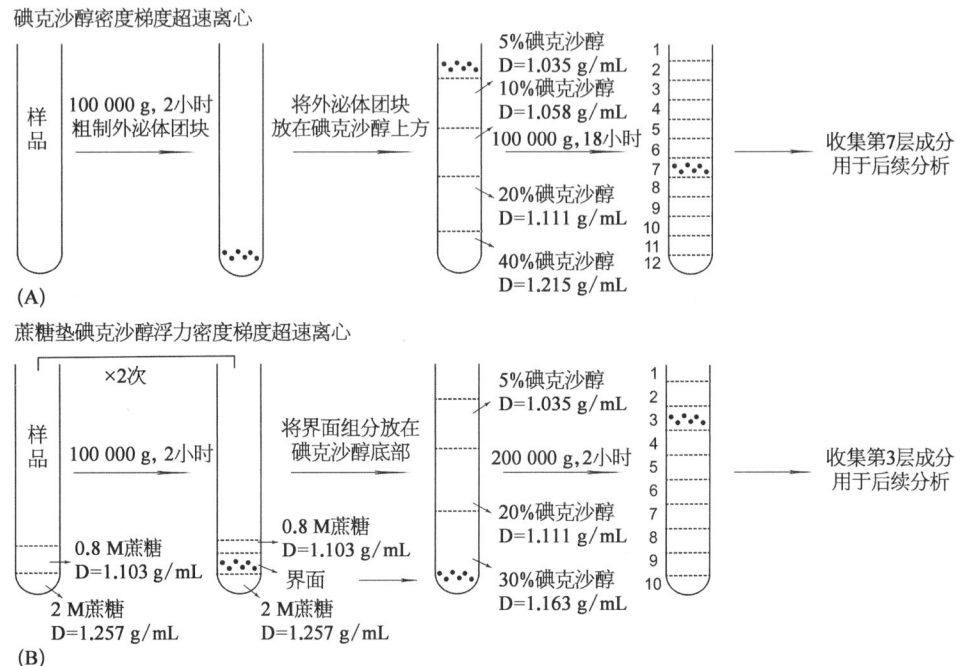

图2-1 A. 碘克沙醇密度梯度超速离心。B. 蔗糖垫碘克沙醇浮力密度梯度超速离心

相反，Choi等报道了一种使用样本底部装载方式进行外泌体分离和下游蛋白质组学分析的方法。这种方法是将实验样品添加到0.8 M和2 M的蔗糖层内并进行超速离心。重复此过程两次后，可以在两个蔗糖缓冲层间的交界面找到外泌体。此交界区溶液会被收集并置入碘克沙醇梯度缓冲液底部。另一超速离心产出了10个分层，外泌体即在从上至下的第3个分层，而后收集这10个分层进行下游分析（图2-1B）。

（四）沉淀

与上述方法相比，外泌体沉淀是一种更快、更有效的外泌体分离方法。这种方法的目的是利用高分子聚合物孵化，并在低速离心分离中与高分子聚合物结合获得外泌体。

此种方法中最常用的聚合物是聚乙二醇（polyethylene glycol，PEG）。ExoQuick外泌体沉淀液（System Biosciences，Palo Alto，CA）和英杰公司Total外泌体分离试剂（Thermo Fisher Scientific，Waltham，MA）是用于外泌体沉淀的两种热门商用产品。根据ExoQuick用户手册，首先对实验样品进行预处理以去除细胞和细胞碎片。清除后的溶液用合适剂量的ExoQuick孵化0.5~12小时，具体时间取决于样品类型。最后在1 500×g下离心分离30分钟以收集外泌体。

(五) 基于免疫俘获的分离方法

无论是超速离心分离还是沉淀法,都无法让外泌体亚型富集。迄今为止,免疫俘获是唯一分离外泌体亚型的方法。在磁珠涂上特定抗体的涂层,可以捕获这些带有表面抗原的外泌体。CD9、CD63 和 CD81 是最常见的标记,并且几乎在所有外泌体中表达[24]。其他标记可以用来分离特殊细胞类型来源的外泌体。例如,硫酸氢酶 4 抗体涂层磁珠可用来捕获黑色素瘤细胞衍生的外泌体[25];而 CD56 或 CD171 抗体涂层的磁珠可用来捕获神经元细胞来源的外泌体[26,27]。

(六) 外泌体分离方法总结

选择合适的外泌体分离方法通常取决于样品的体积、来源及下游分析的目的。为某个特定研究而选择最佳外泌体分离方法的最相关特点是:① 这种方法的外泌体回收率或产量;② 所获得外泌体的纯度;③ 这一方法所用时间和人工成本。我们将重点介绍上述几种方法的这些特征。

1. 回收率

一些研究表明,与其他方法相比,基于 PEG 的沉淀法有最高的回收率,为 80%～90%[28-30]。差速离心和超速离心有低至中的回收率。多项研究表明,由于差速离心在离心过程中失去了一大部分外泌体,而仅有 20%～40% 的回收率[29,31,32]。相比于差速离心,超速离心有更高的回收率,大约 60%[31]。差速离心和超速离心都常用于实验,每个实验室会基于各自的习惯来选择这两种方法。密度梯度超速离心的外泌体回收率最低,在 10% 左右[28]。由于基于 PEG 的沉淀法外泌体回收率最高,此方法通常用于起始样本量小的实验,如涉及临床生物流体样本[如血浆、尿液、羊水、玻璃体和脑脊液(CSF)]的实验。差速离心和超速离心通常用于从细胞培养基中分离外泌体,因为这些研究往往涉及较大的起始样本量。

2. 纯度

目前认为密度梯度超速离心是获得最高纯度外泌体样品的金标准,因为它们从囊泡中去除了非特异性结合蛋白(图 2-2)[28]。因此,密度梯度超速离心通常用于分离外泌体、进行外泌体蛋白质组学和 RNA 测序研究[23]。虽然差速离心和超速离心可以获得相对较高的样品纯度,但外泌体聚团是这些方法中的人为现象。因此,建议对外泌体团块进行充分的重悬。基于 PEG 的沉淀法往往产生纯度最低的外泌体样品。图 2-3 展示了在 TEM 下使用 ExoQuick 从人体玻璃体中分离的外泌体。外泌体很难从结合的聚合物中分离。由于蛋白污染物可能影响实验结果,应谨慎进行下游研究中的数据解释。

3. 时间和人工成本

在这些方法中,密度梯度离心需要的时间和人工最多,须 2～3 天才能完成整个过程。尽管差速离心分离法比超滤法耗时更多,但是如果实验室已具备相应的实验设备,膜过滤法和其他超滤设备需要消耗更多的耗材。基于 PEG 的沉淀法是时间和人力成本最低的方法。

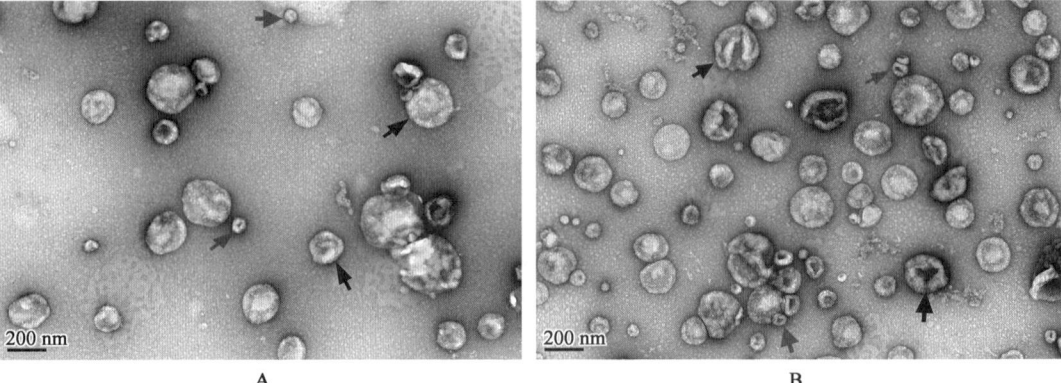

图 2-2　TEM 显示了两个外泌体亚群，使用蔗糖垫碘克沙醇浮力密度梯度超速离心分离出的，从（A）表达野生型腓骨蛋白-3 的视网膜色素上皮细胞和（B）表达 R345W-腓骨蛋白-3 的视网膜色素上皮细胞中分离的小囊泡（灰色箭头）和大囊泡（黑色箭头）

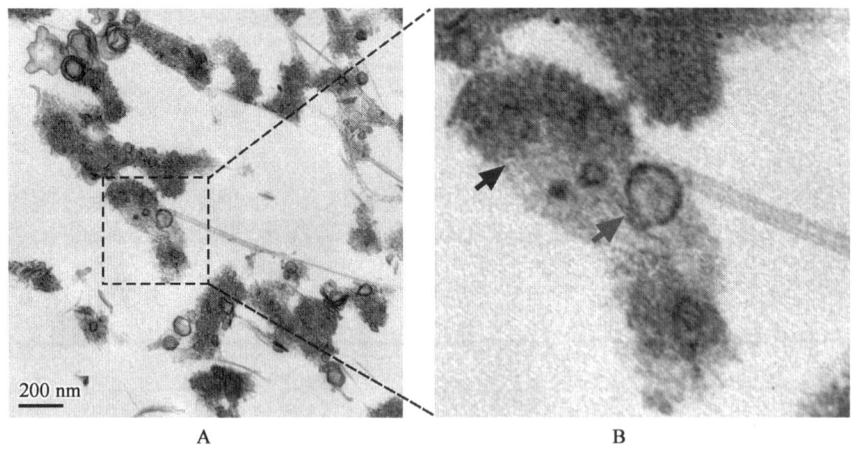

图 2-3　A. 使用 ExoQuick 从人类玻璃体分离出的外泌体 TEM 图像。B. 放大指定区域，显示囊泡（灰色箭头）附着在聚合物上（黑色箭头）

三、外泌体表征方法

（一）超微结构分析

1. TEM

由于外泌体体积小且样品容易制备，TEM 是研究外泌体形态学的金标准。TEM 的分辨率约为 1 nm，负染色过程也简单迅速，总耗时仅 2~3 小时。简言之，将外泌体固定在 2% 的多聚甲醛内，沉积在方华碳膜涂层的 TEM 网上，而后孵育 20 分钟。之后用 PBS 冲洗碳网，用戊二醛孵育，再用水洗涤。此时，囊泡用醋酸铀染色，在室温下风干[33]。常规 TEM 可用于：① 验证溶液中外泌体的存在；② 评估外泌体的质量；③ 研究外泌体的形态。TEM 很少用于外泌体定量，因为可重复性差且效率低下。免疫电镜已用于研究外泌体表面标志物，并可用于通过附着在 5~40 nm 金粒子上的初级抗体和二级抗体来孵育外泌体。

2. 扫描电子显微镜(scanning electron microscopy, SEM)

不同于 TEM 使用宽射束扫描,SEM 使用细点射束以逐线扫描样品。因此,SEM 侧重于根据样品表面提供外泌体的三维图像,而不是 TEM 生成的二维图像。简言之,外泌体用戊二醛固定,用乙醇梯度脱水。样品在室温下风干后,外泌体即准备好进行 SEM 分析[34]。根据 Sharma 等报道,与 TEM 下观察到的杯状形态不同,SEM 显示为圆形凸起且没有中央凹陷的形态。

3. 冷冻电子显微镜(cryogenic electron microscopy, Cryo-EM)

Cryo-EM 是 TEM 的一种类型。与 TEM 和 SEM 的空气干燥样品相比,Cryo-EM 允许样品保存在其原生水环境中。对于 Cryo-EM 分析,将悬浮外泌体放置在一个网格上,然后快速浸入液态乙烷中,从而使样品玻璃化冷冻。样品进行玻璃化冷冻后,可以在 Cryo-EM 下进行分析,或转移到液氮中储存[36]。Yuana 等表明在 Cryo-EM 下,外泌体具有清晰的双层结构,且有时会被较小的囊泡包围[37]。

4. 原子力显微镜(atomic force microscopy, AFM)

AFM 有着约为 1 nm 的高分辨率,且适用于拓扑学研究。Sharma 等使用 AFM 免疫金成像技术,在外泌体上识别出多个 CD63 受体位点[38]。简言之,将外泌体悬液放置在云母基底上,在室温下风干。然后用超纯水清洗样品,用氮气干燥。使用带硅探针的 AFM 查看样品,并使用 AFM 软件进行分析(图 2-4)[5]。

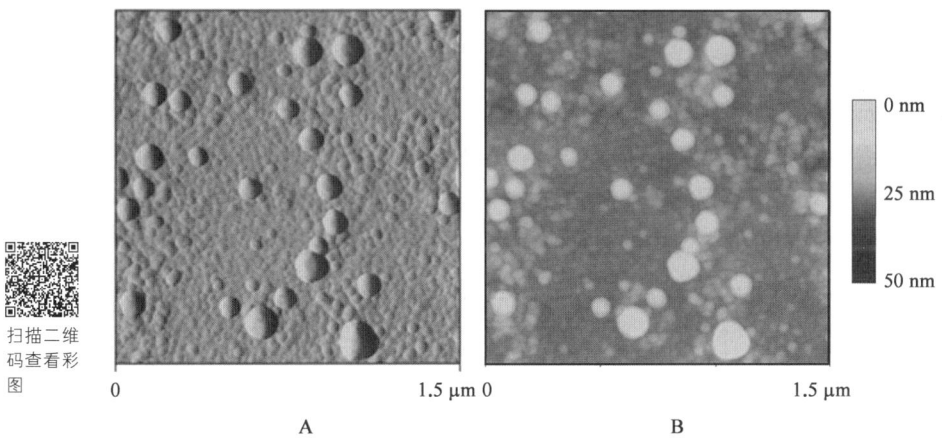

图 2-4 AFM 图像(A)和人玻璃体外泌体 AFM 高度图像(B)

(二) NTA

NTA 是测量外泌体浓度和大小分布的尖端方法。与流式细胞学和 TEM 相比,NTA 有更好的可重复性。NTA 具有高分辨率,能够检测直径为 30~1 000 nm 的囊泡。该技术利用动态光散射和斯托克斯-爱因斯坦方程来量化粒子大小和浓度。根据 NanoSight NS300(Malvern Panalytical,英国,马尔文)用户手册,在离散设置下,每个样品由注射器泵泵入机器中,并生成 5 个 60 秒的视频。样品测量的整个过程大约需要 15 分钟。图 2-5

显示了从 ARPE-19 细胞(人类视网膜色素上皮细胞系)使用过滤或超离提取外泌体的 NTA 结果。

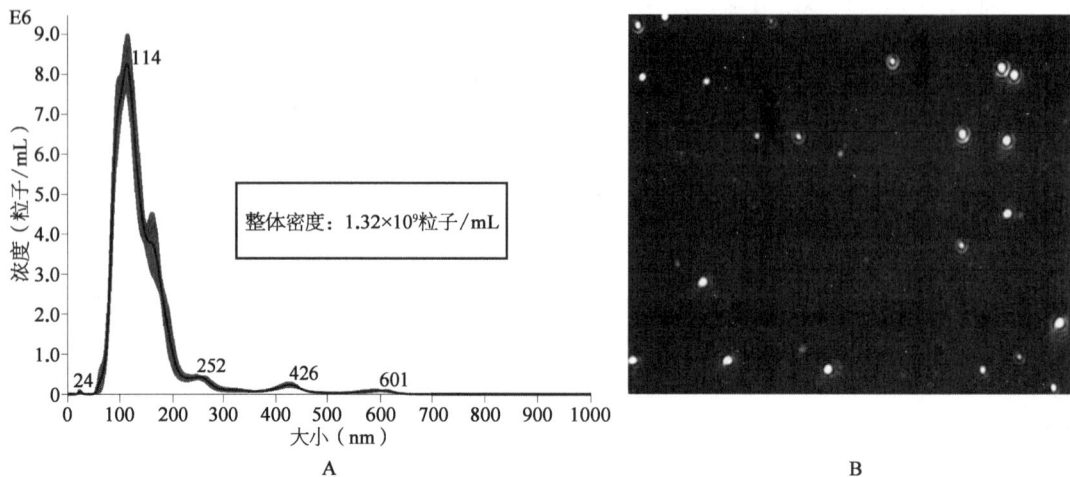

图 2-5 具代表性的 ARPE-19 细胞来源外泌体的 NTA 分布结果,包括(A)粒径分布图和(B)相应的视频截图

(三) AF4

AF4 是少数能够分离 EV 不同子集的方法之一。这项技术基于外泌体的密度和水动力特性进行分离。外泌体流经一个正向的层流通道,根据布朗运动,被分类到不同的种群中。较小的粒子具有较高的扩散率,并且移动更快;相比之下,较大的粒子具有较低的扩散率,并且往往移动较慢。目前,主要有两家公司生产 AF4 系统:怀亚特科技和 Postnova。一些研究针对外泌体定量比较了 AF4 和 NTA。NTA 在先前的研究中只解决了单个从 50～150 nm 的宽峰,但 AF4 能够区分两个独立的外泌体亚型,分别是大小在 90～150 nm 的大型外泌体和大小在 30 nm 左右的小型外泌体[39-41]。因此,AF4 能够更好地解决外泌体样品的大小异质性,并可作为外泌体亚型表征的高级分析技术。

(四) RPS

RPS 根据囊泡通过一个小孔时的电阻测量其大小。RPS 能够探测直径 50～1 000 nm 的囊泡。Spectradyne 有限责任公司是纳米颗粒微流体测量的龙头企业。与动态光散射和 NTA 相比,RPS 在测量粒子尺寸分布时具有更高的分辨率和精度。相比于 NTA,RPS 获得的外泌体浓度更接近从 TEM 获得。Grabarek 等报道,NTA 测量的外泌体浓度比 RPS 高 5～10 倍,因为 NTA 未能区分外泌体与蛋白质聚合体、脂质体和细菌[42]。

(五) 流式细胞学技术

由于外泌体低于标准流式细胞仪的分辨率极限,即 300～500 nm,因此无法通过此方法直接检测外泌体。一些研究报道了通过检测外泌体表面的特定膜标志物来半定量检测外泌体亚群的方法[43,44]。简言之,将外泌体附着在醛/硫酸盐-微球上,进行持续旋转15分钟的孵化。通过添加甘氨酸和牛血清白蛋白(bovine serum albumin,BSA)溶液来停止反应。结合了外泌体的微球用 PBS 洗净,用 BSA 封闭。依次加入一抗和荧光标记的二抗,用于检测特定的膜标记物。通过用相同条件控制以进行阴性对照,即用二抗或缺失一抗对外泌体结合的乳胶珠进行孵化。使用这种方法,Melo 等发现与从非肿瘤细胞中提取的外泌体相比,从胰腺肿瘤细胞中提取的外泌体携带更多的磷脂酰肌醇蛋白聚糖-1[44]。

(六) ExoView 表征平台

最近,Nano View Biosciences 公司开发了基于抗体的外泌体芯片。此方法能够以非常小的样本量对外泌体亚群进行分离。简言之,针对外泌体表面标志物的抗体排列在硅片上。外泌体悬液或含外泌体的体液在此芯片上孵化一晚。孵化之后,用 PBS 在振动器上清洗、风干。而后使用单粒子干涉反射成像传感器技术检测捕获的外泌体。这项技术可以增强粒子的信号对比度。Daaboul 等利用这种方法成功地检测出来自人胚胎肾细胞系的 CD63、CD8和 CD9 阳性的外泌体,以及来自人 CSF 的 CD171 阳性的外泌体[45]。与流式细胞仪相比,此方法需要更小的样品量且耗时更少。

(七) 活体外泌体跟踪

有人认为,外泌体通过在细胞间转运微 RNA 来调理细胞间交流。然而,外泌体执行这一功能的细节在很大程度上是未知的。目前有两种方法可以分析外泌体离开亲代细胞后的命运。这些外泌体标志和跟踪方法包括:① 用亲脂性羰花青染料染色外泌体,包括 PKH67(绿色)和 PKH26(红色)(密理博西格玛,美国)。② 用绿色荧光蛋白(green fluorescent protein,GFP)或荧光探针在细胞内处理外泌体标志,如 CD63[46]。为了研究外泌体内吞的机制,可用共聚焦显微镜观察荧光标记的外泌体与质膜之间的相互作用,以及外泌体与受体细胞细胞体的共定位信息。为了跟踪活体内循环的外泌体,可通过尾静脉将荧光标记的外泌体注射到小鼠体内,并使用小动物活体成像系统进行检测[47]。将 GFP-CD63 融合蛋白转染到大鼠胚胎干细胞[48],可产生 GFP-CD63 转基因大鼠。在这些转基因大鼠中的血清、母乳和羊水中发现了 GDP-CD63 标记的 EV。

四、外泌体货物

(一) 外泌体蛋白

1. 蛋白质组学

由于外泌体的异质性,可用质谱分析技术(mass spectrometry,MS)对几种类型的细胞和体液内的外泌体蛋白进行分析,以更好地了解外泌体,并研究它们是否是潜在的诊断用生物标志物[2,3,49]。外泌体蛋白质信息平台 ExoCarta 已鉴定了与外泌体有关的 9 769 个蛋白质。先进的基因本体分析表明,外泌体蛋白参与了多种生物功能,包括亚细胞定位、蛋白质结合、分子转移等。

MS 有两种常用的样品制备方法：凝胶内酶解和溶液内酶解。与溶液内酶解相比，凝胶内酶解的优点是在电泳过程中可以去除样品中的污染物。凝胶内酶解方法可以通过硫酸钠-聚丙烯酰胺凝胶电泳来分离外泌体蛋白。电泳后，凝胶通道被切成多个大小相等的片段，并用胰蛋白酶进行凝胶内酶解。而后可用 MS 结合高效液相色谱系统对酶解后的多肽进行分析。可用一些生物信息学方法，如通路分析和基因本体论，来进一步分析外泌体蛋白质表达谱[50]。

2. 外泌体蛋白：顶端 vs. 基底

上皮细胞的特定功能高度取决于它们的极性。多项研究比较了上皮细胞顶端与基底分泌产生的外泌体货物。Klingeborn 等发现视网膜上皮细胞顶端释放的外泌体中有 299 种独特的蛋白质，而在基底分泌的外泌体中发现了 94 种独特的蛋白质[51]。在肠道上皮细胞中，发现顶端外泌体携带了参与胞内体运输的蛋白质，而基底外泌体则含有具黏附和刺激作用的蛋白质[52]。这些研究表明，上皮细胞的极性影响外泌体货物，从不同方向分泌的外泌体具有极性特异性的功能。我们需要进行更多研究来阐明这些极性分泌外泌体亚群的功能作用及其潜在机制。

3. 外泌体作为生物标志物

外泌体常被认为是潜在的疾病生物标志物。前列腺肿瘤抗原 3 和跨膜蛋白丝氨酸 2 是两种用于前列腺癌诊断的外泌体蛋白[53]，然而外泌体表皮生长因子受体Ⅷ被证实在胶质母细胞瘤患者体内有较高水平表达[54]。胰腺癌患者体内外泌体蛋白多糖-1 升高[44]，外泌体 CD26 和 CD10 曾被建议用作肝损伤的潜在标志物[55]。蛋白质组学分析结合经蛋白质印迹或酶联免疫吸附测定是发现外泌体生物标志物广泛应用的方法。

4. 外泌体蛋白：表面结合 vs. 封装

与跨膜蛋白和细胞溶质蛋白一样，表面结合和封装的外泌体蛋白应具有不同的生物合成机制，并执行不同的功能。Fitzgerald 等开发了一种系统分析定位外泌体内细胞因子的方法[56]。Triton X-100 和超声处理技术能够裂解外泌体膜。通过比较 Triton X-100 或超声降解处理前后的蛋白质浓度，Fitzgerald 等揭示了 33 个细胞因子和外泌体之间的确切关联。此外，Skliar 等发现使用蛋白酶 K 或胰蛋白酶处理后，由于表面蛋白被酶解，外泌体体积会变得更小[57]。在实验室里，我们发现低浓度的胰蛋白酶（0.1 g 胰蛋白酶/1 g 外泌体蛋白）只酶解位于外泌体外表面的蛋白质，而不会干扰跨膜蛋白或囊泡内蛋白质。相比之下，高浓度的胰蛋白酶（0.3～1 g 胰蛋白酶/1 g 外泌体蛋白）可以破坏外泌体膜的稳定性，从而能够接触到囊泡内部，同时酶解其内外表面的蛋白质（未公布的数据），这为测定某个特定蛋白质与外泌体关联的方式提供了另一种方法。

（二）外泌体微 RNA（miRNA；miR）

与研究外泌体蛋白一样，人们研究了许多病理条件下的外泌体 miRNA，包括肿瘤、炎症和与年龄相关的退变。ExRNA 是一个获取外泌体 RNA 领域最新消息、步骤、近期论文的开放平台。多种肿瘤，包括卵巢癌、肺癌、乳腺癌和食管鳞状细胞癌[58]中都发现了其肿瘤细胞产生的外泌体 miR-21 增加。已证明外泌体 miR-155 可调节炎症反应[59]，外泌体

miR-9、miR-107 和 miR-124 在神经元分化中发挥作用,它们的下调与阿尔茨海默病的发病机制相关[60]。

Tang 等比较了不同的外泌体 RNA 分离方法,发现与 SeraMir Exosome RNA Column Purification Kit(System Biosciences)和 Invitrogen TRIzol LS Reagent(Thermo Fisher Scientific)相比,Invitrogen Total Exosome RNA 和 Protein Isolation kit(Thermo Fisher Scientific)具有更高的提取效率和纯度[29]。下一代测序技术可以生成整体测序数据,标记所有外泌体 miRNA 的位置。miRNA 芯片使用杂交技术来同时检测成百上千的 miRNA。实时聚合酶链反应和商业 miRNA 和抗 miRNA 抗体产品通常用于验证结果和机制研究。

五、总结

总之,最新证据表明外泌体和外泌体货物对细胞间交流的重大作用。本章总结了常用外泌体分离和表征方法的原则、步骤和优缺点。外泌体研究是一个新兴的、进展迅速的领域。新的方法在不断地研发中,并将促进外泌体研究向临床应用的转化。

(高远 李旭冉 张任 吴家琛 陆健 陈书瑶 译,陶诗聪 审校)

参考文献

[1] Thery C, Zitvogel L, Amigorena S. Exosomes: composition, biogenesis and function. Nat Rev Immunol 2002; 2: 569-79.
[2] Kalra H, et al. Comparative proteomics evaluation of plasma exosome isolation techniques and assessment of the stability of exosomes in normal human blood plasma. Proteomics 2013; 13: 3354-64.
[3] Gonzales PA, et al. Large-scale proteomics and phosphoproteomics of urinary exosomes. J Am Soc Nephrol 2009; 20: 363-79.
[4] Stuendl A, et al. Induction of alpha-synuclein aggregate formation by CSF exosomes from patients with Parkinson's disease and dementia with Lewy bodies. Brain 2016; 139: 481-94.
[5] Zhao Y, et al. Liquid biopsy of vitreous reveals an abundant vesicle population consistent with the size and morphology of exosomes. Transl Vis Sci Technol 2018; 7: 6.
[6] Runz S, et al. Malignant ascites-derived exosomes of ovarian carcinoma patients contain CD24 and EpCAM. Gynecol Oncol 2007; 107: 563-71.
[7] Torregrosa Paredes P, et al. Differences in exosome populations in human breast milk in relation to allergic sensitization and lifestyle. Allergy 2014; 69: 463-71.
[8] Colombo M, et al. Analysis of ESCRT functions in exosome biogenesis, composition and secretion highlights the heterogeneity of extracellular vesicles. J Cell Sci 2013; 126: 5553-65.
[9] Katarina Trajkovic CH, Chiantia S, Rajendran L, Wenzel D, Felix Wieland PS, Brügger B, Simons M. Ceramide triggers budding of exosome vesicles into multivesicular endosomes. Science 2008; 319: 1244-7.
[10] Ostrowski M, et al. Rab27a and Rab27b control different steps of the exosome secretion pathway. Nat Cell Biol 2010; 12 (Suppl. 11-13): 19-30.
[11] Bobrie A, Colombo M, Krumeich S, Raposo G, Thery C. Diverse subpopulations of vesicles secreted by different intracellular mechanisms are present in exosome preparations obtained by differential ultracentrifugation. J Extracell Vesicles 2012; 1.
[12] Mittelbrunn M, et al. Unidirectional transfer of microRNA-koaded exosomes from T cells to antigen-presenting cells. Nat Commun 2011; 2: 282.
[13] Azmi AS, Bao B, Sarkar FH. Exosomes in cancer development, metastasis, and drug resistance: a comprehensive review. Cancer Metastasis Rev 2013; 32: 623-42.
[14] Rajendran L, et al. Alzheimer's disease beta-amyloid peptides are released in association with exosomes. Proc Natl Acad Sci U S A 2006; 103: 11172-7.
[15] Alvarez-Erviti L, et al. Lysosomal dysfunction increases exosome-mediated alpha-synuclein release and transmission. Neurobiol Dis 2011; 42: 360-7.
[16] Lin J, et al. Exosomes: novel biomarkers for clinical diagnosis. Scientific World J 2015; 2015: 657086.
[17] Phinney DG, Pittenger MF. Concise review: MSC-derived exosomes for cell-free therapy. Stem Cells 2017; 35: 851-8.
[18] Kamerkar S, et al. Exosomes facilitate therapeutic targeting of oncogenic KRAS in pancreatic cancer. Nature 2017; 546: 498-503.
[19] Johnstone RM, Adam M, Hammond JR, Orr L, Turbide C. Vesicle formation during reticulocyte maturation. Association of plasma membrane activities with released vesicles (exosomes). J Biol Chem 1987; 262: 9412-20.
[20] Kowal J, et al. Proteomic comparison defines novel markers to characterize heterogeneous populations of extracellular

[21] vesicle subtypes. Proc Natl Acad Sci U S A 2016; 113: E968-77.
[21] Van Veldhoven PP, Baumgart E, Mannaerts GP. Iodixanol (Optiprep), an improved density gradient medium for the iso-osmotic isolation of rat liver peroxisomes. Anal Biochem 1996; 237: 17-23.
[22] Greening DW, Xu R, Ji H, Tauro BJ, Simpson RJ. A protocol for exosome isolation and characterization: evaluation of ultracentrifugation, density-gradient separation, and immunoaffinity capture methods. Methods Mol Biol 2015; 1295: 179-209.
[23] Choi D, Gho YS. Isolation of extracellular vesicles for proteomic profiling. Proteomic profiling: methods and protocols. Methods Mol Biol 2016; 1295: 167-77.
[24] Clayton A, et al. Analysis of antigen presenting cell derived exosomes, based on immunomagnetic isolation and flow cytometry. J Immunol Methods 2001; 247: 163-74.
[25] Sharma P, et al. Immunoaffinity-based isolation of melanoma cell-derived exosomes from plasma of patients with melanoma. J Extracell Vesicles 2018; 7: 1435138.
[26] Lugini L, et al. Immune surveillance properties of human NK cell-derived exosomes. J Immunol 2012; 189: 2833-42.
[27] Mustapic M, et al. Plasma extracellular vesicles enriched for neuronal origin: a potential window into brain pathologic processes. Front Neurosci 2017; 11(278).
[28] Van Deun J, et al. The impact of disparate isolation methods for extracellular vesicles on downstream RNA profiling. J Extracell Vesicles 2014; 3.
[29] Tang YT, et al. Comparison of isolation methods of exosomes and exosomal RNA from cell culture medium and serum. Int J Mol Med 2017; 40: 834-44.
[30] Kim J, Shin H, Kim J, Kim J, Park J. Isolation of high-purity extracellular vesicles by extracting proteins using aqueous two-phase system. PLoS ONE 2015; 10: e0129760.
[31] Lobb RJ, et al. Optimized exosome isolation protocol for cell culture supernatant and human plasma. J Extracell Vesicles 2015; 4: 27031.
[32] Yuana Y, et al. Handling and storage of human body fluids for analysis of extracellular vesicles. J Extracell Vesicles 2015; 4: 29260.
[33] Jung MK, Mun JY. Sample preparation and imaging of exosomes by transmission electron microscopy. J Vis Exp 2018.
[34] Sokolova V, et al. Characterisation of exosomes derived from human cells by nanoparticle tracking analysis and scanning electron microscopy. Colloids Surf B Biointerfaces 2011; 87: 146-50.
[35] Sharma S, et al. Structural-mechanical characterization of nanoparticle exosomes in human saliva, using correlative AFM, FESEM, and force spectroscopy. ACS Nano 2010; 4: 1921-6.
[36] Tatischeff I, Larquet E, Falcon-Perez JM, Turpin PY, Kruglik SG. Fast characterisation of cell-derived extracellular vesicles by nanoparticles tracking analysis, cryo-electron microscopy, and Raman tweezers microspectroscopy. J Extracell Vesicles 2012; 1:10.3402/jev.v1i0.19179.
[37] Yuana Y, et al. Cryo-electron microscopy of extracellular vesicles in fresh plasma. J Extracell Vesicles 2013; 2.
[38] Sharma S, Rasool HI, Palanisamy V, Mathisen C, Schmidt M, Wong DT, Gimzewski JK. Structural-mechanical characterization of nanoparticle exosomes in human saliva, using correlative AFM, FESEM, and force spectroscopy. ACSNANO 2010; 4: 1921-6.
[39] Zhang H, Freitas D, Kim HS. Identification of distinct nanoparticles and subsets of extracellular vesicles by asymmetric flow field-flow fractionation. Nat Cell Biol 2018; 20: 332-43.
[40] Petersen KE, et al. A review of exosome separation techniques and characterization of B16-F10 mouse melanoma exosomes with AF4-UV-MALS-DLS-TEM. Anal Bioanal Chem 2014; 406: 7855-66.
[41] Sitar S, et al. Size characterization and quantification of exosomes by asymmetrical-flow field-flow fractionation. Anal Chem 2015; 87: 9225-33.
[42] Grabarek AD, Weinbuch D, Jiskoot W, Hawe A. Critical evaluation of microfluidic resistive pulse sensing for quantification and sizing of nanometer- and micrometer-sized particles in biopharmaceutical products. J Pharm Sci 2019; 108: 563-73.
[43] Suarez H, et al. A bead-assisted flow cytometry method for the semi-quantitative analysis of extracellular vesicles. Sci Rep 2017; 7: 11271.
[44] Melo SA, et al. Glypican-1 identifies cancer exosomes and detects early pancreatic cancer. Nature 2015; 523: 177-82.
[45] Daaboul GG, et al. Digital detection of exosomes by interferometric imaging. Sci Rep 2016; 6: 37246.
[46] Takahashi Y, et al. Visualization and in vivo tracking of the exosomes of murine melanoma B16-BL6 cells in mice after intravenous injection. J Biotechnol 2013; 165: 77-84.
[47] Suetsugu A, et al. Imaging exosome transfer from breast cancer cells to stroma at metastatic sites in orthotopic nude-mouse models. Adv Drug Deliv Rev 2013; 65: 383-90.
[48] Yoshimura A, et al. Generation of a novel transgenic rat model for tracing extracellular vesicles in body fluids. Sci Rep 2016; 6: 31172.
[49] Epple LM, et al. Medulloblastoma exosome proteomics yield functional roles for extracellular vesicles. PLoS ONE 2012; 7: e42064.
[50] Schey KL, Luther JM, Rose KL. Proteomics characterization of exosome cargo. Methods 2015; 87: 75-82.
[51] Klingeborn M, et al. Directional exosome proteomes reflect polarity-specific functions in retinal pigmented epithelium monolayers. Sci Rep 2017; 7: 4901.
[52] van Niel G, Heyman M. The epithelial cell cytoskeleton and intracellular trafficking. II. Intestinal epithelial cell exosomes: perspectives on their structure and function. Am J Physiol Gastrointest Liver Physiol 2002; 283: G251-5.
[53] Nilsson J, et al. Prostate cancer-derived urine exosomes: a novel approach to biomarkers for prostate cancer. Br J Cancer 2009; 100: 1603-7.
[54] Skog J, et al. Glioblastoma microvesicles transport RNA and proteins that promote tumour growth and provide diagnostic biomarkers. Nat Cell Biol 2008; 10: 1470-6.

[55] Momen-Heravi GSF. Extracellular vesicles in liver disease and potential as biomarkers and therapeutic targets. Nat Rev Gastroenterol Hepatol 2017; 14: 455-66.
[56] Fitzgerald W, et al. A system of cytokines encapsulated in extracellular vesicles. Sci Rep 2018; 8: 8973.
[57] Skliar M, et al. Membrane proteins significantly restrict exosome mobility. Biochem Biophys Res Commun 2018; 501: 1055-9.
[58] Taylor DD, Gercel-Taylor C. MicroRNA signatures of tumor-derived exosomes as diagnostic biomarkers of ovarian cancer. Gynecol Oncol 2008; 110: 13-21.
[59] Bala S, et al. Circulating microRNAs in exosomes indicate hepatocyte injury and inflammation in alcoholic, drug-induced, and inflammatory liver diseases. Hepatology 2012; 56: 1946-57.
[60] Van Giau V, An SS. Emergence of exosomal miRNAs as a diagnostic biomarker for Alzheimer's disease. J Neurol Sci 2016; 360: 141-52.

第3章

实体瘤中的外泌体、微泡及其伴侣
Exosomes, microvesicles, and their friends in solid tumors

Denis Corbeila, Aurelio Loricob, c

[a]Biotechnology Center and Center for Molecular and Cellular Bioengineering, Technische Universität Dresden, Dresden, Germany, [b]College of Medicine, Touro University Nevada, Henderson, NV, United States, [c]Mediterranean Institute of Oncology, Viagrande, Italy

一、概述

几乎所有类型的细胞都能将包裹着膜的胞外囊泡(extracellular vesicle, EV)释放到细胞外环境中。对它们功能的初步评价是清除"细胞灰尘",以保持细胞的内稳态。这种清道夫功能并没有引起太多的注意,因此从未得到最终的证实。相比之下,Geuze研究小组在1996年巧妙地证明了由淋巴母细胞释放的EV可诱导抗原特异性的MHCⅡ类限制性T细胞反应,首次证实EV可以参与细胞间的通信[1]。十年后,另有研究证明EV可以包裹不同类型且功能活跃的RNA分子,在细胞间的交流中扮演载体的角色。此外,两个独立的研究小组均在EV中发现了mRNA和miRNA,并揭示了它们被靶细胞或受体细胞摄取后的功能[2,3]。如本书其他章节所述,鉴于越来越多的证据表明EV相关分子在内化后介导表型改变,现在认为,在生理和病理条件下,EV是多细胞生物体在其发育和整个生命周期中可作用于有限范围或长距离的细胞间通信介质[3-6]。此外,宿主细胞核中存在EV衍生的蛋白和核酸表明其内容物可穿梭至细胞核并调节基因表达,从而改变靶细胞的生化特性,尤其是在肿瘤中[7-11]。

通常根据EV的生物合成过程,将其分类为:来源于MVB的外泌体、从质膜直接萌发的核外颗粒体或微泡、由凋亡细胞在死亡过程中细胞破碎后释放的凋亡小体,以及从具有阿米巴样表型的肿瘤细胞非凋亡膜泡中脱落的肿瘤小泡[12-15]。EV的异质性体现在其体积差异很大,这在某种程度上是其形成过程所致的(图3-1)。在指定的类别中,单个EV也区别于其他EV,其组成成分反映着其供体细胞特点及其生理状态。特定成分(可溶性或膜性)可在EV中富集[12]。由于缺乏区分不同EV类别的特异性标记[14],除非作者指出其生物学来源,我们将其统称为EV。

一般而言,肿瘤细胞释放的EV数量多于正常增殖细胞,肿瘤患者血浆中的EV水平通常升高[18,19]。在细胞间通信过程中,EV作为一种载体样结构的作用似乎是肿瘤进展的一个重要的多方面调节因子。例如,肿瘤细胞来源的EV可以在不同水平调节免疫反应,转移致癌蛋白和核酸,重编程基质细胞,促进新生血管生成并转移耐药表型。尽管有大量研究报告突出了肿瘤中EV介导的事件,但关于EV内化后的细胞内通路、载物释放机制及其位于

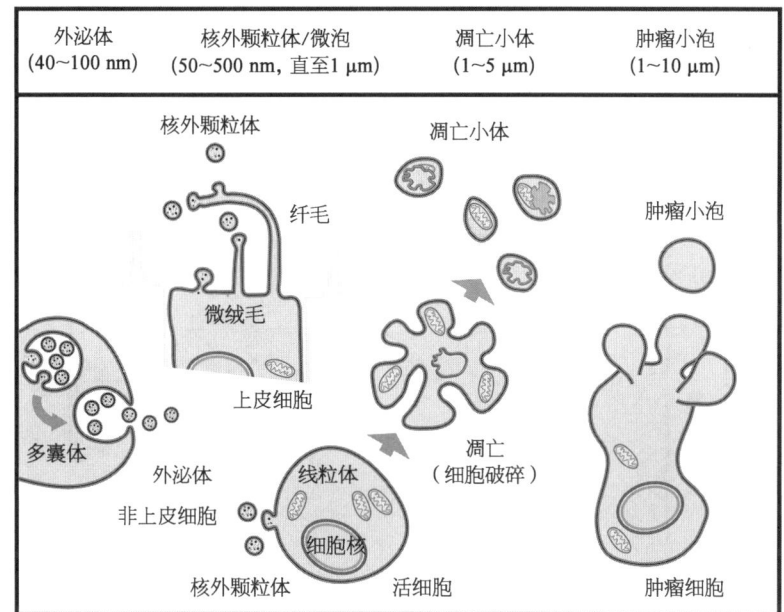

图 3-1 EV 的生物合成和异质性。EV 代表了根据其大小(上图)和细胞来源(下图)分类的不同种类的可溶性颗粒。括号中标明了指定类型 EV 的相对直径。在细胞外环境中可以发现各种类型的 EV,正如在上皮和非上皮细胞中观察到的,MVB 和直接从质膜出芽的核外颗粒体/微泡与质膜及其突起(如微绒毛和纤毛)融合后,单个细胞可以同时将其作为外泌体释放[16,17]。在指定的 EV 类型中,具有不同内容物的各种囊泡也可以共存。各种细胞类型在不同的生物体液中都影响着 EV 的存在,因此体内的 EV 群体尤为复杂。尽管 EV 可携带几种类型的细胞信息,但与细胞(其至病毒)相反,这些个体不能自我更新。EV 的释放可被细胞分化和转化刺激。较大的 EV 被称为凋亡小体和肿瘤小泡,分别由凋亡细胞和肿瘤细胞释放,这一发现使细胞外环境中的 EV 类别变得完整

扫描二维码查看彩图

宿主细胞胞质和核间隔中分子靶标的机制知之甚少[20]。

在本章中,我们将讨论肿瘤细胞来源的 EV 的功能和作用机制、它们与肿瘤微环境中正常细胞及其 EV 的相互作用,以及如何利用越来越多的关于肿瘤相关 EV 的知识优化肿瘤诊断、监测疾病进展和治疗反应,重要的是如何借此开发有效的抗癌策略。

二、(肿瘤)细胞来源胞外囊泡的细胞摄取

人们提出了许多解释 EV 携带的生物活性分子靶向细胞转移的机制,并且这些被肿瘤细胞来源 EV 包裹的分子释放途径与健康细胞释放的生理性 EV 相似[21]。尽管转运机制并不相互排斥,但根据细胞类型和细胞的生理条件,一些机制可能优于其他机制。起初,EV 可以直接与靶细胞的质膜融合,将其可溶性信号和(或)调节分子(蛋白质、脂质和核酸)释放到细胞质中,进而可能引发细胞的级联反应(图 3-2A,i)。在肿瘤微环境中,细胞外环境的酸性 pH 可促进 EV 与细胞融合[23]。在这些硬性条件下,EV 和宿主质膜的膜流动性变化,以

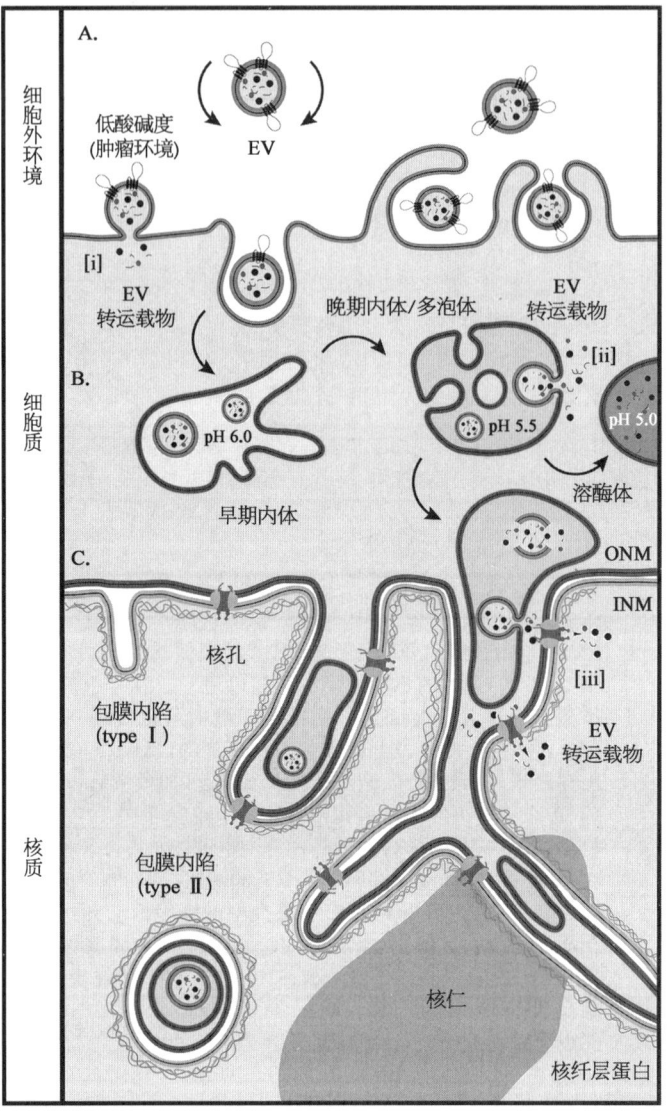

图3-2 EV的内化、细胞内途径及其内容物的运输。A. 描述了各种机制来解释靶细胞中EV载物分子(蛋白质、核酸)的递送。EV的内化可通过各种途径发生,特别是细胞-EV融合,可被肿瘤环境细胞外环境中的低pH、内吞、微胞饮作用和吞噬作用等条件刺激,这些机制并不相互排斥。EV与质膜的直接融合使其将内容物直接递送至靶细胞的细胞质中(i),这可能导致信号转导级联反应。EV与细胞最初的结合可以由特异性受体和(或)黏附蛋白介导,而融合蛋白可能有助于二者的互相融合,这些途径与某些病毒的入侵相似。内吞作用可由网格蛋白依赖性、富含胆固醇的脂筏机制或小窝介导(未显示)。这些不同机制的应用可能与细胞类型有一定的相关性,并且可能同时发生。B. 一旦内化,EV(及其内容物)被递送到内吞通路并在溶酶体中被降解,特别是在早期和晚期内体到溶酶体的"途中"。在晚期内体中,低pH(即约5.5)有利于EV与内体膜融合,并将其内容物释放到细胞质中(ii)。C. 晚期内体的亚细胞定位可能有利于EV内容物的靶向递送。一部分晚期内体群体也可以通过II型核膜内陷的方式转位到核间隔中,II型核膜内陷是由外核膜(outer nuclear membranes, ONM)和内核膜(inner nuclear membranes, INM)内陷共同产生。这些结构不仅可以到达细胞表层,也可以到达细胞核的深部区域。它们通常与核仁密切接触,核仁是负责核糖体生物合成、细胞周期控制和细胞信号传导的细胞器[11,22]。I型核膜内陷仅由INM产生,因此不允许细胞器穿透其中。EV与核内陷相关的晚期内体膜融合后(iii),EV内容物将从细胞质转运到核质,核孔参与其中。正如EV的管腔内容物一样,EV相关膜蛋白(如多次跨膜蛋白CD9、CD133)如何从内体膜中提取并转位到核质中,仍有待确定

及融合蛋白的发现可以解释 EV 与细胞的融合机制。尽管这种选择性细胞靶向的分子基础描述仍不充分[24]，但 EV 与靶细胞最初的相互作用可以通过受体和(或)黏附蛋白以特定的方式完成[21]。同样,关于 EV 细胞融合机制的详细信息需要更多的研究。与 EV 复杂的生物合成机制和载物分选机制相反[25]（另见其他章节），这种递送方式导致生物活性分子在细胞质中随机分布（主要分布在细胞周边），因而可能不足以产生所需的生物学效应。对于需要找到特定 RNA 转录靶标 EV 来源的 miRNA 尤其如此。另外，EV 可以与宿主细胞结合，促进细胞反应而不发生膜融合——这一机制类似于配体-受体相互作用[26]。直接来源于 EV 膜蛋白的可溶性配体在蛋白裂解后也能与宿主细胞受体结合，从而促进下游信号反应[27]。

生物活性分子的转移可以通过 EV 本身的内化发生，也包括各种内吞机制[28]。例如，网格蛋白依赖性或富含胆固醇的膜微区（脂筏）依赖性机制可以介导内吞作用[29]（图 3-2A）。干扰网格蛋白小凹的生物合成和动力学的化学药物或治疗可以阻断 EV 进入，如钾耗竭和胞质酸化[30]。类似地，正如在黑色素瘤来源的 EV 中发现[11]，干扰膜流动性和/或膜微区组织的化合物，如胆固醇螯合剂甲基-β-环糊精[31]可以干扰 EV 的摄取。EV 的内吞作用也可能通过胞膜窖进行，其中胆固醇结合胞膜窖蛋白起主要作用[32]。胞膜窖富含胆固醇和鞘脂，膜胆固醇对其形成至关重要[33]。调节 EV 内吞作用的不同机制可能具有细胞类型依赖性，并且可能在指定细胞中同时存在[34]。最后，巨胞饮和吞噬作用是另外两种机制，可导致 EV 的内化[35,36]（图 3-2A）。

内化后，EV 及其内容物进入内吞途径，开启其在宿主细胞内的旅程。在这一过程中，EV 将被递送到早期内体，这是第一个从质膜接收内化 EV 载物的内吞室[37]（图 3-2B）。这些以细管状伸长出现的动态结构通常作为分选平台，载物蛋白可以通过各种途径转运回质膜或高尔基体，或通过晚期内体转运回溶酶体进行降解[38]。与早期内体相比，后者的 pH 较低、外形更圆、内部囊泡众多，这也解释了为什么它们被称为多囊泡内体或 MVB[39,40]（图 3-2B）。质子泵空泡-ATP 酶，以及可能的管状内体裂变，可能是内体区室逐渐腔内酸化的原因[41,42]。早期和晚期内体不仅在形态和 pH 方面存在差异，而且在蛋白质和脂质组成方面也存在差异[43]。溶酶体含有在酸性条件下完成此类功能所必需的所有酶，在降解进入溶酶体之前，质膜上内化的信号分子及其受体依次分选为早期和晚期内体[44]。内化的 EV 及其载物也可能有类似的命运（图 3-2B）。因其发挥细胞间通信的作用，故 EV 载物的溶酶体降解不会提供任何细胞反应。另外，内化的 EV 可以与晚期内体膜融合，并将其内容物释放到细胞质中（图 3-2B,ii）。与早期内体相比，晚期内体中的酸性微环境可促进 EV 与晚期内体融合。和 EV 与质膜的融合相比，晚期内体的亚细胞定位可能使 EV 内容物易于递送到其分子靶位。位于核周区的晚期内体尤其如此[45,46]（图 3-2C）。晚期内体与不同细胞器的相互作用，如内质网（endoplasmic reticulum，ER）和线粒体也可以将其载物靶向至作用部位[47-49]。最近的研究表明，晚期内体与翻译机制有关，是轴突生长中 RNA 转录本的局部翻译位点，这一发现可能为 EV 及其内化后的命运带来新的时空维度[50]。EV 携带的 mRNA 载物是否可以在 EV 与晚期内体膜融合后立即翻译还有待探索。

（一）早期和晚期内体在细胞外信息核转移中的定位作用

按照内化 EV 的细胞内途径，我们最近观察到一部分载 EV 的晚期内体（存在小 GTP 酶 Rab7）通过侵入核膜内陷到达核间隔的深部区域[11]。描述了两种类型的核膜内陷：Ⅰ型是由 INM 内陷到核质中产生，而Ⅱ型同时含有 ONM 和 INM，后者可承载各种细胞质细胞器[51]。Ⅱ型核膜内陷中晚期内体的存在为 EV 载物靶向到核间隔提供了一条新的途径。已在多种细胞系（包括黑色素瘤细胞和基质细胞）体外研究和乳腺癌样本的体内研究中观察到上述结果[11]。内化的 EV 与晚期内体的膜融合后，EV 载物处于核内陷内的适当位置，通过核孔转运到核质，在那里它们可以进入基因组，并可能调节基因表达[11]。在核膜与核仁（一种亚核结构）内陷的附近[11,51]，EV 载物也可能干扰其活性，如核糖体生物合成和核仁蛋白隔离[52]。核仁经常被肿瘤劫持以促进转化细胞的生长可能不仅仅是巧合[53]，因而可以作为肿瘤干预的靶标[54]。这条新路径至少可以部分解释与 EV 相关的多跨膜蛋白的核定位，如 CD9 和 CD133（参见下文），以及可能存在的 EGFR，尤其是后者的致癌形式[10,55-60]。尽管尚未证实，但不能排除该通路参与质膜蛋白（包括受体）向核间隔的穿梭[61]。在这两种情况下，膜蛋白如何从内体膜中提取并通过核孔仍有待确定。除晚期内体区室外，早期内体（定义为早期内体抗原 1 的存在）与外周核膜的对接和融合也可能参与将细胞外生物材料递送至宿主细胞核[62]。在后者中，核包膜蛋白 SUN1 和 SUN2，以及 Sec61 转座子复合物被发现参与细胞表面蛋白的核转移。总之，核膜相关早期内体（envelope-associated endosome，NAE）[62] 和核膜内陷相关晚期内体（nuclear envelope invagination-associated late endosome，N-ALE）[11]在依靠细胞外信号进入宿主细胞核方面处于战略地位。由于 N-ALE 的外观在鞘内有剑的 Rab7-SUN2 免疫荧光双标记有一定的相似性，因此我们将这种结构命名为"spathasome"，这源于希腊语/拉丁语中的"spathi/spatha"，意为剑[11]。

这两个新发现的细胞内运输途径值得进一步关注，因为它们可以提供潜在的靶标来干扰 EV 介导的肿瘤细胞和健康细胞之间的细胞间通信，特别是那些与肿瘤干细胞微环境相关的细胞。

（二）VOR 蛋白复合物

膜结合细胞器之间的相互作用已成为真核细胞分子生物学的新主题，其通过膜接触的串扰在膜动力学和细胞信号传导中的作用被低估[63,64]。晚期内体与 ER 的相互作用已被充分证实[48]，其相关知识有助于确定调节晚期内体进入核质网及其与 ONM 对接的部分机制[65]。内质网定位的囊泡相关膜蛋白（vesicle associated membrane protein，VAMP）相关蛋白 A（VAMP-associated protein A，VAP-A）是介导晚期内体-核膜相互作用的决定因素。与 R-Ras 相互作用氧化固醇结合蛋白（oxysterol-binding protein，OSBP）相关蛋白 3（OSBP-related protein 3，ORP3）一起，调节细胞黏附并在多种肿瘤中过表达，VAP-A 决定了与晚期内体相关 Rab7 的相互作用[65]。先前已证明 VAP-A-ORP3 复合物可介导 ER 与质膜的膜接触[66,67]。VAP-A/ORP3/Rab7 相互作用形成的三无复合物（命名为 VOR 复合物）对于将 EV 载物转移到核质至关重要。沉默 VAP-A 或 ORP3 阻碍了晚期内体进入核质网[65]，从而阻碍了核 EV 载物的存在[65]。考虑到晚期内体的核转位依赖于微管,未鉴定的运动蛋白应参与该过程[65]。总之,VOR复合体在依赖从EV到靶细胞核区室的信息中发挥重要作用,代表了抑制肿瘤细胞间通信的潜在靶点。VOR复合物在多细胞有机体发育过程中的意义及其参与EV介导的细胞间通信的稳态仍有待研究。

三、胞外囊泡和肿瘤微环境

EV的多效性在致癌作用中得到了很好的阐述,它们促进了健康细胞之间正常细胞间通信的显著改变,进而导致肿瘤生长和转移。在给定的组织或器官中尤其如此,这其中包含许多细胞类型可以释放EV并摄取来自肿瘤细胞的EV。目前认为,EV是肿瘤进展过程中,特别是转移性微环境建立过程中的主要参与者。因此,无论是从细胞生物学的角度,还是作为临床治疗靶点,EV都值得被特别深究。

(一) EV在转移中的作用

肿瘤转移是肿瘤相关的主要死亡原因,是肿瘤细胞脱落后启动的复杂细胞反应的结局。脱落细胞通过淋巴和血液循环播散,并在远离原发肿瘤的部位植入[68-70]。肿瘤细胞与附近以及远处的间充质细胞、内皮细胞和免疫细胞交换生物活性分子,如生长因子、整合素以及编码和非编码RNA,为癌性生长和转移灶的形成建立有利条件[71]。这些分子交换调节信号通路,抑制对抗细胞野蛮生长的免疫反应,招募幼稚的邻近细胞,为肿瘤细胞的局部和远距离扩散提供有利条件[72]。虽然导致肿瘤远处转移的主要因素及其各自效应仍存在争议,但近年来的一些研究已经证实了EV作为微环境调节器的意义,它可以调控对肿瘤生长和远处转移形成至关重要的环节,包括调节血管生成和免疫反应。通过介导肿瘤、间质和免疫细胞之间的间接相互作用,EV似乎在准备转移部位的肿瘤生态位方面起主导作用,这种转化会对在其中发现的天然细胞成分产生负面影响(图3-3)。

肿瘤细胞来源的EV如何定植于特定的器官部位,并在未来转移部位的形成过程中有利于肿瘤生长的肿瘤微环境?根据数据显示,黏附和细胞外基质蛋白(如整合素和张力蛋白分子)可以刺激恶性转化[73,74],EV携带的整合素在这方面可以发挥重要作用[75]。

事实上,EV相关的整合素可以在转移扩散和生物活性分子直接转移到靶细胞的过程中,通过决定靶组织形成新的肿瘤生态位进而促进肿瘤进展[75]。已发现一系列整合素来引导EV到特定的器官。例如,Hoshino等已经证明 $\alpha_6\beta_1$ 和 $\alpha_6\beta_4$ 整联蛋白介导EV在其预测的肺转移部位选择性黏附于细胞外基质,随后被固有成纤维细胞和上皮细胞摄取[76]。同样,据报道,含整合素 $\alpha_v\beta_5$ 的EV与Kupffer细胞特异性结合可介导肝转移[77]。Languino的研究小组描述了在前列腺肿瘤细胞中 $\alpha_v\beta_6$ 和 $\alpha_v\beta_3$ 整联蛋白借助EV的转移[78,79]。$\alpha_v\beta_6$ 是正常前列腺中缺失的整合素,但在前列腺癌的单核细胞M2极化中 $\alpha_v\beta_6$ 是必需的,然而在癌变到非癌变的前列腺细胞中 $\alpha_v\beta_3$ 整合素均可促进其迁移能力[80,81]。总之,循环中EV携带的特殊黏附蛋白可以调控它们的特定扩散,并使特定的组织和(或)器官易于转移。因此在临床上,对EV相关整合素信号的前瞻性分析可以预测其转移倾向。

当他们到达预定的远处转移位时,特定的EV及其载物可促进转移前生态位的形成。因此,它们可以使得正常细胞表型向促转移表型转化,如HSPC所在的骨髓干细胞微环境所示(图3-3)。作为主要靶标,固有细胞如成纤维细胞和 MSC 易转化为 CAF[82,83]。固有和适应性免疫炎症细胞和内皮细胞也有助于肿瘤微环境的形成。此外,肿瘤细胞本身可以交换 EV 进而导致肿瘤细胞异质性。

黑色素瘤细胞来源的 EV 是一个很好的例子,它通过介导癌基因 *c-met* 的转移和将祖细胞重新编程为有利于血管生成的表型,将骨髓生态位向转移表型转化,诱导血管渗漏[84]。尽管该研究的重复实验没有发现表达 c-met 的 EV 的促转移效应具有统计学意义[85],但仍应牢记先前的研究结论。随后,研究发现注射来自高水平 c-met 表达细胞的 EV 增加了低 c-met 表达细胞的转移负担[86]。两个独立的报告发现,肿瘤细胞衍生的 EV 通过调节肝脏微环境并诱发转移前生态位的形成来促进肝脏转移[77,87]。其他几项研究已经证实,在肿瘤细胞注射前,将肿瘤来源的 EV 注射到小鼠身上,可以通过诱导转移前生态位的形成增加转移负担[88-91]。

大量文章已报道关于干性标志物——五次跨膜糖蛋白 CD133(也称为显著蛋白-1)在肿瘤干细胞龛中的意义,其中包括促进肿瘤细胞的侵袭特性和诱导血管生成拟态的形成[92-96]。作为 EV,如核外颗粒体和外泌体的生物标志物[16,97](见参考文献[98]),两项研究报道了从肿瘤细胞(即结肠癌和黑色素瘤)中释放以核外颗粒体和外泌体作为生物标志物的

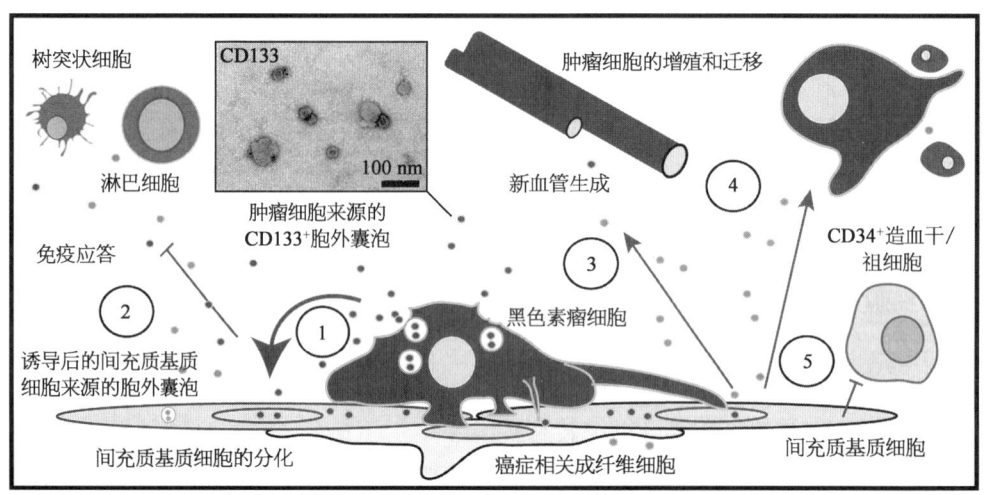

扫描二维码查看彩图

图3-3　EV 在肿瘤条件下对细胞间通信的影响。与其他类型的肿瘤一样,黑色素瘤中的恶性细胞可能会使用 EV 将骨髓造血干细胞龛转化为癌变,特别是那些表达 CD133 的 EV。在骨髓间充质干细胞和其他基质细胞类型(如成纤维细胞)的内吞作用下,肿瘤细胞来源的 EV 可以改变其生化特点,导致其转化为肿瘤相关成纤维细胞(cancer-associated fibroblast, CAF)(♯1)。黑色素瘤衍生的 EV、EV 致敏的基质细胞和(或)其衍生的 EV 也可通过作用于 DC 和淋巴细胞等(♯2)负性调节免疫应答,刺激血管形成(♯3),并通过刺激细胞迁移和增殖增加肿瘤细胞群(♯4)。所有这些 EV 介导的修饰将降低基质细胞对固有 CD34[+] 造血干/祖细胞(hematopoietic stem and progenitor cell, HSPC)的支持能力,同时增加对肿瘤细胞的支持能力(♯5)。一个 CD133 免疫胶体金标记人黑色素瘤来源 EV 的电子显微镜实例(*Micrograph is taken from our previous publication: Rappa G, et al. Wnt interaction and extracellular release of prominin-1/CD133 in human malignant melanoma cells. Exp Cell Res* 2013; 319: 810-9)

CD133[+]EV[16,99](图3-3)。与早期的研究一致,有研究证实 CD133[+]EV 在 FEMX-I 黑色素瘤中的促转移作用[99],该研究表明短干扰(Sh)RNA 介导的 CD133[+]下调会导致黑色素瘤转移潜能的丧失[94]。暴露于 CD133[+]黑色素瘤来源的 EV 增加了骨髓间充质干细胞的侵袭力,这表明 EV 载物改变了靶细胞的生物学特性,从而改变了它们的表型[100]。作为质膜突起(即微绒毛、丝状足、初级纤毛)的组织者,CD133 本身就可以促进这些形态转变[60,101]。与这些观察结果一致,Alessandro 的研究小组巧妙地证明,结肠 SW620 转移细胞释放的 EV 通过 Rac GTPase 激活蛋白 1(Rac GTPase-activating protein 1,RacGAP1)介导的通路调节非转移 SW480 细胞的表面活性、活动性和侵袭性[102]。RacGAP1 是一种 Rho GTP 酶激活蛋白,参与控制胞质分裂、转化、细胞迁移和转移等细胞现象,其可以抑制 Rac1 活性,激活细胞前端的 RhoA 进而促进侵袭性迁移[103]。SW480 和 SW620 细胞系代表肿瘤发展的两个不同阶段,认为是同一患者肿瘤内构成的不同亚克隆的代表。CD133 在 SW620 细胞中高表达,而在 SW480 细胞中不表达[104,105]。同样,活体成像显示侵袭性较弱的乳腺肿瘤细胞内化高度侵袭性肿瘤细胞来源的 EV 后表现出更强的迁移能力,这表明肿瘤细胞来源的 EV 可以充当恶性肿瘤的信使[4](图3-3)。侵袭性表型的转移可能与 EGFR 和 Met 72 肿瘤抗原的致癌形式有关[106,107]。

通过释放细胞因子和细胞外基质(extracellular matrix,ECM)成分,CAF 对于建立转移前的生态位非常重要[108,109](图3-3)。有关转移前生态位形成所涉及的分子和细胞因素的详尽列表,我们邀请读者查阅一篇优秀的综述[110]。如上所述,它们来源于组织内的成纤维细胞和骨髓间充质干细胞,通常对血小板衍生生长因子(platelet-derived growth factor,PDGF)和转化生长因子β(transforming growth factor beta,TGF-β)信号有反应。几个研究小组[113,114]已经证实,与正常驻留细胞相比,CAF 在促进肿瘤生长和转移方面有一定优势[113,114]。有趣的是,来自不同肿瘤类型的肿瘤细胞来源的 EV 已被证实可通过转移 TGF-β、miR-125b 或 miR-155 来促进正常成纤维细胞分化为 CAF。特别是在肿瘤微环境中,EV 介导的 miR-125b 从乳腺肿瘤细胞到正常成纤维细胞的转移有助于其分化,至少部分通过其靶标如肿瘤抑制蛋白 p53(p53;转化相关蛋白53)起作用。类似地,在体内和体外,非小细胞肺癌来源的含双调节蛋白的 EV 通过 EGFR 介导的途径激活 MSC 的破骨细胞生成[118]。黑色素瘤细胞来源的 EV 已被证明可以改变 MSC 的基因表达谱,特别是编码参与炎症过程的基因。EV 介导的 MSC 转化依赖于上述 spathasome 途径[11]。

同时还探讨了 EV 相关的非编码 RNA 在转移和干细胞生态位转化中的作用。在非肿瘤条件下,内源性 RNA 被 RNA 结合蛋白屏蔽[119],据报道,肿瘤细胞在肿瘤微环境中诱导 CAF 产生含有非屏蔽内源性 RNA 的 EV(如 RN7SL1),这反过来又促进了肿瘤的生长、转移和治疗耐药性[120]。Wong 的实验室报道了肿瘤细胞来源的 EV 及其相关 miRNA 对肿瘤干细胞微环境和肿瘤进展的几种影响:① miR-105 诱导 CAFs 的代谢可塑性,将肿瘤产生的代谢废物(如乳酸和氨)转化为富含能量的代谢产物,重新进入肿瘤生物能量循环[121];② 肺成纤维细胞和星形胶质细胞对葡萄糖利用的抑制,促进了肿瘤分泌 miR-122 介导的转移肿瘤细胞摄取葡萄糖[88];③ 肿瘤分泌的 miR-105 引起血管渗漏和转移增强并影响内皮紧密连接[91]。

最近的实验证据表明，在某些情况下转移过程可能不是由肿瘤细胞的迁移决定的，而是由肿瘤细胞源性 EV 中包含的恶性因子靶向转移到非肿瘤细胞引起。因此，肿瘤细胞源性 EV 被上皮和间充质来源的肿瘤抑制突变细胞（oncosuppressor-mutated cell，OMC）摄取，即 BRCA1 突变或磷酸酶和张力蛋白同源物（phosphatase and tensin homolog，PTEN）缺失的细胞发生恶变，产生与 EV 起源的肿瘤细胞表型相容的表型[122-124]。当与肿瘤患者血清、肿瘤细胞条件培养液或肿瘤 EV 接触时，OMC 在体外（锚定非依赖生长实验）和体内（免疫缺陷小鼠肿瘤形成）都表现出转化细胞的特征[122,124]。似乎单一的抑癌基因突变是一个先决条件，并在接触 EV 中的肿瘤因子后，该突变代表着恶性转化后的第一次打击。这些发现、对水平基因转移介导肿瘤进展体内模型的描述[125]和对结直肠癌患者血浆中循环游离核酸介导的致癌转化的观察[126]，支持了基于恶性和非恶性细胞之间肿瘤特征交换的非经典途径的存在，这很可能与肿瘤的进展和转移有关。

虽然所有的肿瘤细胞都会释放小的 EV，但只有某些类型的 EV 会释放被称为肿瘤小泡的非典型的大 EV。它们的首次识别是在体外从间充质迁移模式转变为阿米巴类型的过程中，是 Akt 激活和 diaphanous 相关形成蛋白 3（diaphanous related formin 3，DIAPH3）丢失的结果[127]。后一种蛋白参与肌动蛋白重塑并调节黏附和细胞运动。在转移性前列腺癌患者的肿瘤组织和血浆中相继发现了肿瘤小泡[128]。从技术上讲，肿瘤小泡可以通过差速离心后密度梯度与其他小的 EV 分离。这种方法可以用来识别一组不同的蛋白质[128]。肿瘤小泡内化后进入成纤维细胞将导致转录因子 MYC 激活介导的功能重编程，促进肿瘤细胞生长、反应性基质和管状形态的发生[129]。肿瘤小泡也可以介导功能性 miRNA 的细胞间转移，促进 CAF 迁移到预转移微环境的次级位点[130]。肿瘤小泡在转化肿瘤干细胞龛中的所有方面需要进一步的研究说明。

（二）肿瘤细胞源性 EV 和抗癌免疫应答抑制

对于大多数生物系统来说，EV 与免疫系统之间的相互作用是复杂的。非免疫细胞和免疫细胞产生的 EV 可介导免疫抑制和激活[131]。

在免疫抑制方面，EV 可抑制：① DC 与骨髓前体细胞的分化[132]——DC 是抗原提呈细胞，能够诱导原发性和继发性免疫应答。② 自然杀伤（natural killer，NK）细胞的细胞毒性[133]。③ T 细胞的增殖和细胞毒性[132]。特别是在获得营养后，肠上皮细胞释放表达 Ⅰ、Ⅱ 类 MHC 以及 FasL 的 EV 进而获得抗原，并防止常见的外来抗原引起的慢性炎症和自身免疫[134]。

在免疫刺激方面，EV 可以携带：① DC 的抗原，用于加工并随后提呈给 T 淋巴细胞。② MHC Ⅱ 类分子，用于刺激 T 克隆。③ 促进受体细胞活化为 APC 的信号。④ 调节 T 淋巴细胞和 APC 之间免疫突触的形成[132]。

目前可以肯定的是，肿瘤来源的 EV 是恶性和转化细胞与免疫系统之间串扰的关键因素。在肿瘤细胞自身的生长和转移过程中，它们也是肿瘤细胞抑制免疫监视过程的一部分，即根据肿瘤特异性抗原的表达特异性识别和消除肿瘤细胞[135]。然而在肿瘤微环境中存在来自适应性和先天系统的免疫细胞，这对肿瘤生长和转移的影响更加复杂。事实上，慢性炎症状态可能有利于肿瘤的发生发展,并促进新生血管生成和转移[136],同时,免疫系统也负责肿瘤免疫监视[137,138]。因此,EV 可以通过肿瘤坏死因子(tumor necrosis factor,TNF)-α 途径介导炎症介质的释放从而促进慢性炎症状态[139]。在大多数情况下,肿瘤细胞使用其自分泌的 EV 抑制抗肿瘤免疫应答,例如,诱导抗原提呈缺陷、增加骨髓细胞的免疫抑制活性、增强调节性 T 细胞的功能、抑制 NK 细胞和抑制组织巨噬细胞[140]。多项研究发现,黑色素瘤、卵巢癌和结肠肿瘤细胞来源的 EV 通过自身表面 Fas 配体的表达引起 Fas 配体阳性的淋巴细胞凋亡[141-143]。利用基于 Cre-lox 重组的示踪,Ridder 等在体内实验观察到 EV 介导的 RNA 从肿瘤转移到宿主细胞,并发现 EV 内化后,其免疫抑制表型和 miRNA 谱发生变化。此外,在肿瘤和胶质瘤肿瘤模型中验证了髓源性抑制细胞(myeloid-derived suppressor cell,MDSC)是肿瘤来源 EV 靶向的主要细胞群[144]。这些发现表明,肿瘤 EV 可能负责 MDSC 免疫抑制功能在肿瘤患者中的扩增和激活。

(三) EV、血管生成、内皮细胞和血小板

为了生长和转移,肿瘤往往会形成自己的脉管系统。肿瘤源性 EV 将蛋白质和 RNA 递送至内皮细胞及其祖细胞和支持细胞,从而帮助肿瘤新生血管生成,即在肿瘤团块内部和周围生成新血管。肿瘤源性 EV 还可刺激内皮细胞和血小板的促炎和促凝血活性,这对转移过程的不同步骤,包括肿瘤外渗、肿瘤细胞微血栓形成、细胞外基质重塑以及血小板聚集均有协助作用[145]。除了肿瘤细胞来源的 EV,肿瘤微环境中非肿瘤细胞释放的 EV 也有助于血管生成过程,并最终导致肿瘤转移。血浆中的大多数循环 EV 来源于血小板和内皮细胞[146],血小板源性 EV 的增多与胃癌的严重程度相关[147]。通过这些综述可以更深入地了解肿瘤中的血小板和 EV[148]。内皮细胞来源的 EV 促血管生成或抗血管生成取决于其产生的刺激。

多项研究已经确定,EV 分泌不是组成性的,而是受细胞环境改变的调控。例如,微环境酸性 pH 值的变化和细胞缺氧可影响 EV 的分泌及其摄取[23,149-151]。肿瘤微环境和转移微环境隐藏着的这些恶劣条件与肿瘤密切相关。尤其是在缺氧条件下,肺肿瘤细胞诱导 EV 相关 miR-23a 水平升高,然而其通过抑制靶标脯氨酰羟化酶 1 和 2 以及抑制内皮细胞的紧密连接蛋白 ZO-1 反向促进了肿瘤血管生成并增加血管渗漏[152]。据报道,在肿瘤细胞源性 EV 递送的促血管生成蛋白中,EV 相关 Tspan8 四次跨膜蛋白可触发内皮分支,并促进驱动内皮细胞增殖、迁移、出芽,提高祖细胞成熟的因子水平,包括血管性血友病因子、血管内皮生长因子(vascular endothelial growth factor,VEGF)和 VEGF 受体 2(VEGF receptor 2,VEGF-R2)[153,154]。肺肿瘤细胞源性 EV 将突变 EGFR 递送至内皮细胞,通过丝裂原活化蛋白激酶(mitogen-activated protein kinase,MAPK)和 Akt 驱动自分泌 VEGF 和升高的 VEGF-R2,增强内皮细胞对 VEGF 的反应[106]。肿瘤细胞源性 EV 相关编码和非编码 RNA 的促血管生成作用也在几项研究中得到证实。在胶质母细胞瘤 EV 中发现了与血管生成相关的转录本富集及其随后在靶细胞中的翻译[155]。同样,研究发现,在三维(tri-dimensional,3D)培养系统中,与结肠癌 EV 中细胞周期相关 mRNA 增强了内皮细胞的增殖以及小管的形成[156]。关于 miRNA,白血病细胞源性 EV 将 miR-17-92 簇传递到内皮

细胞导致整合素 α5 下调,从而促进内皮细胞迁移和小管形成[157]。HIF-1 是一种二聚体蛋白复合物,在机体对低氧浓度的反应中发挥作用,而缺氧多发性骨髓瘤细胞分泌的 EV 相关 miR-135b 可以通过靶向缺氧诱导因子(hypoxia-inducible factor,HIF)-1 促进血管生成[158]。在肾癌中,肿瘤细胞源性 EV 同时携带具有促血管生成活性的 mRNA 和 miRNA、刺激新血管的形成并增加转移潜力[159]。由中性鞘磷脂酶 2 调节的特异性 EV 相关 miRNA 的分泌可促进血管生成,随后促进转移的形成[160]。最后,刺激促血管生成活性的长链非编码 RNA[161],例如,肝肿瘤细胞释放的 EV 含有 CD90$^+$ 干细胞样 H19 长链非编码 RNA 分子,被内皮细胞中摄取后诱导促血管表型的生成[161]。关于肿瘤细胞源性 EV 及其组分在血管生成中的更多详细信息以及潜在的分子机制请参见 Song 等最近的综述[162]。

(四) EV 和肿瘤耐药性

恶性肿瘤对目前可用的化疗药物、生物制剂和放射治疗的抗药性限制了肿瘤治疗的效果。除了促进肿瘤生长和转移灶的形成,EV 在促进肿瘤对不同类型的治疗产生抗药性方面发挥着重要作用。它们从耐药细胞将药物输出或将 mRNA/非编码 RNA(包括 miRNA)转移到敏感细胞,这不仅增加它们的表达也实现了肿瘤耐药。或者,它们可以将抗肿瘤单克隆抗体隔离在外周循环中[163],或者在肿瘤细胞脱落过程中排出小分子,形成一种新的药物外排机制[164]。

EV 介导的 P-糖蛋白递送导致 MCF-7 乳腺肿瘤细胞对多西他赛耐药[165],而 ABCA3 转运蛋白的转移导致淋巴瘤对体液免疫疗法耐药[166,167]。在另一项研究中,从阿霉素耐药的 MCF-7 细胞中释放的 EV 通过激活转录因子 NFATc3(活化 T 细胞核因子亚型 c3)诱导 P-糖蛋白表达,将 Ca^{2+} 通透性蛋白通道 TrpC5 转移到与人内皮细胞相关的微血管中[168]。

EV 也可以介导对免疫治疗的耐药。过表达 HER2 的人乳腺肿瘤细胞释放含有 HER2 的 EV,导致对 HER2 抑制剂曲妥珠单抗产生耐药性,诱发恶性肿瘤[169]。这些 EV 的释放受到两种 HER2 受体激活配体(即 EGF 和调蛋白)的调节,这两种配体通常存在于肿瘤细胞外周微环境中。曲妥珠单抗作为一种单克隆抗体,目前用于治疗乳腺癌。因此,来源于 HER2$^+$ SKBR3 和 BT474 细胞系的 EV 隔离了抗 HER2 单克隆抗体,降低了其生物利用度[169]。值得注意的是,晚期乳腺癌患者体内与曲妥珠单抗结合的 HER2$^+$ EV 数量显著高于早期乳腺癌患者,这可能解释了肿瘤转移背景下抗 HER2 治疗的耐药机制[170]。

另有研究发现,在接受过化疗的黑色素瘤和肺肿瘤细胞中,EV 可以清除顺铂[也称为二胺基二氯铂(Ⅱ)][171,172]。顺铂是一种具有方形平面几何形状的金属配合物,其作用是与脱氧核糖核酸(deoxyribonucleic acid,DNA)上的嘌呤碱基交联,从而干扰 DNA 修复机制,导致 DNA 损伤,最终诱导肿瘤细胞凋亡[173]。有趣的是,pH 作为肿瘤细胞外泌体运输的关键因素[23],同样地,研究发现酸性肿瘤微环境导致 EV 相关顺铂的输出增加[171]。通过端粒重复结合因子 1(telomeric repeat-binding factor 1,TERF1)靶向,携带 EV 的 miR-155 在体外和体内均可诱发对顺铂的耐药性,随后增强端粒酶活性。在人骨肉瘤中,miR-221 通过磷酸肌醇 3 激酶/Akt 信号通路诱导顺铂耐药[175]。据报道,通过转移 EV 相关的 miR-221/222[176,177]到敏感的 MCF-7 乳腺肿瘤细胞,从而诱发对其他药物,如他莫昔芬、阿霉素和多西紫杉醇的耐药性。然而，miRNA 诱导抗性的机制尚未阐明。从基质细胞到肿瘤细胞的外泌体交换也可以调控治疗抵抗。基质源性 EV 将非编码 RNA 和转座因子转移到乳腺癌干细胞，刺激维 A 酸诱导基因 1 蛋白（retinoic acid-inducible gene 1 protein，RIG1）样受体表达，进而激活转录因子 STAT1 依赖的抗病毒信号，与 NOTCH3 通路一起诱导化疗药物和放射治疗的耐药[178]。因此，基质细胞借助 EV 与肿瘤细胞进行交流，导致后者抵抗治疗并促进其生长。同样的，头颈部肿瘤细胞系（即 BHY 和 FaDu 细胞）经辐照后释放的 EV 可诱导抗辐射性，同时增加未经辐照靶细胞的增殖[179]。有关 EV 的最新信息和耐药性，我们邀请读者一起阅读一篇优秀且全面的综述[180]。

四、抗肿瘤药物的环境分类和致癌性——对胞外囊泡的影响

大量证据表明，在环境毒素和致癌物诱导的遗传毒性或致突变性变化中可出现 EV 的释放。暴露于环境中的 *noxae* 会触发含有 DNA、编码和非编码 RNA 分子、整合素、细胞因子或趋化因子的 EV 释放，正如在肝癌、肺癌、卵巢癌和气管癌等肿瘤中所证实的结论，这些物质可调节细胞微环境和并具有早期致癌作用[181]。

（一）空气污染物

像烟草烟雾一样，无机砷、氡和石棉等空气污染物是众所周知的致癌物质[182]。吸烟者体内支气管肺泡巨噬细胞释放 EV 诱导肺上皮细胞产生促炎性细胞因子[183]。由于慢性炎症和肿瘤之间有明确的联系[184]，该观察结果说明 EV 可能是烟草烟雾致癌的原因。亚砷酸盐转化的人 L-02 肝上皮细胞的含 EV 培养基将 miR-155 转移到正常肝细胞，进而下调肿瘤抑制基因 QKI[185]。QKI 是一种 RNA 结合蛋白，属于 RNA 信号转导和激活蛋白（signaling transduction and activation of RNA，STAR）家族。这导致了 NF-κB 的激活，并增加了白细胞介素（interleukin，IL）-6 和 IL-8 的产生，从而支持了肿瘤的发生[185]。后一种效应是由 EV 引起的，因为它们从条件培养基中去除后是没有致癌特性的。另一份报告表明，砷在致癌过程中可破坏干细胞动力学[186]。因此，亚砷酸盐转化的前列腺上皮细胞通过 EV 介导的信号募集前列腺干细胞快速获得肿瘤干细胞表型。令人吃惊的是，砷转化的前列腺上皮细胞分泌的 EV 比亲代细胞多 700%，并且富集了致癌因子，包括炎症相关的转录物和肿瘤发生相关 miRNA[186]。

（二）抗肿瘤药物和治疗的致癌潜力

尽管细胞毒性化疗方案在几种类型的肿瘤中具有抗肿瘤和抗转移活性，但许多药物具有致癌潜力，并且在某些情况下可能还具有促转移作用[187-189]。De Palma 的实验室报告称，乳腺癌术前治疗中大量使用的两类细胞毒性药物（紫杉烷和蒽环类药物），在体外和体内两种不同的小鼠乳腺癌模型中诱导产生并释放促乳腺肿瘤细胞转移的 EV[190]。从机制上讲，化疗诱导的 EV 富含膜联蛋白 A6，这是一种 Ca^{2+} 依赖性蛋白，可促进 NF-κB 依赖性内皮细胞活化、C-C 基序趋化因子配体 2（C-C motif chemokine ligand 2，CCL2）诱导和肺转移前微环境中 $Ly6C^+CCR2^+$ 单核细胞扩增，从而促进肺转移[190]。硫化铅量子点可用于声

学应用的荧光生物成像器[191],可以产生活性氧物种,导致氧化应激和细胞死亡。研究发现,它们可以诱导含有 DNA 损伤标志物和促炎因子的 EV 释放,包括 p53、IL-8 和 C-X-C 基序(C-X-C motif,CXC)趋化因子 5,它们是中性粒细胞趋化的有效激活剂,因此在量子点聚集的位置诱发炎症和癌变[192]。

鉴于现有文献报道,暴露于空气污染物和临床使用的致癌物可能影响 EV 的分泌或组成,可以在个体水平和人群中应用 EV 大规模测量其致癌作用。例如,从一组人群中抽血并监测 EV(和相关的载体标志物)的变化可以跟踪与潜在致癌物质或暴露状况相关的肿瘤发展进程[181]。

五、胞外囊泡的临床应用

循环 EV 的临床应用是研究者们十分感兴趣的方向,适当和有效地分离这些颗粒并最终定量的方法正成为各个领域的终极目标,尤其是在肿瘤学领域[193,194]。作为诊断和预测性生物标志物,有必要确定稳定的 EV 标志物、蛋白质和核酸[195],以记录非侵入性诊断背景下患者的现状。当然,这些研究的核心是 EV 检测方法的灵敏度和可用于检测它们的工具。在不久的将来,通过质谱分析对 EV 进行蛋白质组学分析或通过深度测序对其转录组进行蛋白质组学分析可能成为常态[196]。除了利用 EV 及其含量作为生物标志物,这些生物纳米颗粒还可以被设计成用于干扰肿瘤细胞的 EV 或作为药物递送的载体等。我们对 EV 本身的了解及其在不同细胞系统中的参与似乎局限了其应用。在以下小节中,将围绕这些问题展开讨论。

(一)液体活检: 肿瘤细胞源性 EV 相关蛋白和核酸作为生物标志物

EV 的发现提供了易于从给定生物液体中恢复特异性和高度稳定的生物标志物,彻底改变了液体活检与肿瘤患者的相关性。特别是 EV 载物可以反映供体细胞来源的病理状态。液体与组织活检的主要优势是前者是微创,普遍可行,并允许重复采样——这是早期诊断和治疗监测的要点。识别循环肿瘤 EV 中容易获得的材料,如蛋白质和核酸,加上其保护载物的能力,对不同类型肿瘤患者的早期检测、诊断、预后、疾病监测和治疗展示出前所未有的优势[19,197]。在非肿瘤患者中,血液循环中 EV 超过 10^{10}/mL;而在肿瘤患者中,该量可能增加一倍甚至更多[19,198,199]。这可能是因为在肿瘤生长期间常出现可刺激 EV 生产和释放的条件,如遗传毒性、缺氧和代谢应激[200,201]。尽管血浆/血清 EV 不仅包括肿瘤源性 EV,还包括肿瘤微环境中炎性细胞和其他正常细胞释放的 EV,如血细胞、内皮细胞和基质细胞,其行为均因肿瘤发生而改变,但肿瘤细胞对总 EV 群体的分泌和产生具有突出贡献[164]。最近的一项研究表明,将人胶质母细胞瘤细胞原位植入到免疫缺陷小鼠体内,其产生的 EV 占所有循环 EV 的 35%~50%[19]。

1. 蛋白质类

2008 年,在胶质母细胞瘤细胞释放的 EV 中发现 EGFR 的组成型活性形式(EGFRvⅢ),包括细胞外配体结合域中 267 个残基的框内缺失[106],这表明 EV 可能在细胞外携带致肿瘤蛋白,在液体活检中可能具有诊断或预测效用。

在肿瘤患者的循环 EV 中发现了几种具有作为(肿瘤)生物标志物潜在价值的肿瘤相关蛋白。例如,与健康对照组相比,在结直肠癌患者中观察到 CD147$^+$ EV 增加[202],这与另外三项独立研究报告的结果一致,这些研究对磷脂酰肌醇聚糖-1 或一组 29 种 EV 相关蛋白在胰腺癌患者与健康志愿者中的差异调控进行了报道[203-205]。在后一项研究中,18 个外泌体蛋白[如 Tetraspanin 蛋白 CD9、解整联蛋白和金属蛋白酶结构域蛋白 10(disintegrin and metalloproteinase domain-containing protein 10)(ADAM10,CD156c)、整合素 β(CD29)]在患者血清中表达上调,另外 11 个蛋白在患者血清中表达下调。监测它们的表达可能找到应用于肿瘤进展评估的方法。Kimura 等发现,胰腺癌患者血清 EV 中的细胞骨架相关蛋白 4(Dickkopf 相关蛋白 1 的受体)既是一个生物标志物,也是一个潜在的治疗靶点[206]。与前列腺癌相关的活性信号分子,如原癌基因 c-Src、胰岛素样生长因子Ⅰ受体、G 蛋白偶联受体激酶和黏着斑激酶也在 EV 中富集,提示信号网络可能提供液体活检可检测到的、有意义的生物标志物[207]。EV 相关的 α-2-HS-糖蛋白(胎球蛋白-A)、细胞外基质蛋白 1 和癌胚抗原的组合在非小细胞肺癌中有很高的诊断潜力[208]。

如上所述,CD133 作为在细胞外液中发现的 EV 生物标志物值得被特别关注。事实上,在人体尿液、泪液、精液、CSF 中发现了携带 CD133 的核外颗粒体和外泌体[16,209]。近期,在胰腺癌腹水中也发现了 CD133$^+$ EV[210,211]。考虑到肿瘤细胞(包括肿瘤干细胞)表达 CD133,因此特定体液中 CD133$^+$ EV 的上调可能与肿瘤生长和潜在的肿瘤细胞分化有关。事实上,正如神经和造血系统干细胞和结肠肿瘤细胞来源的 EV 一样[16,97],CD133$^+$ EV 的释放与干细胞分化有关。在初步实验筛查中,作者观察到胶质母细胞瘤、正常压力脑积水、帕金森病、复发缓解型和继发性进行性多发性硬化症或其他神经性疾病,如部分性癫痫患者的 CSF 中 CD133$^+$ EV 表达上调[209,212,213]。在胶质母细胞瘤患者中,CD133$^+$ EV 水平的变化与疾病进展有关,这表明其在研究人类疾病方面是有应用价值的[209]。需要更大的具有明确临床和神经放射学参数的患者队列来验证 CD133 可以作为临床公认的 EV 的神经元生物标志物。从每个患者组分离的 CD133$^+$ EV 的详细特征(基因组方法)也可能提供其他标志物(蛋白质、脂质、核酸),并对探究疾病的起源和发展有指导意义[100]。同样,我们应该认识到,CD133$^+$ EV 可以代表不同 EV 的混合物,如从质膜萌发的核外颗粒体或 MVB 与质膜融合后释放的外泌体。

最后,据报道,许多与 EV 相关或与特定的翻译后修饰相关蛋白质,如磷酸化和糖基化,在接触肿瘤细胞的生理液体或条件培养基后有所上调或修饰[214]。例如,腹水源性外泌体 CD133 的差异表达模式被认为是晚期胰腺癌患者潜在的预后生物标志物[210]。从液体活检中发现 EV 相关蛋白作为生物标志物的临床意义,体现在大量关于肿瘤细胞源性 EV 生物标志物信息[PubMed 中使用外泌体/蛋白/肿瘤作为关键词>2 500 个条目(2019 年 6 月 15 日)]和开发可纯化 EV 试剂盒的商业激励。

2. 核酸

由于 RNA 对普遍存在的 RNAses 降解的易感性及其由 EV 脂质双层膜赋予的保护,一些研究者将注意力集中在可作为肿瘤生物标志物的 EV 相关 RNA 上。EV 相关 RNA 通常不受内源性 RNA 污染,如核糖体 RNA[215]。从技术上讲,当 EV 在-20℃下适当保存时,可在数年内保持稳定[216],这使得在启动大型临床筛查时便于储存。作为生物标志物,在不同类型的肿瘤中发现,特定 miRNA 的水平与生产细胞相比有一定变化。例如,与生产细胞中 miRNAome 相比,在黑色素瘤源性 EV 中发现了 20 个具有肿瘤相关功能的 miRNA 特异性积累[100]。在黑色素瘤患者中,低水平的血浆 EV 相关 miR-125b 与疾病进展有关[217]。在卵巢癌中发现 8 个 miRNA 标志物(即 miR-21、miR-141、miR-200a、miR-200b、miR-200c、miR-203、miR-205 和 miR-214),并提出可用于一般人群的肿瘤筛查[218]。类似地,在胰腺导管腺癌、非小细胞肺癌、结肠癌、胶质母细胞瘤、食管癌、前列腺癌、脑膜瘤、肝细胞癌和其他类型肿瘤患者中也报道了潜在的循环 EV 相关 miRNA 标志物[219-230]。从乳腺肿瘤细胞中释放的 EV 展示了 miRNA 生物合成的完整机制,包括 Dicer、TRBP 和 AGO2,这一报道表明某些类型的 EV 可能能够将前 miRNA 转化为成熟的 miRNA[231]。有趣的是,在 HIV-1 感染细胞源性 EV 中也含有 Dicer 和宿主 miRNA 机器的其他成分[232]。

虽然目前大多数 EV 相关 RNA 分子作为肿瘤生物标志物的研究都集中在 miRNA 上,但 EV 中包含的 RNA 大多属于其他种类的非编码 RNA,如信号识别颗粒(signal recognition particle,SRP)RNA、PIWI 相互作用 RNA(p-element-induced wimpy testis-interacting RNA,piRNA)、小核 RNA(small nuclear RNA,snRNA)、小核仁 RNA(small nucleolar RNA,snoRNA)等[120,233,234]。对肿瘤细胞源性 EV 中其他种类非编码 RNA 的系统研究可能会提供更多的标志物并具有一定的临床意义。

最后,EV 作为肿瘤生物标志物,其相关 RNA 转录本也可能对患者(包括转移性乳腺癌患者)的诊断和治疗管理具有潜在价值[235]。例如,在胶质母细胞瘤患者的血浆相关 EV 中,O(6)-甲基鸟嘌呤 DNA 甲基转移酶和烷基嘌呤-DNA-N-糖基化酶(诱导对替莫唑胺耐药的两种酶)的 mRNA 水平和生产细胞中发现的水平有相关性。胶质母细胞瘤接受替莫唑胺治疗后,其转录水平发生显著变化,这可能与治疗反应相关[236]。

(二)基于 EV 的抗肿瘤策略

关于 EV 的异质性、功能、特异性、细胞内途径和调节还有很多有待了解的地方。尽管在肿瘤治疗中合理使用 EV 可能需要我们对其本身及其有效表征深入了解,但几项研究表明,各种治疗方法虽然表面上相互矛盾,但实际上可能在临床上有效[237]。由于其异质性,可以想象通过给予某些 EV 亚类、来源于特定细胞的 EV 或消融特定载物分子可能获得抗癌/抗转移作用。在其他情况下,选择性抑制 EV 生成和(或)靶细胞摄取可能对肿瘤患者有益。干扰肿瘤微环境内或转移前微环境内,靶细胞内化 EV 的细胞内通路可能具有治疗意义。在这方面,最近发现了细胞外载物的新核运输途径涉及早期或晚期内体-核膜的相互作用(参见上文),以及干扰 EV 的内吞作用,这可能为靶向干预打开新的可能性[11,65,238,239]。

在过去的十年中,EV 作为治疗不同医疗状况的天然运载体得到了深入的研究。由于其能够携带生物活性分子并将其转移到靶细胞的细胞内区室,同时保护它们免受蛋白酶/核酸酶降解和作为外来抗原屏蔽免疫检测,脂质双层膜包裹的 EV 成为携带和选择性递送靶向特定肿瘤细胞药物和其他治疗材料(经过筛选的遗传或化学工程)的最佳载体。通过利用内吞-胞吐途径,EV 及其修饰的载物可以以最小的细胞毒性作用绕过免疫系统,从而为控制原发性肿瘤和转移性疾病提供新的治疗机会[240,241]。它们的天然来源和将分子运送到靶细胞的内在功能与迄今为止在抗癌治疗中研究的所有载体(包括脂质体)的人造功能形成了鲜明对比[242]。此外，适当改造过的外泌体或负载治疗分子的核外颗粒体可能被靶向作用于体内的特定组织。鉴于体内注射的治疗药物主要进入肝脏，肝脏是解毒的主要部位，EV 将增加治疗的有效性，同时减少潜在的毒性和其他并发症。到目前为止，尽管一致地将 EV 生物信息转化为治疗信息的最终目标尚未达到，但已经对不同来源、分离 EV 的方法、工程策略和加载技术进行了测试，总体上取得了令人振奋的结果[243]。

总体而言，许多不相互排斥的情况干扰了 EV 在肿瘤进展中的作用。靶向 EV 的生物合成和释放、被特定的细胞类型同化以及抑制载物向靶分子的运送是有待研究的潜在途径。除了临床干预选择，它们还被用作针对和管理选择性抗肿瘤药物的特洛伊木马病毒。以下六个主题可以为利用 EV 抗击肿瘤提供新的见解。

1. 抑制 EV 的产生和释放

外泌体的形成与释放源自一些属于 ESCRT-0、Ⅰ、Ⅱ、Ⅲ 或 ESCRT 相关蛋白质的协同作用。抑制 ESCRT 或 ESCRT 相关蛋白质，如黏结蛋白聚糖、同线蛋白和凋亡诱导因子相互作用蛋白，已被证实可以降低外泌体的产生，并抑制肿瘤的进展[244]。对中性鞘磷脂酶的抑制也观察到了类似的效果，中性鞘磷脂酶是催化鞘磷脂分解为神经酰胺和磷酰胆碱的酶[245]。事实上，同一作者还发现，外泌体所包含的物质在内体膜上被分成不同亚域，并且外泌体相关结构域向内体管腔的转移需要神经酰胺的参与。抑制小分子 GTP 酶 Rab27a，一种调节多囊内体与质膜结合的蛋白质，从而抑制外泌体分泌，引起原发肿瘤生长和转移性乳腺癌的肺转移减慢[246]。

像在 CD133$^+$ 肿瘤细胞中观察的那样，除了阻碍 EV 的产生，还可以通过刺激其释放来限制它们的干预。组蛋白脱乙酰酶 6 (histone deacetylase 6, HDAC6) 抑制剂 tubacin 促进人类转移性黑色素瘤与大肠癌的细胞外 CD133$^+$ EV 的释放，同时伴随着细胞内 CD133 表达的下调。有趣的是，这一作用是 tubacin 所特有的，因为当用另一种选择性的 HDAC6 抑制剂 ACY-1215 或广谱 HDAC 抑制剂曲古柳菌素 A (trichostatin A, TSA) 抑制 HDAC6 的去乙酰化酶活性，或是下调 HDAC6，并不能促进 CD133$^+$ EV 的释放。Tubacin 诱导 EV 释放与细胞脂质成分的改变、克隆形成能力的丧失以及形成多细胞聚集体能力的降低有关，暗示了 tubacin 在表达 CD133 的恶性肿瘤中涉及 EV 一种新的潜在抗肿瘤机制[247]。CD133 与 HDAC6 的相互影响及其在初级纤毛更新和细胞周期中的作用可能在未来值得更多的关注[60,248]。

综上所述，这几个例子表明了深入了解 EV 生物发生机制的重要性，因为在病理状况下，参与其中的所有分子都是干扰 EV 作用的潜在靶点。类似的思路也可以用于内化和 EV 内含物运输到胞内靶点的机制上。之前章节提到的 spathasome 通路的发现可能为抑制 EV 的功能提供了可选择的靶点，进一步的研究将揭示干扰 EV 摄取后细胞内运输的新药物。

2. 抑制 EV 的摄取

已经描述了几种解释 EV 细胞摄取的机制(参见上文)。它们对 EV 内化的作用是可变的，并且是 EV 和靶细胞依赖的。因此，可以想象到一个可行的干预措施，即选择性抑制内化,具有抗肿瘤、防转移功效。例如,一种网格蛋白介导的内吞作用抑制剂氯丙嗪被发现能够通过抑制内吞作用和大型胞饮作用抑制 EV 的摄取,因此用于体外阻止肿瘤的恶性进展[30]。肿瘤源性 EV 表面蛋白质上的特殊糖基化模式被发现参与了靶细胞 EV 摄取的调节,提示 EV 相关蛋白质糖基化的改变可以阻碍肿瘤的进展[249]。所以,识别特定的 EV 相关表面分子以及它们在靶细胞质膜上的受体/黏附伴侣可能是发展这种治疗策略的关键。我们最近提出了一种新的基于针对四次穿膜蛋白 CD9 的小鼠单克隆抗体 5H9 所产生的单价 F(ab)片段(抗原结合片段,以下简称为 CD9 Fab)的免疫治疗方法[250]。CD9(别名四次穿膜蛋白-29,运动相关蛋白-1)是一种参与细胞融合、黏附和运动的穿膜蛋白[251,252]。

根据环境的不同,CD9 具有促进或抑制转移活性的功能(见参考文献[252])。因此,它被广泛认为是一种潜在的治疗靶点。在 EV 与细胞相互作用的环境中,CD9 可以促进初始结合,它的二聚化(顺式或反式)或寡聚化,以及与其他伴侣如黏附性蛋白质的相互作用可以激活自身,促进 EV 的内吞作用(图 3-4A)。CD9 分子与四次穿膜蛋白网络的结合可以促进 CD9 分子空间结构的形成,这也称为富集四次穿膜蛋白的膜性结构域[253]。与该作用一致的是,加入抗 CD9 抗体可以刺激靶细胞摄取黑色素瘤 CD9$^+$EV,而将其在 EV、宿主细胞或两者中的沉默则会阻碍 EV 的内吞[11]。二价抗体会促进宿主细胞和 EV 相关 CD9 蛋白的交联,从而刺激 EV 的内吞作用(图 3-4B)。与全长抗体相比,CD9 Fab 在体内可以达到的剂量下被证明能够阻止 CD9$^+$EV 的内吞[250]。在此情况下,CD9 Fab 可以使位于 EV 和细胞表面的 CD9 分子饱和,从而对其作用产生负性干扰(图 3-4C)。这一假说与一项研究结果相一致,该研究表明 CD9 Fab 可以抑制 CD9$^+$EV(称为附睾小体)与成熟附睾精子之间的生物物质转移[254]。除了调节 EV 黏附到靶细胞及其内化的确切机制,评估其他抗 CD9 抗体是否干扰 EV 的摄取也很重要,如报道的来源于 5H9 抗体的 CD9 Fab 一样[250]。正确定位它们的表位是支持这些效应的关键。对其他 EV 中富含的四次穿膜蛋白,如 CD63 和 CD81,也应该在这方面进行评估。正如之前观察到的,抑制 EV 与精子相互作用的两种抗 CD9 和 CD26 的 Fab 抗体可能产生协同效应[254]。通过阻断肿瘤微环境中的细胞间通信,Fab 介导的抑制 EV 摄取结合肿瘤细胞的直接靶向,可能引领新的抗癌治疗策略的发展。最后,值得一提的是,通过亲和血浆置换将血液循环中的 EV 进行体外血液滤过可能成为干预肿瘤进展的另一种治疗策略[255]。

3. 阻断肿瘤细胞源性 EV 的促血管生成作用

活化的 EGFR 在多种人类恶性肿瘤中起致癌作用,肿瘤细胞释放的致癌 EGFR 与 EV 相关,并且可以与其他细胞(特别是内皮细胞)的相互作用引起细胞反应,尤其是激活 MAPK 和 Akt 信号通路。这一级联反应可以用 EV 表面结合的膜联蛋白 V 同源二聚体阻断,从而阻碍其与内皮细胞的相互作用。这会干扰下游信号通路与后续自分泌 VEGF 的释放并引起 VEGF-R2 的升高,进而导致体内微血管密度的降低和肿瘤生长的减慢[256]。这些现象提供了早期证据,表明靶向 EV 诱导的促血管生成效应在肿瘤中具有治疗潜力,特别是当肿瘤的生长依赖于新血管生成时。

4. 将 EV 介导的免疫应答用于肿瘤治疗

DC 释放抗原提呈外泌体,表达功能性 MHC Ⅰ、Ⅱ类分子和 T 细胞共刺激分子,以 T

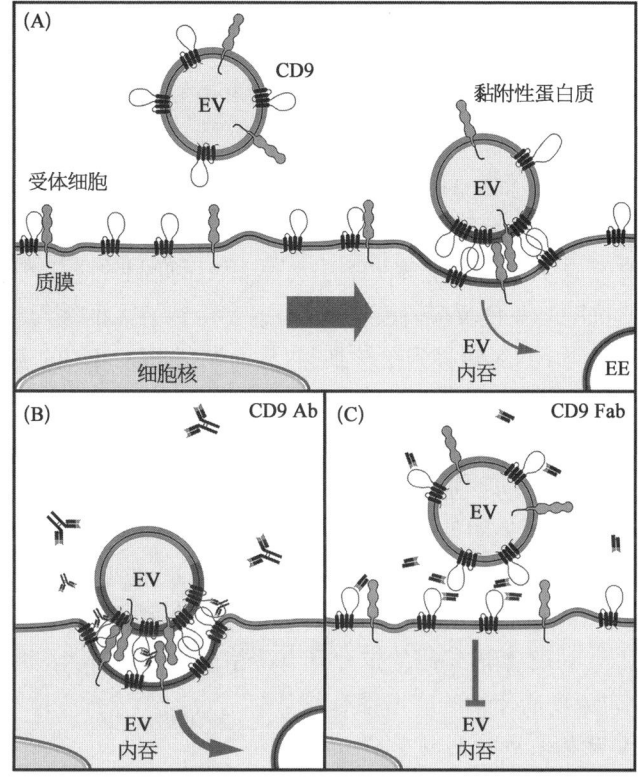

图3-4 抗 CD9 Fab 抑制 EV 的内吞作用与其货物蛋白的细胞核转移。(A) 一个 EV 和一个靶细胞的示意图，它们的膜上都含有 CD9 四次穿膜蛋白，CD9 的相互作用引起 EV 的内吞作用(A，绿色箭头)。在这种环境下，CD9 的顺式和/或反式二聚化、寡聚化和(或)与其他蛋白伴侣的相互作用可能会将宿主细胞质膜的和(或) EV 膜上的蛋白质和脂质成分组织成一个特定的四次穿膜蛋白网(绿色片段)，其成分，特别是潜在的黏附性蛋白质，将调节或利于细胞与 EV 的相互作用，促进 EV 的内吞作用。在内吞作用时，EV 及其内容物将转移到内体腔中，特别是早期内体(early endosomes, EE)和晚期内体(未描绘)，其中一小部分将最终进入细胞核内(见图3-2)。将 CD9 在靶细胞和/或 EV 中沉默会干扰 EV 的内吞，证实了 CD9 在这一细胞过程中的作用[11]。(B,C) 图示表明完整的 CD9 抗体(克隆 5H9)(B)与衍生的 Fab 分别对 CD9⁺ EV 的内吞产生积极与消极的影响。二价 CD9 抗体帮助靶细胞和 EV 通过 CD9 蛋白的相互交联，从而刺激 EV 的内吞作用(B，绿色箭头)[11]。相反，CD9 Fab 会使存在于靶细胞和 EV 表面的 CD9 蛋白饱和，干扰 CD9 的功能，从而阻断 EV 的内吞作用(C，红条)[250]。外核膜(绿色)与内核膜(粉红色)如图所示

细胞依赖的方式抑制肿瘤的进展[257]。发表在 Nature Medicine 上的一项出色的研究证实，利用 EV 的免疫作用达到抗癌、抗转移的目的是可能的。在小鼠动物模型中，搭载肿瘤肽的 DC 源性外泌体诱导细胞毒性 T 淋巴细胞的启动并抑制数种肿瘤的生长。从那时起，一些报道证实，源自 APC 的 EV 含有 MHC 分子，并能够通过激活 T 淋巴细胞来诱导特异性的抗肿瘤免疫反应[258,259]。此外，据报道，在其表面表达热休克蛋白(heat shock protein, Hsp)70 的 EV 通过刺激 NK 细胞和巨噬细胞以及凋亡诱导蛋白酶颗粒酶 B 来诱导抗肿瘤反应[260,261]。

人们正在研究将 EV 作为天然工具，通过 APC 技术开发无细胞的肿瘤疫苗，用于诱导免疫系统识别和杀死肿瘤细胞[262]。在众多的研究中，DC 的免疫原性低，因此被选择作为

EV的供体细胞。它们捕获、加工并提呈肿瘤抗原给同源T细胞,以产生抗肿瘤T细胞反应[263]。它们的特性可以用来产生抗肿瘤细胞的免疫反应。与基于DC的免疫疗法相比,基于EV的免疫疗法的主要优点是EV的稳定性更高,更重要的是,它没有注射材料在体内复制的潜在风险[264]。

免疫检查点蛋白抑制剂,如针对PD-L1和程序性死亡1(programmed death 1,PD-1)受体的抗体,目前在临床上使用,并对黑色素瘤、非小细胞肺癌、肾癌等有效[265]。肿瘤细胞表面的PD-L1与效应T细胞上受体PD-1结合,从而抑制效应T细胞的活性。抗体阻断PD-L1可以激活抗肿瘤免疫反应,使部分肿瘤患者得到持久的缓解。研究发现,肿瘤细胞源性EV可以将非编码RNA转移到单核细胞,从而调节PD-L1的表达和随后的免疫逃逸[266]。EV相关的PD-L1和FasL被发现可以促进免疫细胞凋亡,使肿瘤在未被检测到的情况下生长[267]。同样,它们会抑制引流淋巴结中T细胞的激活。有趣的是,含有PD-L1的外泌体的全身分布会帮助不能自身分泌PD-L1的肿瘤生长,而耗尽含有PD-L1的外泌体可以抑制肿瘤生长,这表明外泌体PD-L1是一个待开发的治疗靶点,可以克服对当前抗体治疗方法的耐药性[268]。值得注意的是,源于自体DC的EV含有黑色素瘤相关抗原(melanoma-associated antigen,MAGE)-3肽,在治疗恶性黑色素瘤方面显示出良好的效果,且毒性最小[241]。MAGE基因编码的抗原具有严格的肿瘤特异性,并且在许多肿瘤中都有表达,因此其在肿瘤免疫治疗中的应用很有前景[269]。

5. 利用工程EV运输抗肿瘤药物

相较于单独使用抗肿瘤药物,工程EV一个重要的优势是可以适当地针对组织特异性靶向进行设计,以达到靶组织中携带药物的最大浓度,同时将整体毒性降至最低。

EV作为包括抗肿瘤药物在内的治疗药物的载体,其另一个潜在优势在于,观察到与化疗化合物一起孵育的细胞可以成功地将分子包装到EV内,这些EV随后可以被收集并用于治疗性输送[270-272]。有趣的是,小的抗肿瘤分子,如紫杉醇和多柔比星(阿霉素),可以在体外被装入来自不同胶质母细胞瘤细胞系的EV中,并通过血脑屏障,成功地输送到斑马鱼胚胎的大脑中,这比单独使用药物的效果显著得多,免疫反应也很低[273]。将药物和EV混合,然后在37℃孵育2小时,制备出载药EV[273,274]。这一实验和其他实验表明,将药物包埋在EV中可以克服溶解性差和毒性差的问题。另一项现有的研究已经证明,阿霉素可以在小鼠肿瘤模型中成功地被运输[275]。有趣的是,含有多柔比星的EV在靶器官特异性积聚,并观察到其大幅度抑制肿瘤生长。在另一篇报道中,姜黄素,一种在姜黄根茎中发现的具有抗肿瘤和抗炎特性的天然多酚,在实验室和肿瘤临床试验中与EV复合以增强其有效性[276,277]。虽然由于姜黄素的疏水性,其生物利用度并不是最佳的,但其疗效和安全性都已被证实[277,278]。

6. 通过生物工程EV运输抗癌蛋白质和RNA

Qian Lu的实验室表明arrestin-domain含有蛋白1(arrestin domain-containing protein 1,ARRDC1)介导的微泡(ARRDC1-mediated microvesicle,ARMM)能将大量的生物活性大分子,包括肿瘤抑制p53蛋白、NOTCH2受体、RNA和基因编辑CRISPR-Cas9指导的RNA复合体选择性地招募、打包和运输到目标细胞[279-281]。ARMM起源于质膜的EV,其出芽需要ARRDC1和ECSCRTI复合物的TSG101蛋白。虽然ARMM的功

能目前尚不清楚，但其在质膜上的战略地位使其成为设计具有治疗目的 EV 的理想生物工具。

例如，p53 通过 ARMM 传递，在小鼠多个组织中诱导 DNA 损伤依赖的凋亡，而外泌体 NOTCH2 在靶细胞中启动一种非常特殊的受体信号传递，这通常需要细胞与细胞接触，促进 NOTCH 受体的长距离信号传递。通过将 ARMM 中的分子与治疗药物交换，这一令人兴奋的发现使 ARMM 成为包装和向细胞内输送治疗性大分子的灵活平台[280]。我们还对正常成纤维细胞样间充质细胞进行了生物设计，使其携带胰腺癌常见的突变 $Kras^{G12D}$ 特异性 shRNA，并在多发胰腺癌小鼠模型中发现其能抑制肿瘤，从而显著提高总生存率[282]。人 O 型红细胞可产生 EV 用于 RNA 治疗。除了可以通过血库大量获取，它们不含 DNA 的这一特点也避免了基因水平转移的风险。通过对针对 miR-125b-2 的反义寡核苷酸或靶向 miR125b-2 人类位点的 Cas9 mRNA 和向导 RNA（guide RNA，gRNA）进行分离和电穿孔后，红细胞源性 EV 能够抑制白血病细胞和乳腺肿瘤细胞的生长[283]。总而言之，这几个例子指出了新的治疗干预措施的出现，在这些干预措施中，生物工程 EV 将作为药物输送载体发挥核心作用。

六、基于胞外囊泡的临床肿瘤治疗研究

随着人们对 EV 及其在细胞间通信中作用的了解不断增加，EV 在肿瘤治疗中的转化应用迅速发展。尽管如此，我们仍处于迈向无细胞疗法这一漫长冒险的开始阶段。评估基于 EV 的肿瘤疫苗的安全性和有效性的第一次临床试验展示了富有希望的数据，这些数据将激励更好的治疗模式发展[237,284,285]。特别是，含有 MHC/肽复合物的 DC 源性 EV 的安全性和有效性已经在晚期恶性肿瘤的Ⅰ期和Ⅱ期临床试验中进行了评估，证明了这种方法的安全性和这些天然粒子在以 T 细胞和 NK 细胞为基础的免疫反应中充当中间体的倾向[241,286,287]。尽管结果令人鼓舞，但仍遇到了一些阻碍，如患者的反应低下或发生变化。进一步研究注射的 EV 在体内的转运和它们的去向将极大地提高 EV 介导的治疗效果。同样重要的是，要注意考虑适当的供体细胞来源和潜在的 EV 修饰或启动，以改善临床结果。联合治疗方案可能会有额外的帮助[288]。最后，在良好操作规范（good manufacturing practices，GMP）的细胞治疗实验室中，EV 准备过程中的质量控制以及其制造所有阶段的质量控制都尤其重要[289]。

七、总结与展望

一项令人印象深刻的、最近迅速增长的证据证明了 EV 与实体肿瘤的关系，确定了它们在肿瘤生长和扩散中的作用，以及利用它们免疫耐受的天然特性和特定细胞、组织或器官的靶向性来设计它们作为抗癌分子载体的可能性。在液体活检的背景下，他们的分析可能对肿瘤的诊断、分类和预后评估有很大的帮助。然而，仍有许多有待发现的地方，特别是关于基于其内容物的 EV 亚类的区别，以及关于它们在目标细胞中的分布和选择性内容释放的理解。未来对它们的产生、摄取和（或）靶向的干扰研究可能导致转移性疾病新的、有效的治疗策略。

致谢

鉴于该领域有大量出版物,由于参考文献的限制,我们向本章未具体引用其研究的个人表示歉意。感谢我们小组的所有成员进行了有意义的讨论和建议,并感谢 Mark F. Santos 帮助编辑了这份手稿。

(周静怡 译,李琦 审校)

参考文献

[1] Raposo G, et al. B lymphocytes secrete antigen-presenting vesicles. J Exp Med 1996; 183: 1161-72.

[2] Ratajczak J, et al. Embryonic stem cell-derived microvesicles reprogram hematopoietic progenitors: evidence for horizontal transfer of mRNA and protein delivery. Leukemia 2006; 20: 847-56.

[3] Valadi H, et al. Exosome-mediated transfer of mRNAs and microRNAs is a novel mechanism of genetic exchange between cells. Nat Cell Biol 2007; 9: 654-9.

[4] Zomer A, et al. In Vivo imaging reveals extracellular vesicle-mediated phenocopying of metastatic behavior. Cell 2015; 161: 1046-57.

[5] van Niel G, D'Angelo G, Raposo G. Shedding light on the cell biology of extracellular vesicles. Nat Rev Mol Cell Biol 2018; 19: 213-28.

[6] Crewe, C. et al. An endothelial-to-adipocyte extracellular vesicle axis governed by metabolic state. Cell 2018 175, 695-708 e613.

[7] Waldenstrom A, Genneback N, Hellman U, Ronquist G. Cardiomyocyte microvesicles contain DNA/RNA and convey biological messages to target cells. PLoS ONE 2012; 7, e34653.

[8] Cai J, et al. Extracellular vesicle-mediated transfer of donor genomic DNA to recipient cells is a novel mechanism for genetic influence between cells. J Mol Cell Biol 2013; 5: 227-38.

[9] Dovrat S, et al. 14-3-3 and beta-catenin are secreted on extracellular vesicles to activate the oncogenic Wnt pathway. Mol Oncol 2014; 8: 894-911.

[10] Read J, et al. Nuclear transportation of exogenous epidermal growth factor receptor and androgen receptor via extracellular vesicles. Eur J Cancer 2017; 70: 62-74.

[11] Rappa G, et al. Nuclear transport of cancer extracellular vesicle-derived biomaterials through nuclear envelope invagination-associated late endosomes. Oncotarget 2017; 8: 14443-61.

[12] Raposo G, Stoorvogel W. Extracellular vesicles: exosomes, microvesicles, and friends. J Cell Biol 2013; 200: 373-83.

[13] Meehan B, Rak J, Di Vizio D. Oncosomes — large and small: what are they, where they came from? J Extracell Vesicles 2016; 5: 33109.

[14] Théry C, et al. Minimal information for studies of extracellular vesicles 2018 (MISEV2018): a position statement of the International Society for Extracellular Vesicles and update of the MISEV2014 guidelines. J Extracell Vesicles 2018; 7: 1535750.

[15] Gyorgy B, et al. Membrane vesicles, current state-of-the-art: emerging role of extracellular vesicles. Cell Mol Life Sci 2011; 68: 2667-88.

[16] Marzesco AM, et al. Release of extracellular membrane particles carrying the stem cell marker prominin-1 (CD133) from neural progenitors and other epithelial cells. J Cell Sci 2005; 118: 2849-58.

[17] Dubreuil V, Marzesco AM, Corbeil D, Huttner WB, Wilsch-Bräuninger M. Midbody and primary cilium of neural progenitors release extracellular membrane particles enriched in the stem cell marker prominin-1. J Cell Biol 2007; 176: 483-95.

[18] Szczepanski MJ, Szajnik M, Welsh A, Whiteside TL, Boyiadzis M. Blast-derived microvesicles in sera from patients with acute myeloid leukemia suppress natural killer cell function via membrane-associated transforming growth factor-beta1. Haematologica 2011; 96: 1302-9.

[19] Osti D, et al. Clinical significance of extracellular vesicles in plasma from glioblastoma patients. Clin Cancer Res 2019; 25: 266-76.

[20] Schneider A, Simons M. Catching filopodia: exosomes surf on fast highways to enter cells. J Cell Biol 2016; 213: 143-5.

[21] Gonda A, Kabagwira J, Senthil GN, Wall NR. Internalization of exosomes through receptormediated endocytosis. Mol Cancer Res 2019; 17: 337-47.

[22] Leung AKL. The Whereabouts of microRNA actions: cytoplasm and beyond. Trends Cell Biol 2015; 25: 601-10.

[23] Parolini I, et al. Microenvironmental pH is a key factor for exosome traffic in tumor cells. J Biol Chem 2009; 284: 34211-22.

[24] Prada I, Meldolesi J. Binding and fusion of extracellular vesicles to the plasma membrane of their cell targets. Int J Mol Sci 2016; 17, pii: E1296.

[25] Colombo M, Raposo G, Théry C. Biogenesis, secretion, and intercellular interactions of exosomes and other extracellular vesicles. Annu Rev Cell Dev Biol 2014; 30: 255-89.

[26] Mulcahy LA, Pink RC, Carter DR. Routes and mechanisms of extracellular vesicle uptake. J Extracell Vesicles 2014; 3: 24641.

[27] Hakulinen J, Junnikkala S, Sorsa T, Meri S. Complement inhibitor membrane cofactor protein (MCP; CD46) is constitutively shed from cancer cell membranes in vesicles and converted by a metalloproteinase to a functionally active soluble form. Eur J Immunol 2004; 34: 2620-9.
[28] McKelvey KJ, Powell KL, Ashton AW, Morris JM, McCracken SA. Exosomes: mechanisms of Uptake. J Circ Biomark 2015; 4: 7.
[29] Lamaze C, et al. Interleukin 2 receptors and detergent-resistant membrane domains define a clathrin-independent endocytic pathway. Mol Cell 2001; 7: 661-71.
[30] Tian T, et al. Exosome uptake through clathrin-mediated endocytosis and macropinocytosis and mediating miR-21 delivery. J Biol Chem 2014; 289: 22258-67.
[31] Klein U, Gimpl G, Fahrenholz F. Alteration of the myometrial plasma membrane cholesterol content with beta-cyclodextrin modulates the binding affinity of the oxytocin receptor. Biochemistry 1995; 34: 13784-93.
[32] Pelkmans L, Burli T, Zerial M, Helenius A. Caveolin-stabilized membrane domains as multifunctional transport and sorting devices in endocytic membrane traffic. Cell 2004; 118: 767-80.
[33] Rothberg KG, et al. Caveolin, a protein component of caveolae membrane coats. Cell 1992; 68: 673-82.
[34] Subtil A, Hemar A, Dautry-Varsat A. Rapid endocytosis of interleukin 2 receptors when clathrin-coated pit endocytosis is inhibited. J Cell Sci 1994; 107: 3461-8.
[35] Fitzner D, et al. Selective transfer of exosomes from oligodendrocytes to microglia by macropinocytosis. J Cell Sci 2011; 124: 447-58.
[36] Feng D, et al. Cellular internalization of exosomes occurs through phagocytosis. Traffic 2010; 11: 675-87.
[37] Gruenberg J, Griffiths G, Howell KE. Characterization of the early endosome and putative endocytic carrier vesicles in vivo and with an assay of vesicle fusion in vitro. J Cell Biol 1989; 108: 1301-16.
[38] Jovic M, Sharma M, Rahajeng J, Caplan S. The early endosome: a busy sorting station for proteins at the crossroads. Histol Histopathol 2010; 25: 99-112.
[39] Piper RC, Luzio JP. Late endosomes: sorting and partitioning in multivesicular bodies. Traffic 2001; 2: 612-21.
[40] Falguieres T, Luyet PP, Gruenberg J. Molecular assemblies and membrane domains in multivesicular endosome dynamics. Exp Cell Res 2009; 315: 1567-73.
[41] Lafourcade C, Sobo K, Kieffer-Jaquinod S, Garin J, van der Goot FG. Regulation of the V-ATPase along the endocytic pathway occurs through reversible subunit association and membrane localization. PLoS ONE 2008; 3, e2758.
[42] Mesaki K, Tanabe K, Obayashi M, Oe N, Takei K. Fission of tubular endosomes triggers endosomal acidification and movement. PLoS ONE 2011; 6, e19764.
[43] Wallroth A, Haucke V. Phosphoinositide conversion in endocytosis and the endolysosomal system. J Biol Chem 2018; 293: 1526-35.
[44] DiCiccio JE, Steinberg BE. Lysosomal pH and analysis of the counter ion pathways that support acidification. J Gen Physiol 2011; 137: 385-90.
[45] Rocha N, et al. Cholesterol sensor ORP1L contacts the ER protein VAP to control Rab7-RILP-p150 Glued and late endosome positioning. J Cell Biol 2009; 185: 1209-25.
[46] Menard L, Parker PJ, Kermorgant S. Receptor tyrosine kinase c-Met controls the cytoskeleton from different endosomes via different pathways. Nat Commun 2014; 5: 3907.
[47] Friedman JR, Dibenedetto JR, West M, Rowland AA, Voeltz GK. Endoplasmic reticulum-endosome contact increases as endosomes traffic and mature. Mol Biol Cell 2013; 24: 1030-40.
[48] Raiborg C, et al. Repeated ER-endosome contacts promote endosome translocation and neurite outgrowth. Nature 2015; 520: 234-8.
[49] Das A, Nag S, Mason AB, Barroso MM. Endosome-mitochondria interactions are modulated by iron release from transferrin. J Cell Biol 2016; 214: 831-45.
[50] Cioni JM, et al. Late endosomes act as mRNA translation platforms and sustain mitochondria in axons. Cell 2019; 176: 56-72, e15.
[51] Malhas A, Goulbourne C, Vaux DJ. The nucleoplasmic reticulum: form and function. Trends Cell Biol 2011; 21: 362-73.
[52] Audas TE, Jacob MD, Lee S. Immobilization of proteins in the nucleolus by ribosomal intergenic spacer noncoding RNA. Mol Cell 2012; 45: 147-57.
[53] Hetman M. Role of the nucleolus in human diseases[Preface]. Biochim Biophys Acta 2014; 1842: 757.
[54] Quin JE, et al. Targeting the nucleolus for cancer intervention. Biochim Biophys Acta 2014; 1842: 802-16.
[55] Zenali MJ, Tan D, Li W, Dhingra S, Brown RE. Stemness characteristics of fibrolamellar hepatocellular carcinoma: immunohistochemical analysis with comparisons to conventional hepatocellular carcinoma. Ann Clin Lab Sci 2010; 40: 126-34.
[56] Rappa G, Green TM, Lorico A. The nuclear pool of tetraspanin CD9 contributes to mitotic processes in human breast carcinoma. Mol Cancer Res 2014; 12: 1840-50.
[57] Cantile M, et al. Nuclear localization of cancer stem cell marker CD133 in triple-negative breast cancer: a case report. Tumori 2013; 99: e245-50.
[58] Nunukova A, et al. Atypical nuclear localization of CD133 plasma membrane glycoprotein in rhabdomyosarcoma cell lines. Int J Mol Med 2015; 36: 65-72.
[59] Huang M, Zhu H, Feng J, Ni S, Huang J. High CD133 expression in the nucleus and cytoplasm predicts poor prognosis in non-small cell lung cancer. Dis Markers 2015; 2015: 986095.
[60] Singer D, et al. Prominin-1 controls stem cell activation by orchestrating ciliary dynamics. EMBO J 2019; 38; e99845.
[61] De Angelis Campos AC, et al. Epidermal growth factor receptors destined for the nucleus are internalized via a clathrin-dependent pathway. Biochem Biophys Res Commun 2011; 412: 341-6.
[62] Chaumet A, et al. Nuclear envelope-associated endosomes deliver surface proteins to the nucleus. Nat Commun 2015; 6:

[63] Schrader M, Godinho LF, Costello JL, Islinger M. The different facets of organelle interplay— an overview of organelle interactions. Front Cell Dev Biol 2015; 3: 56.
[64] Cohen S, Valm AM, Lippincott-Schwartz J. Interacting organelles. Curr Opin Cell Biol 2018; 53: 84-91.
[65] Santos MF, et al. VAMP-associated protein-A and oxysterol-binding protein-related protein 3 promote the entry of late endosomes into the nucleoplasmic reticulum. J Biol Chem 2018; 293: 13834-48.
[66] Lehto M, et al. Targeting of OSBP-related protein 3 (ORP3) to endoplasmic reticulum and plasma membrane is controlled by multiple determinants. Exp Cell Res 2005; 310: 445-62.
[67] Weber-Boyvat M, et al. OSBP-related protein 3 (ORP3) coupling with VAMP-associated protein A regulates R-Ras activity. Exp Cell Res 2015; 331: 278-91.
[68] Jemal A, et al. Global cancer statistics. CA Cancer J Clin 2011; 61: 69-90.
[69] Kim MY, et al. Tumor self-seeding by circulating cancer cells. Cell 2009; 139: 1315-26.
[70] Nguyen DX, Bos PD, Massague J. Metastasis: from dissemination to organ-specific colonization. Nat Rev Cancer 2009; 9: 274-84.
[71] Figueroa J, et al. Exosomes from glioma-associated mesenchymal stem cells increase the tumorigenicity of glioma stem-kike cells via transfer of miR-1587. Cancer Res 2017; 77: 5808-19.
[72] Chiang AC, Massagué J. Molecular basis of metastasis. N Engl J Med 2008; 359: 2814-23.
[73] Weaver VM, et al. Reversion of the malignant phenotype of human breast cells in three-dimensional culture and in vivo by integrin blocking antibodies. J Cell Biol 1997; 137: 231-45.
[74] Oskarsson T, et al. Breast cancer cells produce tenascin C as a metastatic niche component to colonize the lungs. Nat Med 2011; 17: 867-74.
[75] Paolillo M, Schinelli S. Integrins and exosomes, a dangerous liaison in cancer progression. Cancers (Basel) 2017; 9: 95.
[76] Hoshino A, et al. Tumour exosome integrins determine organotropic metastasis. Nature 2015; 527: 329-35.
[77] Costa-Silva B, et al. Pancreatic cancer exosomes initiate pre-metastatic niche formation in the liver. Nat Cell Biol 2015; 17: 816-26.
[78] Fedele C, Singh A, Zerlanko BJ, Iozzo RV, Languino LR. The alphavbeta6 integrin is transferred intercellularly via exosomes. J Biol Chem 2015; 290: 4545-51.
[79] Krishn SR, et al. Prostate cancer sheds the alphavbeta3 integrin in vivo through exosomes. Matrix Biol 2019; 77: 41-57.
[80] Lu H, et al. Exosomal alphavbeta6 integrin is required for monocyte M2 polarization in prostate cancer. Matrix Biol 2018; 70: 20-35.
[81] Singh A, et al. Exosome-mediated transfer of alphavbeta3 integrin from tumorigenic to non-tumorigenic cells promotes a migratory phenotype. Mol Cancer Res 2016; 14: 1136-46.
[82] Ridge SM, Sullivan FJ, Glynn SA. Mesenchymal stem cells: key players in cancer progression. Mol Cancer 2017; 16: 31.
[83] Borriello L, et al. Cancer-associated fibroblasts share characteristics and protumorigenic activity with mesenchymal stromal cells. Cancer Res 2017; 77: 5142-57.
[84] Peinado H, et al. Melanoma exosomes educate bone marrow progenitor cells toward a prometastatic phenotype through MET. Nat Med 2012; 18: 883-91.
[85] Kim J, et al. Replication study: melanoma exosomes educate bone marrow progenitor cells toward a pro-metastatic phenotype through MET. elife 2018; 7, e39944.
[86] Adachi E, et al. Different growth and metastatic phenotypes associated with a cell-intrinsic change of Met in metastatic melanoma. Oncotarget 2016; 7: 70779-93.
[87] Zhang H, et al. Exosome-delivered EGFR regulates liver microenvironment to promote gastric cancer liver metastasis. Nat Commun 2017; 8: 15016.
[88] Fong MY, et al. Breast-cancer-secreted miR-122 reprograms glucose metabolism in premetastatic niche to promote metastasis. Nat Cell Biol 2015; 17: 183-94.
[89] Liu Y, et al. Tumor exosomal RNAs promote lung pre-metastatic niche formation by activating alveolar epithelial TLR3 to recruit neutrophils. Cancer Cell 2016; 30: 243-56.
[90] Plebanek MP, et al. Pre-metastatic cancer exosomes induce immune surveillance by patrolling monocytes at the metastatic niche. Nat Commun 2017; 8: 1319.
[91] Zhou W, et al. Cancer-secreted miR-105 destroys vascular endothelial barriers to promote metastasis. Cancer Cell 2014; 25: 501-15.
[92] Wei Y, et al. Activation of PI3K/Akt pathway by CD133-p85 interaction promotes tumorigenic capacity of glioma stem cells. Proc Natl Acad Sci U S A 2013; 110: 6829-34.
[93] Grosse-Gehling P, et al. CD133 as a biomarker for putative cancer stem cells in solid tumours: limitations, problems and challenges. J Pathol 2013; 229: 355-78.
[94] Rappa G, Fodstad O, Lorico A. The stem cell-associated antigen CD133 (Prominin-1) is a molecular therapeutic target for metastatic melanoma. Stem Cells 2008; 26: 3008-17.
[95] Wang SS, et al. CD133+ cancer stem-kike cells promote migration and invasion of salivary adenoid cystic carcinoma by inducing vasculogenic mimicry formation. Oncotarget 2016; 7: 29051-62.
[96] Liu C, et al. The Interaction between cancer stem cell marker CD133 and Src protein promotes focal adhesion kinase (FAK) phosphorylation and cell migration. J Biol Chem 2016; 291: 15540-50.
[97] Bauer N, et al. Haematopoietic stem cell differentiation promotes the release of prominin-1/CD133-containing membrane vesicles — a role of the endocytic-exocytic pathway. EMBO Mol Med 2011; 3: 398-409.
[98] Marzesco AM. Prominin-1-containing membrane vesicles: origins, formation, and utility. Adv Exp Med Biol 2013; 777: 41-54.

[99] Rappa G, et al. Wnt interaction and extracellular release of prominin-1/CD133 in human malignant melanoma cells. Exp Cell Res 2013; 319: 810-9.
[100] Rappa G, Mercapide J, Anzanello F, Pope RM, Lorico A. Biochemical and biological characterization of exosomes containing prominin-1/CD133. Mol Cancer 2013; 12: 62.
[101] Thamm K, et al. Prominin-1 (CD133) modulates the architecture and dynamics of microvilli. Traffic 2019; 20: 39-60.
[102] Schillaci O, et al. Exosomes from metastatic cancer cells transfer amoeboid phenotype to non-metastatic cells and increase endothelial permeability: their emerging role in tumor heterogeneity. Sci Rep 2017; 7: 4711.
[103] Fackler OT, Grosse R. Cell motility through plasma membrane blebbing. J Cell Biol 2008; 181: 879-84.
[104] Muraro MG, et al. CD133+, CD166+CD44+, and CD24+CD44+ phenotypes fail to reliably identify cell populations with cancer stem cell functional features in established human colorectal cancer cell lines. Stem Cells Transl Med 2012; 1: 592-603.
[105] Wang C, et al. Evaluation of CD44 and CD133 as cancer stem cell markers for colorectal cancer. Oncol Rep 2012; 28: 1301-8.
[106] Al-Nedawi K, et al. Intercellular transfer of the oncogenic receptor EGFRvIII by microvesicles derived from tumour cells. Nat Cell Biol 2008; 10: 619-24.
[107] Hao S, et al. Epigenetic transfer of metastatic activity by uptake of highly metastatic B16 melanoma cell-released exosomes. Exp Oncol 2006; 28: 126-31.
[108] Quail DF, Joyce JA. Microenvironmental regulation of tumor progression and metastasis. Nat Med 2013; 19: 1423-37.
[109] Karagiannis GS, et al. Cancer-associated fibroblasts drive the progression of metastasis through both paracrine and mechanical pressure on cancer tissue. Mol Cancer Res 2012; 10: 1403-18.
[110] Liu Y, Cao X. Characteristics and significance of the pre-metastatic niche. Cancer Cell 2016; 30: 668-81.
[111] Cirri P, Chiarugi P. Cancer-associated-fibroblasts and tumour cells: a diabolic liaison driving cancer progression. Cancer Metastasis Rev 2012; 31: 195-208.
[112] Erez N, Truitt M, Olson P, Arron ST, Hanahan D. Cancer-associated fibroblasts are activated in incipient neoplasia to orchestrate tumor-promoting inflammation in an NF-kappaB-dependent manner. Cancer Cell 2010; 17: 135-47.
[113] Olumi AF, et al. Carcinoma-associated fibroblasts direct tumor progression of initiated human prostatic epithelium. Cancer Res 1999; 59: 5002-11.
[114] LeBleu VS, Kalluri R. A peek into cancer-associated fibroblasts: origins, functions and translational impact. Dis Model Mech 2018; 11, pii: dmm029447.
[115] Pang W, et al. Pancreatic cancer-secreted miR-155 implicates in the conversion from normal fibroblasts to cancer-associated fibroblasts. Cancer Sci 2015; 106: 1362-9.
[116] Webber J, Jenkins RH, Meran S, Phillips A, Steadman R. Modulation of TGFbeta1-dependent myofibroblast differentiation by hyaluronan. Am J Pathol 2009; 175: 148-60.
[117] Vu LT, et al. Tumor-secreted extracellular vesicles promote the activation of cancer-associated fibroblasts via the transfer of microRNA-125b. J Extracell Vesicles 2019; 8, 1599680.
[118] Taverna S, et al. Amphiregulin contained in NSCLC-exosomes induces osteoclast differentiation through the activation of EGFR pathway. Sci Rep 2017; 7: 3170.
[119] Devarkar SC, et al. Structural basis for m7G recognition and 2'-O-methyl discrimination in capped RNAs by the innate immune receptor RIG-I. Proc Natl Acad Sci U S A 2016; 113: 596-601.
[120] Nabet BY, et al. Exosome RNA unshielding couples stromal activation to pattern recognition receptor signaling in cancer. Cell 2017; 170: 352-66, e313.
[121] Yan W, et al. Cancer-cell-secreted exosomal miR-105 promotes tumour growth through the MYC-dependent metabolic reprogramming of stromal cells. Nat Cell Biol 2018; 20: 597-609.
[122] Hamam D, et al. Transfer of malignant trait to BRCA1 deficient human fibroblasts following exposure to serum of cancer patients. J Exp Clin Cancer Res 2016; 35: 80.
[123] Abdouh M, et al. Exosomes isolated from cancer patients' sera transfer malignant traits and confer the same phenotype of primary tumors to oncosuppressor-mutated cells. J Exp Clin Cancer Res 2017; 36: 113.
[124] Abdouh M, et al. Oncosuppressor-mutated cells as a liquid biopsy test for cancer-screening. Sci Rep 2019; 9: 2384.
[125] Trejo-Becerril C, et al. Cancer progression mediated by horizontal gene transfer in an in vivo model. PLoS ONE 2012; 7, e52754.
[126] Garcia-Olmo DC, et al. Cell-free nucleic acids circulating in the plasma of colorectal cancer patients induce the oncogenic transformation of susceptible cultured cells. Cancer Res 2010; 70: 560-7.
[127] Di Vizio D, et al. Oncosome formation in prostate cancer: association with a region of frequent chromosomal deletion in metastatic disease. Cancer Res 2009; 69: 5601-9.
[128] Di Vizio D, et al. Large oncosomes in human prostate cancer tissues and in the circulation of mice with metastatic disease. Am J Pathol 2012; 181: 1573-84.
[129] Minciacchi VR, et al. MYC mediates large oncosome-induced fibroblast reprogramming in prostate cancer. Cancer Res 2017; 77: 2306-17.
[130] Morello M, et al. Large oncosomes mediate intercellular transfer of functional microRNA. Cell Cycle 2013; 12: 3526-36.
[131] Robbins PD, Morelli AE. Regulation of immune responses by extracellular vesicles. Nat Rev Immunol 2014; 14: 195-208.
[132] Bobrie A, Colombo M, Raposo G, Théry C. Exosome secretion: molecular mechanisms and roles in immune responses. Traffic 2011; 12: 1659-68.
[133] Viaud S, et al. Dendritic cell-derived exosomes promote natural killer cell activation and proliferation: a role for NKG2D ligands and IL-15Ralpha. PLoS ONE 2009; 4, e4942.

[134] Ostman S, Taube M, Telemo E. Tolerosome-induced oral tolerance is MHC dependent. Immunology 2005; 116: 464-76.
[135] Zhang HG, Grizzle WE. Exosomes and cancer: a newly described pathway of immune suppression. Clin Cancer Res 2011; 17: 959-64.
[136] Grivennikov SI, Greten FR, Karin M. Immunity, inflammation, and cancer. Cell 2010; 140: 883-99.
[137] de Visser KE, Eichten A, Coussens LM. Paradoxical roles of the immune system during cancer development. Nat Rev Cancer 2006; 6: 24-37.
[138] Vesely MD, Kershaw MH, Schreiber RD, Smyth MJ. Natural innate and adaptive immunity to cancer. Annu Rev Immunol 2011; 29: 235-71.
[139] Obregon C, Rothen-Rutishauser B, Gerber P, Gehr P, Nicod LP. Active uptake of dendritic cell-derived exovesicles by epithelial cells induces the release of inflammatory mediators through a TNF-alpha-mediated pathway. Am J Pathol 2009; 175: 696-705.
[140] Andaloussi ELS, Mager I, Breakefield XO, Wood MJ. Extracellular vesicles: biology and emerging therapeutic opportunities. Nat Rev Drug Discov 2013; 12: 347-57.
[141] Andreola G, et al. Induction of lymphocyte apoptosis by tumor cell secretion of FasL-bearing microvesicles. J Exp Med 2002; 195: 1303-16.
[142] Taylor DD, Gercel-Taylor C, Lyons KS, Stanson J, Whiteside TL. T-cell apoptosis and suppression of T-cell receptor/CD3-zeta by Fas ligand-containing membrane vesicles shed from ovarian tumors. Clin Cancer Res 2003; 9: 5113-9.
[143] Huber V, et al. Human colorectal cancer cells induce T-cell death through release of proapoptotic microvesicles: role in immune escape. Gastroenterology 2005; 128: 1796-804.
[144] Ridder K, et al. Extracellular vesicle-mediated transfer of functional RNA in the tumor microenvironment. Oncoimmunology 2015; 4, e1008371.
[145] Mitrugno A, Tormoen GW, Kuhn P, McCarty OJ. The prothrombotic activity of cancer cells in the circulation. Blood Rev 2016; 30: 11-9.
[146] Berckmans RJ, et al. Cell-derived microparticles circulate in healthy humans and support low grade thrombin generation. Thromb Haemost 2001; 85: 639-46.
[147] Kim HK, et al. Elevated levels of circulating platelet microparticles, VEGF, IL-6 and RANTES in patients with gastric cancer: possible role of a metastasis predictor. Eur J Cancer 2003; 39: 184-91.
[148] Dovizio M, Bruno A, Contursi A, Grande R, Patrignani P. Platelets and extracellular vesicles in cancer: diagnostic and therapeutic implications. Cancer Metastasis Rev 2018; 37: 455-67.
[149] Taraboletti G, et al. Bioavailability of VEGF in tumor-shed vesicles depends on vesicle burst induced by acidic pH. Neoplasia 2006; 8: 96-103.
[150] Ban JJ, Lee M, Im W, Kim M. Low pH increases the yield of exosome isolation. Biochem Biophys Res Commun 2015; 461: 76-9.
[151] Fan GC. Hypoxic exosomes promote angiogenesis. Blood 2014; 124: 3669-70.
[152] Hsu YL, et al. Hypoxic lung cancer-secreted exosomal miR-23a increased angiogenesis and vascular permeability by targeting prolyl hydroxylase and tight junction protein ZO-1. Oncogene 2017; 36: 4929-42.
[153] Gesierich S, Berezovskiy I, Ryschich E, Zoller M. Systemic induction of the angiogenesis switch by the tetraspanin D6.1A/CO-029. Cancer Res 2006; 66: 7083-94.
[154] Nazarenko I, et al. Cell surface tetraspanin Tspan8 contributes to molecular pathways of exosome-induced endothelial cell activation. Cancer Res 2010; 70: 1668-78.
[155] Skog J, et al. Glioblastoma microvesicles transport RNA and proteins that promote tumour growth and provide diagnostic biomarkers. Nat Cell Biol 2008; 10: 1470-6.
[156] Hong BS, et al. Colorectal cancer cell-derived microvesicles are enriched in cell cycle-related mRNAs that promote proliferation of endothelial cells. BMC Genomics 2009; 10: 556.
[157] Umezu T, Ohyashiki K, Kuroda M, Ohyashiki JH. Leukemia cell to endothelial cell communication via exosomal miRNAs. Oncogene 2013; 32: 2747-55.
[158] Umezu T, et al. Exosomal miR-135b shed from hypoxic multiple myeloma cells enhances angiogenesis by targeting factor-inhibiting HIF-1. Blood 2014; 124: 3748-57.
[159] Grange C, et al. Microvesicles released from human renal cancer stem cells stimulate angiogenesis and formation of lung premetastatic niche. Cancer Res 2011; 71: 5346-56.
[160] Kosaka N, et al. Neutral sphingomyelinase 2 (nSMase2)-dependent exosomal transfer of angiogenic microRNAs regulate cancer cell metastasis. J Biol Chem 2013; 288: 10849-59.
[161] Conigliaro A, et al. CD90+ liver cancer cells modulate endothelial cell phenotype through the release of exosomes containing H19 lncRNA. Mol Cancer 2015; 14: 155.
[162] Song W, et al. Tumor-derived extracellular vesicles in angiogenesis. Biomed Pharmacother 2018; 102: 1203-8.
[163] Soekmadji C, Nelson CC. The emerging role of extracellular vesicle-mediated drug resistance in cancers: implications in advanced prostate cancer. Biomed Res Int 2015; 2015: 454837.
[164] Shedden K, Xie XT, Chandaroy P, Chang YT, Rosania GR. Expulsion of small molecules in vesicles shed by cancer cells: association with gene expression and chemosensitivity profiles. Cancer Res 2003; 63: 4331-7.
[165] Lv MM, et al. Exosomes mediate drug resistance transfer in MCF-7 breast cancer cells and a probable mechanism is delivery of P-glycoprotein. Tumour Biol 2014; 35: 10773-9.
[166] Aung T, et al. Exosomal evasion of humoral immunotherapy in aggressive B-cell lymphoma modulated by ATP-binding cassette transporter A3. Proc Natl Acad Sci U S A 2011; 108: 15336-41.
[167] Bebawy M, et al. Membrane microparticles mediate transfer of P-glycoprotein to drug sensitive cancer cells. Leukemia 2009; 23: 1643-9.
[168] Dong Y, et al. Tumor endothelial expression of P-glycoprotein upon microvesicular transfer of TrpC5 derived from

adriamycin-resistant breast cancer cells. Biochem Biophys Res Commun 2014; 446: 85 - 90.
[169] Ciravolo V, et al. Potential role of HER2-overexpressing exosomes in countering trastuzumab-based therapy. J Cell Physiol 2012; 227: 658 - 67.
[170] Tagliabue E, Balsari A, Campiglio M, Pupa SM. HER2 as a target for breast cancer therapy. Expert Opin Biol Ther 2010; 10: 711 - 24.
[171] Federici C, et al. Exosome release and low pH belong to a framework of resistance of human melanoma cells to cisplatin. PLoS ONE 2014; 9, e88193.
[172] Xiao X, et al. Exosomes: decreased sensitivity of lung cancer A549 cells to cisplatin. PLoS ONE 2014; 9: e89534.
[173] Dasari S, Tchounwou PB. Cisplatin in cancer therapy: molecular mechanisms of action. Eur J Pharmacol 2014; 740: 364 - 78.
[174] Challagundla KB, et al. Exosome-mediated transfer of microRNAs within the tumor microenvironment and neuroblastoma resistance to chemotherapy. J Natl Cancer Inst 2015; 107(7).
[175] Zhao G, et al. MicroRNA-221 induces cell survival and cisplatin resistance through PI3K/Akt pathway in human osteosarcoma. PLoS ONE 2013; 8, e53906.
[176] Wei Y, et al. Exosomal miR-221/222 enhances tamoxifen resistance in recipient ER-positive breast cancer cells. Breast Cancer Res Treat 2014; 147: 423 - 31.
[177] Chen WX, et al. Exosomes from drug-resistant breast cancer cells transmit chemoresistance by a horizontal transfer of microRNAs. PLoS ONE 2014; 9, e95240.
[178] Boelens MC, et al. Exosome transfer from stromal to breast cancer cells regulates therapy resistance pathways. Cell 2014; 159: 499 - 513.
[179] Mutschelknaus L, et al. Exosomes derived from squamous head and neck cancer promote cell survival after ionizing radiation. PLoS ONE 2016; 11, e0152213.
[180] Namee NM, O'Driscoll L. Extracellular vesicles and anti-cancer drug resistance. Biochim Biophys Acta Rev Cancer 2018; 1870: 123 - 36.
[181] Harischandra DS, Ghaisas S, Rokad D, Kanthasamy AG. Exosomes in toxicology: relevance to chemical exposure and pathogenesis of environmentally linked diseases. Toxicol Sci 2017; 158: 3 - 13.
[182] Chung JY, Yu SD, Hong YS. Environmental source of arsenic exposure. J Prev Med Public Health 2014; 47: 253 - 7.
[183] Cordazzo C, et al. Rapid shedding of proinflammatory microparticles by human mononuclear cells exposed to cigarette smoke is dependent on Ca^{2+} mobilization. Inflamm Res 2014; 63: 539 - 47.
[184] Chai EZ, Siveen KS, Shanmugam MK, Arfuso F, Sethi G. Analysis of the intricate relationship between chronic inflammation and cancer. Biochem J 2015; 468: 1 - 15.
[185] Chen C, et al. NF-κB-regulated exosomal miR-155 promotes the inflammation associated with arsenite carcinogenesis. Cancer Lett 2017; 388: 21 - 33.
[186] Ngalame NNO, Luz AL, Makia N, Tokar EJ. Arsenic alters exosome quantity and cargo to mediate stem cell recruitment into a cancer stem cell-kike phenotype. Toxicol Sci 2018; 165: 40 - 9.
[187] Shaked Y. Balancing efficacy of and host immune responses to cancer therapy: the yin and yang effects. Nat Rev Clin Oncol 2016; 13: 611 - 8.
[188] Volk-Draper L, et al. Paclitaxel therapy promotes breast cancer metastasis in a TLR4-dependent manner. Cancer Res 2014; 74: 5421 - 34.
[189] Daenen LG, et al. Chemotherapy enhances metastasis formation via VEGFR-1-expressing endothelial cells. Cancer Res 2011; 71: 6976 - 85.
[190] Keklikoglou I, et al. Chemotherapy elicits pro-metastatic extracellular vesicles in breast cancer models. Nat Cell Biol 2019; 21: 190 - 202.
[191] Fang M, Peng CW, Pang DW, Li Y. Quantum dots for cancer research: current status, remaining issues, and future perspectives. Cancer Biol Med 2012; 9: 151 - 63.
[192] Kim JH, et al. Carcinogenic activity of PbS quantum dots screened using exosomal biomarkers secreted from HEK293 cells. Int J Nanomedicine 2015; 10: 5513 - 27.
[193] Witwer KW, et al. Standardization of sample collection, isolation and analysis methods in extracellular vesicle research. J Extracell Vesicles 2013; 2: 20360.
[194] Guo SC, Tao SC, Dawn H. Microfluidics-based on-a-chip systems for isolating and analysing extracellular vesicles. J Extracell Vesicles 2018; 7: 1508271.
[195] Quinn JF, et al. Extracellular RNAs: development as biomarkers of human disease. J Extracell Vesicles 2015; 4: 27495.
[196] Turchinovich A, Drapkina O, Tonevitsky A. Transcriptome of extracellular vesicles: state-ofthe-art. Front Immunol 2019; 10: 202.
[197] Mitchell PS, et al. Circulating microRNAs as stable blood-based markers for cancer detection. Proc Natl Acad Sci U S A 2008; 105: 10513 - 8.
[198] Kalluri R. The biology and function of exosomes in cancer. J Clin Invest 2016; 126: 1208 - 15.
[199] Caradec J, et al. Reproducibility and efficiency of serum-derived exosome extraction methods. Clin Biochem 2014; 47: 1286 - 92.
[200] Webber J, Yeung V, Clayton A. Extracellular vesicles as modulators of the cancer microenvironment. Semin Cell Dev Biol 2015; 40: 27 - 34.
[201] Park JE, et al. Hypoxic tumor cell modulates its microenvironment to enhance angiogenic and metastatic potential by secretion of proteins and exosomes. Mol Cell Proteomics 2010; 9: 1085 - 99.
[202] Tian Y, et al. Protein profiling and sizing of extracellular vesicles from colorectal cancer patients via flow cytometry. ACS Nano 2018; 12: 671 - 80.
[203] Jiao YJ, et al. Characterization and proteomic profiling of pancreatic cancer-derived serum exosomes. J Cell Biochem

2019; 120: 988-99.
[204] Melo SA, et al. Glypican-1 identifies cancer exosomes and detects early pancreatic cancer. Nature 2015; 523: 177-82.
[205] Frampton AE, et al. Glypican-1 is enriched in circulating-exosomes in pancreatic cancer and correlates with tumor burden. Oncotarget 2018; 9: 19006-13.
[206] Kimura H, et al. CKAP4, a DKK1 receptor, is a biomarker in exosomes derived from pancreatic cancer and a molecular target for therapy. Clin Cancer Res 2019; 25: 1936-47.
[207] DeRita RM, et al. c-Src, insulin-kike growth factor I receptor, G-protein-coupled receptor kinases and focal adhesion kinase are enriched into prostate cancer cell exosomes. J Cell Biochem 2017; 118: 66-73.
[208] Niu L, et al. Tumor-derived exosomal proteins as diagnostic biomarkers in non-small cell lung cancer. Cancer Sci 2019; 110: 433-42.
[209] Huttner HB, et al. The stem cell marker prominin-1/CD133 on membrane particles in human cerebrospinal fluid offers novel approaches for studying central nervous system disease. Stem Cells 2008; 26: 698-705.
[210] Sakaue T, et al. Glycosylation of ascites-derived exosomal CD133: a potential prognostic biomarker in patients with advanced pancreatic cancer. Med Mol Morphol 2019; https://doi.org/10.1007/s00795-019-00218-5.
[211] Fargeas CA, Karbanová J, Corbeil D. Assessment of CD133-positive extracellular membrane vesicles in pancreatic cancer ascites and beyond. Med Mol Morphol 2019; https://doi.org/10.1007/s00795-019-00221-w.
[212] Huttner HB, et al. Increased membrane shedding—indicated by an elevation of CD133-enriched membrane particles—into the CSF in partial epilepsy. Epilepsy Res 2012; 99: 101-6.
[213] Bobinger T, et al. CD133-positive membrane particles in cerebrospinal fluid of patients with inflammatory and degenerative neurological diseases. Front Cell Neurosci 2017; 11(77).
[214] Weeraphan C, et al. Phosphoproteome profiling of isogenic cancer cell-derived exosome reveals HSP90 as a potential marker for human cholangiocarcinoma. Proteomics 2019; e1800159.
[215] Cheng L, Sharples RA, Scicluna BJ, Hill AF. Exosomes provide a protective and enriched source of miRNA for biomarker profiling compared to intracellular and cell-free blood. J Extracell Vesicles 2014; 3, 23743.
[216] Sanz-Rubio D, et al. Stability of circulating exosomal miRNAs in healthy subjects. Sci Rep 2018; 8, 10306.
[217] Alegre E, et al. Study of circulating microRNA-125b levels in serum exosomes in advanced melanoma. Arch Pathol Lab Med 2014; 138: 828-32.
[218] Taylor DD, Gercel-Taylor C. MicroRNA signatures of tumor-derived exosomes as diagnostic biomarkers of ovarian cancer. Gynecol Oncol 2008; 110: 13-21.
[219] Madhavan B, et al. Combined evaluation of a panel of protein and miRNA serum-exosome biomarkers for pancreatic cancer diagnosis increases sensitivity and specificity. Int J Cancer 2015; 136: 2616-27.
[220] Dejima H, Iinuma H, Kanaoka R, Matsutani N, Kawamura M. Exosomal microRNA in plasma as a non-invasive biomarker for the recurrence of non-small cell lung cancer. Oncol Lett 2017; 13: 1256-63.
[221] Wang J, et al. Circulating exosomal miR-125a-3p as a novel biomarker for early-stage colon cancer. Sci Rep 2017; 7, 4150.
[222] Manterola L, et al. A small noncoding RNA signature found in exosomes of GBM patient serum as a diagnostic tool. Neuro-Oncology 2014; 16: 520-7.
[223] Alhasan AH, et al. Circulating microRNA signature for the diagnosis of very high-risk prostate cancer. Proc Natl Acad Sci U S A 2016; 113: 10655-60.
[224] Warnecke-Eberz U, Chon SH, Holscher AH, Drebber U, Bollschweiler E. Exosomal oncomiRs from serum of patients with adenocarcinoma of the esophagus: comparison of miRNA profiles of exosomes and matching tumor. Tumour Biol 2015; 36: 4643-53.
[225] Nilsson J, et al. Prostate cancer-derived urine exosomes: a novel approach to biomarkers for prostate cancer. Br J Cancer 2009; 100: 1603-7.
[226] Thind A, Wilson C. Exosomal miRNAs as cancer biomarkers and therapeutic targets. J Extracell Vesicles 2016; 5, 31292.
[227] Sohn W, et al. Serum exosomal microRNAs as novel biomarkers for hepatocellular carcinoma. Exp Mol Med 2015; 47, e184.
[228] Duijvesz D, Luider T, Bangma CH, Jenster G. Exosomes as biomarker treasure chests for prostate cancer. Eur Urol 2011; 59: 823-31.
[229] Huang X, et al. Exosomal miR-1290 and miR-375 as prognostic markers in castration-resistant prostate cancer. Eur Urol 2015; 67: 33-41.
[230] Lai X, et al. A microRNA signature in circulating exosomes is superior to exosomal glypican-1 levels for diagnosing pancreatic cancer. Cancer Lett 2017; 393: 86-93.
[231] Melo SA, et al. Cancer exosomes perform cell-independent microRNA biogenesis and promote tumorigenesis. Cancer Cell 2014; 26: 707-21.
[232] Narayanan A, et al. Exosomes derived from HIV-1-infected cells contain trans-activation response element RNA. J Biol Chem 2013; 288: 20014-33.
[233] Rappa G, Conigliaro A, Santos MF, Alessandro R, Lorico A. Cancer relevance of signal recognition particle and other non-coding RNAs in extracellular vesicles. Transl Cancer Res 2017; 6: S1257-60.
[234] Nolte-'t Hoen EN, et al. Deep sequencing of RNA from immune cell-derived vesicles uncovers the selective incorporation of small non-coding RNA biotypes with potential regulatory functions. Nucleic Acids Res 2012; 40: 9272-85.
[235] Keup C, et al. RNA profiles of circulating tumor cells and extracellular vesicles for therapy stratification of metastatic breast cancer patients. Clin Chem 2018; 64: 1054-62.
[236] Shao H, et al. Chip-based analysis of exosomal mRNA mediating drug resistance in glioblastoma. Nat Commun 2015; 6, 6999.

[237] Tai YL, Chen KC, Hsieh JT, Shen TL. Exosomes in cancer development and clinical applications. Cancer Sci 2018; 109: 2364-74.
[238] Mathieu M, Martin-Jaular L, Lavieu G, Théry C. Specificities of secretion and uptake of exosomes and other extracellular vesicles for cell-to-cell communication. Nat Cell Biol 2019; 21: 9-17.
[239] Heusermann W, et al. Exosomes surf on filopodia to enter cells at endocytic hot spots, traffic within endosomes, and are targeted to the ER. J Cell Biol 2016; 213: 173-84.
[240] Lakhal S, Wood MJ. Exosome nanotechnology: an emerging paradigm shift in drug delivery: exploitation of exosome nanovesicles for systemic in vivo delivery of RNAi heralds new horizons for drug delivery across biological barriers. Bioessays 2011; 33: 737-41.
[241] Escudier B, et al. Vaccination of metastatic melanoma patients with autologous dendritic cell (DC) derived-exosomes: results of the first phase I clinical trial. J Transl Med 2005; 3: 10.
[242] Malam Y, Loizidou M, Seifalian AM. Liposomes and nanoparticles: nanosized vehicles for drug delivery in cancer. Trends Pharmacol Sci 2009; 30: 592-9.
[243] Liu C, Su C. Design strategies and application progress of therapeutic exosomes. Theranostics 2019; 9: 1015-28.
[244] Baietti MF, et al. Syndecan-syntenin-ALIX regulates the biogenesis of exosomes. Nat Cell Biol 2012; 14: 677-85.
[245] Trajkovic K, et al. Ceramide triggers budding of exosome vesicles into multivesicular endosomes. Science 2008; 319: 1244-7.
[246] Bobrie A, et al. Rab27a supports exosome-dependent and -independent mechanisms that modify the tumor microenvironment and can promote tumor progression. Cancer Res 2012; 72: 4920-30.
[247] Chao OS, et al. The HDAC6 inhibitor tubacin induces release of CD133(+) extracellular vesicles from cancer cells. J Cell Biochem 2017; 118: 4414-24.
[248] Mak AB, et al. Regulation of CD133 by HDAC6 promotes beta-catenin signaling to suppress cancer cell differentiation. Cell Rep 2012; 2: 951-63.
[249] Escrevente C, Keller S, Altevogt P, Costa J. Interaction and uptake of exosomes by ovarian cancer cells. BMC Cancer 2011; 11(108).
[250] Santos MF, et al. Anti-human CD9 antibody Fab fragment impairs the internalization of extracellular vesicles and the nuclear transfer of their cargo proteins. J Cell Mol Med 2019; 23: 4408-21.
[251] Schmid E, et al. Antibodies to CD9, a tetraspan transmembrane protein, inhibit canine distemper virus-induced cell-cell fusion but not virus-cell fusion. J Virol 2000; 74: 7554-61.
[252] Zöller M. Tetraspanins: push and pull in suppressing and promoting metastasis. Nat Rev Cancer 2009; 9: 40-55.
[253] Zuidscherwoude M, et al. The tetraspanin web revisited by super-resolution microscopy. Sci Rep 2015; 5, 12201.
[254] Caballero JN, Frenette G, Belleannee C, Sullivan R. CD9-positive microvesicles mediate the transfer of molecules to Bovine Spermatozoa during epididymal maturation. PLoS ONE 2013; 8, e65364.
[255] Marleau AM, Chen CS, Joyce JA, Tullis RH. Exosome removal as a therapeutic adjuvant in cancer. J Transl Med 2012; 10(134).
[256] Al-Nedawi K, Meehan B, Kerbel RS, Allison AC, Rak J. Endothelial expression of autocrine VEGF upon the uptake of tumor-derived microvesicles containing oncogenic EGFR. Proc Natl Acad Sci U S A 2009; 106: 3794-9.
[257] Zitvogel L, et al. Eradication of established murine tumors using a novel cell-free vaccine: dendritic cell-derived exosomes. Nat Med 1998; 4: 594-600.
[258] Théry C, et al. Indirect activation of naive CD4+ T cells by dendritic cell-derived exosomes. Nat Immunol 2002; 3: 1156-62.
[259] Morelli AE, et al. Endocytosis, intracellular sorting, and processing of exosomes by dendritic cells. Blood 2004; 104: 3257-66.
[260] Gastpar R, et al. Heat shock protein 70 surface-positive tumor exosomes stimulate migratory and cytolytic activity of natural killer cells. Cancer Res 2005; 65: 5238-47.
[261] Vega VL, et al. Hsp70 translocates into the plasma membrane after stress and is released into the extracellular environment in a membrane-associated form that activates macrophages. J Immunol 2008; 180: 4299-307.
[262] Tan A, De La Pena H, Seifalian AM. The application of exosomes as a nanoscale cancer vaccine. Int J Nanomedicine 2010; 5: 889-900.
[263] Pitt JM, et al. Dendritic cell-derived exosomes for cancer therapy. J Clin Invest 2016; 126: 1224-32.
[264] Zhang B, Yin Y, Lai RC, Lim SK. Immunotherapeutic potential of extracellular vesicles. Front Immunol 2014; 5 (518).
[265] Salmaninejad A, et al. PD-1/PD-L1 pathway: basic biology and role in cancer immunotherapy. J Cell Physiol 2019; 234: 16824-37.
[266] Haderk F, et al. Tumor-derived exosomes modulate PD-L1 expression in monocytes. Sci Immunol 2017; 2.
[267] Peng P, Yan Y, Keng S. Exosomes in the ascites of ovarian cancer patients: origin and effects on anti-tumor immunity. Oncol Rep 2011; 25: 749-62.
[268] Poggio M, et al. Suppression of exosomal PD-L1 induces systemic anti-tumor immunity and memory. Cell 2019; 177: 414-27.
[269] Schultz ES, et al. A MAGE-3 peptide recognized on HLA-B35 and HLA-A1 by cytolytic T lymphocytes. Tissue Antigens 2001; 57: 103-9.
[270] Ha D, Yang N, Nadithe V. Exosomes as therapeutic drug carriers and delivery vehicles across biological membranes: current perspectives and future challenges. Acta Pharm Sin B 2016; 6: 287-96.
[271] Alvarez-Erviti L, et al. Delivery of siRNA to the mouse brain by systemic injection of targeted exosomes. Nat Biotechnol 2011; 29: 341-5.
[272] Sun D, et al. A novel nanoparticle drug delivery system: the anti-inflammatory activity of curcumin is enhanced when encapsulated in exosomes. Mol Ther 2010; 18: 1606-14.

[273] Yang T, et al. Exosome delivered anticancer drugs across the blood-brain barrier for brain cancer therapy in Danio rerio. Pharm Res 2015; 32: 2003-14.

[274] Jang SC, et al. Bioinspired exosome-mimetic nanovesicles for targeted delivery of chemotherapeutics to malignant tumors. ACS Nano 2013; 7: 7698-710.

[275] Tian Y, et al. A doxorubicin delivery platform using engineered natural membrane vesicle exosomes for targeted tumor therapy. Biomaterials 2014; 35: 2383-90.

[276] Anand P, Sundaram C, Jhurani S, Kunnumakkara AB, Aggarwal BB. Curcumin and cancer: an "old-age" disease with an "age-old" solution. Cancer Lett 2008; 267: 133-64.

[277] Dhillon N, et al. Phase II trial of curcumin in patients with advanced pancreatic cancer. Clin Cancer Res 2008; 14: 4491-9.

[278] Anand P, Kunnumakkara AB, Newman RA, Aggarwal BB. Bioavailability of curcumin: problems and promises. Mol Pharm 2007; 4: 807-18.

[279] Nabhan JF, Hu R, Oh RS, Cohen SN, Lu Q. Formation and release of arrestin domaincontaining protein 1-mediated microvesicles (ARMMs) at plasma membrane by recruitment of TSG101 protein. Proc Natl Acad Sci U S A 2012; 109: 4146-51.

[280] Wang Q, et al. ARMMs as a versatile platform for intracellular delivery of macromolecules. Nat Commun 2018; 9: 960.

[281] Wang Q, Lu Q. Plasma membrane-derived extracellular microvesicles mediate non-canonical intercellular NOTCH signaling. Nat Commun 2017; 8: 709.

[282] Kamerkar S, et al. Exosomes facilitate therapeutic targeting of oncogenic KRAS in pancreatic cancer. Nature 2017; 546: 498-503.

[283] Usman WM, et al. Efficient RNA drug delivery using red blood cell extracellular vesicles. Nat Commun 2018; 9: 2359.

[284] Dai S, et al. Phase I clinical trial of autologous ascites-derived exosomes combined with GMCSF for colorectal cancer. Mol Ther 2008; 16: 782-90.

[285] Pitt JM, Kroemer G, Zitvogel L. Extracellular vesicles: masters of intercellular communication and potential clinical interventions. J Clin Invest 2016; 126: 1139-43.

[286] Morse MA, et al. A phase I study of dexosome immunotherapy in patients with advanced non-small cell lung cancer. J Transl Med 2005; 3: 9.

[287] Besse B, et al. Dendritic cell-derived exosomes as maintenance immunotherapy after first line chemotherapy in NSCLC. Oncoimmunology 2016; 5, e1071008.

[288] Taieb J, et al. Chemoimmunotherapy of tumors: cyclophosphamide synergizes with exosome based vaccines. J Immunol 2006; 176: 2722-9.

[289] Viaud S, et al. Updated technology to produce highly immunogenic dendritic cell-derived exosomes of clinical grade: a critical role of interferon-gamma. J Immunother 2011; 34: 65-75.

第 4 章

血液系统恶性肿瘤：
外泌体在肿瘤进展中的作用

Hematologic malignancies:
The exosome contribution in tumor progression

Stefania Raimondo, Laura Saieva, Riccardo Alessandro

Department of Biomedicine, Neuroscience and Advanced Diagnostics, University of Palermo, Palermo, Italy.

一、血液系统恶性肿瘤与肿瘤微环境

肿瘤受内在和外在信号的调控，这些信号主要通过以下几个阶段促进肿瘤的进展：发生、促进、进展和转移。这些过程是由肿瘤细胞的基因改变以及周围细胞之间不受管制的通信驱动的，这创造了目前我们所知的"肿瘤微环境"[1]。

既往研究主要集中于通过定义肿瘤细胞的遗传和分子特征以确定靶向治疗，但如今我们知道这是不够的。事实上，肿瘤细胞并不是孤立的，它们是一个复杂网络的一部分，在这个网络中，肿瘤细胞和邻近的正常细胞交换信息，促进肿瘤的进展和存活。

因此，针对肿瘤微环境中细胞如何进行沟通的研究是开发新的治疗方法的基础。

微环境在肿瘤发生中扮演的重要角色已经在实体肿瘤[2]和血液肿瘤[3]中被广泛描述。白血病母细胞与内皮细胞和基质细胞的相互作用是肿瘤细胞增殖、存活以及产生耐药性的关键过程[4]，这一机制主要受 CXCL12-CXCR4 轴的调控。事实上，由骨髓微环境中的基质细胞产生的趋化因子 CXCL12 通过与细胞表面受体 CXCR4 相互作用，在白血病母细胞中触发促生长和抗凋亡信号[5]。在多发性骨髓瘤（multiple myeloma，MM）中，浆细胞的增殖和存活受骨髓微环境的调节，特别是血管生成，被认为在疾病的发病和进展中起着关键作用[6]。

在负责血液肿瘤细胞与骨髓微环境之间交互作用的因素中，EV，特别是外泌体，最近在科学界中备受关注。这些脂蛋白结构实际上是微环境细胞成分中细胞信息的容器以及这些信息的载体[7]。在这里，我们将讨论目前关于 EV 介导的肿瘤与正常细胞之间交互作用的知识，以便更好地理解囊泡如何促进肿瘤的进展。

二、胞外囊泡对造血的生理调节和病理改变

造血是血细胞产生的生理过程。造血干细胞（hematopoietic stem cell，HSC）、基质细胞，以及 HSC 生长和分裂所在的细胞外基质是造血的主要参与者。HSC 是一种多能干细胞，可以分化出所有的细胞谱系，包括髓系和淋巴系，并且具有自我更新和分化的能力；血液

和免疫系统的功能需要这两个过程的平衡[8]。

越来越多的证据表明,微环境刺激参与了干性特征的调节。骨髓(bone marrow,BM)由细胞、细胞外基质和一些可溶性因子,如细胞因子、趋化因子、信号分子等组成,为造血干细胞提供良好的微环境,是造血发生的主要场所。不同的机制和因素都在帮助维持造血系统干性的稳定,虽然只有部分为人所知。例如,与BM间充质基质细胞等其他细胞群体的相互作用对HSC的自我更新、存活和行为至关重要[9]。

最近的研究试图阐明BM生态位调节活动的潜在机制,这强调了BM细胞群中存在一个复杂的通信系统。趋化因子、细胞因子、黏附分子、酶、受体和信号转导分子共同构成了这个分子框架。

最近,无论是在生理水平还是在病理水平,普遍认为EV是造血生态位里重要的调节器[10]。研究表明,EV代表了造血生态位里调节细胞稳态的一种新的通信系统(图4-1)。

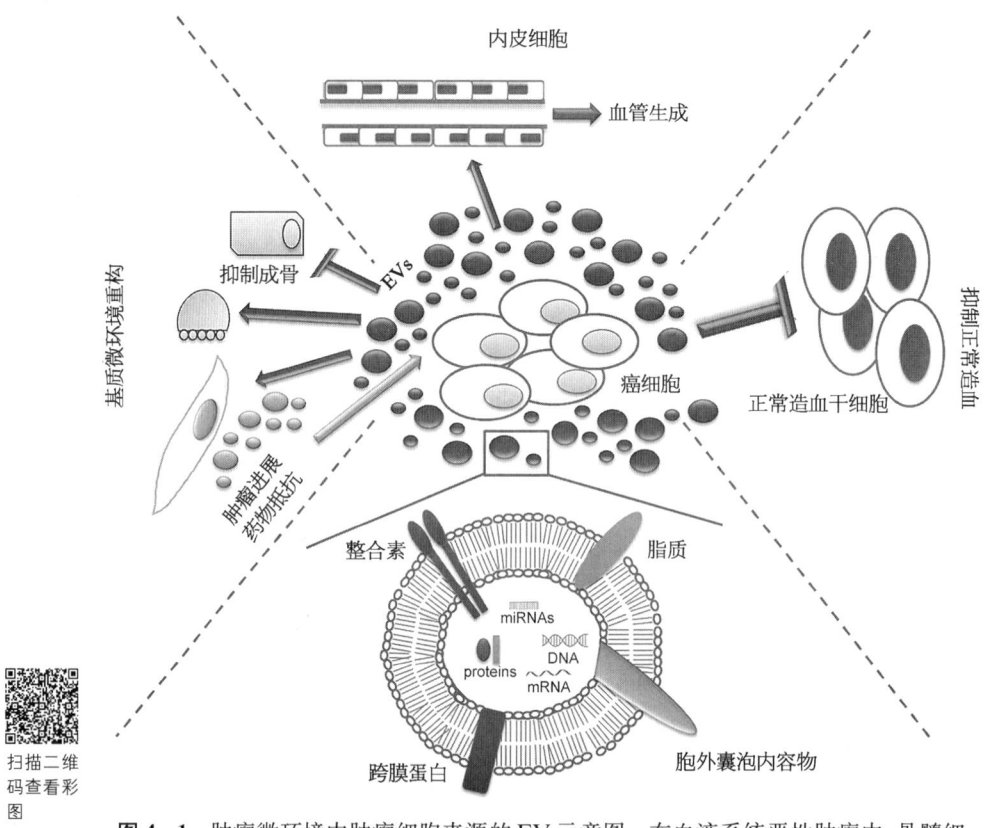

图4-1 肿瘤微环境中肿瘤细胞来源的EV示意图。在血液系统恶性肿瘤中,骨髓细胞和肿瘤细胞之间的交互作用被解除,这有助于为肿瘤创造一个自由生长与发展的微环境

第一个证据在2006年由Ratajczak等发表的一项研究中,作者证实胚胎干细胞向造血干细胞和祖细胞输送外泌体mRNA和蛋白质,增强了它们的多能性[11]。Ekstrom证实,人类肥大细胞来源的外泌体中含有可以穿梭到其他人类肥大细胞和人类$CD34^+$造血祖细胞中的RNA。这些发现表明,外泌体中的穿梭RNA在免疫细胞(包括肥大细胞和$CD34^+$祖

细胞)之间的通信中发挥作用,暗示其在细胞成熟过程中发挥作用[12]。

更多的最新研究阐明了在生态位里,由 BM 基质细胞(包括内皮细胞和 MSC)释放的 EV 的作用。Goloviznina 等发现 MSC 能够通过 EV 的分泌调节造血。特别是,他们观察到造血祖细胞通过体外暴露于 MSC 的 EV 中被激活。事实上,外泌体通过 TLR4 - MyD88 - NF - κB 途径激活髓系祖细胞[13]。此外,Stik 等的一项研究表明,基质细胞来源的 EV 通过维持细胞存活与克隆潜力以及防止细胞凋亡以维持造血干细胞和祖细胞。作者总结,这些效应是由于 EV 中的 miRNA 能够调节靶细胞的表型[14]。

越来越多的证据表明,EV 导致定向祖细胞增殖与分化之间的平衡失调,从而引发血液系统恶性肿瘤。到目前为止,大部分已发表的研究都强调肿瘤外泌体抑制造血的作用源自急性髓细胞性白血病(acute myeloid leukemia,AML)。2015 年,Kurre 团队报道,AML 来源的外泌体能够直接和间接地调节造血干细胞和祖细胞。特别是,他们证明了外泌体治疗下调了基质细胞中 CXCL12 的表达,导致骨髓中造血干细胞的活化。此外,AML 的外泌体还可直接降低造血干细胞和造血祖细胞中 c - Myb、Cebp - β 和 Hoxa - 9 等造血转录因子的表达。通过蛋白质组学的方法,作者确定了参与外泌体介导的干细胞功能调节的候选途径[15]。该团队进一步研究了外泌体介导的造血抑制的分子机制。他们发现 AML 的外泌体中含有针对造血主要调节因子(包括 c - Myb)的 miRNA,其中,外泌体中的 miR - 150 和 miR - 155 足以抑制造血干细胞和造血祖细胞的克隆性[16]。最近,Razmkhah 等从 AML 患者体内分离出微泡,发现将这些 EV 添加到正常造血干细胞中一周就会导致靶细胞中的 oncomiRs,如 miR - 21 和 miR - 29a 过表达[17]。最后,Kumar 等观察到,AML 来源的外泌体减少了造血干细胞支持因子的基质表达,包括 CXCL12、KITL 和 IGF1,从而抑制正常的造血[18]。

除了 AML,已经证实 EV 在骨髓增生异常综合征(myelodysplastic syndromes,MDS)中也会影响造血。事实上,MDS 患者的微泡也会增加造血干细胞的生存力和克隆形成能力[19]。

三、胞外囊泡介导的内皮重构

尽管已认识到血管生成在实体肿瘤中的作用,如今发现其也有助于血液系统疾病的进展[20]。在白血病、MDS 和多发性骨髓瘤等多个血液疾病中,BM 血管密度的增加是刺激血管生成的结果。

血管生成的诱导是骨微环境中激活和抑制的驱动力的结果。越来越多的证据支持了肿瘤细胞释放的 EV 能够刺激内皮细胞重塑 BM 脉管系统的假设,并且这一作用取决于 EV 含量。尤其是当 EV 传递促血管生成蛋白和 miRNA,从而诱导受体细胞发生变化时。Taverna 等的研究调查了慢性髓细胞性白血病(chronic myeloid leukemia,CML)来源的外泌体在血管生成过程中的作用。2012 年,作者首次证实来自 CML 细胞系和患者的外泌体通过增加内皮细胞的能动性、促血管生成细胞因子的分泌和细胞黏附来促进肿瘤血管生成[21]。进一步的研究表明,这种肿瘤与内皮细胞的交互作用是由从 CML 外泌体转移到内皮细胞的 miR - 126 介导的[22]。

同样地，Mineo 等证实了 CML 外泌体介导的血管生成过程的增加，并将其归因于 Src 通路的激活[23]。由于缺氧在肿瘤进展中起着关键作用，Tadokoro 等研究了来自缺氧肿瘤细胞的外泌体调节肿瘤微环境中的能力。研究发现，缺氧 CML 细胞分泌含有促血管生成 miRNA 的外泌体，这些 miRNA 针对受体酪氨酸激酶配体 Ephrin-A3，引起微管的形成增加[24]。同样地，不同的研究强调了多髓细胞来源的外泌体在调节肿瘤血管生成中的作用。Liu 的团队发现 MM 细胞系 RPMI8226 释放直径在 100~1 000 nm 的外泌体，促进了内皮细胞的增殖以及肿瘤细胞的侵袭与迁移。外泌体与内皮细胞的相互作用导致 IL-6 和 VEGF 的分泌增加[25]。2014 年，为了模拟活体骨髓微环境，Umezu 建立了在慢性缺氧条件下持续生长的 MM 细胞系（HR-MM 细胞）模型，证明了 HR-MM 细胞在常氧或急性缺氧条件下比同一细胞系产生更多的外泌体。此外，作者还发现 HR-MM 细胞来源的外泌体促进内皮细胞中微管的形成，这种作用是由外泌体中的 miR-135b 所致[26]。在 AML 患者中，已广泛观察到血管生成的增加。Kurre 的研究组观察到，原代 AML 囊泡中的 RNA 富含胰岛素样生长因子 1 受体（insulin-like growth factor 1 receptor，IGF-IR）mRNA，这导致了基质细胞血管生成的潜力增加[27]。

四、胞外囊泡对骨髓基质细胞的重编程

骨髓微环境在造血干细胞的维持中起着关键作用，特别是在支持细胞更新和分化方面[28]。在血液系统恶性肿瘤中，骨髓基质细胞和肿瘤细胞之间的交互作用被解除，这有助于为肿瘤创造一个自由生长和发展的微环境[29]。

以往认为肿瘤与间质细胞的直接接触是肿瘤微环境形成的唯一原因，现在认识到可溶性因子的释放会影响微环境中的细胞。在这种背景下，肿瘤细胞和基质细胞释放的 EV 被广泛认为是造成 BM 生态位变化的原因[30,31]。尤其是骨髓间充质干细胞（BM mesenchymal stromal cell，BMSC）可以通过释放外泌体支持肿瘤细胞的生长。事实上，BMSC 来源的外泌体可以将核酸和蛋白质运输至受体肿瘤细胞，从而影响肿瘤的生长、转移和治疗反应[31]。

Roccaro 最近证实，与正常 BMSC 相比，MM 中 BMSC 来源的外泌体含有并运输高水平的原癌蛋白，负责肿瘤细胞的黏附和迁移。这些外泌体被 MM 细胞内化，引起肿瘤细胞生长和扩散[32]。Crompot 研究了慢性淋巴细胞白血病（chronic lymphocytic leukemia，CLL）患者 BM 胞外囊泡的作用，结果表明，它们增强了肿瘤细胞的迁移能力和药物抵抗性，并减少了白血病细胞的凋亡[33]。Barrera-Ramirez 等对从 AML 患者与对照组骨髓来源的 MSC 中分离的外泌体 RNA 进行 miRNA 测序。结果发现在 AML 来源的样本中，有两种 miRNA 显著增加，三种 miRNA 显著减少。通过预测分析，作者发现这些 miRNA 能调节与白血病发生相关的基因的表达[34]。

越来越多的证据表明，肿瘤细胞源性外泌体在调节基质细胞表型、为肿瘤进展创造更自由的微环境方面起着重要的作用。

我们已经为慢性粒细胞白血病来源的外泌体对骨髓基质细胞的直接作用提供了证据。我们发现，外泌体刺激骨髓基质细胞产生 IL-8，在体外和体内都能调节白血病细胞的恶性

表型,促进肿瘤细胞的增殖和黏附[7]。进一步研究表明,这些机制是由基质细胞中 EGFR 通路的激活介导的[35]。同样地,Ghosh 等在 B 细胞 CLL 的血浆中发现了促进 BMSC 中 AKT 通路激活和 VEGF 产生的微泡[36]。

Cheng 等发现,MM 来源的外泌体通过传递 miR-21 和 miR146a 促进 MSC 的增殖,并激活 IL-6 的释放[37]。

有趣的是,最近的研究调查了外泌体在重编程基质细胞代谢中的作用[38]。人类黑色素瘤源性外泌体能够重编程基质成纤维细胞的代谢,引起细胞外酸化,这一条件有利于转移前的生态位形成[39]。Johnson 报道,急性淋巴细胞白血病(acute lymphoblastic leukemia,ALL)细胞释放的 EV 被间充质基质细胞内化,这种相互作用导致受体基质细胞中线粒体呼吸减少以及糖酵解率增加。总而言之,作者总结,EV 能够诱导代谢从氧化磷酸化转换为有氧糖酵解以支持肿瘤细胞的需求[40]。

五、胞外囊泡改变骨稳态

骨稳态是由成骨细胞(osteoblast,OB)与破骨细胞(osteoclast,OC)的相反活动维持的动态平衡,这两种细胞都参与骨的重建,包括持续的骨破坏与骨形成。这两个不同的过程受到旁分泌/自分泌因子的分泌精细调控[41]。

骨稳态的失调会引起包括血液系统恶性肿瘤[42]在内的各种疾病的进展,其中吸收大于新生,导致骨量减少、组织微结构损伤和骨折风险增加(图 4-2)。

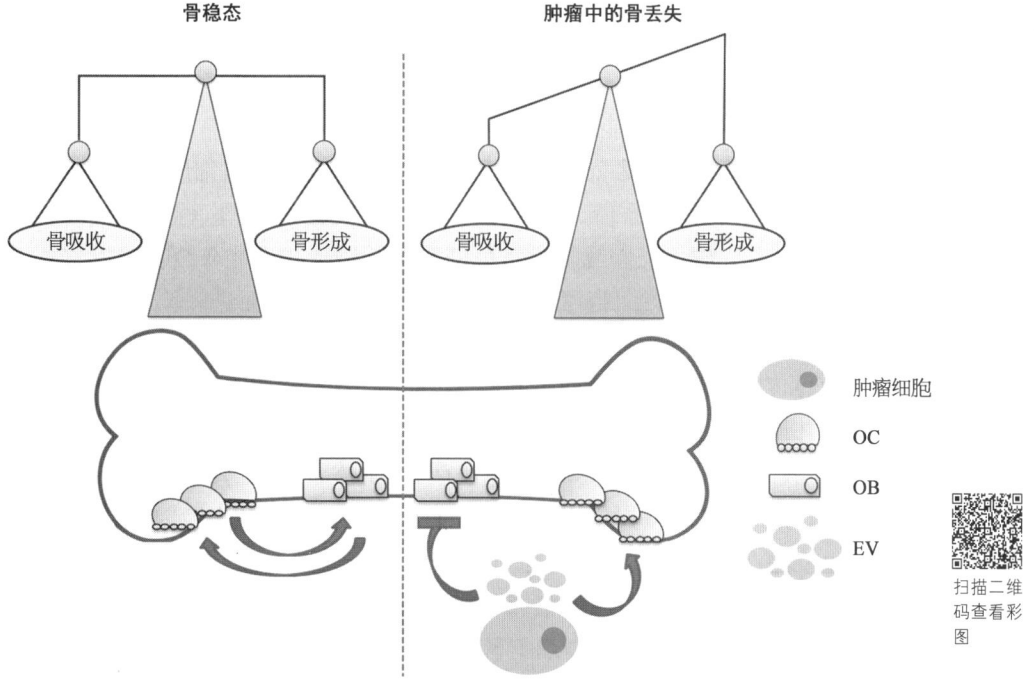

图 4-2 在生理和病理条件下骨稳态的示意图。骨稳态是由 OB 骨形成和 OC 骨吸收的平衡作用维持。在血液系统恶性肿瘤中,EV 会导致骨稳态的失衡,促进骨吸收

近年来,关于 EV 在骨稳态调节中作用的实验证据逐渐增多。研究表明,OC 和 OB 释放的外泌体通过运输参与这两种细胞类型分化的分子调节骨重建。Sun 等报道,破骨细胞分泌富含 miR-214 的外泌体,将这种 microRNA 转移到 OB 中会抑制细胞分化,从而导致体内的骨丢失[43]。另一方面,Cui 等观察到矿化的 OB 释放外泌体,通过激活 Wnt 信号通路促进骨髓基质细胞向 OB 分化[44]。最近的实验证据表明,肿瘤细胞释放的外泌体是导致骨吸收和新骨形成之间失衡的原因,尤其是在 MM[45,46] 和 AML[18] 中。骨病,特别是溶骨性病变,是 MM 患者最常见的并发症。2015 年,我们的团队证实,将破骨前细胞暴露于 MM 细胞系和 MM 患者的外泌体后,其 OC 分化标志物如组织蛋白酶 K(cathepsin K,CTSK)、基质金属蛋白酶 9(matrix metalloproteinases 9,MMP9)和抗酒石酸酸性磷酸酶(tartrate-resistant acid phosphatase,TRAP)增加[45]。此外,我们最近观察到 MM 细胞系和 MM 患者 BM 抽吸物的外泌体中富含 EGFR 配体双调蛋白,其有助于外泌体介导的 OC 形成。我们进一步发现 MM 来源的外泌体阻断了 MSC 的成骨分化。我们的结果与 Li 等提供的数据一致。最近有研究报道,MM 细胞来源的外泌体可以通过运输 lncRNA RUNX2-AS 降低 MSC 的成骨能力。此外,作者在活体小鼠模型中证实了抑制外泌体的分泌可以防止骨丢失[46]。类似地,Kumar 等通过评估 AML 来源的外泌体在重建骨髓生态位中的作用,发现 AML 外泌体抑制了间充质基质祖细胞的成骨分化,降低了骨钙蛋白基因的表达,增加了 OB 分化的负调控因子 DKK1[18]。总体而言,这些近期的证据已经表明了肿瘤外泌体在促进骨丢失中的作用,但还需要进一步的研究以更好地明确导致骨损伤的外泌体的分子成分。

六、胞外囊泡调节免疫细胞的功能

免疫系统在肿瘤进展、调控和杀死肿瘤细胞方面起着至关重要的作用。来自先天性免疫系统和获得性免疫系统的免疫细胞能够识别、攻击和清除肿瘤细胞。它们相互协作和刺激,以诱导针对肿瘤细胞的强大免疫反应。然而,肿瘤仍然会发生。肿瘤细胞可以抵抗或者躲避免疫系统的监视。肿瘤和免疫系统之间的相互作用分为三个阶段,称为肿瘤免疫编辑[47]。在第一阶段(清除或肿瘤免疫监视阶段),免疫系统能够保护宿主免受正在生长的肿瘤的侵袭。然而,一些发生了转变的细胞可能会逃脱免疫的监视,从而进入第二阶段(平衡阶段)。在这段免疫调节的潜伏期内,肿瘤会持续存在并积累新的突变。这可能会使肿瘤进入第三阶段(肿瘤逃逸),在此期间肿瘤开始出现临床表征[48,49]。肿瘤细胞已经发展出来许多方式来改变其表型并误导免疫系统。肿瘤细胞可以改变其细胞表面的表型,从而阻止免疫效应细胞的识别和结合。最近,越来越多的证据表明,外泌体是肿瘤与免疫系统交互作用的主要参与者(图 4-3)。肿瘤来源的外泌体携带多种膜结合因子和可溶性因子,可通过各种不同的机制诱导免疫逃逸。它们可以参与免疫反应的各个阶段,通过影响不同类型的免疫细胞来帮助肿瘤逃避免疫监视,如 NK 细胞、CD8$^+$ T 细胞、调节性 T 细胞、单核细胞和髓样抑制细胞。在实体肿瘤中,外泌体对免疫细胞行为的影响已经得到了广泛的研究,而其在血液系统疾病中的作用还需要进一步的挖掘。

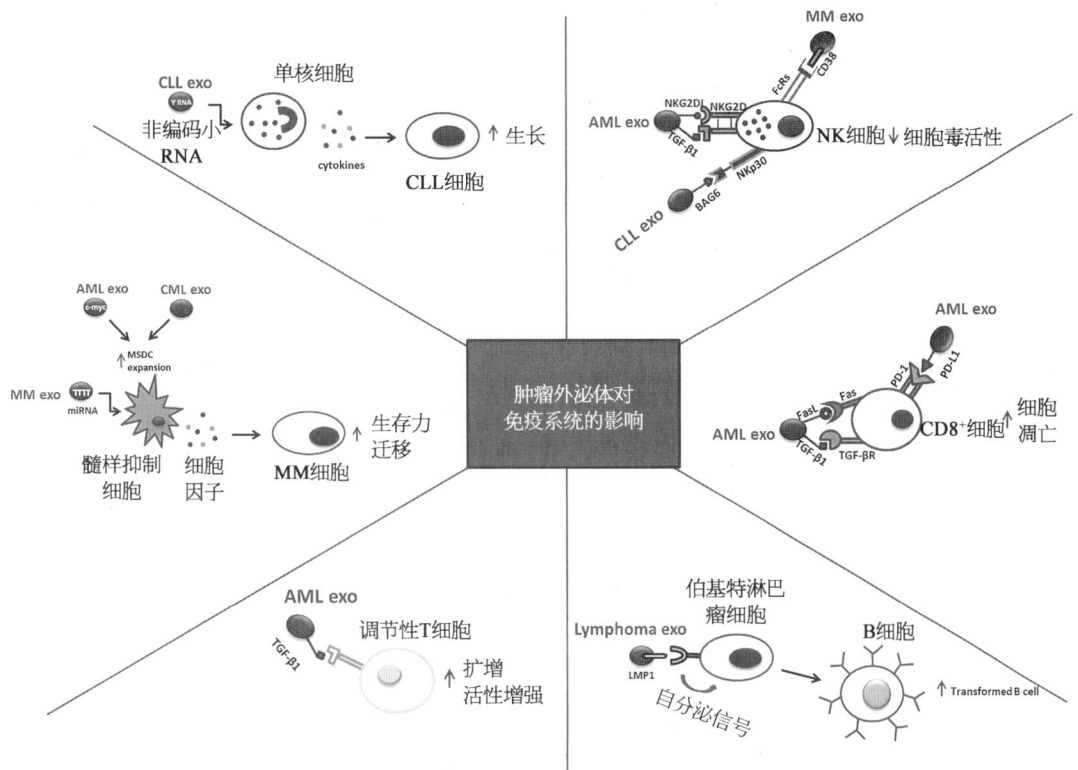

图4-3 肿瘤细胞来源的 EV 在免疫细胞功能调节中的示意图。肿瘤 EV 参与免疫反应的各个阶段，影响不同类型的免疫细胞

（一）外泌体与 NK 细胞

NK 细胞是细胞毒性淋巴细胞，是先天免疫系统的一部分，也是抵御病毒感染细胞和肿瘤细胞的第一道防线。这些细胞的主要特征是它们无须任何启动或预激活即可杀死肿瘤细胞（与需要 APC 启动的细胞毒性 T 细胞相反）。NK 细胞分泌 IFN-γ 和 TNF-α 等细胞因子，作用于巨噬细胞和 DC 等其他免疫细胞，增强免疫应答。这些细胞的另一个关键特征是区分自我和非我的能力。NK 细胞的第一个激活信号是肿瘤细胞表面 MHCⅠ类分子的丢失[50]。MHC Ⅰ类分子可以作为 NK 细胞的抑制信号，因此有 MHC Ⅰ类分子缺陷的肿瘤细胞成为 NK 细胞的靶点。NK 细胞利用其大量的抑制性和激活性受体来检测转化细胞。许多肿瘤细胞在 NK 细胞表面表达 NKG2D 识别的活化 NK 配体（如 MICA 和 MICB），因此它们会被 NK 细胞和 γδT 细胞有效清除[51]。在成功识别肿瘤细胞后，NK 细胞利用成孔蛋白、穿孔素和可以激活胱天蛋白酶的颗粒酶引起肿瘤细胞的凋亡。由效应细胞表达的 TRAIL 或 Fas 配体与其在肿瘤细胞上的同源受体结合也可以激活凋亡程序。这些 NK 细胞可以通过 IFN-γ、TNF-α 和 TNF-β 等细胞因子杀伤肿瘤细胞。肿瘤通过实施不同的免疫逃逸策略使 NK 细胞的功能受损，血液病的免疫逃逸策略导致 NK 细胞功能低下，如 NK 细胞数量减少、细胞毒作用减弱等。越来越多的证据证明了 NKG2D/NKG2DL 系统与白血病/淋巴瘤患者的相关性。细胞表面表达的 NKG2D 配体会标记待 NK 细胞攻击的肿

瘤细胞,但肿瘤细胞利用这些配体的胞外分泌方式逃避免疫系统。事实上,如 Hedlund 等所描述的那样,白血病/淋巴瘤细胞结构性地分泌外泌体,携带 MIC 和 ULBP 家族的 NKG2DL,从而增强对依赖 NKG2D 的 NK 细胞杀伤作用的抑制[52]。从 AML 患者血清中提取的外泌体显示,膜相关 TGF-β1 通过减少 NKG2D 的表达和激活 SMAD 途径削弱 NK 淋巴细胞杀伤白血病细胞的能力[53]。最近,Huang 等证实了来自沉默 TGF-β1 淋系白血病细胞的外泌体通过 $CD4^+$ T 细胞的增殖和细胞毒性 T 淋巴细胞的反应促进 DC 的成熟与免疫功能[54]。

在 CLL 中,由于 NK 细胞上 NKp30 激活受体的配体 BAG6 下调,NK 细胞表现出较低的细胞溶解活性。在生理条件下,BAG6 表达于外泌体表面,与 NKp30 受体结合,激活 NK 细胞的细胞毒活性。CLL 细胞不释放 BAG6 阳性的外泌体,在疾病过程中有助于免疫逃逸的发生[55]。此外,多发性骨髓瘤细胞释放 CD38 阳性的外泌体可能是肿瘤细胞逃避免疫系统的一种策略。MM 外泌体上表达的 CD38 可以通过将核苷酸转化为腺苷而产生一种无功能的免疫系统,腺苷是一种免疫抑制因子,可以降低 NK 细胞对 MM 细胞的细胞毒活性。综上所述,这一证据表明,外泌体介导的 NK 细胞功能障碍破坏了免疫监控,从而消除了各种血液系统恶性肿瘤中的肿瘤细胞。

(二)外泌体与 $CD8^+$ 细胞毒性淋巴细胞

$CD8^+$ 细胞毒性 T 细胞反应是抗肿瘤免疫的关键。$CD8^+$ 细胞与靶细胞结合后,将穿孔素整合到细胞膜上,含有颗粒酶的细胞质颗粒通过 T 细胞的孔道进入靶细胞胞浆,诱导细胞凋亡。$CD8^+$ 细胞也可以通过 FAS/FASL 系统诱导细胞凋亡。肿瘤细胞通过影响 T 细胞的增殖、活化和凋亡等多种机制逃避 $CD8^+$ 细胞的活性。免疫逃逸策略最著名的例子之一是外泌体表面存在的凋亡诱导分子。肿瘤患者循环中的大部分 $CD8^+$ T 淋巴细胞都表达 Fas,也有很多表达程序性死亡受体 1(programmed death 1,PD-1)。因此,它们对膜表面携带 FasL 或程序性死亡配体 1(programmed death igard 1, PD-L1)的外泌体诱导的凋亡很敏感。从 AML 患者血浆中分离出的外泌体富含可以诱导免疫抑制的蛋白,如 TGF-β1、PD-L1 或 FasL[56]。

(三)外泌体与髓样抑制细胞

肿瘤来源的外泌体还有一些其他促进免疫逃逸的机制,如触发 MDSC 的增殖。这些细胞是未成熟的骨髓细胞,大量存在于肿瘤患者的淋巴器官、血液和肿瘤组织中。这些细胞表达髓系标记刺激分子(CD14 和 CD11b),缺乏共刺激分子(HLA DR、CD80、CD86)。它们自发地分泌 TGF-β,并对活化的 T 淋巴细胞具有抑制性,因为它们能够抑制 T 细胞的增殖和溶细胞功能[57]。研究表明,肿瘤来源的外泌体改变了单核细胞的分化和成熟成为 DC,而 DC 是一种能够启动早期的抗肿瘤 T 细胞反应、引起髓系抑制细胞产生的特殊的 APC[57]。此外,研究表明,MDSC 介导的肿瘤进展的促进依赖于外泌体的 TGF-β,也依赖于肿瘤外泌体转运的脂质调节剂前列腺素 E2(prostaglandin E2,PGE2)[58]。特别是,由于与外泌体的肿瘤热休克蛋白 27(heat shock protein 27,HSP27)、髓系 Toll 样受体 2(Toll-like receptor 2，TLR-2)和髓系分化主要反应蛋白 88(myeloid differentiation primary response protein 88，MyD88)之间的相互作用，激活的 MDSC 减少了 CD4$^+$ 和 CD8$^+$ 淋巴细胞以及 NK 细胞的数量，并下调了它们的细胞毒能力[59]。在 CML 中，外泌体促进这些髓样抑制细胞的扩增，这些细胞能够抑制 T 细胞的增殖，从而促进白血病的进展[60,61]。AML 细胞异常表达支持肿瘤细胞增殖和抵抗凋亡的 MUC1 癌基因[62,63]。MUC1 的存在是 AML 中 MSDC 扩增的关键，也是释放含有 c-myc 的外泌体的主要原因。此外，携带 c-myc 的外泌体会引起细胞周期素 D2、细胞周期素 E1 和 c-myc 下游靶点的上调，并驱动 MSDC 的增殖[64]。

最近的研究表明，CLL 来源的外泌体中含有 miR-155，其通过 NF-κB 的激活促进 MSDC 的扩增[65]。多发性骨髓瘤细胞来源的外泌体通过激活 STAT3 通路促进 MDSC 的存活和增殖，并增强其免疫抑制能力。调节这一通路可以诱导高水平的精氨酸酶 1 和 iNOS，从而抑制 T 细胞功能，有助于 MM 细胞的免疫逃避[66]。最后，MM 细胞外泌体中的 miRNA146a 被转移到 MSC 中，诱导其细胞因子的分泌水平升高，从而提升 MM 细胞的生存力和迁移能力[67]。外泌体扩增 MSDC 的能力，创造了一个免疫耐受的环境，导致了 T 细胞的无反应性，促进肿瘤的生长。

（四）外泌体与调节性 T 细胞

CD4$^+$CD25^{high}Foxp3$^+$ 调节性 T 细胞(regulatory T cell，Treg)在维持自身耐受和调节免疫反应方面具有重要的作用[68]。肿瘤细胞可以有效地募集 Treg，并促进其增殖以逃避宿主的免疫反应。肿瘤细胞脱落的外泌体参与了这一机制，特别是通过 TGF-β。研究表明，TGF-β1 在 AML 外泌体中增加，并且已证实其具有促进 Treg 分化和扩增的作用[69]。

（五）外泌体与单核细胞

白血病细胞脱落的外泌体在单核细胞重编程为肿瘤相关巨噬细胞(tumor-associated macrophage，TAM)的过程中起着重要作用[70]。单核细胞进入肿瘤组织，并在那里支持肿瘤的启动、局部进展和远处转移[71]。在 CLL 中，恶性 B 细胞及其外泌体积聚在淋巴结和血液中，引起髓系细胞的慢性刺激与活化。这些外泌体能够将 Y RNA hY4(一种非编码 RNA)转移到单核细胞中，从而诱导细胞因子的释放，支持肿瘤的生长，更重要的是其通过表达免疫抑制蛋白 PD-L1 配体而导致免疫逃逸[72]。淋巴瘤 B 细胞脱落的外泌体包含一个突变的 MYD88 序列，它有助于重编程微环境的细胞如单核巨噬细胞，从而促进促炎信号通路[73]。

（六）外泌体与 B 细胞

众所周知，B 细胞通过产生抗体调节免疫反应和炎症，并通过抗原提呈促进 T 细胞的激活和增殖[74]。最近发现，B 细胞在肿瘤的发生和发展中也起着重要作用。其机制涉及分泌促进肿瘤形成的抗体，以及释放有利于肿瘤细胞生长和转移的促肿瘤因子。肿瘤外泌体帮助 B 细胞发挥免疫抑制功能。B 细胞淋巴瘤细胞脱落的外泌体通过携带促进恶性表型的 Wnt 信号通路的成分促进肿瘤进展[75]。淋巴瘤来源的携带 LMP1 癌基因的外泌体与

Burkitt 淋巴瘤细胞相互作用,触发自分泌信号,使淋巴瘤细胞能够与 B 细胞结合,这种相互作用还会诱导 B 细胞增殖与分化为浆母细胞样表型[76]。此外,有关肿瘤外泌体刺激调节性 B 细胞的能力的研究很少,而调节性 B 细胞反过来抑制 T 细胞的活性,并提供新的免疫逃逸机制。这些多效性的作用引发了假说,即干扰肿瘤细胞释放的外泌体可能代表了一种同时恢复肿瘤患者多种免疫功能的新策略,了解外泌体介导的免疫逃避可能有助于开发成功的、多层次的、多靶点的抗癌治疗。

七、胞外囊泡介导耐药性

尽管传统疗法在治疗实体肿瘤和血液肿瘤方面取得了许多进展,但许多疗法在根除这些疾病方面并不奏效。

抗癌治疗失败的主要原因之一,除了对正常组织的不良反应,还有耐药性的产生[77]。

大量的科学证据表明,肿瘤细胞与微环境细胞之间的双向交互作用在获得药理抗性中起着奠基的作用。事实上,基质细胞受到肿瘤细胞的"教育",帮助建立一个保护肿瘤细胞的环境,使肿瘤细胞在药物治疗过程中得以逃脱。在这种情况下,基质细胞和肿瘤细胞释放的 EV 通过运输核酸和多药耐药蛋白引起药理抗性[78,79]。2009 年,Bebawy 等发表了第一项关于造血系统恶性肿瘤 EV 在诱导耐药性中作用的研究,在这项研究中作者发现耐药 ALL 细胞的微粒含有 P-糖蛋白,这种质膜转运蛋白的过度表达与多重耐药性相关。此外,他们发现,这些微粒被药物敏感的受体细胞内化,它们能够通过转移蛋白质产生抗药性[80]。几年后,同一研究小组观察到,过度表达多药耐药相关蛋白 1(multidrug resistance-associated protein 1,MRP1)的 ALL 细胞释放出富含该蛋白的微粒。此外,他们发现,外泌体上的 MRP1 被对药物敏感的细胞内化之后会导致受体细胞获得 MRP1 介导的多药耐药性[81]。Crompot 等发现,CLL 患者 BM-MSC 释放的 EV 可以保护肿瘤细胞免受自发凋亡的影响,提高细胞的生存力和迁移能力,以及防止常规药物(如克拉屈滨和硼替佐米)诱导的凋亡[33]。

除了蛋白质转移,最近的研究表明,EV 可以通过 microRNA 的转移调节对治疗的反应。Viola 等发现,从 AML 患者骨髓抽提物中提取的外泌体能够通过传递 TGF-β1、miR155 和 miR375 保护肿瘤细胞,并假定它们可以促进 AML 细胞的耐药性[82]。Min 等为慢性粒细胞白血病中外泌体介导耐药性提供依据。他们发现,耐伊马替尼 CLL 细胞释放的外泌体被药物敏感细胞内化,通过传输外泌体的 miR-365 产生耐药性,事实上,miRNA 的转移会导致受体细胞中促凋亡蛋白的抑制[83]。同样地,多发性骨髓瘤患者骨髓中的外泌体通过激活 c-Jun、p38、p53 和 Akt 通路,在 MM 细胞中诱导对硼替佐米治疗的耐药性,从而促进肿瘤细胞的存活[84]。

八、外泌体在疾病诊断和药物治疗监测中的临床意义

在早期阶段检测肿瘤的需要正在推动分子诊断领域的不断进步,以及筛选组织或血液样本中肿瘤特异性基因组、蛋白质组和表观遗传学特征的能力。现代医学的目标是识别肿瘤生物标志物,使其能够以准确和非侵入性的方式在早期发现肿瘤。

最近的研究表明，患者临床资料和 EV 资料的结合可能代表血液系统恶性肿瘤的有效"液体活检"，事实上，EV 通过保护其内容物不被降解，可以提供有关肿瘤分期和治疗结果的临床信息[85]。Caivano 等进行了血浆 EV 数量与血液系统肿瘤之间的相关性研究，作者从不同血液系统肿瘤患者，包括 CLL、MM、AML 和对照组中分离出血清 EV。他们观察到，与正常样本相比，患者样本中的微泡水平更高，这提示了将 EV 作为生物标志物的可能性[86]。

Hong 等比较了新诊断的 AML 患者外泌体中 TGF-β1 的含量与接受了治疗的患者队列中外泌体蛋白的数量。有趣的是，他们发现外泌体 TGF-β1 的水平反映了患者对治疗的反应，并且与健康对照组相比，新诊断患者的水平更高。总体而言，这项研究提供了一个重要证据，证明外泌体相关的 TGF-β1 可以作为 AML 潜在的诊断或预后生物标志物[69]。除了外泌体蛋白，外泌体相关的 microRNA 也被认为可以作为生物标志物[87]。Hornick 等从白血病原始细胞和骨髓基质细胞中鉴定出一组富含 AML 外泌体中的 miRNA，可用于临床诊断[88]。与这些结果相一致，最近 Caivano 观察到与 EV 相关的 miR155 在 CLL 和 AML 中比正常样本更高[89]。

九、总结

对细胞源性 EV 在肿瘤微环境中作用的理解的进展，以及能够快速、准确地分离和鉴定外泌体的新策略的开发，将为识别包括血液系统疾病在内的肿瘤相关生物标志物提供依据。目前已有的和未来的研究结果将使这些囊泡在未来的临床上得以应用，从而改善疾病的结局，提升疾病的存活率。

致谢

Riccardo Alessandro 获得了意大利肿瘤研究协会（Associazione Italiana per la Ricerca sul Cancro，AIRC）的资助（编号 18783）。Stefania Raimondo 获得了意大利肿瘤研究基金会（Fondazione Italiana Ricerca sul Cancro，FIRC）基金的支持。

利益冲突

作者声明没有利益冲突。

（田彬功 译，李琦 审校）

参考文献

[1] Hanahan D, Weinberg RA. Hallmarks of cancer: the next generation. Cell 2011; 144: 646-74.
[2] Belli C, Trapani D, Viale G, D'Amico P, Duso BA, Della Vigna P, Orsi F, Curigliano G. Targeting the microenvironment in solid tumors. Cancer Treat Rev 2018; 65: 22-32.
[3] Sison EAR, Kurre P, Kim YM. Understanding the bone marrow microenvironment in hematologic malignancies: a focus on chemokine, integrin, and extracellular vesicle signaling. Pediatr Hematol Oncol 2017; 34: 365-78.
[4] Sison EA, Brown P. The bone marrow microenvironment and leukemia: biology and therapeutic targeting. Expert Rev Hematol 2011; 4: 271-83.
[5] Cho BS, Kim HJ, Konopleva M. Targeting the CXCL12/CXCR4 axis in acute myeloid leukemia: from bench to bedside. Korean J Intern Med 2017; 32: 248-57.
[6] Hideshima T, Bergsagel PL, Kuehl WM, Anderson KC. Advances in biology of multiple myeloma: clinical applications.

Blood 2004; 104: 607-18.
[7] Corrado C, Raimondo S, Saieva L, Flugy AM, De Leo G, Alessandro R. Exosome-mediated crosstalk between chronic myelogenous leukemia cells and human bone marrow stromal cells triggers an interleukin 8-dependent survival of leukemia cells. Cancer Lett 2014; 348: 71-6.
[8] Arai F, Hirao A, Suda T. Regulation of hematopoiesis and its interaction with stem cell niches. Int J Hematol 2005; 82: 371-6.
[9] Mendelson A, Frenette PS. Hematopoietic stem cell niche maintenance during homeostasis and regeneration. Nat Med 2014; 20: 833-46.
[10] Laurenzana I, Lamorte D, Trino S, De Luca L, Ambrosino C, Zoppoli P, Ruggieri V, Del Vecchio L, Musto P, Caivano A, Falco G. Extracellular vesicles: a new prospective in crosstalk between microenvironment and stem cells in hematological malignancies. Stem Cells Int 2018; 2018: 9863194.
[11] Ratajczak J, Miekus K, Kucia M, Zhang J, Reca R, Dvorak P, Ratajczak MZ. Embryonic stem cell-derived microvesicles reprogram hematopoietic progenitors: evidence for horizontal transfer of mRNA and protein delivery. Leukemia 2006; 20: 847-56.
[12] Ekstrom K, Valadi H, Sjostrand M, Malmhall C, Bossios A, Eldh M, Lotvall J. Characterization of mRNA and microRNA in human mast cell-derived exosomes and their transfer to other mast cells and blood CD34 progenitor cells. J Extracell Vesicles 2012; 1. https://doi.org/10.3402/jev.v1i0.18389.
[13] Goloviznina NA, Verghese SC, Yoon YM, Taratula O, Marks DL, Kurre P. Mesenchymal stromal cell-derived extracellular vesicles promote myeloid-biased multipotent hematopoietic progenitor expansion via toll-kike receptor engagement. J Biol Chem 2016; 291: 24607-17.
[14] Stik G, Crequit S, Petit L, Durant J, Charbord P, Jaffredo T, Durand C. Extracellular vesicles of stromal origin target and support hematopoietic stem and progenitor cells. J Cell Biol 2017; 216: 2217-30.
[15] Huan J, Hornick NI, Goloviznina NA, Kamimae-Lanning AN, David LL, Wilmarth PA, Mori T, Chevillet JR, Narla A, Roberts Jr. CT, et al. Coordinate regulation of residual bone marrow function by paracrine trafficking of AML exosomes. Leukemia 2015; 29: 2285-95.
[16] Hornick NI, Doron B, Abdelhamed S, Huan J, Harrington CA, Shen R, Cambronne XA, Chakkaramakkil Verghese S, Kurre P. AML suppresses hematopoiesis by releasing exosomes that contain microRNAs targeting c-MYB. Sci Signal 2016; 9: ra88.
[17] Razmkhah F, Soleimani M, Mehrabani D, Karimi MH, Amini Kafi-Abad S, Ramzi M, Iravani Saadi M, Kakoui J. Leukemia microvesicles affect healthy hematopoietic stem cells. Tumour Biol 2017; 39: 1010428317692234.
[18] Kumar B, Garcia M, Weng L, Jung X, Murakami JL, Hu X, McDonald T, Lin A, Kumar AR, DiGiusto DL, et al. Acute myeloid leukemia transforms the bone marrow niche into a leukemia-permissive microenvironment through exosome secretion. Leukemia 2018; 32: 575-87.
[19] Muntion S, Ramos TL, Diez-Campelo M, Roson B, Sanchez-Abarca LI, Misiewicz-Krzeminska I, Preciado S, Sarasquete ME, de Las Rivas J, Gonzalez M, et al. Microvesicles from mesenchymal stromal cells are involved in HPC-microenvironment crosstalk in myelodysplastic patients. PLoS One 2016; 11: e0146722.
[20] Moehler TM, Ho AD, Goldschmidt H, Barlogie B. Angiogenesis in hematologic malignancies. Crit Rev Oncol Hematol 2003; 45: 227-44.
[21] Taverna S, Flugy A, Saieva L, Kohn EC, Santoro A, Meraviglia S, De Leo G, Alessandro R. Role of exosomes released by chronic myelogenous leukemia cells in angiogenesis. Int J Cancer 2012; 130: 2033-43.
[22] Taverna S, Amodeo V, Saieva L, Russo A, Giallombardo M, De Leo G, Alessandro R. Exosomal shuttling of miR-126 in endothelial cells modulates adhesive and migratory abilities of chronic myelogenous leukemia cells. Mol Cancer 2014; 13: 169.
[23] Mineo M, Garfield SH, Taverna S, Flugy A, De Leo G, Alessandro R, Kohn EC. Exosomes released by K562 chronic myeloid leukemia cells promote angiogenesis in a Src-dependent fashion. Angiogenesis 2012; 15: 33-45.
[24] Tadokoro H, Umezu T, Ohyashiki K, Hirano T, Ohyashiki JH. Exosomes derived from hypoxic leukemia cells enhance tube formation in endothelial cells. J Biol Chem 2013; 288: 34343-51.
[25] Liu Y, Zhu XJ, Zeng C, Wu PH, Wang HX, Chen ZC, Li QB. Microvesicles secreted from human multiple myeloma cells promote angiogenesis. Acta Pharmacol Sin 2014; 35: 230-8.
[26] Umezu T, Tadokoro H, Azuma K, Yoshizawa S, Ohyashiki K, Ohyashiki JH. Exosomal miR-135b shed from hypoxic multiple myeloma cells enhances angiogenesis by targeting factorinhibiting HIF-1. Blood 2014; 124: 3748-57.
[27] Huan J, Hornick NI, Shurtleff MJ, Skinner AM, Goloviznina NA, Roberts Jr. CT, Kurre P. RNA trafficking by acute myelogenous leukemia exosomes. Cancer Res 2013; 73: 918-29.
[28] Morrison SJ, Scadden DT. The bone marrow niche for haematopoietic stem cells. Nature 2014; 505: 327-34.
[29] Tripodo C, Sangaletti S, Piccaluga PP, Prakash S, Franco G, Borrello I, Orazi A, Colombo MP, Pileri SA. The bone marrow stroma in hematological neoplasms—a guilty bystander. Nat Rev Clin Oncol 2011; 8: 456-66.
[30] Ohyashiki JH, Umezu T, Ohyashiki K. Extracellular vesicle-mediated cell-cell communication in haematological neoplasms. Philos Trans R Soc Lond B Biol Sci 2018; 373(1737).
[31] Zhou J, Tan X, Tan Y, Li Q, Ma J, Wang G. Mesenchymal stem cell derived exosomes in cancer progression, metastasis and drug delivery: a comprehensive review. J Cancer 2018; 9: 3129-37.
[32] Roccaro AM, Sacco A, Maiso P, Azab AK, Tai YT, Reagan M, Azab F, Flores LM, Campigotto F, Weller E, et al. BM mesenchymal stromal cell-derived exosomes facilitate multiple myeloma progression. J Clin Invest 2013; 123: 1542-55.
[33] Crompot E, Van Damme M, Pieters K, Vermeersch M, Perez-Morga D, Mineur P, Maerevoet M, Meuleman N, Bron D, Lagneaux L, Stamatopoulos B. Extracellular vesicles of bone marrow stromal cells rescue chronic lymphocytic leukemia B cells from apoptosis, enhance their migration and induce gene expression modifications. Haematologica 2017; 102: 1594-604.

[34] Barrera-Ramirez J, Lavoie JR, Maganti HB, Stanford WL, Ito C, Sabloff M, Brand M, Rosu-Myles M, Le Y, Allan DS. Micro-RNA profiling of exosomes from marrow-derived mesenchymal stromal cells in patients with acute myeloid leukemia: implications in leukemogenesis. Stem Cell Rev 2017; 13: 817-25.

[35] Corrado C, Saieva L, Raimondo S, Santoro A, De Leo G, Alessandro R. Chronic myelogenous leukaemia exosomes modulate bone marrow microenvironment through activation of epidermal growth factor receptor. J Cell Mol Med 2016; 20: 1829-39.

[36] Ghosh AK, Secreto CR, Knox TR, Ding W, Mukhopadhyay D, Kay NE. Circulating microvesicles in B-cell chronic lymphocytic leukemia can stimulate marrow stromal cells: implications for disease progression. Blood 2010; 115: 1755-64.

[37] Cheng Q, Li X, Liu J, Ye Q, Chen Y, Tan S. Multiple myeloma-derived exosomes regulate the functions of mesenchymal stem cells partially via modulating miR-21 and miR-146a. Stem Cells Int 2017; 2017: 9012152.

[38] Chiarugi P, Cirri P. Metabolic exchanges within tumor microenvironment. Cancer Lett 2016; 380: 272-80.

[39] La Shu S, Yang Y, Allen CL, Maguire O, Minderman H, Sen A, Ciesielski MJ, Collins KA, Bush PJ, Singh P, et al. Metabolic reprogramming of stromal fibroblasts by melanoma exosome microRNA favours a pre-metastatic microenvironment. Sci Rep 2018; 8: 12905.

[40] Johnson SM, Dempsey C, Chadwick A, Harrison S, Liu J, Di Y, McGinn OJ, Fiorillo M, Sotgia F, Lisanti MP, et al. Metabolic reprogramming of bone marrow stromal cells by leukemic extracellular vesicles in acute lymphoblastic leukemia. Blood 2016; 128: 453-6.

[41] Rodan GA. Bone homeostasis. Proc Natl Acad Sci U S A 1998; 95: 13361-2.

[42] Terpos E, Ntanasis-Stathopoulos I, Gavriatopoulou M, Dimopoulos MA. Pathogenesis of bone disease in multiple myeloma: from bench to bedside. Blood Cancer J 2018; 8: 7.

[43] Sun W, Zhao C, Li Y, Wang L, Nie G, Peng J, Wang A, Zhang P, Tian W, Li Q, et al. Osteoclast-derived microRNA-containing exosomes selectively inhibit osteoblast activity. Cell Discov 2016; 2: 16015.

[44] Cui Y, Luan J, Li H, Zhou X, Han J. Exosomes derived from mineralizing osteoblasts promote ST2 cell osteogenic differentiation by alteration of microRNA expression. FEBS Lett 2016; 590: 185-92.

[45] Raimondi L, De Luca A, Amodio N, Manno M, Raccosta S, Taverna S, Bellavia D, Naselli F, Fontana S, Schillaci O, et al. Involvement of multiple myeloma cell-derived exosomes in osteoclast differentiation. Oncotarget 2015; 6: 13772-89.

[46] Li B, Xu H, Han H, Song S, Zhang X, Ouyang L, Qian C, Hong Y, Qiu Y, Zhou W, et al. Exosome-mediated transfer of lncRUNX2-AS1 from multiple myeloma cells to MSCs contributes to osteogenesis. Oncogene 2018; 37: 5508-19.

[47] De La Pena H, Madrigal JA, Rusakiewicz S, Bencsik M, Cave GW, Selman A, Rees RC, Travers PJ, Dodi IA. Artificial exosomes as tools for basic and clinical immunology. J Immunol Methods 2009; 344: 121-32.

[48] Dunn GP, Bruce AT, Ikeda H, Old LJ, Schreiber RD. Cancer immunoediting: from immunosurveillance to tumor escape. Nat Immunol 2002; 3: 991-8.

[49] Dunn GP, Old LJ, Schreiber RD. The immunobiology of cancer immunosurveillance and immunoediting. Immunity 2004; 21: 137-48.

[50] Ljunggren HG, Karre K. Host resistance directed selectively against H-2-deficient lymphoma variants. Analysis of the mechanism. J Exp Med 1985; 162: 1745-59.

[51] Groh V, Rhinehart R, Secrist H, Bauer S, Grabstein KH, Spies T. Broad tumor-associated expression and recognition by tumor-derived gamma delta T cells of MICA and MICB. Proc Natl Acad Sci U S A 1999; 96: 6879-84.

[52] Hedlund M, Nagaeva O, Kargl D, Baranov V, Mincheva-Nilsson L. Thermal- and oxidative stress causes enhanced release of NKG2D ligand-bearing immunosuppressive exosomes in leukemia/lymphoma T and B cells. PLoS One 2011; 6: e16899.

[53] Szczepanski MJ, Szajnik M, Welsh A, Whiteside TL, Boyiadzis M. Blast-derived microvesicles in sera from patients with acute myeloid leukemia suppress natural killer cell function via membrane-associated transforming growth factor-beta1. Haematologica 2011; 96: 1302-9.

[54] Huang F, Wan J, Hao S, Deng X, Chen L, Ma L. TGF-beta1-silenced leukemia cell-derived exosomes target dendritic cells to induce potent anti-keukemic immunity in a mouse model. Cancer Immunol Immunother 2017; 66: 1321-31.

[55] Reiners KS, Topolar D, Henke A, Simhadri VR, Kessler J, Sauer M, Bessler M, Hansen HP, Tawadros S, Herling M, et al. Soluble ligands for NK cell receptors promote evasion of chronic lymphocytic leukemia cells from NK cell anti-tumor activity. Blood 2013; 121: 3658-65.

[56] Hong CS, Sharma P, Yerneni SS, Simms P, Jackson EK, Whiteside TL, Boyiadzis M. Circulating exosomes carrying an immunosuppressive cargo interfere with cellular immunotherapy in acute myeloid leukemia. Sci Rep 2017; 7: 14684.

[57] Gabrilovich DI, Nagaraj S. Myeloid-derived suppressor cells as regulators of the immune system. Nat Rev Immunol 2009; 9: 162-74.

[58] Chen W, Jiang J, Xia W, Huang J. Tumor-related exosomes contribute to tumor-promoting microenvironment: an immunological perspective. J Immunol Res 2017; 2017: 1073947.

[59] Zhang HG, Grizzle WE. Exosomes and cancer: a newly described pathway of immune suppression. Clin Cancer Res 2011; 17: 959-64.

[60] Whiteside TL. Immune modulation of T-cell and NK (natural killer) cell activities by TEXs (tumour-derived exosomes). Biochem Soc Trans 2013; 41: 245-51.

[61] Giallongo C, Parrinello NL, La Cava P, Camiolo G, Romano A, Scalia M, Stagno F, Palumbo GA, Avola R, Li Volti G, et al. Monocytic myeloid-derived suppressor cells as prognostic factor in chronic myeloid leukaemia patients treated with dasatinib. J Cell Mol Med 2018; 22: 1070-80.

[62] Liu S, Yin L, Stroopinsky D, Rajabi H, Puissant A, Stegmaier K, Avigan D, Kharbanda S, Kufe D, Stone R. MUC1-C oncoprotein promotes FLT3 receptor activation in acute myeloid leukemia cells. Blood 2014; 123: 734-42.

[63] Yin L, Kosugi M, Kufe D. Inhibition of the MUC1-C oncoprotein induces multiple myeloma cell death by down-regulating TIGAR expression and depleting NADPH. Blood 2012; 119: 810-6.
[64] Pyzer AR, Stroopinsky D, Rajabi H, Washington A, Tagde A, Coll M, Fung J, Bryant MP, Cole L, Palmer K, et al. MUC1-mediated induction of myeloid-derived suppressor cells in patients with acute myeloid leukemia. Blood 2017; 129: 1791-801.
[65] Bruns H, Bottcher M, Qorraj M, Fabri M, Jitschin S, Dindorf J, Busch L, Jitschin R, Mackensen A, Mougiakakos D. CLL-cell-mediated MDSC induction by exosomal miR-155 transfer is disrupted by vitamin D. Leukemia 2017; 31: 985-8.
[66] Wang J, De Veirman K, Faict S, Frassanito MA, Ribatti D, Vacca A, Menu E. Multiple myeloma exosomes establish a favourable bone marrow microenvironment with enhanced angiogenesis and immunosuppression. J Pathol 2016; 239: 162-73.
[67] De Veirman K, Wang J, Xu S, Leleu X, Himpe E, Maes K, De Bruyne E, Van Valckenborgh E, Vanderkerken K, Menu E, Van Riet I. Induction of miR-146a by multiple myeloma cells in mesenchymal stromal cells stimulates their pro-tumoral activity. Cancer Lett 2016; 377: 17-24.
[68] Sakaguchi S, Yamaguchi T, Nomura T, Ono M. Regulatory T cells and immune tolerance. Cell 2008; 133: 775-87.
[69] Hong CS, Muller L, Whiteside TL, Boyiadzis M. Plasma exosomes as markers of therapeutic response in patients with acute myeloid leukemia. Front Immunol 2014; 5: 160.
[70] Ciardiello C, Cavallini L, Spinelli C, Yang J, Reis-Sobreiro M, de Candia P, Minciacchi VR, Di Vizio D. Focus on extracellular vesicles: new frontiers of cell-to-cell communication in cancer. Int J Mol Sci 2016; 17: 175.
[71] Richards DM, Hettinger J, Feuerer M. Monocytes and macrophages in cancer: development and functions. Cancer Microenviron 2013; 6: 179-91.
[72] Haderk F, Schulz R, Iskar M, Cid LL, Worst T, Willmund KV, Schulz A, Warnken U, Seiler J, Benner A, et al. Tumor-derived exosomes modulate PD-L1 expression in monocytes. Sci Immunol 2017; 2: eaah5509.
[73] Mancek-Keber M, Lainscek D, Bencina M, Chen JG, Romih R, Hunter ZR, Treon SP, Jerala R. Extracellular vesicle-mediated transfer of constitutively active MyD88(L265P) engages MyD88(wt) and activates signaling. Blood 2018; 131: 1720-9.
[74] LeBien TW, Tedder TF. B lymphocytes: how they develop and function. Blood 2008; 112: 1570-80.
[75] Koch R, Demant M, Aung T, Diering N, Cicholas A, Chapuy B, Wenzel D, Lahmann M, Guntsch A, Kiecke C, et al. Populational equilibrium through exosome-mediated Wnt signaling in tumor progression of diffuse large B-cell lymphoma. Blood 2014; 123: 2189-98.
[76] Siravegna G, Marsoni S, Siena S, Bardelli A. Integrating liquid biopsies into the management of cancer. Nat Rev Clin Oncol 2017; 14: 531-48.
[77] Housman G, Byler S, Heerboth S, Lapinska K, Longacre M, Snyder N, Sarkar S. Drug resistance in cancer: an overview. Cancers (Basel) 2014; 6: 1769-92.
[78] Jaiswal R, Raymond Grau GE, Bebawy M. Cellular communication via microparticles: role in transfer of multidrug resistance in cancer. Future Oncol 2014; 10: 655-69.
[79] Gong J, Jaiswal R, Mathys JM, Combes V, Grau GE, Bebawy M. Microparticles and their emerging role in cancer multidrug resistance. Cancer Treat Rev 2012; 38: 226-34.
[80] Bebawy M, Combes V, Lee E, Jaiswal R, Gong J, Bonhoure A, Grau GE. Membrane microparticles mediate transfer of P-glycoprotein to drug sensitive cancer cells. Leukemia 2009; 23: 1643-9.
[81] Lu JF, Luk F, Gong J, Jaiswal R, Grau GE, Bebawy M. Microparticles mediate MRP1 intercellular transfer and the re-templating of intrinsic resistance pathways. Pharmacol Res 2013; 76: 77-83.
[82] Viola S, Traer E, Huan J, Hornick NI, Tyner JW, Agarwal A, Loriaux M, Johnstone B, Kurre P. Alterations in acute myeloid leukaemia bone marrow stromal cell exosome content coincide with gains in tyrosine kinase inhibitor resistance. Br J Haematol 2016; 172: 983-6.
[83] Min QH, Wang XZ, Zhang J, Chen QG, Li SQ, Liu XQ, Li J, Liu J, Yang WM, Jiang YH, et al. Exosomes derived from imatinib-resistant chronic myeloid leukemia cells mediate a horizontal transfer of drug-resistant trait by delivering miR-365. Exp Cell Res 2018; 362: 386-93.
[84] Wang J, Hendrix A, Hernot S, Lemaire M, De Bruyne E, Van Valckenborgh E, Lahoutte T, De Wever O, Vanderkerken K, Menu E. Bone marrow stromal cell-derived exosomes as communicators in drug resistance in multiple myeloma cells. Blood 2014; 124: 555-66.
[85] Marrugo-Ramirez J, Mir M, Samitier J. Blood-based cancer biomarkers in liquid biopsy: a promising non-invasive alternative to tissue biopsy. Int J Mol Sci 2018; 19: E2877.
[86] Caivano A, Laurenzana I, De Luca L, La Rocca F, Simeon V, Trino S, D'Auria F, Traficante A, Maietti M, Izzo T, et al. High serum levels of extracellular vesicles expressing malignancyrelated markers are released in patients with various types of hematological neoplastic disorders. Tumour Biol 2015; 36: 9739-52.
[87] Li Q, Liu L, Li W. Identification of circulating microRNAs as biomarkers in diagnosis of hematologic cancers: a meta-analysis. Tumour Biol 2014; 35: 10467-78.
[88] Hornick NI, Huan J, Doron B, Goloviznina NA, Lapidus J, Chang BH, Kurre P. Serum exosome MicroRNA as a minimally-invasive early biomarker of AML. Sci Rep 2015; 5: 11295.
[89] Caivano A, La Rocca F, Simeon V, Girasole M, Dinarelli S, Laurenzana I, De Stradis A, De Luca L, Trino S, Traficante A, et al. MicroRNA-155 in serum-derived extracellular vesicles as a potential biomarker for hematologic malignancies — a short report. Cell Oncol (Dordr) 2017; 40: 97-103.

第 5 章

前列腺小体的生理和病理功能：
从基础研究到临床应用

Physiological and pathological functions of prostasomes: From basic research to clinical application

Fumihiko Urabe[a, b], Nobuyoshi Kosaka[a, c],
Koji Asano[b], Shin Egawa[b], Takahiro Ochiya[a, c]

[a]Division of Molecular and Cellular Medicine, National Cancer Center Research Institute, Tokyo, Japan, [b]Department of Urology, Jikei University School of Medicine, Tokyo, Japan, [c]Department of Molecular and Cellular Medicine, Institute of Medical Science, Tokyo Medical University, Tokyo, Japan

一、概述

近年来，随着研究的深入，研究人员发现在细胞通信的过程中，除了常规的信号传导机制（直接的细胞接触或间接的可溶性信号传导分子转移），EV 也发挥着重要的作用[1]。1983年，人们第一次发现并报道了 EV。近十年来，科研工作者逐步发现 EV 能够承载 mRNA 和 miRNA，并且转运至受体细胞发挥调控作用。随着 EV 功能的不断发现，其研究热度也急剧升高[2-5]。基于其分泌来源，EV 通常分为外泌体、微泡以及凋亡小体。外泌体即为多囊泡体的腔内囊泡，其在多囊泡体与细胞膜融合时向细胞外释放[6]。微泡通常体积略大于外泌体，在正常生理过程中或应激时可直接从细胞质膜脱落[7]。而凋亡小体则由程序性死亡过程中的细胞形成[8]。通常情况下，区分外泌体、微泡和凋亡小体存在一定困难，因此在文献报道时，依据国际胞外囊泡协会（International Society for Extracellular Vesicles, ISEV）的建议，多使用 EV 一词以全面概括[9]。

除了上述三种 EV，前列腺小体（prostasomes），一种起源于前列腺上皮细胞的 EV，在生殖生物学和泌尿外科学研究领域获得较高的关注度。前列腺是最大的雄性生殖腺，状如核桃，位于男性膀胱和骨盆底之间，在雄性生殖系统中起关键作用。前列腺能够分泌一种乳白状液体，即前列腺液。正常男性 30% 的精液由前列腺液组成，而前列腺小体正存在于该部分的前列腺液中[10]。在最初报道 EV 对细胞间功能相互作用的研究中，人们就发现前列腺上皮细胞分泌的前列腺小体能够增加精子活力[11]。时至今日，越来越多的研究发现前列腺小体在正常的受精过程中发挥着更加多样化的功能。

还有研究发现，前列腺小体不仅参与正常的生理过程，而且还与前列腺癌的发生有关[12]。研究发现，前列腺肿瘤细胞能够分泌前列腺小体，从而促进肿瘤进展。此外，前列腺细胞中的动态分子变化，也能够经由前列腺小体携带并得以表现，从而帮助医师获取有关肿瘤状态的重要信息。因此,前列腺小体具备成为临床生物标志物的巨大潜力。

本章主要论述了来自良性上皮细胞和前列腺肿瘤细胞两种类型的前列腺小体,概述了前列腺小体在生理和病理过程中的主要作用,并且进一步讨论了前列腺小体在诊治前列腺肿瘤方面的临床应用潜力。

二、前列腺上皮细胞:前列腺小体的起源

人类精液和前列腺液中的前列腺小体最早于20世纪70年代被报道[13,14]。前列腺小体直径为30～200 nm,由前列腺的腺泡上皮细胞分泌并储存于前列腺腺腔中,作为前列腺液的组成部分在射精的过程中与精子一起排出,并最终进入精液[15,16]。

前列腺小体与前列腺上皮细胞内所谓贮存囊泡的大小相似[15,17]。贮存囊泡是前列腺小体的来源之一,电子显微镜图像分析显示良性和恶性前列腺上皮细胞都能够产生贮存囊泡[18]。贮存囊泡的功能定位近似于外泌体的前身——MVB。类似地,贮存囊泡能够和细胞质膜融合,在此过程中将前列腺小体释放到前列腺导管中[15,17]。因此,研究人员认为前列腺小体的一个亚群与外泌体具有一定的相似性。同时研究人员还认为,前列腺上皮细胞中的贮存囊泡并非前列腺小体的唯一来源。Zijlstra等认为前列腺小体可以直接由前列腺上皮细胞的质膜脱落而产生。此类型的前列腺小体亚群被认为与微泡具有一定的相似性[19]。

现有研究发现,前列腺小体中含有蛋白质、核酸和脂质等多种分子。以蛋白质为例,蛋白质组学分析发现,前列腺小体中含有的蛋白质多于400种[20,21]。此后,越来越多的研究详尽地报道了前列腺小体中所含蛋白质的种类。其中值得注意的是,多项重复研究证实,前列腺小体中普遍存在EV的标志性蛋白CD9,同时还表达前列腺肿瘤的潜在标志物如前列腺特异性抗原(prostate-specific antigen,PSA)、2型跨膜丝氨酸蛋白酶(type 2 transmembrane serine protease,TMPRSS2)和前列腺干细胞抗原(prostate stem cell antigen,PSCA)[20-22]。

也有报道称在前列腺小体中发现DNA存在。Ronquist等在研究中揭示了人类来源的前列腺小体中含有染色体DNA。通过用核酸酶处理该DNA,他们发现前列腺小体相关的DNA能够免受酶的作用而降解。该发现提示DNA位于前列腺小体的内部并由其携带[23]。同时他们还发现,DNA能够从前列腺小体转移到精子中[24]。而其他类型的核酸,如miRNA或lncRNA,尽管其常在多种肿瘤来源的EV中被发现,但尚无研究表明其存在于正常精液里起源于前列腺上皮细胞的前列腺小体中。

前列腺小体具有特定的脂质成分。通常情况下,哺乳动物细胞的细胞质膜含有较多的磷脂酰胆碱和磷脂酰乙醇胺,但前列腺小体膜的主要磷脂是鞘磷脂。此外,前列腺小体具有高的胆固醇/磷脂比,比例接近2∶1[25]。相比而下,人精子细胞质膜的比率为1∶0.7[26]。这种特殊的脂质成分可能有助于前列腺小体维持极高的膜稳定性[27],也有研究发现其有助于受精[28]。

考虑到前列腺小体较小的尺寸和其中可能携带的较多的分子种类,人们推测前列腺小体中的分子类型与数量可能与其亚群类型有关。研究人员发现不同肿瘤来源的EV具有各

自的异质性[29,30]，同时也发现前列腺小体具有异质性。前列腺小体的异质性最早由 Poliakov 等于 2009 年提出[21]。通过冷冻电子显微镜，他们观察到精液中前列腺体的形态具有多样性[21]。随后，Alberts 等通过电子显微镜和免疫印迹分析蛋白质组成，证实了不同亚群前列腺小体的存在[22]。他们发现了两个前列腺小体的亚群，通过蔗糖梯度分离法，证明了其在尺寸上存在明显差异。虽然这两种亚群都表达 CD9（经典的 EV 标志物）和 PSCA（一种前列腺特异性蛋白），但是其中较小的亚群表达 GLIPR2 蛋白，而较大的亚群则特异性表达膜联蛋白 A1[22]。此项研究证明，前列腺小体的结构异质性可能与其功能上的特异性具有一定联系，即不同亚群的前列腺小体能够发挥不同的特定功能。

三、前列腺小体的生理功能

前列腺小体能够在射精过程中与精细胞接触，如前文所述，前列腺小体中含有多种分子，因此在前列腺小体与精细胞发生接触的同时，对精子的功能可能同时存在刺激或者抑制作用。在本章节中，我们总结了前列腺小体在生殖功能中可能发挥的作用（图 5-1）。

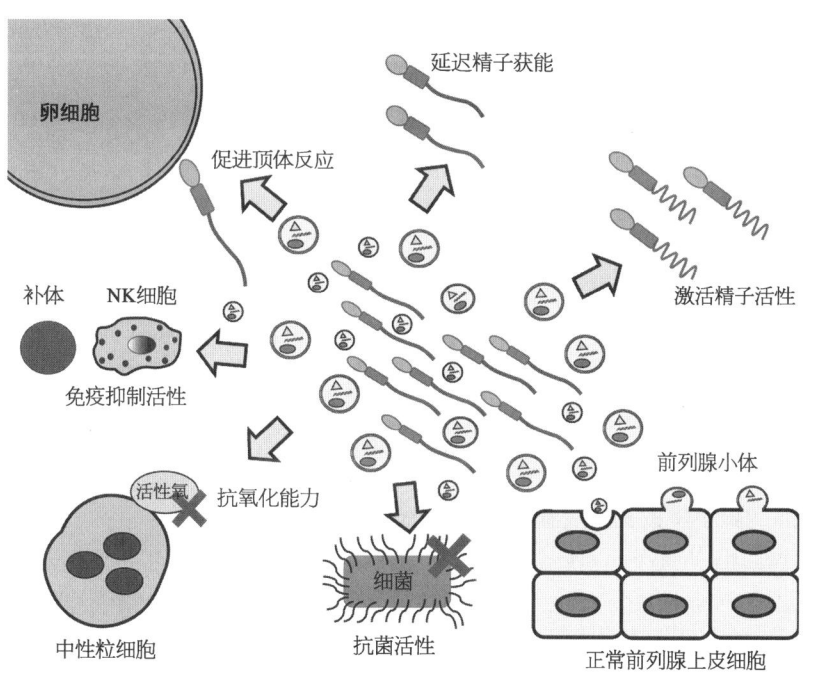

图 5-1　前列腺小体在受精过程中的作用。前列腺小体能够增加精子的活力，同时延迟精子获能，使其在精子接触到卵子后发生，从而提高受精概率。同时前列腺小体具有免疫抑制作用，从而防止女性免疫系统破坏精子。前列腺小体本身还具有抗菌活性。前列腺小体还能够加速顶体反应以促进受精。在适当的时间和位置，前列腺小体与精子之间能够通过一系列复杂的相互作用，从而促进受精及生殖过程

（一）前列腺小体与精子活力

在受精过程中，精子必须穿过女性生殖道，其中最为关键的是通过宫颈黏液并穿过透明

带[31]。因此,精子的活力是评估精液质量的重要因素,精子的活力直接影响精子的受精能力。现有研究发现,前列腺小体可直接黏附于精子表面,并能够与其融合,从而增加精子的整体活动能力[32,33]。

Fabiani 等研究发现,在 37℃下,与白蛋白相比,前列腺小体能够极大地促进精子运动活力[32]。Arienti 等的研究结果显示,即使在低 pH 环境下前列腺小体也能增加活性精子的数量[33]。精子的运动能力受到 Ca^{2+} 信号传导的调节,因此维持精子的活力需要持续的激活 Ca^{2+} 信号。但是精子是极为微小的细胞,其内部细胞器很少,既不产生也不含有 Ca^{2+} 信号传导的相关蛋白。Park 等于 2011 年发现了前列腺小体能够促进精子活力,尽管存在一定争议,但 Park 依然认为前列腺小体能够向精子转移一系列的 Ca^{2+} 信号传导工具来帮助精子获取 Ca^{2+} 信号传导[34]。同时,Park 提出这种 Ca^{2+} 信号传导的获取是维持精子持续运动和雄性生育能力所必需的。

(二) 前列腺小体的免疫抑制活性

女性生殖道具有较为均衡的免疫系统屏障,精子作为外来物会被识别为入侵女性生殖道的病原体而受到攻击。事实上,研究发现巨噬细胞、嗜中性粒细胞和 NK 细胞都会攻击精细胞[35]。因此,精子需要逃避女性免疫系统的攻击以维持生存。多项研究结果表明,前列腺小体具有多种免疫调节能力[36-39]。Skibinsiki 等发现,前列腺小体能够结合中性粒细胞并直接抑制其吞噬能力[36]。根据 Tarazona 等的研究,前列腺小体高水平表达激活受体 CD244 的配体——CD48。进一步研究发现,前列腺小体与 NK 细胞的相互作用导致 CD244 的表达减少,从而抑制 NK 细胞的激活[37]。上述研究结果表明,人前列腺小体能够在女性生殖道中调节嗜中性粒细胞和 NK 细胞的功能。此外,前列腺小体还被发现能够干扰补体系统[38,39]。其含有的 CD46 和 CD59 是补体系统中膜攻击复合物的抑制剂,前列腺小体能够将 CD46 和 CD59 转移至精子,从而干扰补体系统对精子的免疫攻击[38,39]。

(三) 前列腺小体的抗氧化能力

活性氧(reactive oxygen species,ROS)是特发性男性不育症的主要原因之一,ROS 对精子的攻击性极强,能够破坏其细胞膜和 DNA。在 40% 不育男性的精液样本中,ROS 的含量出现非正常升高。但是在正常可育精子的样本中并未发现 ROS[40]。尽管精液中 ROS 的起源仍然存在争议,但主流观点认为精液中的 ROS 主要由细胞渗透而来[41]。Saez 等的研究发现前列腺小体能够抑制 ROS 的产生[42]。他们提出,前列腺小体通过递送脂质到多核中性粒细胞的质膜,抑制 NADPH 氧化酶活性,从而抑制了 ROS 的产生[42]。

(四) 前列腺小体的抗菌活性

现有研究表明,前列腺小体具有类抗生素的作用。Strub 等在前列腺小体中发现了抗菌肽的存在[43]。研究发现,前列腺小体中富含神经内分泌标志物——嗜铬粒蛋白 A 和嗜铬粒蛋白 B,这些嗜铬粒蛋白的含量也异于寻常,嗜铬粒蛋白 B 的含量大大超过嗜铬粒蛋白

A[44]。嗜铬粒蛋白 B 的 C 末端片段肽具有强效的抗菌活性,该肽段形成了一种类似于天蚕素(一种昆虫蛋白质)的三维结构,从而为前列腺小体提供了抗菌活性。另外,Carlsson 等揭示了前列腺小体的抗菌活性与细菌膜变形效应有关[45]。该效应与嗜中性粒细胞的抗菌作用在机制上不尽相同。嗜中性粒细胞的抗菌作用涉及 ROS 的产生,而 ROS 对精子具有极强的破坏能力,因此不会产生 ROS 的前列腺小体比嗜中性粒细胞更适合作为精液中的抗菌成分。

(五) 前列腺小体与精子获能和顶体反应

经由雌性生殖道递送的精子虽然已经成熟,但尚未完全做好受精准备。为了获得受精的能力,精子需要进行一系列的生理修饰,即精子"获能"[46,47]。在获能过程中,精子获得了与卵母细胞透明带结合的能力,从而引起顶体反应[10]。人们对细胞内涉及精子获能的信号通路已经有较为充分的认识,但近年来研究发现,前列腺小体可能也参与了上述过程并影响精子获能。当精子接触卵母细胞后,其细胞膜的胆固醇含量降低,从而引发精子获能。但能够到达卵母细胞的精子数量极少,因此精子过早获能则不利于受精。研究发现,精浆对于精子获能具有抑制作用[48],而精浆中前列腺小体中富含胆固醇,因此前列腺小体对精子获能的抑制作用尤为突出[49]。另一方面,也有研究认为,前列腺小体可以支持顶体反应。正常情况下,卵丘细胞分泌的孕酮是激活顶体反应的主要因素之一[50]。Palmerini 等的研究发现,前列腺小体和精子融合能够使精子对孕酮的作用更加敏感,从而加速顶体反应[51]。此外,Park 等还发现,前列腺小体能够将孕激素受体递送给精子,从而加速顶体反应[34]。

综上所述,前列腺小体与精子的相互作用较为复杂,但又不可或缺。在正常的生理过程中,对精子的正常受精起着重要作用(表 5-1)。

表 5-1 人前列腺小体在促进受精中的作用

功 能	机 制	参考文献
增加精子活力	Ca^{2+} 能够调节精子活力。前列腺小体通过递送 Ca^{2+} 调控信号影响精子活力	[32-34]
免疫抑制	女性生殖道的免疫系统将精子识别为入侵的病原体。而前列腺小体具备多种免疫调节能力,如调节中性粒细胞和 NK 细胞的活性,同时还能够干扰补体系统,从而帮助精子逃避免疫杀伤	[36-39]
抗氧化能力	ROS 是特发性男性不育的主要原因之一。前列腺小体通过向多核中性粒细胞的质膜递送脂质信号,从而减少 ROS 的产生	[42]
抗菌能力	前列腺小体中含有嗜铬粒蛋白 B 的 C 段片段结构,从而形成了类似抗菌蛋白的结构。同时前列腺小体还能够使细菌膜变形,从而发挥抗菌活性	[43-45]
抑制精子获能	前列腺小体通过递送胆固醇阻止精子提前获能	[48,49]
支持顶体反应	卵丘细胞分泌的孕酮是激活顶体反应的主要因素。前列腺小体能够将孕酮的受体蛋白递送至精子,同时增加精子对孕酮的敏感性	[50]

四、前列腺肿瘤来源的前列腺小体

在相当长的一段时间内,EV 被认为是细胞排泄代谢废弃物的工具。直到 2007 年,Valadi 等检测到了 EV 内部携带的 miRNA 和 mRNA,并进一步发现这些 RNA 能够被 EV 递送到受体细胞并发挥潜在的功能。该发现在 2010 年被三项独立进行的研究同时证实,即 EV 中的 miRNA 可以转移到受体细胞中,并进一步发挥调节功能[5,43]。随后,EV 在肿瘤研究领域尤其受到关注,许多研究表明,EV 能够将蛋白质、核酸等细胞内成分从一种细胞转移到另外一种细胞,并影响肿瘤的进展。而近期研究发现,减少肿瘤细胞分泌 EV 的转移,可能成为减少肿瘤扩散和传播概率的新治疗策略[52]。EV 内同时携带各种蛋白质、核酸和脂质,其存在于多种体液如血液、唾液、尿液和精液中,能够反映包括肿瘤在内的多种疾病的动态变化。通过研究 EV,研究人员能够轻松获取有关疾病状况的分子信息[53]。因此,EV 作为临床生物标志物具有巨大的应用潜力。在本节中,作者讲述了前列腺癌来源的前列腺小体在加速肿瘤进展方面的作用,并对前列腺小体靶向疗法的临床应用进行了讨论。同时,还总结了前列腺小体作为肿瘤生物标志物的有效性(图 5-2)。

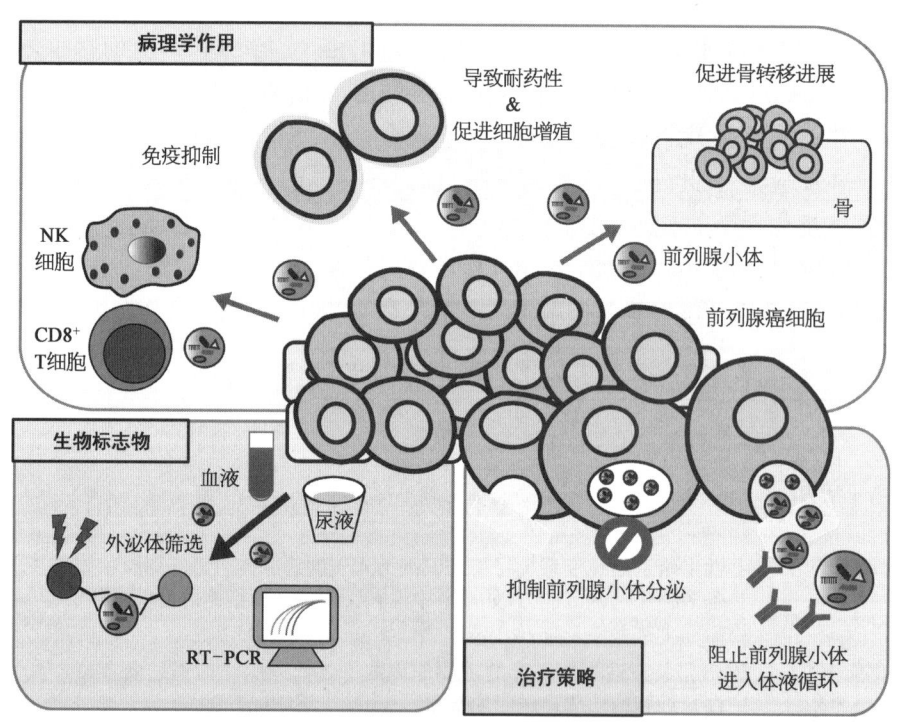

扫描二维码查看彩图

图 5-2 前列腺肿瘤分泌的前列腺小体在病理过程中的作用以及临床应用。前列腺小体能够通过递送生物信号,促进肿瘤的进展。肿瘤来源的前列腺小体可能通过抑制免疫细胞的功能,从而帮助建立肿瘤微环境中的免疫抑制。前列腺肿瘤分泌的前列腺小体能够影响周围的前列腺肿瘤细胞,从而促进其增殖或增加其耐药性。另外,前列腺小体还可以影响骨微环境并促进前列腺癌的骨转移。同时,前列腺小体还具备成为肿瘤生物标志物的潜力。肿瘤不同阶段分泌的前列腺小体能够反映肿瘤自身的状态,并且随着肿瘤的进展而持续反映。因此,抑制前列腺小体介导的细胞间通信,有望成为一种全新的治疗前列腺癌的方法

五、前列腺小体的病理学功能

越来越多的研究发现,EV 在肿瘤的各个阶段都发挥着至关重要的作用。Kosaka 等发现,正常的前列腺上皮细胞能够通过分泌 EV,从而拮抗前列腺肿瘤细胞[54]。进一步研究发现,正常前列腺细胞来源的前列腺小体中含有肿瘤抑制 miRNA。在体内外实验中,其内部的 miR-132 均能够有效阻止前列腺肿瘤细胞的进展[54]。因此他们认为在肿瘤的早期阶段,正常组织细胞能够活跃地分泌富含肿瘤抑制 miRNA 的前列腺小体,从而阻止肿瘤细胞生长,维持健康组织的正常形态。更多的研究发现,在多种肿瘤进展过程中,其分泌的 EV 能够通过多种途径调节肿瘤微环境,以促进肿瘤自身的增殖和扩散。如塑造肿瘤转移前微环境[55]、诱导血管生成[56]、激活肿瘤相关成纤维细胞[57]、破坏血脑屏障[58] 或腹膜[59],以及诱导肿瘤细胞耐药[60] 等。此外,Ono 等发现肿瘤周围骨髓 MSC 来源的 EV 能够有效地帮助乳腺肿瘤细胞进入休眠状态并导致其远期复发[61]。

在美国,前列腺肿瘤是最常见的男性肿瘤,也是第三大肿瘤死亡原因[62]。尽管早期发现并切除的患者 10 年生存率高于 98%,但一旦肿瘤转移,患者的 5 年生存率显著下降至约 30%[62]。雄激素剥夺疗法是转移性前列腺癌的主要治疗手段,尽管早期效果较好,但绝大多数接受雄激素剥夺疗法的转移性前列腺癌患者都会进展为化学去势抵抗型前列腺癌(castration-resistant prostate cancer,CRPC),并在数年内死于肿瘤。目前,前列腺癌进展的机制尚不完全清楚,因此需要进一步的研究来提高患者的生存率。现有报道表明,前列腺癌来源的前列腺小体能够通过调节肿瘤微环境加重肿瘤恶性程度[63-65]。Hosseini-Beheshti 等的研究发现,前列腺肿瘤细胞分泌的前列腺小体能够促进周围前列腺肿瘤细胞的增殖和迁移,从而加速前列腺癌进展[63]。Lundholm 等发现了前列腺小体通过影响 NK 细胞和 $CD8^+$ T 细胞(两种肿瘤免疫中最重要的免疫细胞)导致免疫抑制。前列腺小体在体外还能够选择性地诱导 NK 细胞和 $CD8^+$ T 细胞中 NKG2D 的表达下调。相应地,他们还发现 CRPC 患者血液中的循环 EV 选择性下调了 NKG2D 的表达水平。该研究提示了前列腺小体通过损害淋巴细胞的细胞毒性作用帮助肿瘤细胞实现免疫逃避[64]。多西紫杉醇在临床上常用于治疗 CRPC 患者并能够有效地提高生存率,但该治疗方案同时面临难以避免的肿瘤复发。Corcoran 等的研究发现,前列腺小体在导致前列腺癌的抗药性中起着重要的作用[65]。他们发现由对多西他赛耐药的前列腺肿瘤细胞分泌的前列腺小体,能够将耐药性传递至新产生的前列腺肿瘤细胞,这可能是由前列腺小体将 MDR-1/P-gp 传递至靶细胞所致[65]。

骨转移是晚期前列腺癌的主要转移部位,并且是前列腺癌患者死亡的主要原因[66]。在前列腺癌骨转移病例中,肿瘤细胞与包括 OB、OC 和 MSC 等各种细胞相互作用。前列腺肿瘤细胞常常诱导 OB 型骨转移,较多学者围绕该机制进行了研究。Ito 等首先发现了前列腺肿瘤细胞与 OB 间通过前列腺小体进行细胞间通信。他们发现,激素抵抗型的前列腺肿瘤细胞分泌的前列腺小体中含有 Ets-1 蛋白,而这种蛋白能够促进鼠的 OB 分化[67]。Ye 等在体外实验中发现,前列腺小体中的 miR-141-3p 能够通过靶向 DLC1,促进 OB 增殖和 OPG/RANKL 的表达。在这项研究中,他们发现前列腺肿瘤细胞分泌的前列腺小体能够在内体促进成骨[68]。近年来，Hashimoto 等在前人的基础上，发现前列腺肿瘤细胞分泌的前列腺小体中携带的 miR-940 能够影响 MSC 中 ARHGAP1 和 FAM134A 的表达水平，并诱导 MSC 成骨分化。在体内实验中，他们还发现前列腺小体携带的 miR-190 能够诱导 OB 型骨转移[69]。进一步地，Karlsson 等发现鼠前列腺肿瘤细胞分泌前列腺小体中的 TRAMPC-1 能够减少鼠前体 OC 向成熟多核 OC 的分化，从而促进 OB 的骨转移[70]。尽管前列腺癌进展的机制非常复杂，目前的理论尚难以完全阐释，但上述研究表明了 EV 在前列腺癌的过程中发挥了决定性作用(表 5-2)。

表 5-2 前列腺小体在前列腺癌中的作用

分泌细胞	受体细胞	EV 内容物	功　能	参考文献
前列腺上皮细胞(PNT2)	前列腺肿瘤细胞(PC3M)	miR-143	抑制细胞增殖	[54]
前列腺肿瘤细胞(DU145)	前列腺肿瘤细胞(LNCAP)/前列腺上皮细胞(RWPE-1)	未知	减少细胞凋亡，促进细胞增殖和迁移	[63]
前列腺肿瘤细胞(22RV1)	NK 细胞/CD8+ 细胞(PBMCs 分化而来)	未知	下调 NKG2D 表达，促进免疫抑制	[64]
前列腺肿瘤细胞(22RV1)	多西他赛敏感的前列腺肿瘤细胞(DU145,22RV1)	MDR-1/P-gp	增加多西他赛耐药性	[65]
前列腺肿瘤细胞(PC3,DU145)	小鼠胚胎 OB 前体细胞(MC3T3-E1)	Ets-1	诱导细胞分化	[67]
前列腺肿瘤细胞(MDA PCA 2B)	OB(HFOB1.19)	miR-141-3p	激活 P38-MAPK 通路，调节肿瘤骨转移的微环境	[68]
前列腺肿瘤细胞(C4,C4-2,C4-2B)	MSC(永生化人 MSC 系)	miR-940	下调 ARHGAP1 和 FAM134A，促进成骨分化	[69]
小鼠前列腺肿瘤细胞(Tramp-C1)	小鼠单核巨噬细胞白血病细胞(RAW264.7,小鼠原代骨髓细胞)	未知	减少细胞融合及分化	[70]

六、前列腺小体的临床应用：前列腺癌的生物治疗

正如本文前述，前列腺细胞来源的前列腺小体表型随其细胞微环境的改变而不尽相同，从而在细胞生长或肿瘤转移等方面发挥不同的作用。近年来，研究人员聚焦于前列腺小体的这些特性，并努力将其应用到肿瘤治疗的临床应用中。以肿瘤诊治为例，前列腺小体内的 microRNA 和蛋白质等多种分子能够反映肿瘤进展和机体的实时状态。本节主要阐释前列腺小体在前列腺癌诊断和治疗中的临床应用现状。

（一）前列腺小体靶向治疗前列腺肿瘤的诊疗策略

EV 通过传递信号分子介导了细胞间通信，并在肿瘤的进展中发挥了重要作用[53]。因此，减少肿瘤细胞分泌的 EV 可能在阻滞肿瘤细胞增殖和扩散等方面存在一定临床治疗价

值。相应地,科研人员提出三种潜在的 EV 肿瘤治疗策略:抑制 EV 分泌、阻止 EV 循环和减少 EV 吸收[52]。本章作者对上述策略中的两种进行了研究并认为其具备临床治疗的潜力。首先,Nishida-Aoki 等发现了一种针对肿瘤来源的 EV 进行抗体治疗的新策略。在人乳腺癌的动物模型中,给予了抗 CD9 和 CD63(两种 EV 表面富集蛋白)药物治疗后,研究人员发现尽管肿瘤本身的生长并未受到明显影响,但其转移及扩散概率大大降低[71]。在另一项研究中,Kosaka 等探索了在体内外抑制 EV 产生的可能性和有效性。在乳腺癌的异种移植模型中,研究人员通过抑制体内 nSMase2 减少神经酰胺合成,进一步减少了 EV 的分泌。其递送的 miR-210-3p 也随之减少,肿瘤血管的新生和转移能力也随之降低[56]。但是,由于 DC9 和 CD63 普遍存在于各种 EV,抗 CD9 和抗 CD63 药物无法有选择地针对肿瘤细胞来源的 EV。另外,nSMase2 在正常神经细胞中也有表达[72],而下调 nSMase2 并不能抑制前列腺癌中 EV 的分泌[73]。因此,识别肿瘤特异性的 EV 便显得尤为重要。就前列腺肿瘤而言,鉴别前列腺小体中的肿瘤特异性分子标志物并将其提取是开展有效治疗的前提。2017 年,Datta 等通过筛选两个药物目录文库,检测了各种化学药物对前列腺小体分泌的影响[74]。研究人员使用多种药物干预了携带 CD63-GFP 信号的前列腺小体后,通过定量高通量方法对其进行靶向筛选和检测。他们发现手霉素 A,一种天然的微生物代谢产物,能够特异性抑制前列腺肿瘤来源前列腺小体的合成和分泌,同时对正常前列腺小体没有抑制作用[74]。该研究组还同时发现了其他几种有效的前列腺小体分泌抑制剂和促进剂[75]。上述研究结果为前列腺肿瘤来源前列腺小体的生物靶向治疗应用带来了巨大潜力。

与此同时,研究人员还发现了 EV 的生物学异质性。在 2016 年,Kowal 等发现不同的 EV 组成部分具有不同的 EV 蛋白标志物[29]。次年,Tkach 等又发现不同的 EV 亚群对受体细胞能够产生不同的影响[30]。因此,寻找最易致癌的 EV 亚群是最佳的靶向 EV 进行肿瘤治疗的良好策略。包括前列腺小体在内,EV 的生物起源极为复杂,在进行临床应用前,还需开展进一步的探索性研究。但是 EV 研究领域的巨大进步使人们有望克服 EV 用于肿瘤临床治疗的种种挑战。

(二)前列腺小体相关的前列腺肿瘤生物标志物

目前,前列腺肿瘤的主要诊断标准基于前列腺活检的组织病理学检查,而进行前列腺活检的指征则主要依靠血清 PSA 和直肠指检(digital rectal examination,DRE)。但是,前列腺良性疾病如前列腺炎和前列腺良性增生(benign hyperplasia,BPH)也会导致血清 PSA 改变,因此血清 PSA 难以分辨前列腺疾病的良恶性。而 DRE 检查的准确性又取决于检查者的临床经验[76]。因此,临床上尚缺乏更加特异性的前列腺肿瘤生物标志物。同时,前列腺肿瘤的异质性很大,相应地,其恶性程度也分较多级别[77]。因此,理想的前列腺肿瘤生物标志物不仅能够反映疾病的良恶性,还应该能够预测其恶性程度和日后转移的风险。

根据前列腺小体所反映的前列腺肿瘤情况的特性,其具备成为新型前列腺肿瘤生物标志物的潜力。然而,体液中存在多种不同来源的 EV,因此单独检测前列腺小体还存在一定难度。与此同时,不同的 EV 组合还有可能反映其他不同的疾病,因此在本节中使用 EV 来指代包括前列腺小体在内的所有类型囊泡[9],以给读者全面介绍 EV 作为前列腺肿瘤生物标志物的潜力。

考虑到前列腺的解剖学位置及临床取样的便捷性,尿液是检测前列腺肿瘤的理想基质。Nilsson 等首先从前列腺肿瘤患者尿液分离得到的 EV 中检测到两种已知的前列腺肿瘤标志物:PCA-3 和 TMPRSS2:ERG,证实了尿液 EV 诊断和监测前列腺癌的潜力[78]。Dijkstra 等则发现,DRE 能够增加从尿液检出 EV 生物标志物的准确性。他们发现前列腺按摩后收集的尿液 EV 中,PCA-3 和 TMPRESS2:ERG 的表达水平明显升高,因而建议在行 DRE 之后立刻收集尿液[79]。随后的多项研究也论证了尿液 EV 作为诊断性生物标志物的有效性[80-84]。基于以上理论,McKiernan 等近期开发了一种无创尿液外泌体基因表达测定方法,即 ExoDx 前列腺智能评分尿液外泌体测定法。该方法检测并分析尿液样本中的三种 EV 特征基因(PCA3、ERG 和 SPDEF)并进行对比,随后构建患者的前列腺智能评分。在减少不必要的活检的前提下,该方法不仅能够分辨样本来源的良恶性,还能够区分高度恶性前列腺癌(Gleason 评分≥7 分)和低恶性前列腺癌(Gleason 评分≤6 分)[85]。

血浆也是较为理想的前列腺肿瘤检测基质,研究已经发现血浆的 EV 含有前列腺肿瘤的标志性蛋白。研究人员在前列腺癌患者血浆分离出的 EV 中检测到 PTEN,其表达的减少通常提示前列腺癌进展和转移风险增高,而 PTEN 在正常组织或体液来源的 EV 中并不表达[86]。在另一项研究中,前列腺癌患者血浆 EV 中抗凋亡蛋白 survivin 与 BPH 或健康对照相比也显著增加[87]。随后,Tavoosidana 等开发了"邻位连接"分析,用于检测血浆中的 EV。该方法同时靶向检测一种 EV 表面的多种蛋白质,具有较高的灵敏度和特异性。该方法简述为在 EV 与 CD13 单克隆抗体结合后,用 DNA 偶联抗体探测四种同时表达的 EV 蛋白标志物,并产生可扩增的报告基因。该方法显示,前列腺癌患者,尤其是高度恶性患者(Gleason 评分≥7 分)血浆中的标志性 EV 显著多于健康人和低恶性前列腺癌患者(Gleason 评分≤6 分)[88]。

血清及血浆中的 miRNA 具备前列腺癌的诊断或判断预后的潜力。研究发现并证实,前列腺肿瘤患者血清样品中 miR-141 和 miR-375 的表达水平升高[89-91],这些 miRNA 在前列腺癌患者的血清 EV 中同样也上调。因此,研究人员提出可将其作为诊断前列腺癌的生物标志物[89,92]。在另一项研究中,Bhagirath 等发现血清 EV 中的 miR-1246 可预测前列腺癌的侵袭能力。miR-1246 是一种能够抑制前列腺癌肿瘤的 miRNA,这种 miRNA 通过血清中的 EV 携带并释放,因而其在 EV 中有较高表达水平,但在前列腺肿瘤细胞中的表达水平较低[93]。此外,Huang 等通过 RNA 序列分析发现,血清 EV 中的 miR-375 和 miR-1290 与 CRPC 患者的不良预后显著相关。因此,他们认为这些 miRNA 可以作为潜在的转移性前列腺癌患者的预后生物标志物[94]。

表 5-3 体液中 EV 作为前列腺生物标志物的潜力

用 途	标 志 物	来源	分离方法	分析方法	参考文献
肿瘤诊断	PCA-3 和 TMPRSS2:ERG	尿液	超速离心	RT-PCR	[78,79]
肿瘤诊断	lncRNA-21p	尿液	尿液外泌体 RNA 分离试剂盒	RT-PCR	[80]

续　表

用　途	标　志　物	来源	分离方法	分析方法	参考文献
肿瘤诊断	ERG 和 PCA3（EXO106 score）	尿液	尿液外泌体临床样本浓缩试剂盒	RT-PCR	[81]
肿瘤诊断	PSA、CD9 和 CD63	尿液	超速离心	TR-FIA（时间分辨荧光免疫分析法）	[82]
肿瘤诊断	let-7c、miR-21 和 miR-375	尿液	超速离心	RT-PCR	[83]
肿瘤诊断	miR-196a-5p 和 miR-501-3p	尿液	超速离心	RNA 测序，RT-PCR	[84]
肿瘤诊断	PCA3、ERG 和 SPDEF（ExoDx Prostate IntelliScore）	尿液	EXOPRO 尿液临床样本浓缩试剂盒，超速离心	RT-PCR	[85]
肿瘤诊断	PTEN	血浆	超速离心	Westernblot	[86]
肿瘤诊断	survivin	血浆	超速离心	ELISA，Westernblot	[87]
肿瘤诊断	CD13、mAb78、mAb8H10 和人凝血因子Ⅲ/人体组织	血浆	超速离心，凝胶层析	邻位连接分析	[88]
肿瘤诊断	miR-141，miR-375	血清	ExoMiR	RT-PCR	[89]
肿瘤诊断	miR-141	血清	ExoQuick	RT-PCR	[92]
肿瘤诊断	miR-1246	血清	总外泌体分离试剂，血浆/血清外泌体纯化试剂盒	RT-PCR	[93]
预后判断	miR-1290，miR-375	血浆	ExoQuick	RNA 测序，RT-PCR	[94]
肿瘤诊断及预后判断	CD9	血浆	超速离心	TR-FIA	[95,96]
预后判断	AR-V7	血浆	exoRNeasy 试剂盒	RT-PCR	[99]

尽管 CD9 一直作为经典的 EV 标志物存在，但是有研究发现，EV 中的 CD9 也具备诊断和预测前列腺癌预后的潜力。Soekmadji 等发现，与 BPH 患者相比，前列腺癌患者血浆中 CD9 阳性的 EV 明显增多[95]。在他的另一项研究中发现，前列腺癌患者血液循环肿瘤细胞中 CD9 阳性的 EV 与对照组相比明显增多。该研究提示，CD9 阳性 EV 的数量也可能是晚期前列腺癌的诊断指标之一[96]。

自 2014 年以来，随着恩杂鲁胺和乙酸阿比特龙酯等新药的问世，CRPC 的治疗策略发生了巨大变化。尽管这些药物带来了 CRPC 治疗的突破，但不幸的是，20%~40%的患者对这些药物无反应[97]。AR-V7 是雄激素受体的 V7 剪接变体，由除去配体结合结构域后由剩下的活性 N 端组成[98]。临床治疗发现，AR-V7 的表达通常意味着前列腺癌向 CRPC 转变，并且产生了恩杂鲁胺和乙酸阿比特龙酯耐药性。在此基础上，Del 等揭示了血浆 EV 中 AR-V7 核酸作为预测 CRPC 患者产生激素治疗耐药性的生物标志物的潜在可能[99]。

如前文所述，EV 在作为前列腺癌生物标志物方面具有极大的发展潜力（表 5-3）。而逐渐简单易行的 EV 提取和检测方法使其临床应用逐渐成为可能。Yoshioka 等发明了一种名为"ExoScreen"的全新 EV 检测方法[100]。该方法能够靶向检测 EV 的膜蛋白，通过使用光敏剂珠及两种 EV 表面抗原，进行邻近荧光扩增均相测定，能够检测培养基或者血清中的循环 EV。该方法只需要少量样品（最低 5 μL）且不需要任何纯化步骤，并能够进行高通量分析。在他们的研究中，血浆来源的 EV 比传统的肿瘤标志物——如癌胚抗原（carcinoembryonic antigen，CEA）和糖类抗原 19-9（carbohydrate antigen 19-9，CA19-9）——能够更加有效地用于诊断结肠癌。类似的膜蛋白靶向筛选方法使得通过高通量检测 EV 成为更加便捷有效的选项。

与膜蛋白检测相比，捕获或提纯 EV 的内部物质仍然是非常规的方法。EV 由双层脂质膜构成，可以保护其内容物不被降解。尽管人类体液中 RNA 酶的含量很高，但是 EV 的膜结构仍然能够有效保护其内部的 RNA 稳定存在。在使用 EV 作为生物标志物时，这种保护带来极大的优势，如稳定性、可存储性和可重复性。而现有的核酸检测技术，如定量逆转录聚合酶链反应（quantitative reverse transcription polymerase chain reaction，qRT-PCR）和微阵列 RNA 分析等，可有效且客观地评估 EV 内核酸的表达水平。基于以上优势，EV 内部携带的核酸便成为了前列腺癌生物诊断标志物的理想来源。为了更加充分地满足医学上对于 EV 内核酸的应用需要，需要研发易推广的新型高通量检测方法。在未来，肿瘤特异性蛋白分子靶向捕获 EV 可能与肿瘤特异性 miRNA 的 qRT-PCR 相结合，成为 EV 生物标志物的标准研究策略。

七、总结

在本章中，作者总结了前列腺小体在人体内的生理和病理作用。一方面，前列腺小体能够增加精子活力，诱导生殖道内的受精过程；另一方面，前列腺癌来源的前列腺小体能够加速肿瘤的进展，并可能作为生物治疗靶点而存在。此外，包括前列腺小体在内的 EV 极有可能发展成为前列腺癌的诊断和（或）预后标志物。随着对 EV 研究的深入，人们对前列腺小体特征和功能的认知也会不断加深，并为临床应用带来极大的希望和可能。

致谢

本章得到了 Practical Research for Innovative Cancer Control（17ck0106366h001）from Japan Agency for Medical Research and Development（AMED）的支持。

我们感谢 Dr. Takahiro Kimura（Department of Urology，Jikei University School of Medicine）和 Ari Miura（Boston University）对本章的批判性讨论。

利益冲突

作者声明没有利益冲突。

（吴若愚　译，郑军华　审校）

参考文献

[1] Raposo G, Stoorvogel W. Extracellular vesicles: exosomes, microvesicles, and friends. J Cell Biol 2013; 200: 373-83.
[2] Valadi H, Ekstrom K, Bossios A, et al. Exosome-mediated transfer of mRNAs and microRNAs is a novel mechanism of genetic exchange between cells. Nat Cell Biol 2007; 9: 654-9.
[3] Pegtel DM, Cosmopoulos K, Thorley-Lawson DA, et al. Functional delivery of viral miRNAs via exosomes. Proc Natl Acad Sci U S A 2010; 107: 6328-33.
[4] Kosaka N, Iguchi H, Yoshioka Y, et al. Secretory mechanisms and intercellular transfer of microRNAs in living cells. J Biol Chem 2010; 285: 17442-52.
[5] Zhang Y, Liu D, Chen X, et al. Secreted monocytic miR-150 enhances targeted endothelial cell migration. Mol Cell 2010; 39: 133-44.
[6] Yanez-Mo M, Siljander PR, Andreu Z, et al. Biological properties of extracellular vesicles and their physiological functions. J Extracell Vesicles 2015; 4: 27066.
[7] Cocucci E, Racchetti G, Meldolesi J. Shedding microvesicles: artefacts no more. Trends Cell Biol 2009; 19: 43-51.
[8] Bergsmedh A, Szeles A, Henriksson M, et al. Horizontal transfer of oncogenes by uptake of apoptotic bodies. Proc Natl Acad Sci U S A 2001; 98: 6407-11.
[9] Gould SJ, Raposo G. As we wait: coping with an imperfect nomenclature for extracellular vesicles. J Extracell Vesicles 2013; 2; . 20389.
[10] Aalberts M, Stout TA, Stoorvogel W. Prostasomes: extracellular vesicles from the prostate. Reproduction 2014; 147: R1-14.
[11] Stegmayr B, Ronquist G. Promotive effect on human sperm progressive motility by prostasomes. Urol Res 1982; 10: 253-7.
[12] Urabe F, Kosaka N, Kimura T, et al. Extracellular vesicles: toward a clinical application in urological cancer treatment. Int J Urol 2018; 25: 533-43.
[13] Ronquist G, Brody I, Gottfries A, et al. An Mg^{2+} and Ca^{2+}-stimulated adenosine triphosphatase in human prostatic fluid: part I. Andrologia 1978; 10: 261-72.
[14] Ronquist G, Brody I, Gottfries A, et al. An Mg^{2+} and Ca^{2+}-stimulated adenosine triphosphatase in human prostatic fluid-part II. Andrologia 1978; 10: 427-33.
[15] Ronquist G, Brody I. The prostasome: its secretion and function in man. Biochim Biophys Acta 1985; 822: 203-18.
[16] Ronquist GK, Larsson A, Stavreus-Evers A, et al. Prostasomes are heterogeneous regarding size and appearance but affiliated to one DNA-containing exosome family. Prostate 2012; 72: 1736-45.
[17] Brody I, Ronquist G, Gottfries A. Ultrastructural localization of the prostasome — an organelle in human seminal plasma. Ups J Med Sci 1983; 88: 63-80.
[18] Sahlen GE, Egevad L, Ahlander A, et al. Ultrastructure of the secretion of prostasomes from benign and malignant epithelial cells in the prostate. Prostate 2002; 53: 192-9.
[19] Zijlstra C, Stoorvogel W. Prostasomes as a source of diagnostic biomarkers for prostate cancer. J Clin Invest 2016; 126: 1144-51.
[20] Utleg AG, Yi EC, Xie T, et al. Proteomic analysis of human prostasomes. Prostate 2003; 56: 150-61.
[21] Poliakov A, Spilman M, Dokland T, et al. Structural heterogeneity and protein composition of exosome-kike vesicles (prostasomes) in human semen. Prostate 2009; 69: 159-67.
[22] Aalberts M, van Dissel-Emiliani FM, van Adrichem NP, et al. Identification of distinct populations of prostasomes that differentially express prostate stem cell antigen, annexin A1, and GLIPR2 in humans. Biol Reprod 2012; 86: 82.
[23] Ronquist KG, Ronquist G, Carlsson L, et al. Human prostasomes contain chromosomal DNA. Prostate 2009; 69: 737-43.
[24] Ronquist GK, Larsson A, Ronquist G, et al. Prostasomal DNA characterization and transfer into human sperm. Mol Reprod Dev 2011; 78: 467-76.
[25] Arienti G, Carlini E, Polci A, et al. Fatty acid pattern of human prostasome lipid. Arch Biochem Biophys 1998; 358: 391-5.
[26] Carlini E, Palmerini CA, Cosmi EV, et al. Fusion of sperm with prostasomes: effects on membrane fluidity. Arch Biochem Biophys 1997; 343: 6-12.
[27] Arvidson G, Ronquist G, Wikander G, et al. Human prostasome membranes exhibit very high cholesterol/phospholipid ratios yielding high molecular ordering. Biochim Biophys Acta 1989; 984: 167-73.
[28] Cross NL. Human seminal plasma prevents sperm from becoming acrosomally responsive to the agonist, progesterone: cholesterol is the major inhibitor. Biol Reprod 1996; 54: 138-45.
[29] Kowal J, Arras G, Colombo M, et al. Proteomic comparison defines novel markers to characterize heterogeneous populations of extracellular vesicle subtypes. Proc Natl Acad Sci U S A 2016; 113; E968-77.
[30] Tkach M, Kowal J, Zucchetti AE, et al. Qualitative differences in T-cell activation by dendritic cell-derived extracellular vesicle subtypes. EMBO J 2017; 36: 3012-28.
[31] Saez F, Frenette G, Sullivan R. Epididymosomes and prostasomes: their roles in posttesticular maturation of the sperm cells. J Androl 2003; 24: 149-54.
[32] Fabiani R, Johansson L, Lundkvist O, et al. Promotive effect by prostasomes on normal human spermatozoa exhibiting no forward motility due to buffer washings. Eur J Obstet Gynecol Reprod Biol 1994; 57: 181-8.
[33] Arienti G, Carlini E, Nicolucci A, et al. The motility of human spermatozoa as influenced by prostasomes at various pH levels. Biol Cell 1999; 91: 51-4.
[34] Park KH, Kim BJ, Kang J, et al. Ca^{2+} signaling tools acquired from prostasomes are required for progesterone-induced sperm motility. Sci Signal 2011; 4: ra31.
[35] Matthijs A, Engel B, Woelders H. Neutrophil recruitment and phagocytosis of boar spermatozoa after artificial

insemination of sows, and the effects of inseminate volume, sperm dose and specific additives in the extender. Reproduction 2003; 125: 357 - 67.

[36] Skibinski G, Kelly RW, Harkiss D, et al. Immunosuppression by human seminal plasma — extracellular organelles (prostasomes) modulate activity of phagocytic cells. Am J Reprod Immunol 1992; 28: 97 - 103.

[37] Tarazona R, Delgado E, Guarnizo MC, et al. Human prostasomes express CD48 and interfere with NK cell function. Immunobiology 2011; 216: 41 - 6.

[38] Rooney IA, Atkinson JP, Krul ES, et al. Physiologic relevance of the membrane attack complex inhibitory protein CD59 in human seminal plasma: CD59 is present on extracellular organelles (prostasomes), binds cell membranes, and inhibits complement-mediated lysis. J Exp Med 1993; 177: 1409 - 20.

[39] Kitamura M, Namiki M, Matsumiya K, et al. Membrane cofactor protein (CD46) in seminal plasma is a prostasome-bound form with complement regulatory activity and measles virus neutralizing activity. Immunology 1995; 84: 626 - 32.

[40] Iwasaki A, Gagnon C. Formation of reactive oxygen species in spermatozoa of infertile patients. Fertil Steril 1992; 57: 409 - 16.

[41] Ronquist G. Prostasomes are mediators of intercellular communication: from basic research to clinical implications. J Intern Med 2012; 271: 400 - 13.

[42] Saez F, Motta C, Boucher D, et al. Prostasomes inhibit the NADPH oxidase activity of human neutrophils. Mol Hum Reprod 2000; 6: 883 - 91.

[43] Strub JM, Garcia-Sablone P, Lonning K, et al. Processing of chromogranin B in bovine adrenal medulla. Identification of secretolytin, the endogenous C-terminal fragment of residues 614-626 with antibacterial activity. Eur J Biochem 1995; 229: 356 - 68.

[44] Stridsberg M, Fabiani R, Lukinius A, et al. Prostasomes are neuroendocrine-kike vesicles in human semen. Prostate 1996; 29: 287 - 95.

[45] Carlsson L, Pahlson C, Bergquist M, et al. Antibacterial activity of human prostasomes. Prostate 2000; 44: 279 - 86.

[46] Bailey JL. Factors regulating sperm capacitation. Syst Biol Reprod Med 2010; 56: 334 - 48.

[47] Fraser LR. The "switching on" of mammalian spermatozoa: molecular events involved in promotion and regulation of capacitation. Mol Reprod Dev 2010; 77: 197 - 208.

[48] Cross NL. Role of cholesterol in sperm capacitation. Biol Reprod 1998; 59: 7 - 11.

[49] Pons-Rejraji H, Artonne C, Sion B, et al. Prostasomes: inhibitors of capacitation and modulators of cellular signalling in human sperm. Int J Androl 2011; 34: 568 - 80.

[50] Osman RA, Andria ML, Jones AD, et al. Steroid induced exocytosis: the human sperm acrosome reaction. Biochem Biophys Res Commun 1989; 160: 828 - 33.

[51] Palmerini CA, Saccardi C, Carlini E, et al. Fusion of prostasomes to human spermatozoa stimulates the acrosome reaction. Fertil Steril 2003; 80: 1181 - 4.

[52] Kosaka N, Yoshioka Y, Fujita Y, et al. Versatile roles of extracellular vesicles in cancer. J Clin Invest 2016; 126: 1163 - 72.

[53] Urabe F, Kosaka N, Yoshioka Y, et al. The small vesicular culprits: the investigation of extracellular vesicles as new targets for cancer treatment. Clin Transl Med 2017; 6: 45.

[54] Kosaka N, Iguchi H, Yoshioka Y, et al. Competitive interactions of cancer cells and normal cells via secretory microRNAs. J Biol Chem 2012; 287: 1397 - 405.

[55] Peinado H, Aleckovic M, Lavotshkin S, et al. Melanoma exosomes educate bone marrow progenitor cells toward a pro-metastatic phenotype through MET. Nat Med 2012; 18: 883 - 91.

[56] Kosaka N, Iguchi H, Hagiwara K, et al. Neutral sphingomyelinase 2 (nSMase2)-dependent exosomal transfer of angiogenic microRNAs regulate cancer cell metastasis. J Biol Chem 2013; 288: 10849 - 59.

[57] Pang W, Su J, Wang Y, et al. Pancreatic cancer-secreted miR-155 implicates in the conversion from normal fibroblasts to cancer-associated fibroblasts. Cancer Sci 2015; 106: 1362 - 9.

[58] Tominaga N, Kosaka N, Ono M, et al. Brain metastatic cancer cells release microRNA-181ccontaining extracellular vesicles capable of destructing blood-brain barrier. Nat Commun 2015; 6: 6716.

[59] Yokoi A, Yoshioka Y, Yamamoto Y, et al. Malignant extracellular vesicles carrying MMP1 mRNA facilitate peritoneal dissemination in ovarian cancer. Nat Commun 2017; 8: 14470.

[60] Wei F, Ma C, Zhou T, et al. Exosomes derived from gemcitabine-resistant cells transfer malignant phenotypic traits via delivery of miRNA-222-3p. Mol Cancer 2017; 16: 132.

[61] Ono M, Kosaka N, Tominaga N, et al. Exosomes from bone marrow mesenchymal stem cells contain a microRNA that promotes dormancy in metastatic breast cancer cells. Sci Signal 2014; 7: ra63.

[62] Siegel RL, Miller KD, Jemal A. Cancer Statistics, 2017. CA Cancer J Clin 2017; 67: 7 - 30.

[63] Hosseini-Beheshti E, Choi W, Weiswald LB, et al. Exosomes confer pro-survival signals to alter the phenotype of prostate cells in their surrounding environment. Oncotarget 2016; 7: 14639 - 58.

[64] Lundholm M, Schroder M, Nagaeva O, et al. Prostate tumor-derived exosomes down-regulate NKG2D expression on natural killer cells and CD8+ T cells: mechanism of immune evasion. PLoS One 2014; 9: e108925.

[65] Corcoran C, Rani S, O'Brien K, et al. Docetaxel-resistance in prostate cancer: evaluating associated phenotypic changes and potential for resistance transfer via exosomes. PLoS One 2012; 7: e50999.

[66] Ottewell PD, Wang N, Meek J, et al. Castration-induced bone loss triggers growth of disseminated prostate cancer cells in bone. Endocr Relat Cancer 2014; 21: 769 - 81.

[67] Itoh T, Ito Y, Ohtsuki Y, et al. Microvesicles released from hormone-refractory prostate cancer cells facilitate mouse pre-osteoblast differentiation. J Mol Histol 2012; 43: 509 - 15.

[68] Ye Y, Li SL, Ma YY, et al. Exosomal miR-141-3p regulates osteoblast activity to promote the osteoblastic metastasis of prostate cancer. Oncotarget 2017; 8: 94834 - 49.

[69] Hashimoto K, Ochi H, Sunamura S, et al. Cancer-secreted hsa-miR-940 induces an osteoblastic phenotype in the bone

metastatic microenvironment via targeting ARHGAP1 and FAM134A. Proc Natl Acad Sci U S A 2018; 115: 2204-9.
[70] Karlsson T, Lundholm M, Widmark A, et al. Tumor cell-derived exosomes from the prostate cancer cell line TRAMP-C1 impair osteoclast formation and differentiation. PLoS One 2016; 11: e0166284.
[71] Nishida-Aoki N, Tominaga N, Takeshita F, et al. Disruption of circulating extracellular vesicles as a novel therapeutic strategy against cancer metastasis. Mol Ther 2017; 25: 181-91.
[72] Yuyama K, Sun H, Mitsutake S, et al. Sphingolipid-modulated exosome secretion promotes clearance of amyloid-beta by microglia. J Biol Chem 2012; 287: 10977-89.
[73] Phuyal S, Hessvik NP, Skotland T, et al. Regulation of exosome release by glycosphingolipids and flotillins. FEBS J 2014; 281: 2214-27.
[74] Datta A, Kim H, Lal M, et al. Manumycin A suppresses exosome biogenesis and secretion via targeted inhibition of Ras/Raf/ERK1/2 signaling and hnRNP H1 in castration-resistant prostate cancer cells. Cancer Lett 2017; 408: 73-81.
[75] Datta A, Kim H, McGee L, et al. High-throughput screening identified selective inhibitors of exosome biogenesis and secretion: a drug repurposing strategy for advanced cancer. Sci Rep 2018; 8: 8161.
[76] Varenhorst E, Berglund K, Lofman O, et al. Inter-observer variation in assessment of the prostate by digital rectal examination. Br J Urol 1993; 72: 173-6.
[77] Boyd LK, Mao X, Lu YJ. The complexity of prostate cancer: genomic alterations and heterogeneity. Nat Rev Urol 2012; 9: 652-64.
[78] Nilsson J, Skog J, Nordstrand A, et al. Prostate cancer-derived urine exosomes: a novel approach to biomarkers for prostate cancer. Br J Cancer 2009; 100: 1603-7.
[79] Dijkstra S, Birker IL, Smit FP, et al. Prostate cancer biomarker profiles in urinary sediments and exosomes. J Urol 2014; 191: 1132-8.
[80] Isin M, Uysaler E, Ozgur E, et al. Exosomal lncRNA-p21 levels may help to distinguish prostate cancer from benign disease. Front Genet 2015; 6: 168.
[81] Donovan MJ, Noerholm M, Bentink S, et al. A molecular signature of PCA3 and ERG exosomal RNA from non-DRE urine is predictive of initial prostate biopsy result. Prostate Cancer Prostatic Dis 2015; 18: 370-5.
[82] Duijvesz D, Versluis CY, van der Fels CA, et al. Immuno-based detection of extracellular vesicles in urine as diagnostic marker for prostate cancer. Int J Cancer 2015; 137: 2869-78.
[83] Foj L, Ferrer F, Serra M, et al. Exosomal and non-exosomal urinary miRNAs in prostate cancer detection and prognosis. Prostate 2017; 77: 573-83.
[84] Rodriguez M, Bajo-Santos C, Hessvik NP, et al. Identification of non-invasive miRNAs biomarkers for prostate cancer by deep sequencing analysis of urinary exosomes. Mol Cancer 2017; 16: 156.
[85] McKiernan J, Donovan MJ, O'Neill V, et al. A novel urine exosome gene expression assay to predict high-grade prostate cancer at initial biopsy. JAMA Oncol 2016; 2: 882-9.
[86] Gabriel K, Ingram A, Austin R, et al. Regulation of the tumor suppressor PTEN through exosomes: a diagnostic potential for prostate cancer. PLoS One 2013; 8: e70047.
[87] Khan S, Jutzy JM, Valenzuela MM, et al. Plasma-derived exosomal survivin, a plausible biomarker for early detection of prostate cancer. PLoS One 2012; 7: e46737.
[88] Tavoosidana G, Ronquist G, Darmanis S, et al. Multiple recognition assay reveals prostasomes as promising plasma biomarkers for prostate cancer. Proc Natl Acad Sci U S A 2011; 108: 8809-14.
[89] Bryant RJ, Pawlowski T, Catto JW, et al. Changes in circulating microRNA levels associated with prostate cancer. Br J Cancer 2012; 106: 768-74.
[90] Yaman Agaoglu F, Kovancilar M, Dizdar Y, et al. Investigation of miR-21, miR-141, and miR-221 in blood circulation of patients with prostate cancer. Tumour Biol 2011; 32: 583-8.
[91] Haldrup C, Kosaka N, Ochiya T, et al. Profiling of circulating microRNAs for prostate cancer biomarker discovery. Drug Deliv Transl Res 2014; 4: 19-30.
[92] Li Z, Ma YY, Wang J, et al. Exosomal microRNA-141 is upregulated in the serum of prostate cancer patients. Onco Targets Ther 2016; 9: 139-48.
[93] Bhagirath D, Yang TL, Bucay N, et al. microRNA-1246 is an exosomal biomarker for aggressive prostate cancer. Cancer Res 2018; 78: 1833-44.
[94] Huang X, Yuan T, Liang M, et al. Exosomal miR-1290 and miR-375 as prognostic markers in castration-resistant prostate cancer. Eur Urol 2015; 67: 33-41.
[95] Soekmadji C, Riches JD, Russell PJ, et al. Modulation of paracrine signaling by CD9 positive small extracellular vesicles mediates cellular growth of androgen deprived prostate cancer. Oncotarget 2017; 8: 52237-55.
[96] Soekmadji C, Corcoran NM, Oleinikova I, et al. Extracellular vesicles for personalized therapy decision support in advanced metastatic cancers and its potential impact for prostate cancer. Prostate 2017; 77: 1416-23.
[97] Antonarakis ES, Lu C, Wang H, et al. AR-V7 and resistance to enzalutamide and abiraterone in prostate cancer. N Engl J Med 2014; 371: 1028-38.
[98] Chan SC, Dehm SM. Constitutive activity of the androgen receptor. Adv Pharmacol 2014; 70: 327-66.
[99] Del Re M, Biasco E, Crucitta S, et al. The detection of androgen receptor splice variant 7 in plasma-derived exosomal RNA strongly predicts resistance to hormonal therapy in metastatic prostate cancer patients. Eur Urol 2017; 71: 680-7.
[100] Yoshioka Y, Kosaka N, Konishi Y, et al. Ultra-sensitive liquid biopsy of circulating extracellular vesicles using ExoScreen. Nat Commun 2014; 5: 3591.

第6章

外泌体在细菌感染中的作用和治疗应用

The function and therapeutic use of exosomes in bacterial infections

Yong Cheng, Jeffery S. Schorey

Department of Biological Sciences, Eck Institute for Global Health, Center for Rare and Neglected Diseases, University of Notre Dame, Notre Dame, IN, United States

一、概述

众所周知,细菌性病原体释放的毒力因子以宿主细胞或先天和特异性免疫反应组件为攻击目标。不同菌种,甚至同一菌种的不同菌株,其作用靶点不同,一般都能限制或抑制免疫反应的激活。阻断补体激活的蛋白质(如金黄色葡萄球菌的 SCIN-B)[1]或灭活趋化因子(如金黄色葡萄球菌的 β-溶血素)[2]已证实上述机制。细菌还能释放诱导细胞裂解或阻断吞噬作用的因子(如化脓性链球菌分泌的 M 蛋白)[3]。这些破坏免疫的方法可以通过诸如巨噬细胞和中性粒细胞产生和释放活性氧和氮等机制来阻断。激活吞噬细胞并杀死摄入的细菌是控制细菌感染的另一种机制。吞噬细胞的活化由释放经模式识别受体作用的细菌产物,即病原体相关分子模式(pathogen-associated molecular pattern,PAMP)促进。活化 Th1 细胞释放的 IFN-γ 等细胞因子进一步诱导吞噬细胞的活化。刺激 T 细胞和 B 细胞则需要接触细菌抗原。对于 T 细胞,这需要 APC 摄取抗原,并在 MHC Ⅱ类或 CD1 分子上提呈,以便与 T 细胞受体结合。对于金黄色葡萄球菌等细胞外的细菌病原体,细菌 PAMP 和抗原的释放发生在组织中的细菌生长或裂解过程中。对于细胞内病原体,由于 PAMP 和抗原存在于细胞内,其暴露于吞噬细胞、B 细胞、T 细胞或其他免疫细胞的机制尚不清楚。最近的研究发现,将这些细菌成分输送到免疫系统的一个机制是通过释放 EV,如外泌体。然而,研究也表明,EV 可携带毒力因子促进细菌的存活和复制。因此,在感染过程中,这些 EV(包括宿主和细菌来源)的成分对于免疫系统和病原体之间的斗争有着重要的影响。除了调节宿主免疫应答,在细菌感染的情况下,EV 还可作为疾病的生物标志物、疫苗和药物传递系统用于治疗,这将在本章的最后进行讨论(图 6-1)。

二、胞外囊泡

在细菌感染的情况下,可以从宿主和细菌中获得 EV,广泛定义为细胞释放的膜结合囊泡。细菌产生的 EV 包括革兰阴性菌产生的外膜囊泡和革兰阳性菌产生的膜囊泡。许多文章总结了细菌源性囊泡领域的最新进展,因此本章将不予讨论[4-6]。这些囊泡可能在细胞外

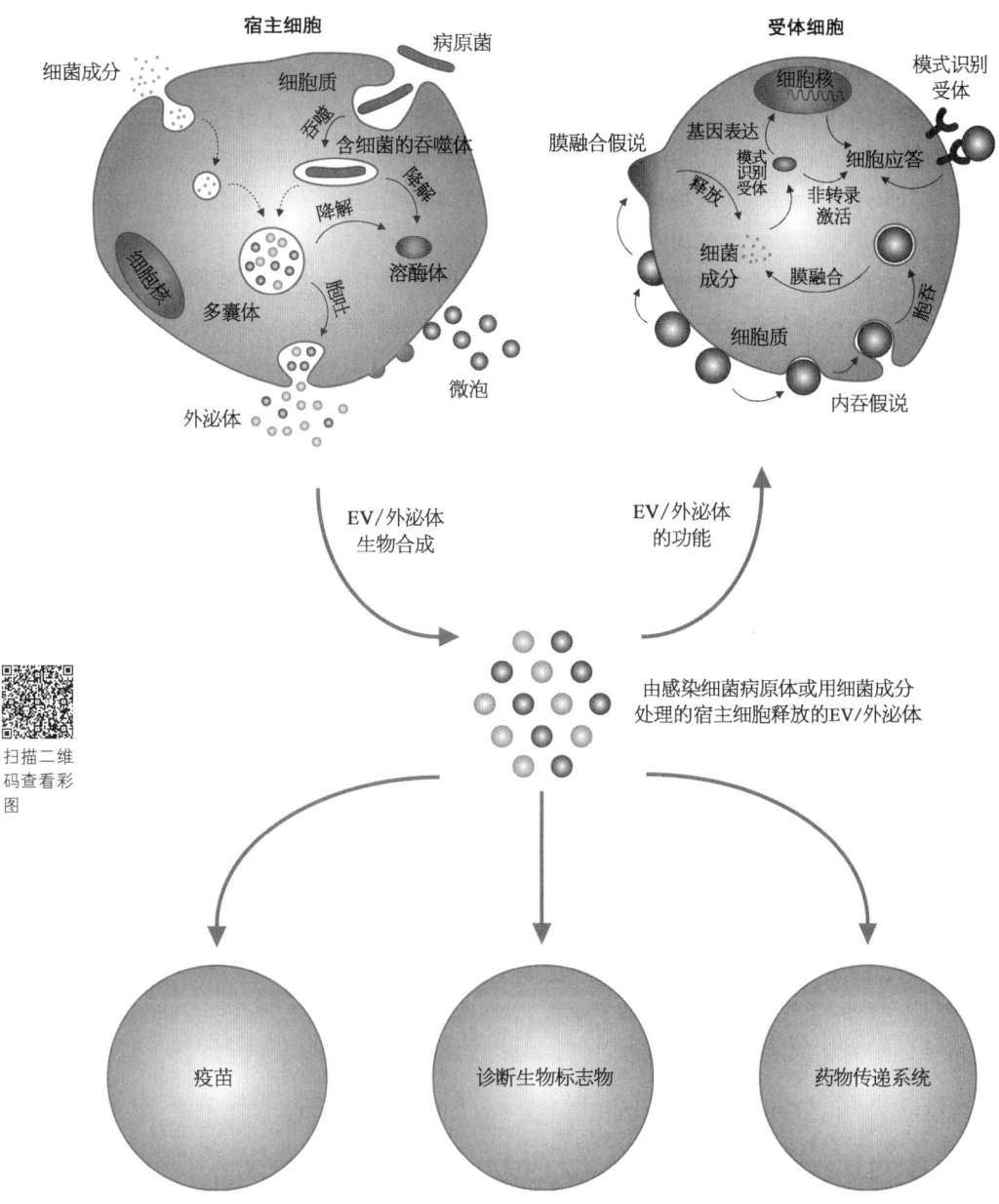

图6-1 受体细胞产生和摄取 EV 的一般机制及其治疗潜力

感染过程中发挥重要作用,但它们在细胞内病原体感染的作用尚不清楚,因为囊泡转运到宿主细胞外的机制仍有待确定。根据 EV 的合成方式和组成的不同,将 EV 分成三大类:凋亡小体、外泌体和微泡。三种囊泡都被脂质双分子层包围,但大小和组成各不相同。与从质膜出芽产生的微泡不同[7],外泌体来自内溶酶体途径,具有独特的脂质和蛋白质组成。外泌体是研究最多的感染因子。然而,外泌体的纯度并不一致,而且由于外泌体和微泡的大小和密度部分重叠,囊泡群可能同时包含外泌体和微泡。在讨论结果时,我们将使用原论文中定义的术语。

三、外泌体合成

外泌体是 MVB 与质膜融合并通过 ILV 释放形成[8]。外泌体为 30～150 nm 的脂质双层囊泡，密度为 1.13～1.19 g/mL。在生物物理学上，外泌体相当于被脂质双分子层包裹的细胞质，它的跨膜蛋白外部区域暴露在细胞外环境中。已有研究表明，外泌体可以从造血干来源的细胞中释放，包括 B 细胞[9]、肥大细胞[10]、树突状细胞（dendritic cell，DC）[11,12]、血小板[13]、巨噬细胞[14]，以及非造血干来源的细胞如神经元和上皮细胞[15-17]。外泌体可在局部器官发挥作用，也可在包括血液和淋巴液在内的各种体液中循环，从而引起全身反应[18]。外泌体最早在网织红细胞的培养基中被发现[19,20]。然而，在过去的三十年里，外泌体的研究已经扩展到涵盖了大多数细胞类型，以及它们从单细胞真核生物在内的不同生物体中分离出来的情况。进化过程中外泌体产生和功能的保存表明了这种细胞通信机制是一种的强有力的选择。另外，利用外泌体进行细胞间通信的优势在于其结构的复杂性，可以对通信过程进行更多的控制。此外，信号脂质、蛋白质和不同种类的 RNA 在单一结构的存在可以引起靶细胞快速和深刻的变化，从而对细胞干扰产生快速响应。这些干扰可能是在生理或病理条件下发生的。虽然外泌体结构的复杂性对产生外泌体的生物体有明显的好处，但对其功能的研究仍具有挑战性，因为外泌体或外泌体池包含多种成分，其中许多成分可以诱导靶细胞的细胞反应。此外，我们在体内和体外调节外泌体产生和组成的工具有限，阻碍了我们在正常和疾病状态下定义外泌体功能的能力。然而，在过去的十年里，我们已经对外泌体的合成、组成和功能有了重要的了解；近十年来，关于外泌体和其他 EV 的论著也显著增加。

去除质膜受体的一个重要机制是通过内吞作用并转运到 MVB，随后 MVB 与溶酶体的融合导致内吞受体降解[21]。然而，并不是所有与溶酶体融合的 MVB 都能与质膜融合，导致 ILV 的细胞外释放。目前尚不清楚与溶酶体融合的 MVB 是否由与质膜融合的 MVB 组成不同的亚群，或者在适当的条件下，特定 MVB 是否可以遵循任一条路径。MHC 分子转运的数据表明，可能确实存在不同的亚群[22]。尽管最近有这些研究，但在 MVB 合成和外泌体释放的认识仍存在巨大空白。有几种模型已经提出了 ILV 形成的机制。在酵母中的初步研究表明，转运蛋白所需的 ESCRT 的作用[23]。虽然研究 ESCRT 机制的主要目的是其在核内体分选和蛋白质降解中的作用，但更多的研究暗示了 ESCRT 蛋白在膜内陷中的作用[24,25]。通过泛素相互作用结合域，ESCRT-0 聚集泛素蛋白并将其传递到 MVB 中[26]。然后，ESCRT-0 将 ESCRT-Ⅰ 招募到内体膜，后者随后招募 ESCRT 家族的剩余成员，分别为 ESCRT-Ⅱ 和 ESCRT-Ⅲ[27,28]。通过 ESCRT-Ⅲ 介导聚合丝的产生，膜内陷导致 ILV 形成[29]（最近的综述发现[30]）。为了证明 ESCRT 参与 ILV 的形成，对外泌体的蛋白质组学研究已经确定了外泌体中 ESCRT 蛋白的存在，并且敲除 ESCRT 机制的关键成分可以阻止 ILV 的形成和外泌体释放[31]，当然，这可能是细胞特异性的[32,33]。虽然已经发表的结果支持这种 MVB 合成的模型，但尚不清楚这是否是 MVB 形成的主要机制，因为已有研究表明在 MVB 的合成和外泌体释放中存在与 ESCRT 无关的机制。为了寻找其他机制，Stuffers 等发现从 4 个 ESCRT 复合物中去除特定亚基并不能完全抑制 MVB 的形成[32]。Van Niel 等发现了四次穿膜蛋白 CD63，这是一种在外泌体上发现的高浓度蛋白质，可以促进产物分类和 ILV 的形成[34]。此外，尽管这种四次穿膜蛋白的敲除似乎不会改变 MVB 的形态或外泌体的释放，但是 CD81 已被证明可以影响四次穿模蛋白配体(如 Rac GTP 酶)的产物分类[35]。总之，研究表明，有多种机制可以促进 MVB 的合成和外泌体的产生以及装载。这些机制可能因细胞类型而异，甚至可能因细胞内 MVB 的不同亚群而异。为了支持后者，Buschow 等证明在未成熟的 DC 中，低胆固醇但富含溶二磷脂的 MVB 的 MHC 分子注定会被溶酶体降解。而在成熟的 DC 中，富含 CD9 和胆固醇的 MVB 的 MHC 分子则与质膜融合[22]。

　　MVB 与质膜的融合是由细胞骨架、融合机制（如 SNARE）和分子开关（即小分子量 GTP 酶）介导的[36]。Rab GTP 酶是 Ras GTP 酶超家族成员，在膜转运过程中调控四个步骤：囊泡形成、囊泡转运、停靠和与靶细胞器融合。目前，在哺乳动物细胞中发现了近 70 种不同的 Rab GTP 酶[37]，一些在外泌体中发现，包括 Rab5、Rab11、Rab27 和 Rab35。其中一些 Rab 效应因子已经被实验证明在外泌体释放中起作用。初步的研究发现了 Rab11 在 K562 红细胞白血病细胞系中 MVB 与质膜融合中的作用[38]。另外有研究表明，Rab35 介导 MVB 与神经细胞的质膜结合，Rab35 的缺失导致这些细胞释放的外泌体显著减少[39]。最近的研究证实了 Rab27a 和 Rab27b 在 MVB 合成中的作用。数据表明，Rab27a 和 Rab27b 在 MVB 合成途径中功能不同但有时是重合的，其中 Rab27a 在介导 MVB 与质膜的融合中发挥了更为突出的作用[40]。虽然 Rab-GTP 酶参与了 MVB 的转运和融合，但需要注意的是，它们在这一过程中的具体作用仍有待确定，而且很可能依赖于细胞类型以及细胞的生理/病理状态。

四、胞外囊泡、病原体和感染性疾病

　　外泌体和其他 EV 已经在包括病毒、寄生虫、真菌和细菌在内的所有已知病原体类别中被分离和鉴定。然而，这些 EV 的组成和活性在不同类群之间，甚至在同一属的病原体之间都存在显著差异。此外，所使用的动物模型、实验设计、为感染选择的细胞类型以及靶向的受体细胞等多种因素都会影响观察结果。

　　在细菌感染期间，宿主的免疫系统暴露于完整的细菌和微生物组分，这两者都是控制感染和病原体破坏免疫系统的关键。许多已知参与免疫反应的激活或破坏有关的细菌成分都是在感染期间被分泌或释放出来的。了解这些细菌因子以及它们在感染期间如何传播，对于我们理解疾病以及免疫系统如何应对感染是十分必要的。EV 是一种新发现的细菌成分扩散的机制（表 6-1）。关于外泌体/EV 在细菌感染后的产生和功能的大部分知识来自对分枝杆菌的研究，我们将首先对此进行讨论，然后分析在其他细菌背景下的外泌体/EV。

表 6-1　细菌感染后宿主细胞产生外泌体

细菌病原体	宿主来源	参考文献
沙眼衣原体	成纤维细胞	[41]
肺炎衣原体	ECV304 细胞	[42]
结核分枝杆菌	巨噬细胞,血浆	[14,43-49]
牛分枝杆菌	巨噬细胞,血浆,BALF	[48,50]
耻垢分枝杆菌	巨噬细胞	[51]
鸟分枝杆菌	巨噬细胞	[51-53]
鼠伤寒沙门氏菌	巨噬细胞	[14,54]
支原体	肿瘤细胞	[55]
炭疽芽孢杆菌	视网膜色素上皮细胞	[56]
假单胞菌	Ⅰ型肺泡上皮细胞	[57]

五、外泌体和胞外囊泡在分枝杆菌感染中的组成和功能

Russell 等观察到,结核分枝杆菌(*Mycobacterium tuberculosis*,*M.tb*)的 LAM 和 PIM 在巨噬细胞感染期间从吞噬体转运到 MVB。这些分枝杆菌成分也存在于感染巨噬细胞释放的 EV 中,并且在邻近未感染细胞内也可以检测到[44]。这些囊泡具有晚期核内体/溶酶体的标志,并以钙依赖的方式向外分泌[45]。

我们在这些原始观察的基础上进行了更多的研究(图 6-2)。我们发现,鸟分枝杆菌感染的巨噬细胞释放囊泡可刺激非感染或"旁观者"巨噬细胞的促炎症反应[52]。Wang 等也报道了类似的结果[53]。另外的研究发现,与未感染的细胞相比,感染鸟分枝杆菌和耻垢分枝杆菌的巨噬细胞释放更多的外泌体,并且感染巨噬细胞释放的外泌体中宿主蛋白 HSP70 的水平也有所提高。Anand 等进一步证明,HSP70 是体外巨噬细胞的激活剂[51]。*M.tb* 或牛分枝杆菌(*M. bovis* BCG)感染的巨噬细胞释放的外泌体也可刺激促炎反应[52]。随后发现,*M.tb* 感染细胞释放的外泌体上的分枝杆菌 19-kDa 脂蛋白是导致这一炎症反应的主要因素,这是通过 TLR/MyD88 途径介导[58]。感染巨噬细胞释放的其他类型的 EV 也可能刺激靶细胞的促炎反应[59,60]。此外,从 *M. bovis* BCG 感染小鼠的支气管肺泡灌洗液(bronchoalveolar lavage fluid,BALF)中分离的 EV 含有包括 19 kDa 脂蛋白的分枝杆菌成分,并且在体外是促炎的。此外,*M. bovis* BCG 或 *M.tb* 感染巨噬细胞释放的外泌体在体内可以产生促炎反应,如小鼠鼻内注射可诱导 TNF-α 和 IL-12 产生,以及招募巨噬细胞和中性粒细胞到肺[52]。

用 *M.tb* 感染的巨噬细胞外泌体处理的巨噬细胞分泌趋化因子,在体外可诱导幼稚巨噬细胞和 T 细胞迁移。综上所述,这些结果表明,来自分枝杆菌感染细胞的外泌体在体内和体外都能促进免疫细胞的募集和激活,并可能在促进分枝杆菌感染后的固有免疫反应中发挥作用。然而,外泌体上/内存在的分枝杆菌成分也可以抑制免疫应答[47]。需要进一步的研究来确定外泌体-巨噬细胞相互作用所引起的受体和信号反应,以及这些相互作用/反应

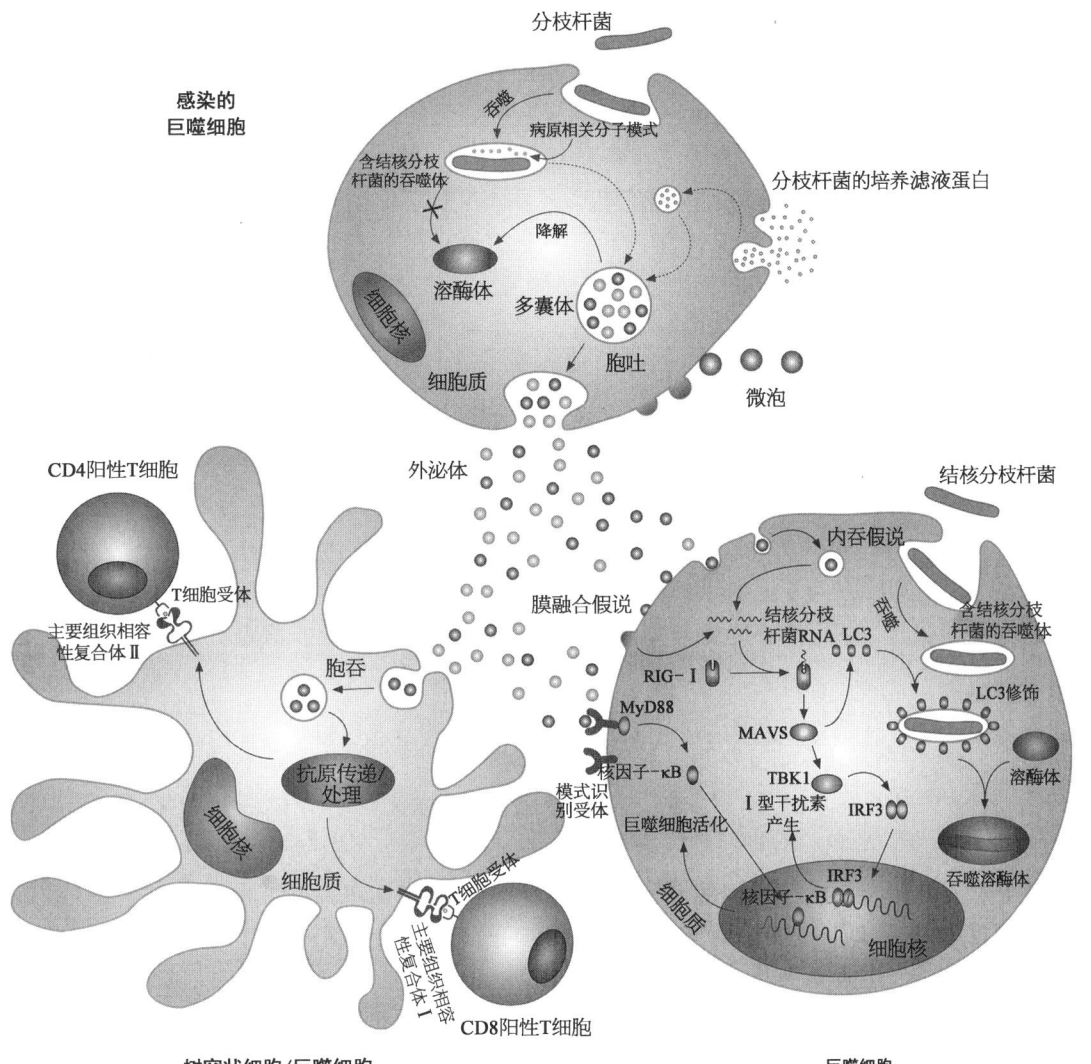

图 6-2 由感染分枝杆菌的巨噬细胞释放的外泌体刺激先天和适应性免疫反应

如何随着感染期间外泌体成分的改变而改变。除了对巨噬细胞活化的影响,*M.tb* 感染的细胞外泌体可以通过增加黏附分子如 ICAM-1 的表达来激活内皮细胞[61]。外泌体还可以通过 PE 家族的一员诱导 Jurkat T 细胞凋亡[62]。这些结果表明,外泌体的作用靶点可以扩展到免疫细胞和非免疫细胞。

(一) M.tb 感染与外泌体和 EV 的性质

从 *M.tb* 感染巨噬细胞中释放的外泌体上存在分枝杆菌 19 kDa 脂蛋白,这提示分枝杆菌的其他成分也可能通过外泌体和其他 EV 释放。事实上,许多研究已经发现了几种分枝杆菌蛋白,包括诱发小鼠和人类免疫反应的关键抗原[14,43,63,64]。此外,在感染小鼠和结核病患者血清中分离出的 EV 中也检测到分枝杆菌蛋白[14,63,64]。感染和未感染的巨噬细胞外泌体上的宿主蛋白质含量也存在差异，Diaz 等发现从 M.tb 感染和未感染的 THP-1 细胞释放的外泌体中有 41 个蛋白质发生显著变化[65]。Hare 等还发现 M.tb 感染和未感染巨噬细胞释放的 EV 蛋白质组存在差异，其中许多不同的结合蛋白与免疫功能相关[66]。随后的研究还发现，糖源寡糖基转移酶复合物和葡糖苷酶在 EV 中的差异结合[67]。尽管还没有直接检验，但他们的数据表明，靶细胞可能在摄取不同 EV 群体时发生不同的糖基化。

众所周知，外泌体和其他 EV 含有不同种类的 RNA，包括 miRNA，目前的研究已经解决了分枝杆菌感染的囊泡与未感染细胞释放的 RNA 成分之间的差异。Singh 等的研究表明，大约有 100 个转录物富集或独特于 M.tb 感染小鼠巨噬细胞释放的外泌体中，其中许多参与调节免疫应答[68]。在同一项研究中，他们还发现大量 miRNA 在感染和未感染巨噬细胞释放的外泌体中差异表达。总之，数据表明，与未感染细胞的外泌体相比，M.tb 感染的巨噬细胞的外泌体含有 RNA，能在靶细胞中诱导更多促炎反应，这与之前的激活研究相匹配。与未感染细胞相比，尽管所涉及的 miRNA 在每个研究中都是独特的，但是研究也观察到感染 M.bovis BCG 的人类单核细胞来源巨噬细胞释放的外泌体中 miRNA 的差异表达[69]。Singh 等的研究中更令人惊讶的结果之一是发现感染巨噬细胞来源的外泌体中的 M.tb RNA[68]。目前，分枝杆菌 RNA 转运到 MVB/外泌体所需的宿主机制尚不清楚。然而，最近的一项研究表明，它的释放需要分枝杆菌 SecA2 分泌系统的表达[70]。有趣的是，这个研究发现中的分枝杆菌 RNA 存在于 EV，并激活巨噬细胞中的 RIG-I/MAVS RNA 传感通路，导致 I 型干扰素（interferon，IFN）的生成增加[70]。这些 EV 也促进了巨噬细胞的活化，从而增加了吞噬细胞 M.tb 的杀伤作用，这同样依赖于分枝杆菌 RNA 的存在和 RIG-I/MAVS 传感通路的激活。EV 中微生物 RNA 的存在提示了一种以前未被认识的改变宿主免疫反应的机制，激活核酸传感器，这一机制通常与控制病毒感染有关。然而，值得注意的是，I 型 IFN 在 M.tb 感染中促进细菌存活和疾病发病进展[71,72]。除 I 型 IFN 产生外，M.tb 感染的巨噬细胞释放的 EV 也被发现可以促进一个非典型的自噬途径，并通过 RIG-I RNA 传感器途径杀死细胞内 M.tb[72]。当巨噬细胞被从 M.tb 感染的中性粒细胞释放的 EV 处理时，也发现了类似的机制[73]。通过 EV 传播的细菌 RNA 提示了另一种免疫监测途径，因此有必要对分枝杆菌和其他细菌性病原体进行更多的研究。

（二）分枝杆菌感染时 EV 对适应性免疫反应的调节作用

从感染 M.tb 或 M.bovis BCG 细胞和 M.tb 培养滤液蛋白（culture filtrate protein，CFP）处理的巨噬细胞中释放出的外泌体，也能在体内激活抗原特异性 $CD4^+$ 和 $CD8^+$ T 细胞，并促进骨髓来源的树突状细胞（bone marrow-derived dendritic cell，BMDC）的活化和成熟[49,50]。这些外泌体可诱导 Th1 免疫应答，使抗原特异性 T 细胞产生 IFN-γ。此外，用经 CFP 处理的巨噬细胞释放的外泌体接种小鼠可保护小鼠免受低剂量雾化结核分枝杆菌接种的影响，相当于接种卡介苗的小鼠[49]。从感染的巨噬细胞释放分枝杆菌抗原并不局限于外泌体。Ramachandra 等观察到 M.tb 或 M.bovis BCG 感染会导致外泌体和微泡释放增加，这两者都能刺激抗原特异性 T 细胞应答[46]。综上所述，这些结果表明，外泌体和其他 EV 可以作为刺激获得性免疫应答的抗原来源。然而，也有人提出了分枝杆菌感染期间抗原传递的其他机制，包括坏死细胞、凋亡小体和游离抗原的释放[74-76]。$M.tb$ 抗原很可能是通过多种途径提供给 MHC 提呈。不幸的是，因为缺乏分子工具来阻止巨噬细胞和 DC 的外泌体产生而不影响其他方面的囊泡运输，也不阻止其他细胞类型的外泌体产生，我们检测外泌体/EV 在抗原传递中重要性的能力有限。

六、外泌体和胞外囊泡在其他细菌感染中的组成和功能

尽管与分枝杆菌感染相比，我们对其他细菌的了解更少，但是许多研究已经证明外泌体和 EV 中细菌成分的存在及其可能引起细菌感染的宿主反应（图 6-3）。来自沙门菌感染巨噬细胞的外泌体被发现可以通过诱导人类单核细胞产生 TNF-α 促进炎症反应[52]。此外，鼠伤寒沙门菌感染巨噬细胞的外泌体可刺激 RANTES、IL-1Ra、MIP-2 和 G-CSF 等细胞因子和生长因子的产生，这依赖于靶细胞中 TLR4 的表达[54]。TLR4 的依赖性可能是由于这些外泌体上脂多糖（lipopolysaccharide，LPS）的存在，这是一种存在于沙门菌和其他革兰阴性菌上 TLR4 配体。Hui 等的研究还发现，受沙门菌感染的巨噬细胞产生外泌体 CD63$^+$ 和 CD9$^+$ 亚群，这符合最近的数据，表明即使从单细胞系释放，外泌体的蛋白质组成也是不同的[54]。这些不同的 EV 亚群对免疫应答的影响尚不清楚。革兰阴性细菌感染引起的 EV 促炎性质并不限于这些体外研究，在急性肺损伤和急性呼吸窘迫综合征相关的炎症反应中发现，从肺炎假单胞菌感染小鼠的 BALF 分离出来的 EV 刺激 TNF-α、IL-6 和 IL-1β 的产生[57]。有趣的是，肺氧化应激后从 BALF 中分离出的 EV 也促炎，但这些 EV 主要是从 I 型肺泡上皮细胞释放出来的，而肺炎假单胞菌感染后的活动性 EV 主要来自肺泡巨噬细胞。这说明多种细胞可产生促炎 EV，这些 EV 可能与不同病理条件下的组织损伤有关，以这些促炎 EV 为靶向的研究可能有利于治疗一些过度炎症引起的疾病。

支原体感染细胞的外泌体可以诱导多种细胞因子反应，包括 B 细胞 IFN-γ 和 IL-10 的产生。然而，这些外泌体的作用主要是抑制，至少对 T 细胞的激活是如此[55]。Abrami 等发现，外泌体也可以是毒素的载体，如致死因子（lethal factor，LF）是炭疽杆菌产生的一种特征性毒素，当在人上皮细胞系中表达时，将被包装成腔内囊泡并在外泌体上释放[56]。包裹在外泌体中的 LF 可被保护，不受抗体等细胞外因子的中和作用，并可被靶细胞吸收。当用完整的白喉类毒素处理 DC 时，在 DC 分泌的外泌体上也发现白喉毒素[77]。有趣的是，这些外泌体被发现可以诱导白喉类毒素特异性抗体免疫应答，这表明包裹外泌体的外源蛋白可以激活 B 细胞。这可能发生在外泌体进入淋巴结的过程中，但有待实验验证。Colino 和 Snapper 继续了这项工作，并证明了外泌体诱导的抗肺炎链球菌 14 型荚膜多糖的抗体免疫应答可以保护小鼠免受肺炎链球菌的致命感染[78]。Ettelaie 等报道，肺炎衣原体感染的细胞释放出的"微粒"含有一种凝血蛋白 TF，它也与细胞增殖、迁移和凋亡有关。TF 阳性的微粒激活 NF-κB，这是一种调节内皮细胞 TF 表达的转录因子。肺炎衣原体也被认为以微粒的形式释放，在通过血管系统的传播中可能起到了作用。这些发现在控制宿主感染方面有一定的意义，但也可能与炎症性疾病（如动脉粥样硬化）相关的心血管后果有关[42]。尽管肺炎衣原体囊泡被称为微粒，但用于分离的程序会富集出外泌体。一些细胞毒蛋白和分泌蛋白也与沙眼衣原体释放的宿主囊泡有关，这些蛋白可能在毒力因子的鉴别中发挥作用[41]。

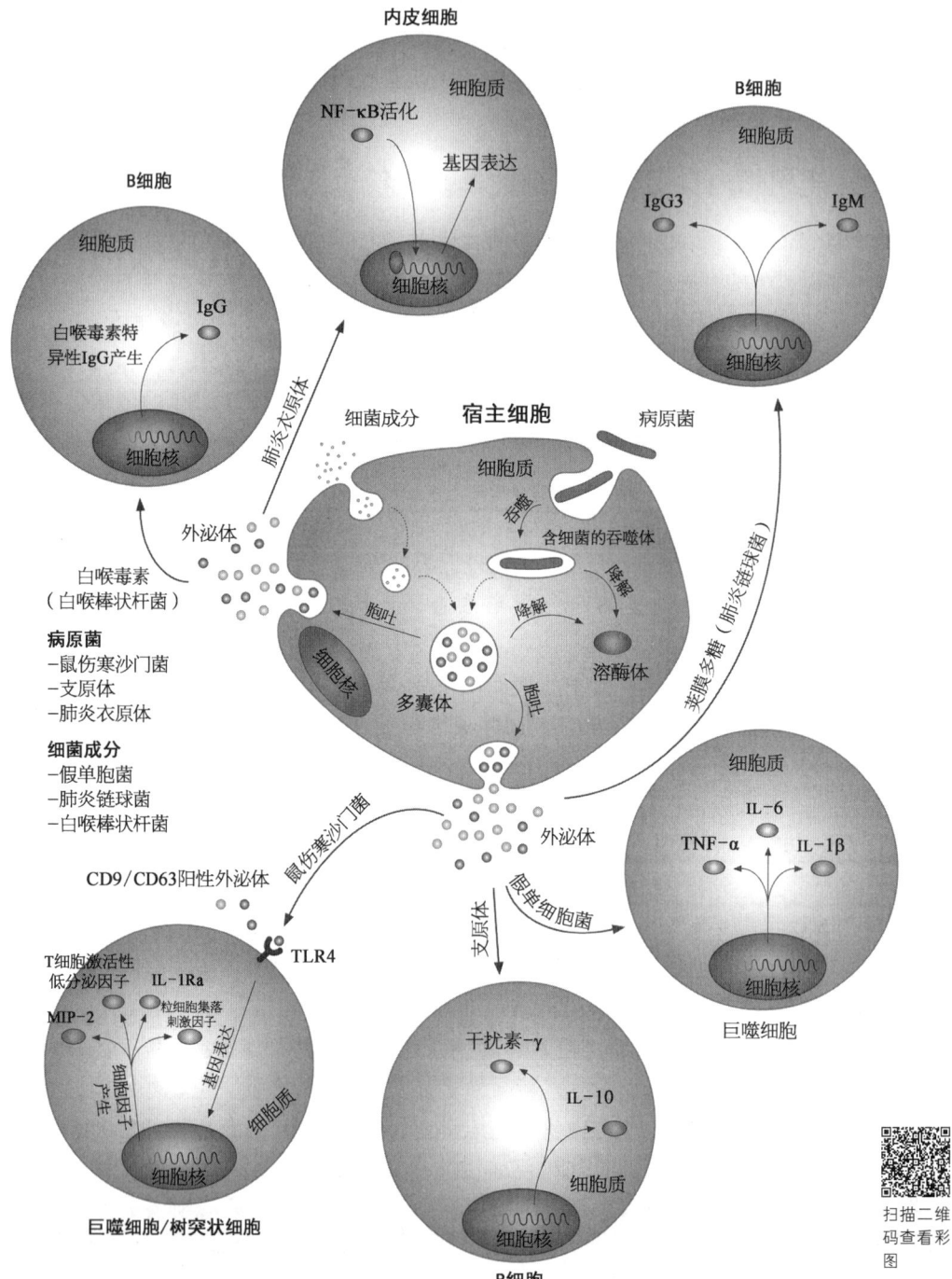

图 6-3 不同受体细胞对感染细菌病原体的宿主细胞释放外泌体的反应

总之,已有研究表明,在活跃的细胞感染或被免疫细胞(如巨噬细胞和 DC)内吞噬时,各种细菌成分可以被包装。然而,这些成分被运送到 EV 的机制和这种运输的特殊性仍然是一个悬而未决的问题。为了解决这个问题,Smith 等研究了将分枝杆菌蛋白运输到外泌体需要的宿主因子。他们发现,感染过程或巨噬细胞内吞时释放的分枝杆菌蛋白需要单泛素化才能被转运到 MVB 并进入腔内小泡[79,80]。然而,泛素化是否是细菌蛋白转运到 MVB 的一般机制,或者是否有其他机制在起作用尚不清楚。此外,目前仍不清楚其他细菌成分如脂质和核酸如何被运输到外泌体或其他 EV 中。

七、胞外囊泡作为预防细菌感染的疫苗

从 EBV 转化的 B 淋巴细胞外泌体携带 MHCⅡ复合物,可以在缺乏 APC 的情况下激活抗原特异性 MHCⅡ限制的 T 淋巴细胞,这一发现启发了将外泌体作为疫苗的研究[9]。在过去的二十年里,许多创新性的研究着眼于开发基于外泌体的疫苗在动物模型上治疗肿瘤,最近则在人类患者身上进行。根据良好生产规范(good manufacturing,GMP),外泌体已经被成功生产出来,在晚期肿瘤患者的Ⅰ期临床试验中,对三种基于外泌体的疫苗候选物进行了评价。其中一种候选药物正在进行非小细胞肺癌患者的Ⅱ期临床试验[81-84]。在细菌感染领域,来自病原体感染宿主细胞的 EV 也为开发新型无细胞抗菌疫苗提供了新的思路。越来越多的证据强调了 EV 作为疫苗的独特优势:① EV 由细菌感染的宿主细胞释放,并继承了亲代细胞的一些特性。这包括来自 APC 的囊泡,可能携带 MHC Ⅰ/Ⅱ抗原复合物、游离抗原、辅助分子和其他调节宿主因子;② EV 作为内源性成分,比大多数外源性疫苗更稳定;③ 与传统疫苗不同的是,几乎在所有体液中都检测到 EV。这表明 EV 携带的抗原可以到达远端器官或区域,而这些器官或区域可能被传统疫苗错过,但对保护性免疫反应很重要。

如上所述,APC 来源的 EV 在基于 EV 的抗菌疫苗研究中尤其具有吸引力。Colino 等发现,用白喉毒素(diphtheria toxin,DT)或肺炎链球菌 14 型(*Streptococcus pneumoniae* type 14,Cps14)荚膜多糖预处理的小鼠 BMDC 释放的外泌体在幼稚受体小鼠中诱导抗原(DT/CPs14)特异性抗体反应[77,78]。有趣的是,来自 DT 处理的 BMDC 的外泌体也刺激了游离 DT 激发小鼠的次级抗 DT 抗体反应。与游离 DT 主要诱导 2 型抗 DT 反应不同,来自 DT 处理 BMDC 的外泌体优先刺激 1 型抗 DT 反应[77]。小鼠存活实验进一步表明,来自 Cps14 处理的 BMDC 的外泌体可以使小鼠在肺炎链球菌 14 型活菌株的致命感染中存活下来,但缺少 Cps14 的菌株则不然[77]。

M. tb 是传染性疾病死亡的第一大原因,全世界每年约有 170 万人死亡[85]。*M. bovis* BCG 是目前唯一获批的抗结核疫苗,但其效力随时间而波动,对青少年和成人的保护作用有限。外泌体为抗结核疫苗接种提供了一种新的替代策略。来自 *M. bovis* BCG 感染或 *M. tb* CFP 预处理巨噬细胞的外泌体诱导幼稚小鼠产生抗原特异性 $CD4^+$ 和 $CD8^+$ T 细胞应答[49,50]。与来自经 DT 处理的 BMDC 的外泌体相似,来自经 CFP 处理的巨噬细胞的外泌体在接种了 *M. bovis* BCG 的小鼠中促进了次级 T 细胞反应,这为外泌体作为增强疫苗与 *M. bovis* BCG 联合接种提供证据。与 *M. bovis* BCG 不同,来自经 CFP 处理的巨噬细胞的外泌体在接种疫苗的小鼠中显示了对 Th1 免疫应答的偏向激活,这对控制患者的结核病是必要的[49,86]。此外,研究表明,与接受未经处理的巨噬细胞的外泌体或单剂量 *M. bovis* BCG 的小鼠相比,经 CFP 处理巨噬细胞的外泌体免疫的小鼠 *M. tb* 感染被明显抑

制。作为一种增强疫苗,外泌体表现出与 M. bovis BCG 相当或更高剂量依赖性的抗菌效果[49]。

外泌体疫苗的一个局限性是将体外抗原 APC 作为外泌体的来源,而这种方法不适用于大规模 GMP 生产外泌体。此外,研究表明,抗原进入外泌体依赖于抗原中包含的传递到 MVB 和腔内小泡的"信号"。因此,需要一种简单而有效的方法将抗原靶向到外泌体中,而不考虑内在的分选"信号",并且对于大规模生产外泌体是可行的。一种可能的策略是设计一种转基因哺乳动物细胞系,该细胞系持续性地释放携带选择抗原的外泌体。研究发现,单泛素修饰在分枝杆菌和宿主蛋白进入宿主来源的外泌体中发挥关键作用[80]。利用这一信息设计了一种转基因 HEK 293T 细胞系,在该细胞系中引入一个单泛素标记作为蛋白质进入外泌体的信号[87]。为了优化这种方法,对四个不同版本的单泛素修饰进行了测试,结果表明,在将 GFP、M. tb Ag85B - EAST6 融合蛋白和宿主 HER2 蛋白转运至外泌体的过程中,C 端野生型单泛素修饰是最有效的。然而,与 CFP 处理或 M. bovis BCG 感染巨噬细胞释放的外泌体不同,在没有佐剂的情况下,HEK 293T 细胞的外泌体不能诱导 Ag85B 或 ESAT6 特异性 T 细胞活化。这表明,经过改造的外泌体缺少一个存在于 CFP 处理/BCG 感染释放的外泌体中分枝杆菌成分,而这种成分可以作为疫苗接种后的佐剂。通过使用细胞膜 C1C2 结构域内乳糖贴壁蛋白或将 HIV Nef 蛋白作为外泌体靶向信号序列的策略已经被测试[88-92]。然而,这些外泌体的免疫原性仍有待确定。

八、胞外囊泡作为药物传递系统

外泌体可以与受体细胞结合,激活细胞表面受体,并将其内容物释放到宿主细胞中。研究表明,外泌体对受体细胞有一定的特异性,这是其由细胞来源决定的[14,70]。与传统的药物传递系统不同,外泌体被认为具有更高的治疗活性[93]。外泌体被广泛研究,以了解其作为无细胞治疗剂和调控受体细胞过程的药物传递系统的潜力。其中,作为核酸类药物载体的外泌体尤其具有吸引力,因为包括 miRNA、发夹 RNA 和 mRNA 在内的核酸可以通过产生外泌体的亲本细胞内源装载,也可以通过电穿孔外源装载[94]。例如,DC 的外泌体被设计成表达 Lamp2b(一种外泌体膜蛋白,可融合到神经元特异性 RVG 肽中),可以穿过血脑屏障(blood-brain barrier,BBB),将外源装载的 BACE1 特异性 siRNA 送入大脑。结果,BACE1 的表达在 mRNA 水平被抑制了 60%,在蛋白质水平被抑制了 62%,这表明外泌体可能用于治疗阿尔茨海默病[95]。在另一项研究中,我们发现细胞类型靶向外泌体具有显著的高治疗活性。HEK 293 细胞预先负载合成的抑癌基因 let - 7a miRNA,并表达与 GE11 肽融合的血小板源生长因子受体的跨膜结构域,从这些细胞中分离出的外泌体通过 GE11 - EGFR 相互作用特异性地靶向异种移植乳腺肿瘤细胞,可减少 $RAG2^{-/-}$ 小鼠肿瘤细胞的恶性生长[96]。

EV 作为药物传递系统或用于加强传染病的药物治疗还有许多未被探索。但是,最近的一项研究在 M. tb 抗生素治疗的背景下观察 EV。如前所述,M. tb 通过依赖 SecA2 的途径将其 RNA 释放到细胞外环境,其中一些释放的 RNA 被包装到宿主来源的外泌体中[70,72]。这些外泌体诱导 I 型 IFN 的产生,并激活感染巨噬细胞中含有 M. tb 的吞噬体的泛素非依赖性 LC3 相关修饰。吞噬溶酶体的成熟度限制了 M.tb 在宿主细胞中的复制。无论是 I 型 IFN 的产生，还是 LC3 对含有 M.tb 的吞噬体的非典型修饰，都依赖于宿主 RIG-I/MAVS 依赖的途径，该途径是由 EV 结合的 M.tb RNA 激活。在同一研究中发现，当在气管内给药时，从 M.tb 感染的 BMMS 中发现的外泌体抑制了 M.tb 在受感染小鼠肺和脾脏中的存活，这提示 M.tb 感染的 BMMS 的外泌体可以作为暴露前或暴露后的抗菌制剂，来控制结核分枝杆菌在宿主细胞中的存活。此外，与单用莫西沙星或外泌体相比，联合使用第二种抗结核抗生素莫西沙星时，肺和脾脏的 M.tb 负荷明显下降。小鼠外泌体摄取试验表明，气管内或鼻内给药主要针对肺泡巨噬细胞和 DC[14,70]。这表明，来自 M.tb 感染的巨噬细胞的外泌体可能作为靶向抗结核药物的替代机制，如增强抗结核药物的抗菌活性。在抗结核治疗方面，外泌体可用于补充二线抗生素，治疗单用抗生素难以治疗的耐多药和广泛耐药结核病（multidrug-resistant and extensively drug-resistant TB，M/XDR-TB）[70]。然而，与基于外泌体的疫苗相似，仍存在安全问题和开发的治疗性外泌体是否符合 GMP 标准等实用性问题。

九、外泌体作为传染病诊断的生物标志物

外泌体作为亲本细胞核酸和蛋白质天然载体的发现，引起了人们对基于外泌体的生物标志物的极大兴趣。许多研究表明，在健康个体和有潜在疾病（包括肿瘤和肾脏疾病）的个体之间，外泌体的组成存在定量和定性差异[81]。此外，与来自健康个体的外泌体相比，患者释放的外泌体（如活动性结核病患者）不仅表现出宿主分子的变化，而且还携带细菌成分，包括蛋白质、核酸和脂质[64,97]。这为诊断提供了一个明显的优势，因为细菌大分子的存在使得与宿主分子的定量变化相比具有更高的特异性。然而，令人惊讶的是，没有更多的工作投入到开发基于外泌体的传染病诊断。但这种潜力以前已经被注意到，因为一些出版物鼓励基于外泌体的细菌感染诊断技术的发展，特别是对那些难以诊断的疾病，如结核病[98]。结核病的典型诊断方法包括分枝杆菌培养或使用患者的痰液进行 PCR 检测。这些检测的敏感性和特异性受多种因素的影响。例如，在痰液中很少甚至没有 M.tb 的结核病患者和不能产生痰液的患者中，基于痰液的检测往往失败。此外，M.tb 生长缓慢，分枝杆菌培养试验需要 3~4 周。然而，目前培养试验是诊断 M/XDR-TB 的唯一可用方法。

为了探讨 EV 能否作为结核病诊断的生物标志物，采用 LC-MS-MS 分析了 M.tb 感染的 J774 巨噬细胞或 Balb/c 小鼠释放的 EV 的 M.tb 蛋白谱，从 M.tb 感染的 J774 巨噬细胞中鉴定了 41 种分枝杆菌蛋白，并从感染 M.tb H37RV 的小鼠 BALF 中分离出 69 种细菌蛋白[43,63]。在小鼠 M.tb 感染过程中观察到 BALF 外泌体中分枝杆菌蛋白的动态变化，表明 M.tb 蛋白可被用作基于外泌体的结核病诊断的生物标志物。在活动性结核病患者的血清外泌体中也发现了类似的结果[64]。在 41 名活动性肺结核患者中，所有 EV 样本均未发现常见的 M.tb 蛋白/肽。然而，数据表明，83% 的活动性肺结核病例可以通过生物标志物候选集（由活动性结核病患者特有的 7 种蛋白质组成）进行阳性诊断，与活动性结核不同的是，在潜伏结核患者的血清外泌体中没有发现这些独特的 M.tb 蛋白。考虑到在这项研究中只测试了一小部分潜伏性患者（$n=9$），因此需要更多的该队列成员来潜在地识别基于外

泌体的生物标志物,以区分活动性结核病和潜伏性结核病。除了 *M. tb* 蛋白生物标志物,在结核病患者 EV 中发现潜在的 *M. tb* RNA 生物标志物有重要意义。利用 Illumina RNA 测序技术,从 *M. tb* 感染的 RAW264.7 巨噬细胞和小鼠骨髓源性肥大细胞(bone marrow-derived mast cell,BMM)的外泌体[68,70]和活动性结核病患者的血清外泌体中分离鉴定出了一些 *M. tb* RNA[97]。

除了外泌体生物标志物,基于外泌体的诊断的一个关键步骤是找到一种简单而经济有效的从患者体液中富集外泌体的方法。对于以外泌体蛋白为基础的检测,宿主血浆蛋白如白蛋白和球蛋白的高浓度显著干扰了检测的敏感性和特异性。在体液中富集外泌体有一些成熟的方法,这些方法可以与基于外泌体的诊断相结合,包括外泌体抗体获取,如使用商用的抗 CD63 抗体的外泌体分离试剂。其他方法包括尺寸排除,该方法的优点是开发了基于 Capto Core 700 的分子排阻色谱方法,可以去除分子量小于 700 kDa 的游离蛋白,同时允许 EV 通过[99]。蛋白质定量证实该方法去除了超过 99% 的宿主血浆蛋白,LC-MS-MS 比较分析表明该方法显著提高了检测灵敏度[99,100]。除了这些方法,还有其他的外泌体纯化方法,包括聚合沉淀法、密度梯度离心法和差速超速离心法。然而,这些方法的缺点是显而易见的。聚合沉淀法非特异性地沉淀囊泡和大量的游离蛋白。当使用血液样本时,缺陷就更明显了。而对于依赖离心的方法,需要一个设备齐全的实验室,而在结核病流行的资源匮乏的环境中,往往很难获得这种设备。对于 RNA 的外泌体诊断,游离蛋白的水平不像基于蛋白质的外泌体检测那样是一个重要因素,但下游 RNA 富集/纯化方法将是至关重要的。

十、总结

很明显,EV 与宿主对细菌感染的反应密切相关,包括蛋白质、脂质和 RNA 在内的细菌成分都可以驻留在 EV 中。然而,它们的释放是促进还是阻碍免疫反应尚未明确。很可能两者都发生在感染的过程中,这取决于细菌的种类/菌株,以及在感染过程中免疫反应的时间。回答这个问题需要更好地理解哪些细菌成分被运输到 EV、哪些宿主因素调控着这一过程,以及这些细菌成分对受体细胞有什么影响。目前,我们缺乏许多必要的工具,包括在时间和空间上调节外泌体合成的方法。然而,目前的理解使我们能够探索外泌体和其他 EV 在疫苗、药物传递系统和诊断标志物开发中的应用,以更好地抗击细菌性疾病。随着我们对细菌性疾病中 EV 的生产、功能和组成了解得更多,其在治疗方面的应用将继续发展。

(陈金梅 译,陈小华 审校)

参考文献

[1] Laarman A, Milder F, van Strijp J, Rooijakkers S. Complement inhibition by gram-positive pathogens: molecular mechanisms and therapeutic implications. J Mol Med 2010; 88: 115-20. https://doi.org/10.1007/s00109-009-0572-y.

[2] Tajima A, Iwase T, Shinji H, Seki K, Mizunoe Y. Inhibition of endothelial interleukin-8 production and neutrophil transmigration by staphylococcus aureus beta-hemolysin. Infect Immun 2009; 77: 327-34. https://doi.org/10.1128/IAI.00748-08.

[3] Frost HR, Sanderson-Smith M, Walker M, Botteaux A, Smeesters PR. Group A streptococcal M-kike proteins: from pathogenesis to vaccine potential. FEMS Microbiol Rev 2018; 42: 193-204. https://doi.org/10.1093/femsre/fux057.

[4] Acevedo R, Fernández S, Zayas C, Acosta A, Sarmiento ME, Ferro VA, Rosenqvist E, Campa C, Cardoso D, Garcia L, Perez JL. Bacterial outer membrane vesicles and vaccine applications. Front Immunol 2014; 5: 121. https://doi.org/10.3389/fimmu.2014.00121.

[5] Deatherage BL, Cookson BT. Membrane vesicle release in bacteria, eukaryotes, and archaea: a conserved yet underappreciated aspect of microbial life. Infect Immun 2012; 80: 1948-57. https://doi.org/10.1128/IAI.06014-11.

[6] Kulp A, Kuehn MJ. Biological functions and biogenesis of secreted bacterial outer membrane vesicles. Annu Rev Microbiol 2010; 64: 163-84. https://doi.org/10.1146/annurev.micro.091208.073413.

[7] D'Souza-Schorey C, Clancy JW. Tumor-derived microvesicles: shedding light on novel microenvironment modulators and prospective cancer biomarkers. Genes Dev 2012; 26: 1287-99. https://doi.org/10.1101/gad.192351.112.

[8] Schorey JS, Cheng Y, Singh PP, Smith VL. Exosomes and other extracellular vesicles in host-pathogen interactions. EMBO Rep 2015; 16: 24-43. https://doi.org/10.15252/embr.201439363.

[9] Raposo G, Nijman HW, Stoorvogel W, Liejendekker R, Harding CV, Melief CJ, Geuze HJ. B lymphocytes secrete antigen-presenting vesicles. J Exp Med 1996; 183: 1161-72.

[10] Raposo G, Tenza D, Mecheri S, Peronet R, Bonnerot C, Desaymard C. Accumulation of major histocompatibility complex class II molecules in mast cell secretory granules and their release upon degranulation. Mol Biol Cell 1997; 8: 2631-45.

[11] Théry C, Regnault A, Garin J, Wolfers J, Zitvogel L, Ricciardi-Castagnoli P, Raposo G, Amigorena S. Molecular characterization of dendritic cell-derived exosomes. Selective accumulation of the heat shock protein hsc73. J Cell Biol 1999; 147: 599-610.

[12] Zitvogel L, Regnault A, Lozier A, Wolfers J, Flament C, Tenza D, Ricciardi-Castagnoli P, Raposo G, Amigorena S. Eradication of established murine tumors using a novel cell-free vaccine: dendritic cell derived exosomes. Nat Med 1998; 4: 594-600. https://doi.org/10.1038/nm0598-594.

[13] Heijnen HF, Schiel AE, Fijnheer R, Geuze HJ, Sixma JJ. Activated platelets release two types of membrane vesicles: microvesicles by surface shedding and exosomes derived from exocytosis of multivesicular bodies and alpha-granules. Blood 1999; 94: 3791-9.

[14] Bhatnagar S, Shinagawa K, Castellino FJ, Schorey JS. Exosomes released from macrophages infected with intracellular pathogens stimulate a proinflammatory response in vitro and in vivo. Blood 2007; 110: 3234-44. https://doi.org/10.1182/blood-2007-03-079152.

[15] Fauré J, Lachenal G, Court M, Hirrlinger J, Chatellard-Causse C, Blot B, Grange J, Schoehn G, Goldberg Y, Boyer V, Kirchhoff F, Raposo G, Garin J, Sadoul R. Exosomes are released by cultured cortical neurones. Mol Cell Neurosci 2006; 31: 642-8. https://doi.org/10.1016/j.mcn.2005.12.003.

[16] Guescini M, Genedani S, Stocchi V, Agnati LF. Astrocytes and Glioblastoma cells release exosomes carrying mtDNA. J Neural Transm (Vienna) 2010; 117: 1-4. https://doi.org/10.1007/s00702-009-0288-8.

[17] Marzesco A-M, Janich P, Wilsch-Bräniger M, Dubreuil V, Langenfeld K, Corbeil D, Huttner WB. Release of extracellular membrane particles carrying the stem cell marker prominin-1 (CD133) from neural progenitors and other epithelial cells. J Cell Sci 2005; 118: 2849-58. https://doi.org/10.1242/jcs.02439.

[18] Zhu M, Li Y, Shi J, Feng W, Nie G, Zhao Y. Exosomes as extrapulmonary signaling conveyors for nanoparticle-induced systemic immune activation. Small 2012; 8: 404-12. https://doi.org/10.1002/smll.201101708.

[19] Harding C, Heuser J, Stahl P. Endocytosis and intracellular processing of transferrin and colloidal gold-transferrin in rat reticulocytes: demonstration of a pathway for receptor shedding. Eur J Cell Biol 1984; 35: 256-63.

[20] Johnstone RM, Adam M, Hammond JR, Orr L, Turbide C. Vesicle formation during reticulocyte maturation. Association of plasma membrane activities with released vesicles (exosomes). J Biol Chem 1987; 262: 9412-20.

[21] Woodman PG, Futter CE. Multivesicular bodies: co-ordinated progression to maturity. Curr Opin Cell Biol 2008; 20: 408-14. https://doi.org/10.1016/j.ceb.2008.04.001.

[22] Buschow SI, Nolte-'t Hoen ENM, van Niel G, Pols MS, ten Broeke T, Lauwen M, Ossendorp F, Melief CJM, Raposo G, Wubbolts R, Wauben MHM, Stoorvogel W. MHC II in dendritic cells is targeted to lysosomes or T cell-induced exosomes via distinct multivesicular body pathways. Traffic 2009; 10: 1528-42. https://doi.org/10.1111/j.1600-0854.2009.00963.x.

[23] Hurley JH. The ESCRT complexes. Crit Rev Biochem Mol Biol 2010; 45: 463-87. https://doi.org/10.3109/10409238.2010.502516.

[24] Davies BA, Lee JRE, Oestreich AJ, Katzmann DJ. Membrane protein targeting to the MVB/lysosome. Chem Rev 2009; 109: 1575-86. https://doi.org/10.1021/cr800473s.

[25] Metcalf D, Isaacs AM. The role of ESCRT proteins in fusion events involving lysosomes, endosomes and autophagosomes. Biochem Soc Trans 2010; 38: 1469-73. https://doi.org/10.1042/BST0381469.

[26] Raiborg C, Stenmark H. Hrs and endocytic sorting of ubiquitinated membrane proteins. Cell Struct Funct 2002; 27: 403-8.

[27] Babst M, Katzmann DJ, Snyder WB, Wendland B, Emr SD. Endosome-associated complex, ESCRT-II, recruits transport machinery for protein sorting at the multivesicular body. Dev Cell 2002; 3: 283-9.

[28] Katzmann DJ, Babst M, Emr SD. Ubiquitin-dependent sorting into the multivesicular body pathway requires the function of a conserved endosomal protein sorting complex, ESCRT-I. Cell 2001; 106: 145-55.

[29] Wollert T, Wunder C, Lippincott-Schwartz J, Hurley JH. Membrane scission by the ESCRTIII complex. Nature 2009; 458: 172-7. https://doi.org/10.1038/nature07836.

[30] Hanson PI, Cashikar A. Multivesicular body morphogenesis. Annu Rev Cell Dev Biol 2012; 28: 337-62. https://doi.org/10.1146/annurev-cellbio-092910-154152.

[31] Tamai K, Tanaka N, Nakano T, Kakazu E, Kondo Y, Inoue J, Shiina M, Fukushima K, Hoshino T, Sano K, Ueno Y, Shimosegawa T, Sugamura K. Exosome secretion of dendritic cells is regulated by Hrs, an ESCRT-0 protein. Biochem Biophys Res Commun 2010; 399: 384-90. https://doi.org/10.1016/j.bbrc.2010.07.083.

[32] Stuffers S, Sem Wegner C, Stenmark H, Brech A. Multivesicular endosome biogenesis in the absence of ESCRTs. Traffic 2009; 10: 925-37. https://doi.org/10.1111/j.1600-0854.2009.00920.x.

[33] Trajkovic K, Hsu C, Chiantia S, Rajendran L, Wenzel D, Wieland F, Schwille P, Brügger B, Simons M. Ceramide

triggers budding of exosome vesicles into multivesicular endosomes. Science 2008; 319: 1244 - 7. https://doi.org/10.1126/science.1153124.

[34] van Niel G, Charrin S, Simoes S, Romao M, Rochin L, Saftig P, Marks MS, Rubinstein E, Raposo G. The tetraspanin CD63 regulates ESCRT-independent and -dependent endosomal sorting during melanogenesis. Dev Cell 2011; 21: 708 - 21. https://doi.org/10.1016/j.devcel.2011.08.019.

[35] Perez-Hernandez D, Gutiérrez-Vázquez C, Jorge I, López-Martín S, Ursa A, Sánchez-Madrid F, Vázquez J, Yáñez-Mó M. The intracellular interactome of tetraspanin-enriched microdomains reveals their function as sorting machineries toward exosomes. J Biol Chem 2013; 288: 11649 - 61. https://doi.org/10.1074/jbc.M112.445304.

[36] Colombo M, Raposo G, Théry C. Biogenesis, secretion, and intercellular interactions of exosomes and other extracellular vesicles. Annu Rev Cell Dev Biol 2014; 30: 255 - 89. https://doi.org/10.1146/annurev-cellbio-101512-122326.

[37] Schwartz SL, Cao C, Pylypenko O, Rak A, Wandinger-Ness A. Rab GTPases at a glance. J Cell Sci 2007; 120: 3905 - 10. https://doi.org/10.1242/jcs.015909.

[38] Savina A, Vidal M, Colombo MI. The exosome pathway in K562 cells is regulated by Rab11. J Cell Sci 2002; 115: 2505 - 15.

[39] Hsu C, Morohashi Y, Yoshimura S-I, Manrique-Hoyos N, Jung S, Lauterbach MA, Bakhti M, Grønborg M, Möbius W, Rhee J, Barr FA, Simons M. Regulation of exosome secretion by Rab35 and its GTPase-activating proteins TBC1D10A-C. J Cell Biol 2010; 189: 223 - 32. https://doi.org/10.1083/jcb.200911018.

[40] Ostrowski M, Carmo NB, Krumeich S, Fanget I, Raposo G, Savina A, Moita CF, Schauer K, Hume AN, Freitas RP, Goud B, Benaroch P, Hacohen N, Fukuda M, Desnos C, Seabra MC, Darchen F, Amigorena S, Moita LF, Thery C. Rab27a and Rab27b control different steps of the exosome secretion pathway. Nat Cell Biol 2010; 12: 19 - 30. Sup. pp 1 - 13, https://doi.org/10.1038/ncb2000.

[41] Frohlich K, Hua Z, Wang J, Shen L. Isolation of *Chlamydia* trachomatis and membrane vesicles derived from host and bacteria. J Microbiol Methods 2012; 91: 222 - 30. https://doi.org/10.1016/j.mimet.2012.08.012.

[42] Ettelaie C, Collier MEW, James NJ, Li C. Induction of tissue factor expression and release as microparticles in ECV304 cell line by *Chlamydia pneumoniae* infection. Atherosclerosis 2007; 190: 343 - 51. https://doi.org/10.1016/j.atherosclerosis.2006.04.005.

[43] Giri PK, Kruh NA, Dobos KM, Schorey JS. Proteomic analysis identifies highly antigenic proteins in exosomes from *M. tuberculosis*-infected and culture filtrate protein-treated macrophages. Proteomics 2010; 10: 3190 - 202. https://doi.org/10.1002/pmic.200900840.

[44] Beatty WL, Russell DG. Identification of mycobacterial surface proteins released into subcellular compartments of infected macrophages. Infect Immun 2000; 68: 6997 - 7002.

[45] Beatty WL, Ullrich HJ, Russell DG. Mycobacterial surface moieties are released from infected macrophages by a constitutive exocytic event. Eur J Cell Biol 2001; 80: 31 - 40. https://doi.org/10.1078/0171-9335-00131.

[46] Ramachandra L, Qu Y, Wang Y, Lewis CJ, Cobb BA, Takatsu K, Boom WH, Dubyak GR, Harding CV. Mycobacterium tuberculosis synergizes with ATP to induce release of microvesicles and exosomes containing major histocompatibility complex class II molecules capable of antigen presentation. Infect Immun 2010; 78: 5116 - 25. https://doi.org/10.1128/IAI.01089-09.

[47] Singh PP, LeMaire C, Tan JC, Zeng E, Schorey JS. Exosomes released from *M. tuberculosis* infected cells can suppress IFN-γ mediated activation of naïve macrophages. PLoS ONE 2011; 6: e18564. https://doi.org/10.1371/journal.pone.0018564.

[48] Singh PP, Smith VL, Karakousis PC, Schorey JS. Exosomes isolated from mycobacteriainfected mice or cultured macrophages can recruit and activate immune cells in vitro and in vivo. J Immunol 2012; 189: 777 - 85. https://doi.org/10.4049/jimmunol.1103638.

[49] Cheng Y, Schorey JS. Exosomes carrying mycobacterial antigens can protect mice against *Mycobacterium tuberculosis* infection. Eur J Immunol 2013; 43: 3279 - 90. https://doi.org/10.1002/eji.201343727.

[50] Giri PK, Schorey JS. Exosomes derived from *M. bovis* BCG infected macrophages activate antigen-specific CD4+ and CD8+ T cells in vitro and in vivo. PLoS ONE 2008; 3: e2461. https://doi.org/10.1371/journal.pone.0002461.

[51] Anand PK, Anand E, Bleck CKE, Anes E, Griffiths G. Exosomal Hsp70 induces a pro-inflammatory response to foreign particles including mycobacteria. PLoS ONE 2010; 5: e10136. https://doi.org/10.1371/journal.pone.0010136.

[52] Bhatnagar S, Schorey JS. Exosomes released from infected macrophages contain *Mycobacterium avium* glycopeptidolipids and are proinflammatory. J Biol Chem 2007; 282: 25779 - 89. https://doi.org/10.1074/jbc.M702277200.

[53] Wang J, Chen C, Xie P, Pan Y, Tan Y, Tang L. Proteomic analysis and immune properties of exosomes released by macrophages infected with mycobacterium avium. Microbes Infect 2014; 16: 283 - 91. https://doi.org/10.1016/j.micinf.2013.12.001.

[54] Hui WW, Hercik K, Belsare S, Alugubelly N, Clapp B, Rinaldi C, Edelmann MJ. *Salmonella enterica* serovar typhimurium alters the extracellular proteome of macrophages and leads to the production of proinflammatory exosomes. Infect Immun 2018; 86 https://doi.org/10.1128/IAI.00386-17.

[55] Yang C, Chalasani G, Ng Y-H, Robbins PD. Exosomes released from mycoplasma infected tumor cells activate inhibitory B cells. PLoS ONE 2012; 7 https://doi.org/10.1371/journal.pone.0036138.

[56] Abrami L, Brandi L, Moayeri M, Brown MJ, Krantz BA, Leppla SH, van der Goot FG. Hijacking multivesicular bodies enables long-term and exosome-mediated long-distance action of anthrax toxin. Cell Rep 2013; 5: 986 - 96. https://doi.org/10.1016/j.celrep.2013.10.019.

[57] Lee H, Zhang D, Laskin DL, Jin Y. Functional evidence of pulmonary extracellular vesicles in infectious and noninfectious lung inflammation. J Immunol 2018; 201: 1500 - 9. https://doi.org/10.4049/jimmunol.1800264.

[58] Schorey JS, Bhatnagar S. Exosome function: from tumor immunology to pathogen biology. Traffic 2008; 9: 871 - 81. https://doi.org/10.1111/j.1600-0854.2008.00734.x.

[59] Athman JJ, Wang Y, McDonald DJ, Boom WH, Harding CV, Wearsch PA. Bacterial membrane vesicles mediate the release of *Mycobacterium tuberculosis* lipoglycans and lipoproteins from infected macrophages. J Immunol 2015; 195: 1044 – 53. https://doi.org/10.4049/jimmunol.1402894.

[60] Walters SB, Kieckbusch J, Nagalingam G, Swain A, Latham SL, Grau GER, Britton WJ, Combes V, Saunders BM. Microparticles from mycobacteria-infected macrophages promote inflammation and cellular migration. J Immunol 2013; 190: 669 – 77. https://doi.org/10.4049/jimmunol.1201856.

[61] Li L, Cheng Y, Emrich S, Schorey J. Activation of endothelial cells by extracellular vesicles derived from *Mycobacterium tuberculosis* infected macrophages or mice. PLoS ONE 2018; 13: e0198337. https://doi.org/10.1371/journal.pone.0198337.

[62] Balaji KN, Goyal G, Narayana Y, Srinivas M, Chaturvedi R, Mohammad S. Apoptosis triggered by Rv1818c, a PE family gene from *Mycobacterium tuberculosis* is regulated by mitochondrial intermediates in T cells. Microbes Infect 2007; 9: 271 – 81. https://doi.org/10.1016/j.micinf.2006.11.013.

[63] Kruh-Garcia NA, Schorey JS, Dobos KM. Exosomes: new tuberculosis biomarkers — prospects from the bench to the clinic. In: Understanding tuberculosis — global experiences and innovative approaches to the diagnosis. 2012. https://doi.org/10.5772/30720.

[64] Kruh-Garcia NA, Wolfe LM, Chaisson LH, Worodria WO, Nahid P, Schorey JS, Davis JL, Dobos KM. Detection of *Mycobacterium tuberculosis* peptides in the exosomes of patients with active and latent *M. tuberculosis* infection using MRM-MS. PLoS ONE 2014; 9: e103811. https://doi.org/10.1371/journal.pone.0103811.

[65] Diaz W, Wolfe LM, Kruh-Garcia NA, Dobos KM. Changes in the membrane-associated proteins of exosomes released from human macrophages after *Mycobacterium tuberculosis* infection. Sci Rep 2016; 6: 37975. https://doi.org/10.1038/srep37975.

[66] Hare NJ, Chan B, Chan E, Kaufman KL, Britton WJ, Saunders BM. Microparticles released from *Mycobacterium tuberculosis*-infected human macrophages contain increased levels of the type I interferon inducible proteins including ISG15. Proteomics 2015; 15: 3020 – 9. https://doi.org/10.1002/pmic.201400610.

[67] Hare NJ, Lee LY, Loke I, Britton WJ, Saunders BM, Thaysen-Andersen M. *Mycobacterium tuberculosis* infection manipulates the glycosylation machinery and the N-glycoproteome of human macrophages and their microparticles. J Proteome Res 2017; 16: 247 – 63. https://doi.org/10.1021/acs.jproteome.6b00685.

[68] Singh PP, Li L, Schorey JS. Exosomal RNA from *Mycobacterium tuberculosis*-infected cells is functional in recipient macrophages. Traffic 2015; 16: 555 – 71. https://doi.org/10.1111/tra.12278.

[69] Alipoor SD, Mortaz E, Tabarsi P, Farnia P, Mirsaeidi M, Garssen J, Movassaghi M, Adcock IM. Bovis Bacillus Calmette-Guerin (BCG) infection induces exosomal miRNA release by human macrophages. J Transl Med 2017; 15: 105. https://doi.org/10.1186/s12967-017-1205-9.

[70] Cheng Y, Schorey JS. Extracellular vesicles deliver *Mycobacterium* RNA to promote host immunity and bacterial killing. EMBO Rep 2019. https://doi.org/10.15252/embr.201846613.

[71] Berry MPR, Graham CM, McNab FW, Xu Z, Bloch SAA, Oni T, Wilkinson KA, Banchereau R, Skinner J, Wilkinson RJ, Quinn C, Blankenship D, Dhawan R, Cush JJ, Mejias A, Ramilo O, Kon OM, Pascual V, Banchereau J, Chaussabel D, O'Garra A. An interferoninducible neutrophil-driven blood transcriptional signature in human tuberculosis. Nature 2010; 466: 973 – 7. https://doi.org/10.1038/nature09247.

[72] Cheng Y, Schorey JS. *Mycobacterium tuberculosis*-induced IFN-β production requires cytosolic DNA and RNA sensing pathways. J Exp Med 2018; 215: 2919 – 35. https://doi.org/10.1084/jem.20180508.

[73] Alvarez-Jiménez VD, Leyva-Paredes K, García-Martínez M, Vázquez-Flores L, García-Paredes VG, Campillo-Navarro M, Romo-Cruz I, Rosales-García VH, Castañeda-Casimiro J, González-Pozos S, Hernández JM, Wong-Baeza C, García-Pérez BE, Ortiz-Navarrete V, Estrada-Parra S, Serafín-López J, Wong-Baeza I, Chacón-Salinas R, Estrada-García I. Extracellular vesicles released from mycobacterium tuberculosis-infected neutrophils promote macrophage autophagy and decrease intracellular mycobacterial survival. Front Immunol 2018; 9. https://doi.org/10.3389/fimmu.2018.00272.

[74] Behar SM, Martin CJ, Nunes-Alves C, Divangahi M, Remold HG. Lipids, apoptosis, and cross-presentation: links in the chain of host defense against *Mycobacterium tuberculosis*. Microbes Infect 2011; 13: 749 – 56. https://doi.org/10.1016/j.micinf.2011.03.002.

[75] Sridharan H, Upton JW. Programmed necrosis in microbial pathogenesis. Trends Microbiol 2014; 22: 199 – 207. https://doi.org/10.1016/j.tim.2014.01.005.

[76] Srivastava S, Ernst JD. Cell-to-cell transfer of *M. tuberculosis* antigens optimizes CD4 T cell priming. Cell Host Microbe 2014; 15: 741 – 52. https://doi.org/10.1016/j.chom.2014.05.007.

[77] Colino J, Snapper CM. Exosomes from bone marrow dendritic cells pulsed with diphtheria toxoid preferentially induce type 1 antigen-specific IgG responses in naive recipients in the absence of free antigen. J Immunol 2006; 177: 3757 – 62.

[78] Colino J, Snapper CM. Dendritic cell-derived exosomes express a *Streptococcus pneumoniae* capsular polysaccharide type 14 cross-reactive antigen that induces protective immunoglobulin responses against pneumococcal infection in mice. Infect Immun 2007; 75: 220 – 30. https://doi.org/10.1128/IAI.01217-06.

[79] Smith VL, Cheng Y, Bryant BR, Schorey JS. Exosomes function in antigen presentation during an in vivo *Mycobacterium tuberculosis* infection. Sci Rep 2017; 7: 43578. https://doi.org/10.1038/srep43578.

[80] Smith VL, Jackson L, Schorey JS. Ubiquitination as a mechanism to transport soluble mycobacterial and eukaryotic proteins to exosomes. J Immunol 2015; 195: 2722 – 30. https://doi.org/10.4049/jimmunol.1403186.

[81] Chaput N, Théry C. Exosomes: immune properties and potential clinical implementations. Semin Immunopathol 2011; 33: 419 – 40. https://doi.org/10.1007/s00281-010-0233-9.

[82] Dai S, Wei D, Wu Z, Zhou X, Wei X, Huang H, Li G. Phase I clinical trial of autologous ascites-derived exosomes combined with GM-CSF for colorectal cancer. Mol Ther 2008; 16: 782 – 90. https://doi.org/10.1038/mt.2008.1.

[83] Escudier B, Dorval T, Chaput N, André F, Caby M-P, Novault S, Flament C, Leboulaire C, Borg C, Amigorena S,

Boccaccio C, Bonnerot C, Dhellin O, Movassagh M, Piperno S, Robert C, Serra V, Valente N, Le Pecq J-B, Spatz A, Lantz O, Tursz T, Angevin E, Zitvogel L. Vaccination of metastatic melanoma patients with autologous dendritic cell (DC) derived-exosomes: results of thefirst phase I clinical trial. J Transl Med 2005; 3: 10. https://doi.org/10.1186/1479-5876-3-10.

[84] Morse MA, Garst J, Osada T, Khan S, Hobeika A, Clay TM, Valente N, Shreeniwas R, Sutton MA, Delcayre A, Hsu D-H, Le Pecq J-B, Lyerly HK. A phase I study of dexosome immunotherapy in patients with advanced non-small cell lung cancer. J Transl Med 2005; 3: 9. https://doi.org/10.1186/1479-5876-3-9.

[85] WHO. WHO | Global tuberculosis report, http://www.who.int/tb/publications/global_report/en/; 2018. [accessed 2 March 2019].

[86] O'Garra A, Redford PS, McNab FW, Bloom CI, Wilkinson RJ, Berry MPR. The immune response in tuberculosis. Annu Rev Immunol 2013; 31: 475–527. https://doi.org/10.1146/annurev-immunol-032712-095939.

[87] Cheng Y, Schorey JS. Targeting soluble proteins to exosomes using a ubiquitin tag. Biotechnol Bioeng 2016; 113: 1315–24. https://doi.org/10.1002/bit.25884.

[88] Delcayre A, Estelles A, Sperinde J, Roulon T, Paz P, Aguilar B, Villanueva J, Khine S, Le Pecq J-B. Exosome display technology: applications to the development of new diagnostics and therapeutics. Blood Cells Mol Dis 2005; 35: 158–68. https://doi.org/10.1016/j.bcmd.2005.07.003.

[89] Hartman ZC, Wei J, Glass OK, Guo H, Lei G, Yang X-Y, Osada T, Hobeika A, Delcayre A, Le Pecq J-B, Morse MA, Clay TM, Lyerly HK. Increasing vaccine potency through exosome antigen targeting. Vaccine 2011; 29: 9361–7. https://doi.org/10.1016/j.vaccine.2011.09.133.

[90] Lattanzi L, Federico M. A strategy of antigen incorporation into exosomes: comparing crosspresentation levels of antigens delivered by engineered exosomes and by lentiviral virus-kike particles. Vaccine 2012; 30: 7229–37. https://doi.org/10.1016/j.vaccine.2012.10.010.

[91] Rountree RB, Mandl SJ, Nachtwey JM, Dalpozzo K, Do L, Lombardo JR, Schoonmaker PL, Brinkmann K, Dirmeier U, Laus R, Delcayre A. Exosome targeting of tumor antigens expressed by cancer vaccines can improve antigen immunogenicity and therapeutic efficacy. Cancer Res 2011; 71: 5235–44. https://doi.org/10.1158/0008-5472.CAN-10-4076.

[92] Zeelenberg IS, Ostrowski M, Krumeich S, Bobrie A, Jancic C, Boissonnas A, Delcayre A, Le Pecq J-B, Combadière B, Amigorena S, Théry C. Targeting tumor antigens to secreted membrane vesicles in vivo induces efficient antitumor immune responses. Cancer Res 2008; 68: 1228–35. https://doi.org/10.1158/0008-5472.CAN-07-3163.

[93] Tian Y, Li S, Song J, Ji T, Zhu M, Anderson GJ, Wei J, Nie G. A doxorubicin delivery platform using engineered natural membrane vesicle exosomes for targeted tumor therapy. Biomaterials 2014; 35: 2383–90. https://doi.org/10.1016/j.biomaterials.2013.11.083.

[94] EL Andaloussi S, Mäger I, Breakefield XO, Wood MJA. Extracellular vesicles: biology and emerging therapeutic opportunities. Nat Rev Drug Discov 2013; 12: 347–57. https://doi.org/10.1038/nrd3978.

[95] Alvarez-Erviti L, Seow Y, Yin H, Betts C, Lakhal S, Wood MJA. Delivery of siRNA to the mouse brain by systemic injection of targeted exosomes. Nat Biotechnol 2011; 29: 341–5. https://doi.org/10.1038/nbt.1807.

[96] Ohno S, Takanashi M, Sudo K, Ueda S, Ishikawa A, Matsuyama N, Fujita K, Mizutani T, Ohgi T, Ochiya T, Gotoh N, Kuroda M. Systemically injected exosomes targeted to EGFR deliver antitumor microRNA to breast cancer cells. Mol Ther 2013; 21: 185–91. https://doi.org/10.1038/mt.2012.180.

[97] Schorey JS, Singh PP, Cheng Y. Exosomal biomarkers diagnostic of tuberculosis. 2017. US20170253916A1.

[98] Sheridan C. Exosome cancer diagnostic reaches market. Nat Biotechnol 2016; 34: 359–60. https://doi.org/10.1038/nbt0416-359.

[99] Schorey JS, Cheng Y. Particle size purification method and devices. 2019. US20190011342A1.

[100] Diaz G, Bridges C, Lucas M, Cheng Y, Schorey JS, Dobos KM, Kruh-Garcia NA. Protein digestion, ultrafiltration, and size exclusion chromatography to optimize the isolation of exosomes from human blood plasma and serum. J Vis Exp 2018. https://doi.org/10.3791/57467.

第 7 章

外泌体在 HIV-1 感染中的新兴治疗作用
Emerging therapeutic roles of exosomes in HIV-1 infection

Siew-Wai Pang, Sin-Yeang Teow

Department of Medical Sciences, School of Healthcare and Medical Sciences, Sunway University, Petaling Jaya, Malaysia

一、概述

人类免疫缺陷病毒 1 型（human immunodeficiency virus type 1，HIV-1）和 HIV-2 是引起获得性免疫缺陷综合征（acquired immunodeficiency syndrome，AIDS）的逆转录病毒[1]。病毒通常通过性接触传播，也可以通过共用针头或者母乳喂养从母亲传染给孩子[1]。HIV-1 进入宿主后通过多种途径进行扩散，而 30～100 nm 的外泌体在 HIV-1 的扩散中起着重要作用。膜结合外泌体来源于内体，广泛存在于各种细胞和体液中，如血浆[2]、唾液[3]、尿液[4]、腹水[5]、精液[6]、母乳[7]、CSF[8]、支气管肺泡灌洗（bronchoalveolar lavage，BAL）[9] 和羊水[10] 等。这些纳米大小的囊泡也可由免疫细胞分泌，这些细胞包括但不限于巨噬细胞、B 细胞、T 细胞、DC 和肿瘤细胞[11,12]。外泌体被用于细胞间通信，其所携带的信息可以调节各种细胞的基因表达、细胞增殖和侵袭以及免疫调节[4,11,12]。这些在 30 多年前就被发现了，而且自从发现 B 细胞的外泌体可以将 MHC-II 转运到 T 细胞后，外泌体就成为许多学者研究的课题[13]。2007 年，人类肥大细胞的外泌体就被发现含有 mRNA 和 miRNA，并且这些 RNA 可以对受体细胞产生生物学效应[14,15]。在这篇文章中，我们将回顾外泌体在 HIV-1 发病机制中的影响，以及对外泌体的深入了解如何有助于更好的临床判断。

二、外泌体与 HIV-1：鸡还是蛋？

有趣的是，外泌体的理化性质与 HIV-1 粒子非常相似[16]。所以，外泌体是进化成逆转录病毒还是正好相反的问题就成了该领域科学家们争论的焦点。特洛伊外泌体假说模型认为，外泌体向逆转录病毒的进化是在 gag 基因突变后发生的[17,18]。这一观点得到了这样一个事实的支持，即病毒可以通过预先存在的外泌体途径将病毒传播到缺乏 Env 和受体的细胞[19]。相比之下，第二种理论认为逆转录病毒可能已经进化为利用外泌体途径进行细胞-细胞通信，进而加重病毒的感染[20]。已经证实特洛伊外泌体假说是有误的，因为 HIV-1 的出芽类似于胞外体，这是一种生物化学上不同于外泌体的 EV[21]。虽然这两个理论的结果不一样，但都认为外泌体在 HIV-1 的发病机制中起着至关重要的作用，因为病毒颗粒和外泌体之间的脂质、蛋白质、糖类，甚至 RNA 组成相似。

从物理性质上说，外泌体和HIV-1颗粒有相似的大小和密度，而且都被一个脂质双分子层所包裹。就成分而言，两者都含有胆固醇和鞘糖脂[22]、糖类（高甘露糖和复合N-连接聚糖）[23]和蛋白质（MHC、四次穿膜蛋白、肌动蛋白和TSG101）[24]。外泌体和HIV-1颗粒中RNA含量的类型也十分相似。最近的一项研究还表明，DC分泌外泌体高度依赖于DC的免疫受体，而DC的免疫受体是HIV病毒与DC和CD4+T细胞相互作用的受体。这种受体的抑制减少了外泌体的分泌，这表明HIV-1和外泌体所使用的机制相似[25]。因此，人们认为HIV-1粒子是通过与外泌体合成相同的途径产生[20]。在这个过程中，免疫应答相关分子如MHC-Ⅱ，也可并入病毒颗粒中，以此逃避宿主免疫监视[17]。

外泌体是人类、其他动物和微生物（包括细菌[26]、真菌[27]和原生动物[27]）分泌的EV。除外泌体外，EV可以是凋亡小体或微泡（如外胚体）的形式。外泌体与其他形式的EV（如外胚体）的区别在于囊泡产生的方式及其内含物的不同。外泌体通常由质膜、胞浆或内吞室组装而成，而不存在细胞器和血清蛋白中[28]。它的内容物包括蛋白质、脂类、糖类、小分子和各种类型的RNA，但这些物质如何被装载到外泌体的分子机制仍有待阐明。目前已知的是，转运所需的ESCRT在腔内囊泡形成和外泌体出芽中起重要作用，此外，ESCRT相关蛋白，TSG101也有助于肿瘤细胞外泌体的分泌[15,29]。有趣的是，据报道，外泌体可以通过与ESCRT无关的方式分泌，这种方式涉及四次穿膜蛋白[30,31]。除四次穿膜蛋白外，一组属于小GTP酶家族的蛋白质也被证明参与了囊泡运输的几个过程，包括囊泡的对接、出芽、膜融合和释放。在肿瘤细胞中，RAB家族几个成员的丢失可以迅速消耗完外泌体，充分说明了其在外泌体分泌途径中的重要性[15,32]。

虽然外泌体和病毒颗粒具有许多共同的生化特性，但有几个关键的不同。在结构上，外泌体可能因来源细胞的类型而有很大差异，而HIV颗粒通常是相同的，与受感染细胞的类型无关[33]；在生化上，外泌体的内容物与细胞类型有很大的相关性，而HIV-1颗粒始终携带相同的内容物，例如，HIV-1感染细胞的外泌体富含病毒RNA和Nef等蛋白质[34]。

三、外泌体对HIV-1的双刃剑作用

体液中的外泌体成分差异很大，可以促进或抑制病毒的发病。究竟被抑制还是促进在很大程度上取决于外泌体的细胞来源。例如，来自HIV-1感染细胞的外泌体通常表现出强大的致病性[35]，而来自其他来源的外泌体（如唾液、眼泪、母乳和精液）则具有保护性[4]。图7-1总结了可能促进或抑制HIV-1发病机制的外泌体相关分子。

血液是HIV-1的寄居地，也是HIV-1的传播方式。血液中含有各种类型的细胞，因此也充满了大量不同性质的外泌体[4]。如前所述，感染HIV-1的细胞会分泌外泌体，从而促进病毒的扩散。这些外泌体含有趋化因子受体如CCR5和CXCR4，被传递到受体细胞，通过病毒包膜蛋白与这些受体的结合使HIV-1进入细胞[36]。受感染细胞分泌的含有Nef的外泌体也可诱导T细胞凋亡[34]，下调CD4和MHC-Ⅰ等免疫细胞分子的表达[37]，并抑制各种RNA[38]。而且Nef可以促进外泌体分泌，病毒颗粒的扩散也被增强[34]。病毒逃避免疫的另一种方式是通过外泌体去除一些细胞表面分子，如CD45、CD86和MHC-Ⅱ。此外，病毒颗粒还可以和多种宿主细胞分子结合，从而使其不受如NK细胞等免疫监视细胞的

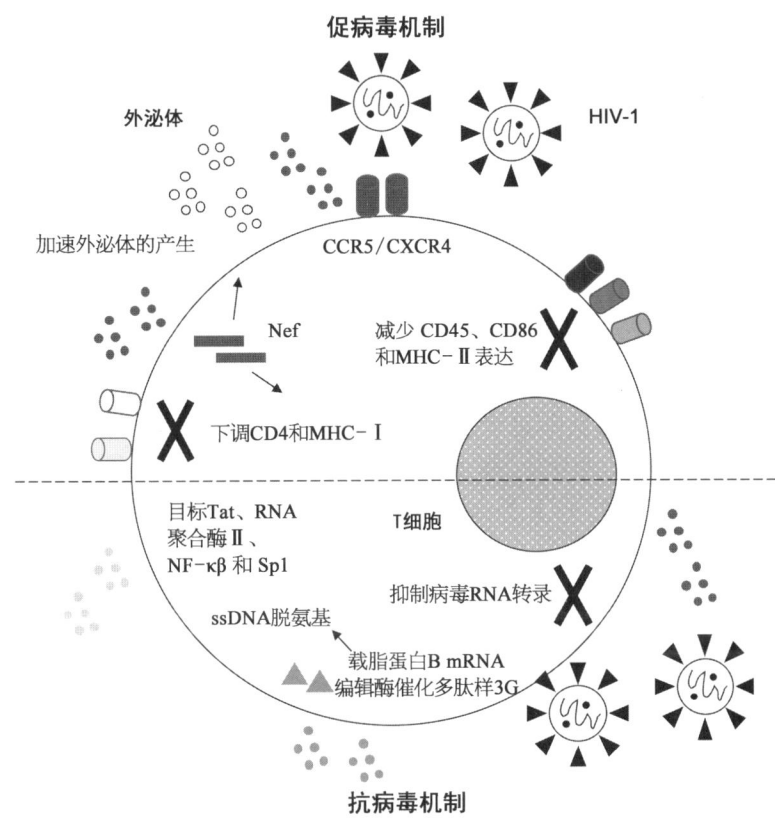

图7-1 外泌体对HIV-1的双刃剑作用。外泌体发挥什么样的作用与细胞类型密切相关。Nef能促进HIV-1相关外泌体的产生,从而促进病毒的进展。Nef还下调宿主免疫防御机制中的关键表面分子,如MHC-Ⅰ和CD4。同样,HIV-1相关的外泌体能够减少CD45、CD86和MHC-Ⅱ表面分子的表达。同时,外泌体上调共同受体CCR5和CXCR4的表达,以促进HIV-1的进入细胞。相反地,外泌体也表现出抗病毒活性。它们能抑制病毒RNA的转录,干扰Tat,RNA聚合酶Ⅱ、NF-κβ和Sp1的功能。外泌体还携带宿主来源的APOBEG3G,抑制HIV-1复制未感染的细胞

影响[4,39]。病毒通过不依赖Env和受体的传播也对当前针对病毒与受体细胞融合的抗病毒策略的发展提出了巨大挑战[19,40]。最近的一项研究提出了这样一种观念,即联合了抗反转录病毒疗法,含有HIV-1病毒产物的EV仍然可以持续释放,从而导致神经认知免疫紊乱[41]。

相比之下,在母乳和精液中发现的外泌体则具有抗病毒特性。虽然如人们期望的一样,母乳的外泌体含有抗病毒特性,能为婴儿提供自然免疫,但令人惊讶的是,精液来源的外泌体也具有抗病毒特性。研究发现精液中的外泌体可以抑制病毒RNA的反转录[28]。然而,这似乎不足以有效地阻止HIV-1的传播,因为性接触仍然是HIV-1感染的主要原因[4]。这些保护特性所涉及的确切机制尚不清楚,但值得研究。2018年,Jennifer Welch及其团队通过生化和功能研究表明,精液外泌体可以在多个转录检查点阻断HIV-1的前病毒转录,包括转录因子向长串联重复序列(long-tandem repeats,LTR)的募集、转录起始和延伸。凝

胶转移分析和 qPCR 技术揭示了精液外泌体的作用靶点,包括病毒蛋白 Tat、人 RNA 聚合酶Ⅱ和人类转录因子 NF-κβ 和 Sp1。本质上说,精液外泌体直接抑制 NF-κβ、RNA 聚合酶Ⅱ和 Sp1 与 LTR 的结合,而 LTR 是 HIV-1 生命周期的组成部分[42]。因此,更多地了解精液的保护特性,有助于预防 HIV-1 的传播。

集体研究也证实了外泌体可以调节免疫系统。例如,NK 细胞的功能是通过外泌体以一种不同于巨噬细胞激活的方式间接增强。据记载,乙型肝炎病毒(hepatitis B virus,HBV)[43]和丙型肝炎病毒(hepatitis C virus,HCV)[44]可以激活 NK 细胞诱导,而且在 HBV 感染的情况下,外泌体的耗竭显著降低了 NK 细胞激活的重要配体的表达[43]。外泌体还通过诱导细胞成熟和增加炎症细胞因子的表达来促进 T 细胞活性,这在细胞免疫和体液免疫中都很重要[45]。巨噬细胞和 DC 是 APC,通过 MHC-Ⅰ和 MHC-Ⅱ向 T 细胞提呈抗原。因此,这两个 APC 的外泌体表面都有 MHC-Ⅰ、MHC-Ⅱ和 T 细胞共刺激分子,这一事实强烈表明,外泌体在抗原提呈过程中非常重要[45,46]。在一定程度上,外泌体可以诱导免疫系统对 HIV-1 产生应答。

载脂蛋白 B mRNA 编辑酶催化多肽样 3G(apolipoprotein B mRNA-editing enzyme-catalytic polypeptide-like 3G,APOBEC3G)是一种宿主细胞蛋白,可以通过外泌体细胞-细胞转移保护受体细胞免受 HIV-1 感染[47,48]。除反转录病毒外,它还被证明能抵抗疱疹病毒、细小病毒、乙型肝炎病毒、乳头状瘤病毒和逆转录转座子[49]。APOBEC3G 是一种腺苷脱氨酶,通过 DNA 编辑或者编辑无关的活动来抑制 HIV-1 的复制[50,51]。前一种机制涉及在反转录过程中单链 DNA(-)胞嘧啶脱氨基为尿嘧啶[49],这可能导致复制子的降解。此外,Bishop 等报道反转录的抑制是通过限制延伸而不是降解[52]。脱氨作用由保守的锌结合结构域催化,但进一步的研究表明,脱氨酶的活性对 APOBEC3G 的抑制作用不是必需的。APOBEC3G 的功能只有在 N-末端和锌结合域都不起作用时才丧失。这表明只要有一个结构域存在对 HIV-1 的抑制作用就足够[51]。值得注意的是,APOBEC3G 的保护作用只有在 HIV-1 的辅助蛋白 Vif 缺失的情况下才明显。在 Vif 存在的情况下,APOBEC3G 被多泛素化并定向用于蛋白酶体降解[53]。此外,APOBEC3G 与 ssDNA 复合物的晶体结构最近才被阐明[54]。这是一个重要的发现,阐述了在原子水平上 APOBEC3G 与 ssDNA 的相互作用。

四、外泌体与自噬

自噬,有时被称为自体吞噬,来源于希腊语中的"自食"。它是一个进化保守的过程,通过溶酶体途径降解半衰期稳定的蛋白质和清除细胞质细胞器,维持细胞水平的稳态和新陈代谢。在某些情况下,不需要或受损的 RNA 和蛋白质通过外泌体释放到细胞外环境中。当这些外泌体被邻近的细胞吸收时,将对宿主产生影响。外泌体分泌有时依赖于自噬系统,自噬的激活可以抑制或促进外泌体的释放[55]。蛋白质的降解和再循环已经被证明可以促进细胞正常发育、死亡、衰老,甚至保护细胞免受感染。肿瘤、炎症、神经退行性疾病和代谢性疾病都可能是自噬途径失调的结果[56]。在 HIV-1 相关的神经退行性疾病中,许多自噬调节基因失调,这反过来可能影响外泌体[55]。

由于外泌体在 HIV-1 的发病机制中起着重要作用,因此了解自噬作用如何影响外泌体的释放是非常重要的。自噬是由 HIV-1 诱导的,但在不同细胞类型和感染状态下,自噬与 HIV-1 的相互作用是十分复杂的[55]。HIV-1 Tat 蛋白能刺激人类胶质细胞自噬,其与溶酶体相关膜蛋白 2A(lysosome associated membrane protein 2A,LAMP2A)的相互作用表明 Tat 促进了神经元自噬体的形成和与溶酶体的融合[57]。此外,在感染 HIV-1 相关脑炎的患者的死后大脑中也观察到自噬活动的增加[58]。这些结果表明尽管确切的机制可能取决于细胞类型,仍有待阐明,但 HIV-1 成分可以诱导自噬[55]。

虽然确切的机制尚不清楚,但已经证明自噬在一定程度上提供了抗 HIV-1 的免疫力。例如,在一项研究中,Espert 和同事观察到 HIV-1 病毒没有在有大量自噬体的巨噬细胞中检测到,而是出现在自噬活性较弱的巨噬细胞中[59]。Sagnier 等推测这可能是由于 Tat 蛋白与自噬蛋白复合物 p62/SQSTM1 之间的相互作用,后者通过溶酶体介导的 $CD4^+$ T 细胞降解来引导 Tat 选择性自噬。此外,Tat 的降解不仅发现在新感染的细胞,还有未受感染的邻近细胞[60]。在另一项研究中,Nardacci 等报道了 HIV-1 感染的长期非进展期患者以及严格控制患者的外周血单个核细胞(peripheral blood mononuclear cell,PBMC)的自噬体和相关标记物与正常进展者相比显著增加[61]。

尽管自噬途径激活并通过溶酶体降解病毒成分可以产生对 HIV-1 的免疫,但是 HIV-1 已经进化出了抗自噬的机制。Nef[62]、Vif[63]和 Tat[64]等病毒蛋白都被证实能抑制自噬途径。在 DC 中,HIV-1 介导 Akt 激活,导致 MHC-Ⅱ 对 $CD4^+$ T 细胞的病毒抗原提呈减少[55]。在自噬受损的情况下,外泌体的形成和释放可作为维持细胞内稳态和改善细胞压力的替代方案。因此,当自噬体的降解被 HIV-1 抑制时,宿主将外泌体转运作为清除病毒成分的另一种方法[34]。简言之,HIV-1 有可能故意破坏自噬,激活外泌体释放,从而使病毒向邻近细胞传播。因此,在受感染细胞中诱导自噬可能会阻止外泌体的产生,从而减少依赖于外泌体的病毒传播[55]。

由于外泌体对 HIV-1 既有致病性又有抗病毒作用,它们在 HIV-1 的治疗中扮演着不同的角色,即要么使治疗更具挑战性,要么提高治疗效果。目前的抗 HIV-1 治疗策略可将致病性外泌体或相关蛋白作为治疗靶点,而抗病毒外泌体则有可能发展成为一种新的抗病毒治疗方式。第 6 章中讨论外泌体的治疗潜力。根据目前已知的线索,探索一种针对 HIV-1 依赖的外泌体途径的抗病毒策略,对于开发新的抗 HIV-1 治疗方法具有很大的潜力。

五、外泌体作为 HIV-1 的生物标志物

以肿瘤患者为例,在体液中发现了携带肿瘤特异性分子的外泌体,其作为肿瘤生物标志物的潜力正在被评估中。虽然外泌体与肿瘤相关的诊断和治疗潜力正在迅速发展中,但 HIV-1 的情况却并非如此。除了传统的抗原-抗体筛选试验,含有 HIV-1 RNA 和其他病毒相关分子的外泌体也可以成为潜在的疾病生物标志物(表 7-1)。这得到了含 HIV-1 RNA 和蛋白质的外泌体存在于 HIV-1 阳性患者血液中这一事实的支持。此外,收集这些外泌体,可以与病毒载量监测一起,评估抗反转录病毒治疗的疗效[15]。

表 7-1　外泌体中可以作为 HIV-1 生物标志物的潜在分子

分　子	生物标志物	功　能	参考文献
MHC Ⅱ	诊断	抗原提呈	[4]
Nef	诊断	病毒复制,免疫逃逸	[65,66]
Vif	诊断	病毒复制,抑制 APOBEC3G	[67]
Vpu	诊断	病毒复制,增强病毒释放	[68]
Vpr	诊断	病毒复制,免疫逃逸	[69]
Gag	诊断	核心结构蛋白	[70]
Tat	诊断	增强病毒转录	[71]
Pol(反转录酶,整合酶,蛋白酶)	诊断	病毒复制	[72]
Env	诊断	包膜蛋白	[72]
Rev	诊断	基因表达	[72]
miRNA	诊断	RNA 沉默和基因表达的转录后调节	[73]
HMGB1	预后	DAMP,alarmin	[74]
NF-L	预后	轴突变性标志物	[74]
Aβ 蛋白	预后	神经炎症、氧化性应激,细胞信号	[74]

　　大量的实验还发现了母乳[53,75]和精液[20,40]中 HIV-1 感染的外泌体对机体有保护作用。当用母乳和精液处理体外细胞时,细胞不易受到感染,这表明这些外泌体可以作为一种预防手段,甚至可以是治疗。2015 年,Madison 等用小鼠艾滋病(murine AIDS,mAIDS)和人类的精液外泌体共同感染小鼠阴道,发现病毒复制受到抑制,病毒的全身播散和载量都降低[21]。虽然我们现在已经知道了外泌体具有保护特性,但其保护特性的机制大多还不清楚[4,15]。

　　近年来,HIV-1 阳性患者尿液中的 EV 被发现是一种非侵入性生物标志物来源。一般来说,蛋白质在健康人的尿液中非常稀少(0.01%),但在某些疾病情况下,蛋白质和 EV 的含量会升高[76]。在感染 HIV-1 的患者中,HIV-1 蛋白包括但不限于 Gag、Pol、Tat、Vif、Vpu、Vpr 等,其中 Nef[77]可以在尿液的 EV 中检测到[78]。所有 HIV-1 阳性的尿样都含有至少一种 HIV-1 相关蛋白的外泌体,而所有 HIV-1 阴性的尿样都不含 HIV-1 蛋白的外泌体。虽然 HIV-1 病毒在尿液中有报道,但其检测的敏感性极低。因此,尿液中的 EV 更加可靠,并有可能用于多种疾病的诊断[78]。Nef 也被证明持续存在于瞬时转染细胞的 EV 中,随体液全身循环,并可通过外泌体转移到未受感染的细胞中,甚至包括缺乏 CD4 的非感染细胞[65]。

　　除尿液外,神经源性外泌体(neuron-derived exosome,NDE)也是 HIV-1 引起认知障碍的潜在生物标志物。神经系统中的许多细胞,包括星形胶质细胞、神经元、小胶质细胞和少突胶质细胞,在正常和病理条件下也会释放出外泌体,这些神经源性外泌体可以穿过血脑屏障进入身体的其他部位,所以可以从大脑[79]、CSF[8]甚至血浆中分离出来[80]。Sun 等研究发现,认知障碍患者的 NDE,无论其 HIV-1 状态如何,HMGB1、NF-L 和 Aβ 蛋白等的含量都会显著增加。虽然 NDE 并不是 HIV-1 特异性的，但 NDE 对于患有 HIV-1 相关认知障碍的患者"实时"监测神经元健康非常有用[74]。

外泌体不仅可以作为 HIV-1 的生物标志物，还可以携带与免疫应答和氧化应激有关的信息。总的来说，HIV-1 阳性患者的血浆外泌体数量高于 HIV-1 阴性对照组，还有氧化应激标志物（如胱氨酸、氧化半胱氨酰甘氨酸、PRDX1、PRDX2、CAT 和 TXN）的增加，以及 EPA、DHA 和 DPA 等多不饱和脂肪酸的减少。免疫激活标志物如 CD14、HLA-A、HLA-B 和 CRP 也被检测到[81]。Chettimada 等发现接受抗反转录病毒治疗（antiretroviral therapy，ART）的 HIV-1 患者的外泌体携带免疫激活和氧化应激蛋白，这些外泌体能够对髓系细胞产生免疫调节作用，也有可能在发病过程中影响促炎和氧化还原反应[81]。

六、靶向外泌体的治疗潜力

（一）以病毒蛋白为靶向

潜在的靶点包括酶（脂肪酶、核糖核酸酶和蛋白酶）、细胞质蛋白（TSG101、MHC-Ⅱ、四次穿膜蛋白和亲环蛋白）和 HIV-1 蛋白（CCR5、CXCR4 和 Nef）[4]。Gag、Pol、Tat、Vif、Vpu 和 Vpr 也是在外泌体中发现的 HIV-1 蛋白，它们也可以成为治疗靶点[78]（图 7-2）。有研究还发现，外泌体抑制剂可以降低 Env 依赖性的感染[28,75]，因此，在当前的抗病毒疗法基础上增加外泌体抑制剂可能可以提高治疗效果。此外，具有抗病毒特性的外泌体可以被提纯，并被开发为治疗手段。

如前所述，外泌体途径中涉及的几种胞质蛋白是潜在的治疗靶点。TSG101，又称抑癌基因 101，是 HIV-1 复制和出芽所需的细胞 ESCRT 的一个组成部分[82]。MHC-Ⅱ是细胞表面蛋白，其通过与 T 细胞相互作用和提呈抗原的能力参与免疫反应的调节[83]。虽然 MHC-Ⅱ在调节对病原体的免疫反应中很重要，但研究发现，MHC-Ⅱ在 T 细胞中的高表达与 HIV-1 的表达增加有关[84,85]。MHC-Ⅱ的高表达促进 HIV-1 颗粒的组装和释放。尽管 MHC-Ⅱ是一个的治疗靶点，但需要注意的是，它的抑制会导致抗原提呈

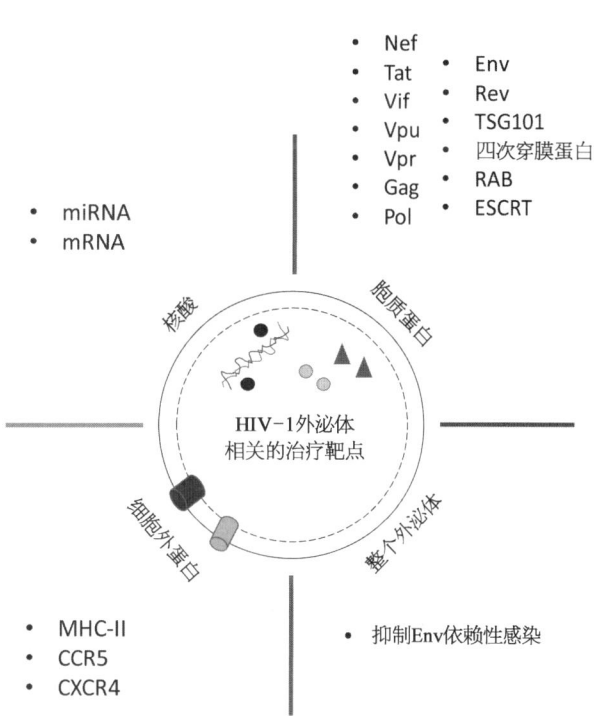

图 7-2　外泌体对 HIV-1 的治疗应用。有多种外泌体相关的分子可能成为抗病毒治疗的靶点。这些包括细胞外蛋白（如 MHC-Ⅱ、CCR5 和 CXCR4）、细胞质蛋白（如 HIV 蛋白、TSG101、ESCRT、RAB 等）、核酸（如 mRNA 和 miRNA）以及整个外泌体

能力的丧失,从而导致对其他病原体的易感性增加[84]。

CCR5 和 CXCR4 是相关 G 蛋白偶联趋化因子受体,HIV-1 利用这些受体进入细胞。CCR5 缺陷个体对 CCR5 依赖性的 HIV-1 感染具有高度的抵抗力,但由于病毒可通过 CXCR4 进入细胞而不能完全抵抗[86]。HIV-1 感染细胞也能通过外泌体将这些受体输出到受体细胞,从而扩大感染范围[4]。因此,可以把这些受体和包含受体的外泌体作为治疗靶点[86]。有两种方法可以阻止受体配体的结合:第一,根据这些受体的生物学表现和作用机制,使用药物诱导硬脂酸封锁 CCR5/CXCR4 结合域。第二,药物可以作为这些受体内化或再循环的诱导剂,从而在病毒面前掩蔽受体细胞。这两种方法都可以抑制 HIV-1 进入细胞[87-89]。尽管如此,但因为 CCR5 在宿主免疫系统中起非常重要的作用,抑制 CCR5 可能会产生很多不良反应。

Nef 蛋白是由灵长类慢病毒(包括 HIV-1、HIV-2 和 SIV)表达的辅助蛋白。Nef 蛋白对病毒的生存必不可少,它通过下调重要的细胞表面分子来促进病毒的复制和感染。这些表面分子包括 MHC-Ⅰ、MHC-Ⅱ、CD4 和 CD28,都对抗病毒的免疫反应至关重要。这就使得疫苗的研制变得困难,因为没有 APC 的正常工作,免疫系统就无法消灭受感染的细胞。Geyer 等详细研究了 Nef 蛋白的功能基序和结构,可以作为药物和治疗发展的参考[90]。最近,Dekaban 和 Dikakos 发现 Nef 抑制剂,这是一种可以阻断 Nef MHC-Ⅰ的下调功能的 2c 样化合物[91],从而导致免疫细胞抗原提呈功能的恢复并允许细胞毒性 T 细胞介导的杀伤受感染细胞作用。因此,这种抑制剂有可能作为疫苗的免疫佐剂。然而,Dekaban 也强调目前的 2c 样 Nef 抑制剂只恢复细胞表面的 MHC-Ⅰ,所以需要开发第二代 2c 类的 Nef 抑制剂来阻断 Nef 的其他有害功能[91]。

除了 Nef 蛋白,Gag、Pol 和 Env 也是在外泌体中发现的病毒蛋白,也可能被用于治疗。HIV-1 Gag 是病毒组装的主要协调器,对感染性颗粒的形成和释放至关重要。这使得它成为药物开发的一个十分有吸引力的目标。到目前为止,已经有了针对 Gag 的药物,其他新型抗病毒药物也正在开发中[92]。Env 蛋白通过与 CD4 和 CCR5/CXCR4 共受体的相互作用介导病毒进入宿主细胞。进入的过程十分复杂,容易受到小分子的抑制。Herschhorn 等已经发现几种潜在的 Env 抑制剂,并确定一种新化合物 18A,但仍需要进一步研究[93]。HIV-1 编码的包含逆转录酶的聚合酶是复制所必需的。以聚合酶为靶点的核苷类似物是最早显示临床疗效的几种药物之一,同时被广泛用于治疗 HIV-1、肝炎和单纯疱疹病毒[94]。

Vpr、Vpu 和 Vif 是参与病毒复制的病毒蛋白,也存在于外泌体中。Vpr 蛋白可被苏木精及其衍生物抑制[95]。Vpu 是另一个潜在的治疗靶点,因为它下调宿主蛋白 BST-2,而 BST-2 可以抑制病毒颗粒释放[96]。此外,Vif 以其抑制 APOBEC3G 的能力而闻名,APOBEC3G 是一种通过诱导高频突变来抑制 HIV-1 复制的蛋白质。Pery 等发现了一种可以抑制 Vif-APOBEC3G 相互作用,同时提高细胞 APOBEC3G 水平,减少病毒颗粒的化合物[97]。

Tat 和 Rev 都是对病毒基因表达很重要的蛋白质。如果没有 Tat 参与病毒转录,HIV-1 将大部分停留在潜伏期[71]。Balachandran 等最近的一项研究揭示了一些小分子不仅可以抑制 Tat 和 Rev,还可以抑制 Gag 和 Env 的蛋白表达。虽然这些分子显示出巨大的潜力,但其生物效应仅在体内得到证实[98]。

CD4⁺T 细胞的丧失是 HIV-1 感染的标志性特征之一,HIV-1 感染的 DC 存在于黏膜组织中,并通过外泌体促进 HIV-1 的传播和存在。与此相反,一项研究表明,与对照组相比,在 HIV-1 存在的情况下,DC 有更多的外泌体生成。通过上调促调亡蛋白如 Apaf-1 和 Dap-3,外泌体的大量产生使得病毒感染性降低和 CD4 细胞凋亡率下降。然而,这些蛋白质在多大程度上影响细胞凋亡尚不清楚。通过这项研究,现在已经知道,感染 HIV-1 的 DC 可以显著提高外泌体分泌[99]。另一个研究小组还发现,外泌体释放是通过与调节免疫系统相关的特定受体来刺激[100]。根据这些结果,我们可以得知,外泌体很可能通过调节免疫系统来发挥细胞因子的作用。有趣的是,Subra 还发现成熟的 DC 与未成熟 DC 相比,外泌体释放更多,这表明外泌体可能在炎症反应中起重要作用。总之,DC 来源的外泌体具有免疫调节特性,有助于抵抗 HIV-1。然而,由于 HIV-1 容易适应其微环境,将 DC 衍生的外泌体作为治疗工具存在一些挑战[101]。

有趣的是,HIV-1 蛋白 Tat 最近被证明可以激活原代静止 CD4⁺T 细胞中潜伏的 HIV-1,使 HIV-1 mRNA 表达增加 30 倍以上。Tang 等将这些蛋白质包装成外泌体,并以最小的细胞毒性处理受感染的静止 CD4⁺T 细胞,发现这是一种特定的 HIV-LTR 激活,而不是普通的免疫刺激[71]。Tat 蛋白激活已经开始转录的前病毒 DNA 的 LTR 区域的 HIV-1 启动子,其在动物模型和人类身上的安全性和耐受性已得到充分的证明[102,103]。也就是说,Tat 不太可能重新激活所有潜伏的病毒,而是先激活已经开始转录的前病毒。此外,含有 Tat 的外泌体生成可能比较烦琐,暂时不适合临床应用[71]。

(二)以病毒 RNA 为靶向

在过去的 30 年里,基于 RNA 的 *HIV-1* 基因治疗取得了显著进展,其中包括反义-单链 RNA(single-stranded RNA,ssRNA)[104,105]、核酶[104]、RNA 诱饵[106]、RNA 干扰(RNA interference,RNAi)[107]以及涉及 Cas9 和单导 RNA 的 CRISPR[108]。这些 RNA 靶点抑制活跃的复制和消除隐藏感染库的能力也得到充分的证明[109]。为了使以 RNA 为靶向的治疗成功,它们必须被送到靶组织,并且在有效的时间内达到并稳定在足够的剂量。而 RNA 具有不稳定性,很容易被宿主的免疫系统通过 RNA 酶清除掉。此外,RNA 的亲水性降低了它对受体细胞脂质膜的亲和力,相对较大的 RNA 也不易穿过细胞膜。因此,细胞对 RNA 的吸收效果不佳,从而降低抗病毒效果。种种局限性要求更有效的 RNA 传递系统来提高药物的生物利用度。传统的药物传递方法,如病毒载体、脂质体、纳米聚合物和靶肽都很常用,但即使不断地改进,它们也不能满足有效基因治疗的要求[104]。

外泌体将是这些药物传递系统的替代品,因为外泌体是人体自然产生的,而 RNA(如 mRNA 和 miRNA)从一个细胞传递到另一个细胞在许多物种不同情况下都会发生[4]。前面提到的 RNA 可以被装载在外泌体上,通过不同的机制特异性识别和靶向病毒蛋白或核酸。反义 ssRNA 可通过与 HIV-1 RNA 形成互补碱基对或阻断核糖体结合,来诱导 RNA 酶 H 降解 RNA[105]。核酶,特别是锤头状核酶和发夹状核酶,是具有催化活性的小 RNA 分子,可被设计成切割病毒 RNA 的特定序列[104]。RNA 诱饵也是 ssRNA,其序列与病毒

RNA相似。因此,它与病毒RNA竞争结合复制的相关调节蛋白,如核糖体[106]。另一方面,RNAi是一种自然发生的现象[110],它可以通过组装RNA诱导沉默复合体(RNA-induced silencing complex,RISC)使HIV-1基因的表达沉默,导致mRNA在严格调控中降解。RISC可以以双链siRNA或者短发夹RNA的形式引入[107]。最后,CRISPR是一种相对较新的技术,被认为是分子生物学的未来。它是从化脓性链球菌[111]对抗噬菌体[112]的过程中发现的适应性免疫系统。它由Cas9蛋白和一种短导RNA组成,该RNA具有针对要切割的目标DNA设计的特定序列[108]。目前,已经成功地通过大量的切割使HIV-1的整合DNA永久失活。但目前的治疗方法仍无法有效地抑制整合前病毒DNA的活性[113]。

外泌体是抗HIV-1 RNA的理想纳米载体。原因包括:第一,单核吞噬细胞系统通常清除直径大于100 nm的颗粒,而外泌体体积小,可以逃脱单核吞噬细胞系统的吞噬作用。这样就可以在体内保留携带RNA的外泌体。第二,外泌体是由人体内的细胞产生的,因此细胞毒性较小,与免疫系统的生物相容性更强。事实上,一些外泌体具有特殊的免疫状态,可以逃脱免疫。第三,外泌体能够跨越生物屏障,如黏膜屏障和血脑屏障,而人工纳米载体和其他药物传递系统则不能。特别是,来源于精液的外泌体已经被证明能够自然地穿过黏膜屏障[15],大脑内皮细胞衍生的外泌体可以穿过血脑屏障[114]。第四,外泌体对受体细胞具有很高的亲和力,可以通过膜融合、吞噬或内吞作用促进其与细胞充分融合[115-117]。最后,外泌体对肝脏的亲和力很低,不用经过肝脏加工运输,因而外泌体毒性较低[118]。因此,外泌体以最小的损耗被有效地运输到其预定的接收单元。

在过去的20年里,治疗性外泌体在体内的应用已经取得了成功,并且这种外泌体在肿瘤治疗中的应用也在蓬勃发展中[119]。虽然外泌体在HIV-1治疗中的应用仍处于初级阶段,但通过治疗性RNA外泌体在肿瘤治疗中所收集的结果和数据有助于开发类似的HIV-1治疗系统。三种不同的方法可用于HIV-1治疗的外泌体和RNA的装载。第一种方法是直接用RNA装载从亲代细胞中分离出的外泌体,这个过程包括冻融、超声、渗透和转染等步骤。这种方法是将RNA负载到外泌体的最方便、最直接的方法,可以在几次分离的过程中产生大量的RNA外泌体。并且,几种不同细胞类型的外泌体可以同时装载[104,120]。第二种方法是将外源RNA装载到亲代细胞中,然后在外泌体合成时,通过向内出芽将RNA包裹在外泌体中,然后释放和分离外泌体。这种方法不常用,但是有效。但Qazi等研究发现,仅仅通过使用RNA装载方法,在体内和体外对免疫反应的激发可能会有所不同[104,121]。第三种方法需要用可以转录成具有治疗能力RNA的DNA转染或感染亲代细胞,然后将其包裹在外泌体中。这种方法产生的RNA具有很好的完整性,但价格昂贵,需要专门的设备。此外,MSC能产生大量的外泌体,Yeo等建议将它们作为临床上外泌体的体外生产者[122]。这种方法的另一个优点是可以使用转染的永生化MSC获得连续的外泌体供应[123],与第一种装载分离外泌体的方法相比,该方法的合理性已经被证实。也有证据表明,在小鼠模型中,转基因巨噬细胞能够持续产生负载RNA的外泌体,所以产生这种外泌体的细胞可以帮助减轻40天以上的神经炎症[124]。虽然这三种方法在产生和分离RNA外泌体方面有着相同的目的,但具体使用哪种方法将取决于设备、设施、亲本细胞类型以及实验的总体目标和设计[104]。虽然我们现有的技术和手段可以将抗HIV-1 RNA装载到外泌体中,但下一步能否将外泌体有效地运输到其预期的受体细胞也是关键。外泌体通常通过表面黏附蛋白或其他分子与受体细胞结合。为了最大限度地提高外泌体转运的效率,需要使外泌体的表面蛋白与受体细胞具有高亲和力。但是,外泌体靶向 CD4 T 细胞的表面修饰过程尚未建立。Yong 等建议将 gp-120 的 DNA 与外泌体蛋白 Lamp2b(gp-120 fused with exosomal protein Lamp2b,Lamp2b-gp120)融合在一个能同时表达抗 HIV 短发夹 RNA 的多顺反子质粒中,并将其转染到亲代细胞中[104]。

虽然外泌体的 RNA 负载和表面修饰给 HIV-1 治疗带来了巨大希望,但总的来说仍存在许多障碍和不确定性。目前已知的蛋白质家族包括 RAB[125]、四次穿膜蛋白[31]和 ESCRT[29]都参与了外泌体装载过程。外泌体装载及其背后的精确机制仍不清楚,需要进一步阐明[126]。由于种种原因,目前尚不清楚通过转染/感染的 RNA 是否能够被有效地输送,并且质粒表达的表面蛋白能否被成功地装配到外泌体上。更重要的是,外泌体先天地承载着大量的内源性物质,这些物质来源于亲本细胞,可能抑制人工合成的物质或对受体细胞产生毒性。现有内源性物质也可能限制外泌体储存更多的外源性物质。如何选择获得外泌体的亲本细胞也是至关重要的,这将决定外泌体的产量[104]。最后,如果一切顺利,外泌体的生产需要扩大到临床应用。Hupfeld 和 Mitchell 等已经证明,与培养瓶法相比,专门设计的生物反应器系统具有更优越的外泌体产量[127,128]。

七、经验教训

(一)了解外泌体通路在修订病毒治疗策略中的作用

随着外泌体研究的不断深入,特别是在肿瘤领域,外泌体在病毒发病过程中的途径、机制、理化结构、介质和信号级联反应等方面的研究已成为研究病毒致病机制的重要关注点。研究表明,肿瘤细胞和病毒都可以利用外泌体作为免疫逃避的手段,其包括但不限于下调表面分子[4,129],以及将有害分子从细胞中输出[4,130]。此外,外泌体也可以改善肿瘤和病毒的进展[4,130]。随着外泌体的作用逐渐阐明,我们发现病毒和肿瘤在外泌体合成方面具有相似性,可以考虑在 HIV-1 感染的细胞中寻找针对肿瘤的潜在治疗药物。

如前所述,一些用于治疗 HIV-1 的抗反转录病毒药物通过抑制病毒-细胞融合来阻止病毒进入细胞。HIV-1 可以通过外泌体进行不依赖 Env 和受体的传播,因此,需要一种更好的治疗策略,这种策略可能是外泌体抑制药物和核苷逆转录酶抑制剂的结合。此外,从精液中纯化的外泌体也被发现可以抑制 HIV-1 复制[42]。了解诱导外泌体释放的刺激物也变得很有趣,也许这种外泌体可以在 HIV-1 感染的高危个体中被人为刺激释放。

介质也可以用于治疗。例如,外泌体可以被设计包含这些特定的介质,或者可以设计出更有效的类似物以获得更好的抗病毒性能。可以设计一种类似精液外泌体的纳米颗粒输送系统,其能被有效地运输到其受体部位,并且能够穿过其他囊泡系统无法克服的黏膜屏障[15]。

(二)外泌体检测与表征技术进展

1. 一般方法

外泌体和细胞源性囊泡在体液中含量丰富,可以携带有关个人健康和疾病状况的重要信息。正因为如此,囊泡的检测在临床和科研上都引起了广泛的兴趣。多年来,世界各地的研究人员开发了许多技术来检测和/或量化囊泡,但这些技术仍不完善,因为它们通常很难检测到极小尺寸的囊泡(小于 100 nm)。而当这些囊泡的折射率较低、形状和大小不同时,就更具挑战性[131]。传统的方法是通过超速离心法分离外泌体,但这需要长时间的分离、设备昂贵、产量低、回收率低、纯度不高和特异性低。等密度离心法是超速离心法的一个改进版本,可以以更高的纯度和产量回收外泌体,但在时间和设备方面,它与超离心法有相同的局限性。这使得这两种技术在临床环境中都不实用[132]。考虑到这些问题,科学家们通过囊泡的其他特性,设想出了几种检测方法[131]。几种相对高通量的囊泡检测方法包括流式细胞术、RPS 和 NTA。

2. 流式细胞术

流式细胞术早在 2 000 年以前就已经被用于研究囊泡,但这种方法已经到了检测小颗粒的极限,因此很难避免假阳性或伪影小泡的出现。这种方法通过前向散射和侧散射来检测和量化囊泡,类似于细胞如何通过"流"进行排序和量化。

随着 NTA 和 RPS 等其他技术的出现,人们知道流式细胞术在检测单个颗粒的极小囊泡时不够敏感,从而引发了人们对更好检测方法的研究。同时,也有人试图使囊泡的测量标准化。然而,到目前为止,还没有检测囊泡的金标准[131]。2017 年,Suarez 和他的研究小组展示了一种改进的流式细胞术,这种方法可以通过使用涂有抗囊泡蛋白(如四次穿膜蛋白、MHC 分子和 CD59)抗体的微珠,进行 EV 的半定量分析,并且在大多数实验室中轻松应用,同时具有足够的准确度[133]。

3. RPS

RPS 是一种利用 Coulter 原理检测和测量大于 50 nm 纳米颗粒的方法[134,135]。它在分析过程中观察电流的变化,变化越大,囊泡的体积就越大。这样可以精确测量单个囊泡的大小[134]。

这种技术的局限性通常取决于所使用的仪器,由于 qNano(新西兰基督城 Izon 公司)仪器中孔隙的堵塞会阻碍结果的周转时间,其不适合作为临床诊断工具[131]。

4. NTA

NTA 是一种由 Nanosight 公司(英国埃姆斯伯里)商业化的技术,与 RPS 类似,它测量悬浮液中囊泡的分布,范围大于 50 nm。与前者的区别在于,囊泡在激光照射下散射光或发射荧光,然后通过暗视野显微镜跟踪由布朗运动引起的囊泡的位置,并测量每个小泡的均方速度。布朗运动的均方速度由囊泡的直径决定,因此将得知囊泡的绝对大小分布[132,134,136]。NTA 还可以通过荧光标记来测量囊泡亚群的大小[131,137]。就其在临床诊断中的应用而言,NTA 使用方便,因为它只需几分钟进行分析。样本可视化的实时反馈也有助于识别囊泡分离后细胞的存在。

这种方法的限制是每次测量生成的每个视频数据的大小可以达到 2 GB,因此需要相当大的存储空间和强大的处理硬件。由于数据涉及多个操作和变量,还需要熟练的操作员来处理[131]。

5. 免疫测定

酶联免疫吸附试验(enzyme-linked immunosorbent assay,ELISA)是一种利用特异性

抗体固定靶抗原,然后用含有荧光团/发色团的二级抗体检测荧光的方法。一些研究人员通过囊泡蛋白,如四次穿膜蛋白、CD9、CD63 和 CD81 来检测外泌体[138]。用这种方法发出的信号与样本中的外泌体蛋白量成正比。另一方面,侧流免疫层析法(lateral flow immunoassay,LFIA)与 ELISA 有相似的原理,它也利用抗体捕捉抗原。然而,这些样本首先与附着在金纳米粒子上的检测抗体混合,以便于观察。使用 LFIA 时,检测信号与样本中的外泌体蛋白量成反比。这是因为外泌体可以被抗体完全覆盖,产生强烈的硬脂酸障碍,从而阻止抗体捕获抗原。

如前所述,在临床诊断中使用 ELISA 或 LFIA 需要谨慎,因为这两种方法对于外泌体蛋白的丰度给出完全不同的结果。此外,由于不同患者的丰度差异很大,目前临床上可能不适合使用 ELISA 或 LFIA。当然,由于免疫分析在大多数研究和临床实验室都很容易获得,它在临床诊断方面的潜力仍有待探索[138]。

6. 其他方法

近年来,外泌体和囊泡检测技术有了很大的进展。许多技术还没有商业化,但很有可能在临床应用中快速准确地测量外泌体。它们包括但不限于 Liu 小组的微柱上的纳米线[139]、Lee 和 Weissleder 小组的声学分类[140]、Trau 小组的交流电流体动力学诱导的纳米剪切[141]、Ozcan 小组的芯片上纳米生物成像[142]、Lee 和 Weissleder 小组的磁共振[143]、Grigorenko 小组的表面等离子体共振[144,145]、无标记频率锁定微环光学谐振器[146]等。

(三)外泌体临床应用的挑战

如前面几节所述,外泌体应用于临床需要克服一些挑战。为了使外泌体应用于临床,必须大规模生产。1 mL 培养基一般产生少于 1 μg 的外泌体蛋白,而大多数研究的有效剂量为 10~100 μg。外泌体通常是通过在培养基中培养产生外泌体的细胞来制备的,这个过程长达几天,但是 Richies 和 Yamashita 等发现这取决于不同的细胞类型,外泌体的产生在孵育 12 小时后就结束[73,147]。如前所述,使用生物反应器可能有助于提高外泌体产量[127]。此外,在低 pH、抗癌药物治疗和缺氧等应激条件下,外泌体的产量也是增加的[148]。然而,这些情况下产生的外泌体组成发生了变化,应仔细评估这些应激诱导的外泌体的潜在有害影响。此外,应激诱导的外泌体可能含有高水平的凋亡小体,这可能产生不良影响和高估外泌体计数[73]。外泌体的有效分离是另一种有待探索的方法。如前所述,超速离心法是一种分离外泌体的方法,对该方法进行一些改进可以提高分离率。此外,分子排阻色谱法[149]、双水相系统[150]、聚合物沉淀法[151]和超滤[152]等可用于大规模的外泌体生产[73]。然而,值得注意的是,这些不同方法在外泌体产量、资源、时间和效率方面的差异尚未得到适当的比较和评估,因此需要进一步关注。

与外泌体的临床应用相关的另一个挑战是收集统一和高质量的外泌体。如前所述,有许多方法可以分离和纯化外泌体。分离方法将极大地影响外泌体的理化性质和纯度[153]。具体地说,有三种不同的超速离心方法可用于外泌体纯化,包括简单造粒法、密度缓冲法和密度梯度法[153]。简单的造粒方法易于进行,运行成本相对较低,但分离出的外泌体可能受到蛋白质的高度污染。密度缓冲法和密度梯度法均能得到高纯度的外泌体,后者对外泌体比较温和,但样品容量较低。由于缺乏效率,超速离心可能不是临床分离外泌体的理想方法。另一方面,聚合物沉淀法会导致污染和严重聚合,因此不适合用于临床[151]。根据大小的分离,如超滤[152]和大小排阻色谱[149]也有各自的优缺点。前一种方法非常有效,但产生低纯度的外泌体,并且可能受到剪切应力的破坏;而色谱法产生的外泌体纯度较高,但样品容量较低[149,152]。

另一个需要考虑的因素是外泌体亚群的存在,它们的大小和组成各不相同[154]。不同的分离方法将分离出不同的亚群[155]。这使得外泌体在治疗中的应用更加复杂,因为具有不同理化性质的亚群可能会产生不同的生物学效应。综上所述,不同的分离方法会产生不同纯度、不同理化性质和组成的外泌体。为了使其在治疗应用中产生疗效,必须对分离方法进行最好的优化,以保持外泌体的特性,并确保每个生产批次外泌体含量的一致性[73]。

在成功分离提纯外泌体后,下一个挑战是如何保存外泌体。外泌体可在−80℃下储存在 PBS 中[156]。海藻糖的添加已经被证明可以保护外泌体免受低温伤害[157]。较高的温度会导致外泌体减少[80],但在临床中是可以接受的,因此它不需要专门的设备。虽然有一项明确的证据表明,心脏来源细胞的外泌体可以在生物活性损失最小的情况下冻干[158],但没有其他的证据表明这将适用于其他来源的外泌体。冻干外泌体的保质期尚不清楚,需要进行更多的研究来回答这些不确定性[73]。

现在我们讨论了在治疗应用中使用外泌体的策略,无论是否经过修饰,我们都将纯化的外泌体输送到患者体内。外泌体的生物学效应只有在被预期的受体细胞吸收后才能知道,因此控制外泌体的体内分布是非常重要的。Takahashi 等报道静脉注射的外泌体在脾、肝和肺中快速积聚[159]。而在肝脏和脾脏中,这些外泌体最终被巨噬细胞吞噬,这可能是因为外泌体膜中含磷脂酰丝氨酸[160]。由于 Wiklander 等的研究,我们现在知道注射的途径会影响外泌体的体内分布[161]。特别是,腹腔注射导致胃肠道和胰腺外泌体积聚,而皮下注射导致所有测量器官都有少量外泌体积聚。一般来说,无论细胞来源和给药途径如何,大多数注射的外泌体最终进入网状内皮系统的巨噬细胞中[161]。血液中外泌体的快速清除将限制全身给药,因此需要研究外泌体在宿主体内更好的输送和生物稳定性。

当涉及以外泌体内容物为治疗靶向或抑制外泌体内容物时,也具有挑战性。如前所述,Balachandran 等已经确定了几个小分子,它们在阻断 Tat、Rev、Env 和 Gag 的蛋白表达方面表现出巨大的潜力[98]。虽然这些药物在非外泌体环境下可能有效,但在穿透外泌体方面可能没有那么有效。研究表明,外泌体与其内容物的装载需要几个蛋白质的参与,如 RAB[125]、ESCRT[29]和四次穿膜蛋白[31],但确切的机制仍不清楚[104]。此外,由于外泌体的生物理化性质因细胞来源而异[33],外泌体表面分子可能会有所不同,这可能会限制小分子通过硬脂酸阻碍进入。此外,外泌体的表面通常带有负电荷[104],这可能使一些药物或分子由于静电排斥而失效。

(四)提高外泌体治疗效果

由于在临床应用中生成外泌体很难,一个可能的解决方案是提高其治疗潜力。治疗分子或蛋白质的过度表达是提高疗效的一种简单方法。Zhang 和 Qu 等发现 miRNA 的过度表达增加了外泌体的治疗效果[162,163]，其中增加 miRNA 表达谱的过表达也是另一种有效的方法[164,165]。另一种方法是用功能分子修饰外泌体。Morishita 等通过用免疫佐剂 CpG-DNA 修饰 B16BL6 衍生的外泌体，将诱导肿瘤抗原特异性免疫反应所需的外泌体剂量减少了 100 倍[166]。此外，缺氧也被报道可以改变外泌体成分，从而改善外泌体的生物效应[167,168]。虽然将这些修饰应用于临床应用是很有吸引力的，但是外泌体结构和成分的改变可能会导致未知的不良反应。因此，必须单独评估外泌体修饰的安全性和效果[73]。

（五）展望

我们现在知道，HIV-1 的进展可以通过外泌体在宿主的合成途径而大大增强，并且可以通过外泌体以不依赖受体和 Env 的途径传播。此外，从母乳和精液中提取的外泌体的抗病毒特性已在多个论著中得到证实，其中部分还解释了精液外泌体的作用机制[42]。考虑到这些矛盾，现有的 HIV-1 治疗的策略需要重新评估，找到更好的治疗方法。由于我们现在知道 HIV-1 可以通过受体和 Env 非依赖性途径中的外泌体进行传播，一个更明智的方法是研究先前讨论过的外泌体抑制剂。也就是说，治疗的特异性必须相当高，因为外泌体不仅在其他生理功能中起着重要作用，还携带着宿主丰富的遗传和蛋白质组学信息。随着技术的不断进步，在没有昂贵设备的情况下，在临床中准确地检测和测量外泌体开始慢慢实现。对检测外泌体和囊泡的方法进行简单的文献检索，可以得到从 ELISA、LFIA 和流式细胞术到能够检测单个外泌体的先进技术。这是因为外泌体不仅与 HIV-1 和其他病毒（如 HBV[16]、HCV[169] 和 HSV[170]）感染有关，它们也是肿瘤发病和进展的主要因素[132]。在临床中进行外泌体检测和测量设备将有可能改进和补充现有的 HIV-1、其他病毒和肿瘤检测。除检测外，含有抗病毒特性的纯化外泌体还可能用于高危人群的预防或 HIV-1 感染患者的治疗。随着对精液外泌体抑制机制的最新发现，外泌体可以被改造成含有类似抑制作用的介质或蛋白质。

八、总结

总的来说，宿主外泌体可以通过细胞间传播和免疫逃避来促进 HIV-1 的发病，而一些研究表明，来自母乳和精液的外泌体具有抗病毒的特性。这表明，外泌体的性质取决于细胞来源、受体细胞及其内含物。由于 HIV-1 可以通过外泌体进行传播，深入了解外泌体在 HIV-1 发病机制中的作用将有助于制订更全面的治疗策略。目前，检测、测量和纯化外泌体的方法仍然需要大量的操作，不适合临床应用。然而，这在未来将发生变化，因为可以看到关于外泌体和囊泡检测方法更新的文章越来越多。具有抗病毒特性的外泌体也是潜在的治疗方法，能够补充现有的治疗方法。最后，即使在肿瘤研究领域，我们对外泌体生物学及其在肿瘤中所起作用的理解也仅仅停留在表面。关于 HIV-1 外泌体的研究要少得多，如果我们要实现一个没有 HIV-1 的世界，需要不停地改进。随着外泌体的发现越来越多，无论是对肿瘤或 HIV-1，这将推动发展强大和敏感的测试，以帮助临床决策。

（陈金梅　译，陈小华　审校）

参考文献

[1] Mabuka J, Nduati R, Odem-Davis K, Peterson D, Overbaugh J. HIV-specific antibodies capable of ADCC are common in breastmilk and are associated with reduced risk of transmission in women with high viral loads. PLoS Pathog 2012; 8(6): e1002739.

[2] Caby MP, Lankar D, Vincendeau-Scherrer C, Raposo G, Bonnerot C. Exosomal-kike vesicles are present in human blood plasma. Int Immunol 2005; 17(7): 879–87.

[3] Michael A, Bajracharya SD, Yuen PST, Zhou H, Star RA, Illei GG, Alevizos I. Exosomes from human saliva as a source of microRNA biomarkers. Oral Dis 2010; 16(1): 34–8.

[4] Teow SY, Nordin AC, Ali SA, Khoo AS. Exosomes in human immunodeficiency virus type I pathogenesis: threat or opportunity? Adv Virol 2016; 2016: 9852494.

[5] Andre F, Schartz NEC, Movassagh M, Flament C, Pautier P, Morice P, et al. Malignant effusions and immunogenic tumour-derived exosomes. Lancet 2002; 360(9329): 295–305.

[6] Sullivan R, Saez F, Girouard J, Frenette G. Role of exosomes in sperm maturation during the transit along the male reproductive tract. Blood Cells Mol Dis 2005; 35(1): 1–10.

[7] Admyre C, Johansson SM, Qazi KR, Filen J-J, Lahesmaa R, Norman M, et al. Exosomes with immune modulatory features are present in human breast milk. J Immunol 2007; 179(3): 1969–78.

[8] Street JM, Barran PE, Mackay CL, Weidt S, Balmforth C, Walsh TS, et al. Identification and proteomic profiling of exosomes in human cerebrospinal fluid. J Transl Med 2012; 10(1): 5.

[9] Admyre C, Grunewald J, Thyberg J, Gripenbäck S, Tornling G, Eklund A, et al. Exosomes with major histocompatibility complex class II and co-stimulatory molecules are present in human BAL fluid. Eur Respir J 2003; 22(4): 578–83.

[10] Keller S, Rupp C, Stoeck A, Runz S, Fogel M, Lugert S, et al. CD24 is a marker of exosomes secreted into urine and amniotic fluid. Kidney Int 2007; 72(9): 1095–102.

[11] Teow SY, Peh SC. Exosomes as the promising biomarker of Epstein-Barr virus (EBV)-associated cancers. In: Novel implications of exosomes in diagnosis and treatment of cancer and infectious diseases. vol. 5; 2017. p. 97–114.

[12] Teow SY, Liew K, Khoo ASB, Peh SC. Pathogenic role of exosomes in Epstein-Barr virus (EBV)-associated cancers. Int J Biol Sci 2017; 13(10): 1276–86.

[13] Raposo G, Nijman HW, Stoorvogel W, Liejendekker R, Harding CV, Melief CJ, Geuze HJ. B lymphocytes secrete antigen-presenting vesicles. J Exp Med 1996; 183(3): 1161–72.

[14] Lotvall J, Valadi H. Cell to cell signalling via exosomes through esRNA. Cell Adh Migr 2007; 1(3): 156–8.

[15] Madison MN, Okeoma CM. Exosomes: implications in HIV-1 pathogenesis. Viruses 2015; 7(7): 4093–118.

[16] Meckes DG, Raab-Traub N. Microvesicles and viral infection. J Virol 2011; 85(24): 12844–54.

[17] Gould SJ, Booth AM, Hildreth JEK. The Trojan exosome hypothesis. Proc Natl Acad Sci U S A 2003; 100(19): 10592–7.

[18] Izquierdo-Useros N, Naranjo-Gómez M, Erkizia I, Puertas MC, Borràs FE, Blanco J, Martinez-Picado J. HIV and mature dendritic cells: Trojan exosomes riding the Trojan horse? PLoS Pathog 2010; 6(3): e1000740.

[19] Chow Y, Yu D, Zhang JY, Xie Y, Wei OLC, Chiu C, et al. Gp120-independent infection of CD4- epithelial cells and CD4+ T-cells by HIV-1. J Acquir Immune Defic Syndr 2002; 30(1): 1–8.

[20] Izquierdo-Useros N, Puertas MC, Borràs FE, Blanco J, Martinez-Picado J. Exosomes and retroviruses: the chicken or the egg? Cell Microbiol 2011; 13(1): 10–7.

[21] Madison MN, Jones PH, Okeoma CM. Exosomes in human semen restrict HIV-1 transmission by vaginal cells and block intravaginal replication of LP-BM5 murine AIDS virus complex. Virology 2015; 482: 189–201.

[22] Wubbolts R, Leckie RS, Veenhuizen PTM, Schwarzmann G, Möbius W, Hoernschemeyer J, et al. Proteomic and biochemical analyses of human B cell-derived exosomes: potential implications for their function and multivesicular body formation. J Biol Chem 2003; 278(13): 10963–72.

[23] Krishnamoorthy L, Bess JW, Preston AB, Nagashima K, Mahal LK. HIV-1 and microvesicles from T cells share a common glycome, arguing for a common origin. Nat Chem Biol 2009; 5(4): 244–50.

[24] Théry C, Zitvogel L, Amigorena S. Exosomes: composition, biogenesis and function. Nat Rev Immunol 2002; 2(8): 569–79.

[25] Mfunyi CM, Vaillancourt M, Vitry J, Nsimba Batomene TR, Posvandzic A, Lambert AA, Gilbert C. Exosome release following activation of the dendritic cell immunoreceptor: a potential role in HIV-1 pathogenesis. Virology 2015; 484: 103–12.

[26] Lee JC, Lee EJ, Lee JH, Jun SH, Choi CW, Kim SI, et al. *Klebsiella pneumoniae* secretes outer membrane vesicles that induce the innate immune response. FEMS Microbiol Lett 2012; 331(1): 17–24.

[27] Oliveira DL, Nakayasu ES, Joffe LS, Guimarães AJ, Sobreira TJP, Nosanchuk JD, et al. Characterization of yeast extracellular vesicles: evidence for the participation of different pathways of cellular traffic in vesicle biogenesis. PLoS ONE 2010; 5(6): e11113.

[28] Madison MN, Roller RJ, Okeoma CM. Human semen contains exosomes with potent anti-HIV-1 activity. Retrovirology 2014; 11(1): 102.

[29] Colombo M, Moita C, van Niel G, Kowal J, Vigneron J, Benaroch P, et al. Analysis of ESCRT functions in exosome biogenesis, composition and secretion highlights the heterogeneity of extracellular vesicles. J Cell Sci 2013; 126(24): 5553–65.

[30] Stuffers S, Sem Wegner C, Stenmark H, Brech A. Multivesicular endosome biogenesis in the absence of ESCRTs. Traffic 2009; 10(7): 925–37.

[31] van Niel G, Charrin S, Simoes S, Romao M, Rochin L, Saftig P, et al. The tetraspanin CD63 regulates ESCRT-independent and -dependent endosomal sorting during melanogenesis. Dev Cell 2011; 21(4): 708–21.

[32] Ostrowski M, Carmo NB, Krumeich S, Fanget I, Raposo G, Savina A, et al. Rab27a and Rab27b control different steps

[33] of the exosome secretion pathway. Nat Cell Biol 2010; 12(1): 19-30.

[33] Cantin R, Diou J, Bélanger D, Tremblay AM, Gilbert C. Discrimination between exosomes and HIV-1: purification of both vesicles from cell-free supernatants. J Immunol Methods 2008; 338(1-2): 21-30.

[34] Lenassi M, Cagney G, Liao M, Vaupotič T, Bartholomeeusen K, Cheng Y, et al. HIV Nef is secreted in exosomes and triggers apoptosis in bystander CD4+ T cells. Traffic 2010; 11(1): 110-22.

[35] Kadiu I, Narayanasamy P, Dash PK, Zhang W, Gendelman HE. Biochemical and biologic characterization of exosomes and microvesicles as facilitators of HIV-1 infection in macrophages. J Immunol 2012; 189(2): 744-54.

[36] Mack M, Kleinschmidt A, Brühl H, Klier C, Nelson PJ, Cihak J, et al. Transfer of the chemokine receptor CCR5 between cells by membrane-derived microparticles: a mechanism for cellular human immunodeficiency virus 1 infection. Nat Med 2000; 6(7): 769-75.

[37] Gray LR, Gabuzda D, Cowley D, Ellett A, Chiavaroli L, Wesselingh SL, et al. CD4 and MHC class 1 down-modulation activities of nef alleles from brain-and lymphoid tissue-derived primary HIV-1 isolates. J Neurovirol 2011; 17(1): 82-91.

[38] Aqil M, Naqvi AR, Bano AS, Jameel S. The HIV-1 Nef protein binds argonaute-2 and functions as a viral suppressor of RNA interference. PLoS ONE 2013; 8(9): e74472.

[39] Esser MT, Graham DR, Coren LV, Trubey CM, Bess JW, Arthur LO, et al. Differential incorporation of CD45, CD80 (B7-1), CD86 (B7-2), and major histocompatibility complex class I and II molecules into human immunodeficiency virus type 1 virions and microvesicles: implications for viral pathogenesis and immune regulation. J Virol 2001; 75(13): 6173-82.

[40] Marras D, Bruggeman LA, Gao F, Tanji N, Mansukhani MM, Cara A, et al. Replication and compartmentalization of HIV-1 in kidney epithelium of patients with HIV-associated nephropathy. Nat Med 2002; 8(5): 522-6.

[41] Demarino C, Pleet ML, Cowen M, Barclay RA, Akpamagbo Y, Erickson J, et al. Antiretroviral drugs alter the content of extracellular vesicles from HIV-1-infected cells. Sci Rep 2018; 8(1): 7653.

[42] Welch JL, Kaddour H, Schlievert PM, Stapleton JT, Okeoma CM. Semen exosomes promote transcriptional silencing of HIV-1 by disrupting NF-kB/Sp1/Tat circuitry. J Virol 2018; 92: 00731-18.

[43] Kouwaki T, Fukushima Y, Daito T, Sanada T, Yamamoto N, Mifsud EJ, et al. Extracellular vesicles including exosomes regulate innate immune responses to hepatitis B virus infection. Front Immunol 2016; 7: 335.

[44] Nakai M, Oshiumi H, Funami K, Okamoto M, Matsumoto M, Seya T, Sakamoto N. Interferon (IFN) and cellular immune response evoked in RNA-pattern sensing during infection with hepatitis C virus (HCV). Sensors (Basel) 2015; 15(10): 27160-73.

[45] Zhang W, Jiang X, Bao J, Wang Y, Liu H, Tang L. Exosomes in pathogen infections: a bridge to deliver molecules and link functions. Front Immunol 2018; 9: 90.

[46] Schorey JS, Cheng Y, Singh PP, Smith VL. Exosomes and other extracellular vesicles in host-pathogen interactions. EMBO Rep 2015; 16(1): 24-43.

[47] Kulkarni R, Prasad A. Exosomes derived from HIV-1 infected DCs mediate viral trans-infection via fibronectin and galectin-3. Sci Rep 2017; 7(1): 14787.

[48] Wang X, Ao Z, Chen L, Kobinger G, Peng J, Yao X. The cellular antiviral protein APOBEC3G interacts with HIV-1 reverse transcriptase and inhibits its function during viral replication. J Virol 2012; 86(7): 3777-86.

[49] Stavrou S, Ross SR. APOBEC3 proteins in viral immunity. J Immunol 2015; 195(10): 4565-70.

[50] Holmes RK, Koning FA, Bishop KN, Malim MH. APOBEC3F can inhibit the accumulation of HIV-1 reverse transcription products in the absence of hypermutation: comparisons with APOBEC3G. J Biol Chem 2007; 282(4): 2587-95.

[51] Schumacher AJ, Hache G, MacDuff DA, Brown WL, Harris RS. The DNA deaminase activity of human APOBEC3G is required for Ty1, MusD, and human immunodeficiency virus type 1 restriction. J Virol 2008; 82(6): 2652-60.

[52] Bishop KN, Verma M, Kim EY, Wolinsky SM, Malim MH. APOBEC3G inhibits elongation of HIV-1 reverse transcripts. PLoS Pathog 2008; 4(12): e1000231.

[53] Khatua AK, Taylor HE, Hildreth JEK, Popik W. Exosomes packaging APOBEC3G confer human immunodeficiency virus resistance to recipient cells. J Virol 2009; 83(2): 512-21.

[54] Maiti A, Myint W, Kanai T, Delviks-Frankenberry K, Sierra Rodriguez C, Pathak VK, et al. Crystal structure of the catalytic domain of HIV-1 restriction factor APOBEC3G in complex with ssDNA. Nat Commun 2018; 9(1): 2460.

[55] Ojha CR, Lapierre J, Rodriguez M, Dever SM, Zadeh MA, Demarino C, et al. Interplay between autophagy, exosomes and HIV-1 associated neurological disorders: new insights for diagnosis and therapeutic applications. Viruses 2017; 9(7): E176.

[56] Mizushima N, Komatsu M. Autophagy: renovation of cells and tissues. Cell 2011; 147(4): 728-41.

[57] Fields J, Dumaop W, Elueteri S, Campos S, Serger E, Trejo M, et al. HIV-1 Tat alters neuronal autophagy by modulating autophagosome fusion to the lysosome: implications for HIVassociated neurocognitive disorders. J Neurosci 2015; 35(5): 1921-38.

[58] Zhou D, Masliah E, Spector SA. Autophagy is increased in postmortem brains of persons with HIV-1-associated encephalitis. J Infect Dis 2011; 203(11): 1647-57.

[59] Espert L, Varbanov M, Robert-Hebmann V, Sagnier S, Robbins I, Sanchez F, et al. Differential role of autophagy in CD4 T cells and macrophages during X4 and R5 HIV-1 infection. PLoS ONE 2009; 4: e5787.

[60] Sagnier S, Daussy CF, Borel S, Robert-Hebmann V, Faure M, Blanchet FP, et al. Autophagy restricts HIV-1 infection by selectively degrading Tat in CD4+ T lymphocytes. J Virol 2015; 89(1): 615-25.

[61] Nardacci R, Amendola A, Ciccosanti F, Corazzari M, Esposito V, Vlassi C, et al. Autophagy plays an important role in the containment of HIV-1 in nonprogressor-infected patients. Autophagy 2014; 10(7): 1167-78.

[62] Campbell GR, Rawat P, Bruckman RS, Spector SA. Human immunodeficiency virus type 1 Nef inhibits autophagy through transcription factor EB sequestration. PLoS Pathog 2015; 11(6): e1005018.

[63] Borel S, Robert-Hebmann V, Alfaisal J, Jain A, Faure M, Espert L, et al. HIV-1 viral infectivity factor interacts with microtubule-associated protein light chain 3 and inhibits autophagy. AIDS 2014; 29(3): 275-86.

[64] Li JCB, Au KY, Fang JW, Yim HC, Chow KH, et al. HIV-1 trans-activator protein dysregulates IFN-γ signaling and contributes to the suppression of autophagy induction. AIDS 2011; 25(1): 15-25.

[65] McNamara RP, Costantini LM, Myers TA, Schouest B, Maness NJ, Griffith JD, et al. Nef secretion into extracellular vesicles or exosomes is conserved across human and simian immunodeficiency viruses. MBio 2018; 9(1): e02344-17.

[66] Das SR, Jameel S. Biology of the HIV Nef protein. Indian J Med Res 2005; 121(4): 315-32.

[67] Miller JH, Presnyak V, Smith HC. The dimerization domain of HIV-1 viral infectivity factor Vif is required to block virion incorporation of APOBEC3G. Retrovirology 2007; 4: 81.

[68] Andrew AJ, Miyagi E, Strebel K. Differential effects of human immunodeficiency virus type 1 Vpu on the stability of BST-2/tetherin. J Virol 2011; 85(6): 2611-9.

[69] Kogan M, Rappaport J. HIV-1 accessory protein Vpr: relevance in the pathogenesis of HIV and potential for therapeutic intervention. Retrovirology 2011; 8: 25.

[70] Bell NM, Lever AML. HIV Gag polyprotein: processing and early viral particle assembly. Trends Microbiol 2013; 21(3): 136-44.

[71] Tang X, Lu H, Dooner M, Chapman S, Quesenberry PJ, Ramratnam B. Exosomal Tat protein activates latent HIV-1 in primary, resting CD4+ T lymphocytes. JCI Insight 2018; 3(7): e95676.

[72] Nagata S, Imai J, Makino G, Tomita M, Kanai A. Evolutionary analysis of HIV-1 pol proteins reveals representative residues for viral subtype differentiation. Front Microbiol 2017; 8: 2151.

[73] Yamashita T, Takahashi Y, Takakura Y. Possibility of exosome-based therapeutics and challenges in production of exosomes eligible for therapeutic application. Biol Pharm Bull 2018; 41(6): 835-42.

[74] Sun B, Dalvi P, Abadjian L, Tang N, Pulliam L. Blood neuron-derived exosomes as biomarkers of cognitive impairment in HIV. AIDS 2017; 31(14): F9-17.

[75] Näslund TI, Paquin-Proulx D, Paredes PT, Vallhov H, Sandberg JK, Gabrielsson S. Exosomes from breast milk inhibit HIV-1 infection of dendritic cells and subsequent viral transfer to CD4+ T cells. AIDS 2014; 28(2): 171-80.

[76] Salih M, Zietse R, Hoorn EJ. Urinary extracellular vesicles and the kidney: biomarkers and beyond. Am J Physiol Renal Physiol 2014; 306(11): F1251-9.

[77] Ellwanger JH, Veit TD, Chies JAB. Exosomes in HIV infection: a review and critical look. Infect Genet Evol 2017; 53: 146-54.

[78] Anyanwu SI, Doherty A, Powell MD, Obialo C, Huang MB, Quarshie A, et al. Detection of HIV-1 and human proteins in urinary extracellular vesicles from HIV+ patients. Adv Virol 2018; 2018: 7863412.

[79] Banigan MG, Kao PF, Kozubek JA, Winslow AR, Medina J, Costa J, et al. Differential expression of exosomal microRNAs in prefrontal cortices of schizophrenia and bipolar disorder patients. PLoS ONE 2013; 8(1): e48814.

[80] Fiandaca MS, Kapogiannis D, Mapstone M, Boxer A, Eitan E, Schwartz JB, et al. Identification of preclinical Alzheimer's disease by a profile of pathogenic proteins in neurally derived blood exosomes: a case-control study. Alzheimers Dement 2015; 11(6): 600-607.e1.

[81] Chettimada S, Lorenz DR, Misra V, Dillon ST, Reeves RK, Manickam C, et al. Exosome markers associated with immune activation and oxidative stress in HIV patients on antiretroviral therapy. Sci Rep 2018; 8(1): 7227.

[82] Strickland M, Ehrlich LS, Watanabe S, Khan M, Strub MP, Luan CH, et al. Tsg101 chaperone function revealed by HIV-1 assembly inhibitors. Nat Commun 2017; 8(1): 1391.

[83] Fridkis-Hareli M. Design of peptide immunotherapies for MHC class-II-associated autoimmune disorders. Clin Dev Immunol 2013; 2013: 826191.

[84] Finzi A, Brunet A, Xiao Y, Thibodeau J, Cohen EA. Major histocompatibility complex class II molecules promote human immunodeficiency virus type 1 assembly and budding to late endosomal/multivesicular body compartments. J Virol 2006; 80(19): 9789-97.

[85] Saifuddin M, Spear GT, Chang C, Roebuck KA. Expression of MHC class II in T cells is associated with increased HIV-1 expression. Clin Exp Immunol 2000; 121(2): 324-31.

[86] Alkhatib G. The biology of CCR5 and CXCR4. Curr Opin HIV AIDS 2009; 4(2): 96-103.

[87] Alkhatib G, Locati M, Kennedy PE, Murphy PM, Berger EA. HIV-1 coreceptor activity of CCR5 and its inhibition by chemokines: independence from G protein signaling and importance of coreceptor downmodulation. Virology 1997; 234(2): 340-8.

[88] Amara A, Gall SL, Schwartz O, Salamero J, Montes M, Loetscher P, et al. HIV coreceptor downregulation as antiviral principle: SDF-1alpha-dependent internalization of the chemokine receptor CXCR4 contributes to inhibition of HIV replication. J Exp Med 1997; 186(1): 139-46.

[89] Signoret N, Oldridge J, Pelchen-Matthews A, Klasse PJ, Tran T, Brass LF, et al. Phorbol esters and SDF-1 induce rapid endocytosis and down modulation of the chemokine receptor CXCR4. J Cell Biol 1997; 139(3): 651-64.

[90] Geyer M, Fackler OT, Peterlin BM. Structure-function relationships in HIV-1 Nef. EMBO Rep 2001; 2(7): 580-5.

[91] Dekaban GA, Dikeakos JD. HIV-I Nef inhibitors: a novel class of HIV-specific immune adjuvants in support of a cure. AIDS Res Ther 2017; 14: 53.

[92] Spearman P. HIV-1 Gag as an antiviral target: development of assembly and maturation inhibitors. Curr Top Med Chem 2016; 16(10): 1154-66.

[93] Herschhorn A, Gu C, Espy N, Richard J, Finzi A, Sodroski JG. A broad HIV-1 inhibitor blocks envelope glycoprotein transitions critical for entry. Nat Chem Biol 2014; 10(10): 845-52.

[94] von Kleist M, Metzner P, Marquet R, Schütte C. HIV-1 polymerase inhibition by nucleoside analogs: cellular- and kinetic parameters of efficacy, susceptibility and resistance selection. PLoS Comput Biol 2012; 8(1): e1002359.

[95] Hagiwara K, Ishii H, Murakami T, Takeshima SN, Chutiwitoonchai N, Kodama EN, et al. Synthesis of a Vpr-binding derivative for use as a novel HIV-1 inhibitor. PLoS ONE 2015; 10(12): e0145573.

[96] Mi Z, Ding J, Zhang Q, Zhao J, Ma L, Yu H, et al. A small molecule compound IMB-LA inhibits HIV-1 infection by preventing viral Vpu from antagonizing the host restriction factor BST-2. Sci Rep 2015; 5: 18499.

[97] Pery E, Sheehy A, Nebane NM, Brazier AJ, Misra V, Rajendran KS, et al. Identification of a novel HIV-1 inhibitor targeting Vif-dependent degradation of human APOBEC3G protein. J Biol Chem 2015; 290(16): 10504-17.

[98] Balachandran A, Wong R, Stoilov P, Pan S, Blencowe B, Cheung P, et al. Identification of small molecule modulators of HIV-1 Tat and Rev protein accumulation. Retrovirology 2017; 14(1): 7.

[99] Wolfson B, Yu JE, Zhou Q. Exosomes may play a crucial role in HIV dendritic cell immunotherapy. Ann Transl Med 2017; 5(16): 337.

[100] Théry C, Regnault A, Garin J, Wolfers J, Zitvogel L, Ricciardi-Castagnoli P, et al. Molecular characterization of dendritic cell-derived exosomes: selective accumulation of the heat shock protein hsc73. J Cell Biol 1999; 147(3): 599-610.

[101] Chistiakov DA, Grechko AV, Orekhov AN, Bobryshev YV. An immunoregulatory role of dendritic cell-derived exosomes versus HIV-1 infection: take it easy but be warned. Ann Transl Med 2017; 5(17): 362.

[102] Chang HC, Samaniego F, Nair BC, Buonaguro L, Ensoli B. HIV-1 Tat protein exits from cells via a leaderless secretory pathway and binds to extracellular matrix-associated heparan sulfate proteoglycans through its basic region. AIDS 1997; 11(12): 1421-31.

[103] Lin X, Irwin D, Kanazawa S, Huang L, Romeo J, Yen TSB, Peterlin BM. Transcriptional profiles of latent human immunodeficiency virus in infected individuals: effects of Tat on the host and reservoir. J Virol 2003; 77(15): 8227-36.

[104] Yong Q, Jing M, Yi Z. Therapeutic potential of anti-HIV RNA-koaded exosomes. Biomed Environ Sci 2018; 31(3): 215-26.

[105] Zeller SJ, Kumar P. RNA-based gene therapy for the treatment and prevention of HIV: from bench to bedside. Yale J Biol Med 2011; 84(3): 301-9.

[106] Strayer DS, Akkina R, Bunnell BA, Dropulic B, Planelles V, Pomerantz RJ, et al. Current status of gene therapy strategies to treat HIV/AIDS. Mol Ther 2005; 11(6): 823-42.

[107] Bobbin ML, Burnett JC, Rossi JJ. RNA interference approaches for treatment of HIV-1 infection. Genome Med 2015; 7(1): 50.

[108] Mali P, Yang L, Esvelt KM, Aach J, Guell M, DiCarlo JE, et al. RNA-guided human genome engineering via Cas9. Science 2013; 339(6121): 823-6.

[109] Hu W, Kaminski R, Yang F, Zhang Y, Cosentino L, Li F, Luo B, Alvarez-Carbonell D, Garcia-Mesa Y, Karn J, Mo X, Khalili K. RNA-directed gene editing specifically eradicates latent and prevents new HIV-1 infection. Proc Natl Acad Sci U S A 2014; 111(31): 11461-6.

[110] Swaminathan G, Navas-Martín S, Martín-García J. MicroRNAs and HIV-1 infection: antiviral activities and beyond. J Mol Biol 2014; 426(6): 1178-97.

[111] Ran FA, Hsu PD, Wright J, Agarwala V, Scott DA, Zhang F. Genome engineering using the CRISPR-Cas9 system. Nat Protoc 2013; 8(11): 2281-308.

[112] Horvath P, Barrangou R. CRISPR/Cas, the immune system of bacteria and archaea. Science 2010; 327(5962): 167-70.

[113] Huang Z, Tomitaka A, Raymond A, Nair M. Current application of CRISPR/Cas9 geneediting technique to eradication of HIV/AIDS. Gene Ther 2017; 24(7): 377-84.

[114] Yang T, Martin P, Fogarty B, Brown A, Schurman K, Phipps R, et al. Exosome delivered anticancer drugs across the blood-brain barrier for brain cancer therapy in *Danio rerio*. Pharm Res 2015; 32(6): 2003-14.

[115] Feng D, Zhao WL, Ye YY, Bai XC, Liu RQ, Chang LF, et al. Cellular internalization of exosomes occurs through phagocytosis. Traffic 2010; 11(5): 675-87.

[116] Morelli AE, Larregina AT, Shufesky WJ, Sullivan MLG, Stolz DB, Papworth GD, et al. Endocytosis, intracellular sorting, and processing of exosomes by dendritic cells. Blood 2004; 104(10): 3257-66.

[117] Svensson KJ, Christianson HC, Wittrup A, Bourseau-Guilmain E, Lindqvist E, Svensson LM, et al. Exosome uptake depends on ERK1/2-heat shock protein 27 signaling and lipid raft-mediated endocytosis negatively regulated by caveolin-1. J Biol Chem 2013; 288(24): 17713-24.

[118] Alvarez-Erviti L, Seow Y, Yin H, Betts C, Lakhal S, Wood MJA. Delivery of siRNA to the mouse brain by systemic injection of targeted exosomes. Nat Biotechnol 2011; 29(4): 341-5.

[119] Zhou Y, Zhou G, Tian C, Jiang W, Jin L, Zhang C, Chen X. Exosome-mediated small RNA delivery for gene therapy. Wiley Interdiscip Rev RNA 2016; 7(6): 758-71.

[120] Quah BJC, O'Neill HC. The immunogenicity of dendritic cell-derived exosomes. Blood Cells Mol Dis 2005; 35(2): 94-110.

[121] Qazi KR, Gehrmann U, Jordö ED, Karlsson MCI, Gabrielsson S. Antigen-koaded exosomes alone induce Thl-type memory through a B cell dependent mechanism. Blood 2009; 113(12): 2673-83.

[122] Yeo RWY, Lai RC, Zhang B, Tan SS, Yin Y, Teh BJ, Lim SK. Mesenchymal stem cell: an efficient mass producer of exosomes for drug delivery. Adv Drug Deliv Rev 2013; 65(3): 336-41.

[123] Chen TS, Arslan F, Yin Y, Tan SS, Lai RC, Choo ABH, et al. Enabling a robust scalable manufacturing process for therapeutic exosomes through oncogenic immortalization of human ESC-derived MSCs. J Transl Med 2011; 9: 47.

[124] Haney MJ, Zhao Y, Harrison EB, Mahajan V, Ahmed S, He Z, et al. Specific transfection of inflamed brain by macrophages: a new therapeutic strategy for neurodegenerative diseases. PLoS ONE 2013; 8(4): e61852.

[125] Savina A, Fader CM, Damiani MT, Colombo MI. Rab11 promotes docking and fusion of multivesicular bodies in a calcium-dependent manner. Traffic 2005; 6(2): 131-43.

[126] Janas T, Janas MM, Sapoń K, Janas T. Mechanisms of RNA loading into exosomes. FEBS Lett 2015; 589(13): 1391-8.

[127] Hupfeld J, Gorr IH, Schwald C, Beaucamp N, Wiechmann K, Kuentzer K, et al. Modulation of mesenchymal stromal cell characteristics by microcarrier culture in bioreactors. Biotechnol Bioeng 2014; 111(11): 2290–302.

[128] Mitchell JP, Court J, Mason MD, Tabi Z, Clayton A. Increased exosome production from tumour cell cultures using the Integra CELLine culture system. J Immunol Methods 2008; 335(1–2): 98–105.

[129] Barros FM, Carneiro F, Machado JC, Melo SA. Exosomes and immune response in cancer: friends or foes? Front Immunol 2018; 9: 730.

[130] Yang C, Robbins PD. The roles of tumor-derived exosomes in cancer pathogenesis. Clin Dev Immunol 2011; 2011: 842849.

[131] van der Pol E, Coumans F, Varga Z, Krumrey M, Nieuwland R. Innovation in detection of microparticles and exosomes. J Thromb Haemost 2013; 1: 36–45.

[132] Ko J, Carpenter E, Issadore D. Detection and isolation of circulating exosomes and microvesicles for cancer monitoring and diagnostics using micro-/nano-based devices. Analyst 2016; 141(2): 450–60.

[133] Suárez H, Gámez-Valero A, Reyes R, López-Martín S, Rodríguez MJ, Carrascosa JL, et al. A bead-assisted flow cytometry method for the semi-quantitative analysis of extracellular vesicles. Sci Rep 2017; 7(1): 11271.

[134] Ahmad MA. Electrical detection, identification and quantification of exosomes. IEEE Access 2018; 6.

[135] Vogel R, Willmott G, Kozak D, Roberts GS, Anderson W, Groenewegen L, et al. Quantitative sizing of nano/microparticles with a tunable elastomeric pore sensor. Anal Chem 2011; 83(9): 3499–506.

[136] Dragovic RA, Gardiner C, Brooks AS, Tannetta DS, Ferguson DJP, Hole P, et al. Sizing and phenotyping of cellular vesicles using nanoparticle tracking analysis. Nanomed Nanotechnol Biol Med 2011; 7(6): 780–8.

[137] Braeckmans K, Buyens K, Bouquet W, Vervaet C, Joye P, De Vos F, et al. Sizing nanomatter in biological fluids by fluorescence single particle tracking. Nano Lett 2010; 10(11): 4435–42.

[138] López-Cobo S, Campos-Silva C, Moyano A, Oliveira-Rodríguez M, Paschen A, Yáñez-Mó M, et al. Immunoassays for scarce tumour-antigens in exosomes: detection of the human NKG2D-kigand, MICA, in tetraspanin-containing nanovesicles from melanoma. J Nanobiotechnol 2018; 16(1): 47.

[139] Wang Z, Wu HJ, Fine D, Schmulen J, Hu Y, Godin B, et al. Ciliated micropillars for the microfluidic-based isolation of nanoscale lipid vesicles. Lab Chip 2013; 13(15): 2879–82.

[140] Lee K, Shao H, Weissleder R, Lee H. Acoustic purification of extracellular microvesicles. ACS Nano 2015; 9(3): 2321–7.

[141] Vaidyanathan R, Naghibosadat M, Rauf S, Korbie D, Carrascosa LG, Shiddiky MJA, Trau M. Detecting exosomes specifically: a multiplexed device based on alternating current electrohydrodynamic induced nanoshearing. Anal Chem 2014; 86(22): 11125–32.

[142] McLeod E, Dincer TU, Veli M, Ertas YN, Nguyen C, Luo W, et al. High-throughput and label-free single nanoparticle sizing based on time-resolved on-chip microscopy. ACS Nano 2015; 9(3): 3265–73.

[143] Issadore D, Min C, Liong M, Chung J, Weissleder R, Lee H. Miniature magnetic resonance system for point-of-care diagnostics. Lab Chip 2011; 11(13): 2282–7.

[144] Im H, Lee K, Weissleder R, Lee H, Castro CM. Novel nanosensing technologies for exosome detection and profiling. Lab Chip 2017; 17(17): 2892–8.

[145] Kravets VG, Schedin F, Jalil R, Britnell L, Gorbachev RV, Ansell D, et al. Singular phase nano-optics in plasmonic metamaterials for label-free single-molecule detection. Nat Mater 2013; 12(4): 304–9.

[146] Su J. Label-free single exosome detection using frequency-kocked microtoroid optical resonators. ACS Photonics 2015; 2(9): 1241–5.

[147] Riches A, Campbell E, Borger E, Powis S. Regulation of exosome release from mammary epithelial and breast cancer cells — a new regulatory pathway. Eur J Cancer 2014; 50(5): 1025–34.

[148] Harmati M, Tarnai Z, Decsi G, Kormondi S, Szegletes Z, Janovak L, et al. Stressors alter intercellular communication and exosome profile of nasopharyngeal carcinoma cells. J Oral Pathol Med 2017; 46(4): 259–66.

[149] Böing AN, van der Pol E, Grootemaat AE, Coumans FAW, Sturk A, Nieuwland R. Singlestep isolation of extracellular vesicles by size-exclusion chromatography. J Extracell Vesicles 2014; 3(1): 23430.

[150] Shin H, Han C, Labuz JM, Kim J, Kim J, Cho S, et al. High-yield isolation of extracellular vesicles using aqueous two-phase system. Sci Rep 2015; 5: 13103.

[151] Weng Y, Sui Z, Shan Y, Hu Y, Chen Y, Zhang L, Zhang Y. Effective isolation of exosomes with polyethylene glycol from cell culture supernatant for in-depth proteome profiling. Analyst 2016; 141(15): 4640–6.

[152] Heinemann ML, Ilmer M, Silva LP, Hawke DH, Recio A, Vorontsova MA, et al. Benchtop isolation and characterization of functional exosomes by sequential filtration. J Chromatogr A 2014; 1371: 125–35.

[153] Yamashita T, Takahashi Y, Nishikawa M, Takakura Y. Effect of exosome isolation methods on physicochemical properties of exosomes and clearance of exosomes from the blood circulation. Eur J Pharm Biopharm 2016; 98: 1–8.

[154] Willms E, Johansson HJ, Mäger I, Lee Y, Blomberg KEM, Sadik M, et al. Cells release subpopulations of exosomes with distinct molecular and biological properties. Sci Rep 2016; 6: 22519.

[155] Tauro BJ, Greening DW, Mathias RA, Ji H, Mathivanan S, Scott AM, Simpson RJ. Comparison of ultracentrifugation, density gradient separation, and immunoaffinity capture methods for isolating human colon cancer cell line LIM1863-derived exosomes. Methods 2012; 56(2): 293–304.

[156] Witwer KW, Buzás EI, Bemis LT, Bora A, Lässer C, Lötvall J, et al. Standardization of sample collection, isolation and analysis methods in extracellular vesicle research. J Extracell Vesicles 2013; 2(1): 20360.

[157] Bosch S, De Beaurepaire L, Allard M, Mosser M, Heichette C, Chrétien D, et al. Trehalose prevents aggregation of exosomes and cryodamage. Sci Rep 2016; 6: 36162.

[158] Kreke, M., Smith, R., Hanscome, P., Peck, K., Ibrahim, A., 2016. Processes for producing stable exosome formulations. US Patent 20160158291A1.

[159] Takahashi Y, Nishikawa M, Shinotsuka H, Matsui Y, Ohara S, Imai T, Takakura Y. Visualization and in vivo

[160] tracking of the exosomes of murine melanoma B16-BL6 cells in mice after intravenous injection. J Biotechnol 2013; 165 (2): 77-84.
[160] Imai T, Takahashi Y, Nishikawa M, Kato K, Morishita M, Yamashita T, et al. Macrophagedependent clearance of systemically administered B16BL6-derived exosomes from the blood circulation in mice. J Extracell Vesicles 2015; 4: 26238.
[161] Wiklander OPB, Nordin JZ, O'Loughlin A, Gustafsson Y, Corso G, Mäger I, et al. Extracellular vesicle in vivo biodistribution is determined by cell source, route of administration and targeting. J Extracell Vesicles 2015; 4: 26316.
[162] Qu Y, Zhang Q, Cai X, Li F, Ma Z, Xu M, Lu L. Exosomes derived from miR-181-5p-modified adipose-derived mesenchymal stem cells prevent liver fibrosis via autophagy activation. J Cell Mol Med 2017; 21(10): 2491-502.
[163] Zhang J, Ma J, Long K, Qiu W, Wang Y, Hu Z, et al. Overexpression of exosomal cardioprotective miRNAs mitigates hypoxia-induced H9c2 cells apoptosis. Int J Mol Sci 2017; 18(4): 711.
[164] Yang MQ, Du Q, Varley PR, Goswami J, Liang Z, Wang R, et al. Interferon regulatory factor 1 priming of tumour-derived exosomes enhances the antitumour immune response. Br J Cancer 2018; 118(1): 62-71.
[165] Yu B, Kim HW, Gong M, Wang J, Millard RW, Wang Y, et al. Exosomes secreted from GATA-4 overexpressing mesenchymal stem cells serve as a reservoir of anti-apoptotic microRNAs for cardioprotection. Int J Cardiol 2015; 182 (C): 349-60.
[166] Morishita M, Takahashi Y, Matsumoto A, Nishikawa M, Takakura Y. Exosome-based tumor antigens – adjuvant co-delivery utilizing genetically engineered tumor cell-derived exosomes with immunostimulatory CpG DNA. Biomaterials 2016; 111: 55-65.
[167] Cui GH, Wu J, Mou FF, Xie WH, Wang FB, Wang QL, et al. Exosomes derived from hypoxia-preconditioned mesenchymal stromal cells ameliorate cognitive decline by rescuing synaptic dysfunction and regulating inflammatory responses in APP/PS1 mice. FASEB J 2018; 32(2): 654-68.
[168] Lamichhane TN, Leung CA, Douti LY, Jay SM. Ethanol induces enhanced vascularization bioactivity of endothelial cell-derived extracellular vesicles via regulation of microRNAs and long non-coding RNAs. Sci Rep 2017; 7(1): 13794.
[169] Bukong TN, Momen-Heravi F, Kodys K, Bala S, Szabo G. Exosomes from hepatitis C infected patients transmit HCV infection and contain replication competent viral RNA in complex with Ago2-miR122-HSP90. PLoS Pathog 2014; 10 (10): e1004424.
[170] Wurdinger T, Gatson NN, Balaj L, Kaur B, Breakefield XO, Pegtel DM. Extracellular vesicles and their convergence with viral pathways. Adv Virol 2012; 2012: 767694.

第 8 章

寄生虫病胞外囊泡

Extracelluar vesicels in parasitic disease

Patricia Xander, André Cronemberger-Andrade, and Ana Claudia Torrecilhas

Laboratory of Cellular Immunology and Biochemistry of Fungi and Protozoa, Department of Pharmaceutical Sciences, Federal University of São Paulo (UNIFESP), Diadema, SP, Brazil

一、胞外囊泡和寄生虫

病原体在宿主微环境中脱落 EV。病原体释放的 EV 和宿主产生的 EV 已从多种微生物中分离并鉴定,并在病原体和宿主之间的细胞内的通信中发挥重要作用[1-4]。

病毒、细菌、真菌、原虫和蠕虫不断地向细胞外环境释放 EV[1-3],其直径在 20~200 nm 之间,包含蛋白质、糖复合物、脂质、核酸(RNA、非转录 RNA 和 miRNA)。EV 可在各种体液(血清、血浆、唾液、尿液和母乳等)中被检测到,调控与宿主间的交流和相互作用,也可传递毒力因子和抗原。事实上,从寄生虫中分离到的 EV 可作为信使启动宿主细胞进行特定的相互作用,促进病原体侵入,或者激活宿主的天然免疫和获得性免疫[1,2,5,6]。

一些研究表明,寄生虫释放的 EV 可影响宿主细胞,如寄生虫 EV 与宿主的相互作用可改变巨噬细胞释放的外泌体组分。病原体还可刺激宿主释放含有蛋白质或寄生虫其他组分的 EV,作为这些微生物转运其所携带物质的机制。此外,一些病原体释放 EV,可作为适应宿主的一种机制,从而促进其感染或逃避宿主免疫系统。

在本章中,我们将介绍一些重要原虫释放的 EV 作用的最新研究进展。

二、利什曼原虫

利什曼病是被忽视的疾病[World Health Organization(WHO),2015 年],其在一些国家流行。该病由利什曼属原虫感染引起,根据不同的临床表现可分为:① 局限性皮肤利什曼病;② 黏膜皮肤利什曼病;③ 弥漫性皮肤利什曼病;④ 内脏利什曼病。据估计,目前有 5.56 亿和近 3.99 亿人生活在内脏利什曼病和局限性皮肤利什曼病的风险地区,而这些地区大多在高负担国家[7,7a,7b]。

利什曼原虫的生活史为在哺乳动物宿主和白蛉科昆虫媒介之间世代交替[8]。在吸血过程中,雌性白蛉摄取被利什曼原虫感染的哺乳动物宿主体内的无鞭毛体,无鞭毛体进入白蛉体内后发育为梭形的前鞭毛体。当白蛉再次吸食新鲜血液时,前鞭毛体随即被排出并被宿主的巨噬细胞吞噬,随后在巨噬细胞内分化成无鞭毛体并繁殖,进而导致宿主细胞膜的破裂并感染新的巨噬细胞[9]。

利什曼原虫感染中天然免疫起重要作用[10],在接触到或感染利什曼原虫时,中性粒细胞、巨噬细胞和 DC 均可被识别和激活[11]。巨噬细胞是利什曼病感染免疫和致病的主要细胞。利什曼原虫通过结合其表面分子如磷酸酯多糖(lipophosphoglycan，LPG)，与巨噬细胞表面表达的受体如补体 1 和补体 3 的受体(complement 1 and 3 receptors，CR1 和 CR3)、甘露糖受体(mannose receptor，MR)、Fc 受体(Fc receptors，FcR)和纤维连接蛋白受体结合[12]。激活的巨噬细胞释放 ROS，使一氧化氮合酶(nitric oxide synthase，iNOS)的表达升高，产生一氧化氮(nitric oxide，NO)。ROS 和 NO 对利什曼原虫具有高度毒性[10]。

天然免疫细胞表达模式识别受体(pattern recognition receptor，PRR)识别病原体相关分子模式(pathogen-associated molecular pattern，PAMP)。这些受体包括 toll 样受体(Toll-like receptor，TLR)、胞质 DNA 传感器(cytosolic DNA sensors，CDS)、nod 样受体(NOD-like receptor，NLR)、rig-I 样受体(RIG-I-like receptors，RLR)和 C 型凝集素受体(C-type lectin receptor，CLR)。TLR2 和 TLR4 识别细胞外利什曼原虫，而 TLR3 和 TLR9 则识别胞内利什曼原虫。每种 TLR 在利什曼原虫防御或持续感染中的作用取决于利什曼原虫的种类[13]。然而，NLRP3 炎症小体的功能仍存在争议。一些研究表明，NLRP3 可被利什曼原虫激活，导致促炎细胞因子 IL-1β 和 IL-18 的产生(见综述[10])；另一方面，杜氏利什曼原虫利用巨噬细胞刺激 A20 的表达，这种分子抑制 NLRP3 炎症小体的激活和 IL-1β 的表达[14]。

利什曼原虫感染的适应性免疫有助于宿主清除虫体或参与致病进程[15]。利什曼虫的保护性免疫需适当激活天然免疫细胞。活化的 DC 产生 IL-12、IL-18 和 IL-27 细胞因子，可进一步刺激 IFN-γ 的分泌及 CD4$^+$T 细胞 Th1 分化。一方面，Th1 型应答产生细胞因子(尤其是 IFN-α 可增强巨噬细胞的活化，产生更多的 NO 和 ROS，从而有助于清除虫体)(见综述[16])；另一方面，Th2 型应答高表达 IL-4 和 IL-13，以及与 TNF-α 高表达相关的超炎症反应，有助于促进 DCL 的易感性或发展[17]。其他 Th 亚细胞的作用尚未被阐明，Th17 T 细胞在虫种间的特有作用尚存在争议[18]。在利什曼原虫感染中 Treg 细胞产生 IL-10，与虫体发育迟缓、耐药性和疾病复发有关[19]。

尽管宿主免疫系统有清除虫体的机制，但利什曼原虫亦已形成了逃避宿主免疫应答的策略。利什曼原虫产生的分子可干扰细胞信号通路，改变促炎受体和细胞因子的表达，从而促进虫体存活[20]。GP63 是一种含量丰富的重要的表面蛋白酶，被认为是一种毒力因子，通过改变补体介导的裂解参与虫体侵入，并干扰巨噬细胞的 PKC 信号，参与利什曼原虫与宿主细胞及细胞外基质的相互作用[21]。利什曼原虫的表面还含有一种 LPG，保护虫体免受补体介导的裂解作用。而 LPG 诱导补体活化，伴随着吞噬溶酶体的延迟形成，促进利什曼原虫的吞噬作用，使虫体分化为增生性无毛鞭毛体[22]。

寄生虫释放的组分可调节和活化吞噬细胞的功能以及免疫应答。一些研究表明，寄生虫的分泌物含有潜在的可调节免疫细胞的分子[23]。除分泌分子外，利什曼原虫还会自发释放 EV(图 8-1)，这些囊泡在感染免疫和疾病进程中具有生物学作用[24,25]。

Silverman 等首次报道了婴儿利什曼原虫前鞭毛体的发育过程，从鞭毛囊到稳定期细胞均可释放 EV[26]。另有研究表明，利什曼原虫的 EV 中含有毒力因子(如 *GP63* 和 LPG)以

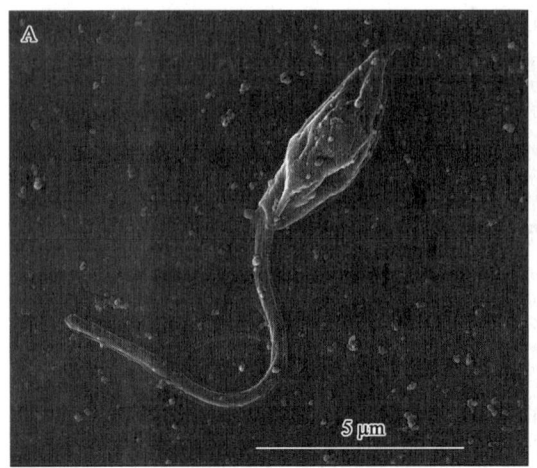 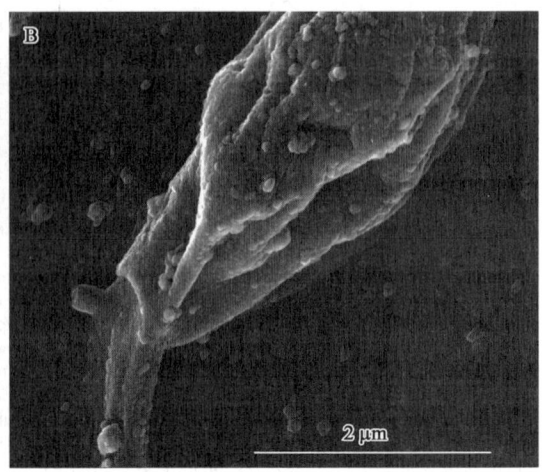

图 8-1 亚马孙利什曼原虫 MHOM/BR/1973/M2269 株的 SEM 显示 EV 脱落。在含有 2%葡萄糖的 DMEM 中培养的前鞭毛体,黏附在含有多聚赖氨酸的盖玻片上,随后进行固定和 SEM 观察。简单地说,将样品按照已建立的实验方案操作。2.5%戊二醛溶液固定后用 0.1 M 碳酸钙溶液洗涤,再用鞣酸处理的四氧化锇固定,乙醇脱水,然后在 CPD 030 临界点干燥仪中干燥。最后采用溅射方法(sputtering,© Leica EM 500 SCD, Germany)将样品镀上金层,然后在 FEI Quanta 250 FEG 的 SEM 下进行场发射观察。每个图像中都用标尺显示大小

及参与利什曼原虫致病的多种分子[25,27],提示这些 EV 可能参与了利什曼病感染和疾病的进程。在前鞭毛体培养的上清液中检测到其释放的 EV,在白蛉肠腔内也检测到利什曼原虫,表明利什曼原虫可能参与宿主的感染进程[27]。培养的巨噬细胞通过表面结合、与细胞膜融合或内吞作用吞噬利什曼原虫的外泌体[25,28]。杜氏利什曼原虫释放的 EV 通过 THP-1 巨噬细胞的分化,可提高 IL-8 的产生[25]。而人单核细胞暴露于杜氏利什曼原虫的 EV 后可感染该虫,经 IFN-γ 处理后,IL-8、TNF-α 表达水平显著降低,而 IL-10 表达水平升高,表明杜氏利什曼原虫释放的 EV 对人单核细胞具有免疫抑制作用[29]。

小鼠模型实验也有助于更好地理解利什曼原虫释放的 EV 在疾病进程中的作用。与未处理组小鼠相比,杜氏利什曼原虫 EV 处理的 C57Bl/6 小鼠显示出更高的虫荷和 IL-10 表达[25]。在硕大利什曼原虫 EV 处理的 BALB/c 小鼠实验中也得到了相同结果。与对照组相比,经两次注射 15 μg 利什曼原虫 EV 的小鼠表现 Th2 极化优势,病变体积(mm)增大,病情加重[25]。此外,对 BALB/c 小鼠足底同时注射虫体和 EV 对感染部位的影响也进行了评估。硕大利什曼原虫 EV 通过促进虫体复制和增强细胞因子的表达,尤其是 IL-17a 的表达(一种促炎细胞因子),显著促进了病变的发展[27]。因此,利什曼原虫 EV 可能是利什曼原虫建立感染的一种机制,有利于其生存和促进疾病进程。

被利什曼原虫感染的细胞释放的 EV 中已鉴定到病原体组分[30]。因此,已有一些研究对利什曼原虫感染细胞释放的 EV 进行了评估[29,31]。蛋白质组学分析表明,感染墨西哥利什曼原虫的 J774 细胞释放的 EV 中存在 GP63[31]。研究发现,感染墨西哥利什曼原虫的 J774 细胞释放的 EV 可诱导幼稚 naïve 型巨噬细胞,导致 MAP 激酶磷酸化[31]。原代培养的小鼠骨髓巨噬细胞经亚马孙利什曼原虫前鞭毛体感染的巨噬细胞释放的 EV 处理后,其炎性细胞因子的产生显著增加,这有助于清除病原体[32]。除了病原体分子,EV 还含有细胞

免疫分子,如 MHC 抗原肽复合物、游离抗原、细胞因子和共刺激分子,这些均有助于其参与免疫调节作用[30]。因此,利什曼原虫感染细胞的 EV 被认为与细胞-细胞间通信有关,影响免疫细胞的抗原提呈和免疫激活。

三、克氏锥虫

克氏锥虫也是一种原虫,是恰加斯病或南美洲锥虫病的病原体,是拉丁美洲和中美洲最致命的传染病之一。据估计,有 600 万~800 万人被感染,约 2 500 万人处于该病的危险中。超过 500 万人不知道自己患有该病。恰加斯病在美国和欧洲国家也是一种新现疾病,原因是流行区国家慢性感染者迁移,以及这些地区的血库和医院均没有定期筛查。这种原虫经昆虫媒介在伤口和黏膜内沉积,或通过被昆虫污染的食物经口传播给人类,如在巴西莓或甘蔗汁中发现该虫。该原虫还可通过输血、器官移植以及妊娠和(或)分娩时通过胎盘传播。虫媒介导的传播始于克氏锥虫粪便中由锥虫衍生的循环后期锥鞭毛体,随后进入哺乳动物宿主,并通过形成纳虫空泡入侵宿主细胞,进而开始虫媒传播。在宿主细胞内,锥鞭毛体转换为无鞭毛体,在细胞质中自由繁殖。在细胞内,无鞭毛体分化为感染性的锥鞭毛体,突破细胞膜,到达细胞外基质,随后随血流侵入周围的细胞和组织[33]。随后,虫媒接触到含有感染性锥鞭毛体的血液,或传播给其他宿主。

在人体中,恰加斯病的特点为急性期伴随慢性期。急性期表现为显微镜下可检测到血液寄生虫血症,并可在初次接触后持续 8 周。慢性期的诊断依赖血清学分析,因为此时只能应用高度敏感的 PCR 技术才能检测到。慢性克氏锥虫感染患者没有恰加斯病体征或临床症状,故认为具有不确定性。据估计,最初血清学检测呈阳性的患者中,有 20%~30% 的患者在数年或数十年内发展为临床症状明显的心肌病或严重胃肠道疾病,或两者兼有。

克氏锥虫利用一种非常精细的分子阵列和策略入侵广泛的宿主细胞[34,35],并逃避宿主免疫防御机制[36]。侵入和免疫抵御都是克氏锥虫在哺乳动物宿主体内成功生存、增殖和永存所必需的重要过程。一些寄生虫表面分子与宿主细胞侵入和(或)宿主免疫调节有关[37]。60%~80% 的锥鞭毛体表面由糖复合物组成,主要为黏蛋白样糖蛋白、黏蛋白相关表面蛋白(mucin-associated surface proteins,MASP)和 gp85/反式-唾液酸酶样糖蛋白超家族成员[38,39]。所有这些糖蛋白都通过糖基磷脂酰肌醇(glycosylphosphatidyl inositol,GPI)脂与细胞膜相联系,而虫体表面也有被称为糖基磷脂酰肌醇脂(glycosylphospholipid,GPIL)的糖基磷脂[37]。当虫体进入宿主细胞,巨噬细胞被激活,级联反应达到高潮:细胞因子产生,白细胞被吸引和激活,IL-12、IL-10 的表达升高。巨噬细胞和 NK 细胞产生的 IL-12 和 IFN-γ 影响巨噬细胞效应因子的功能,导致向促炎反应的极化,相对于有利于寄生虫生存的 Th2 型反应,这有助于消除虫体[37]。

一些研究对诱导这些细胞因子和 NO 产生的寄生虫组分进行研究。锥鞭毛体中含量最为丰富的表面蛋白、黏蛋白样糖蛋白可激活促炎反应,这归因于 GPI 锚点中独一无二的不饱和脂肪酸[37]。然而,目前尚不清楚这些表面蛋白及其他表面蛋白,以及 GPI 锚定分子是如何传递的? 它们如何通过同源受体触发特定的信号通路发挥作用的? 预测有两种可能性:① 作为可溶性分子释放;② EV。在原虫中已发现酶介导或自发释放 GPI 锚定组分[37]。在克氏锥虫中,抗原脱落也是非常重要的现象[1,40]。然而,这些研究并没有揭示这些抗原是否以可溶性和(或)膜结合的形式释放。

与此同时,电子扫描显微镜显示,锥鞭毛体自发释放 20~200 nm 的 EV(图 8-2)。不同克氏锥虫在分离株释放 EV 的过程中不会丧失其感染性,表明细胞死亡并不发生在囊泡分泌过程中。经凝胶过滤纯化的 EV 的主要成分为含有替代 α-半乳糖残基的黏蛋白样糖蛋白,包含 TS 样糖蛋白家族成员,并具有强免疫原性[40,41]。这些 α-半乳糖富集(α-galactosyl-enriched, α-Gal)的 EV,通过 TLR2 依赖的通路,强有力地触发小鼠巨噬细胞的促炎反应[42]。克氏锥虫的 EV 与宿主 TLR2 相互作用导致炎症反应和细胞侵袭增强,这可能有利于虫体在宿主内的长期生存(未发表数据)。的确,在感染锥鞭毛体前用这些 EV 预处理的 BALB/c 小鼠,可产生更严重的心脏病变,并伴随强烈的炎症反应,以及增加心脏组织细胞内无鞭毛体巢的数量[4]。

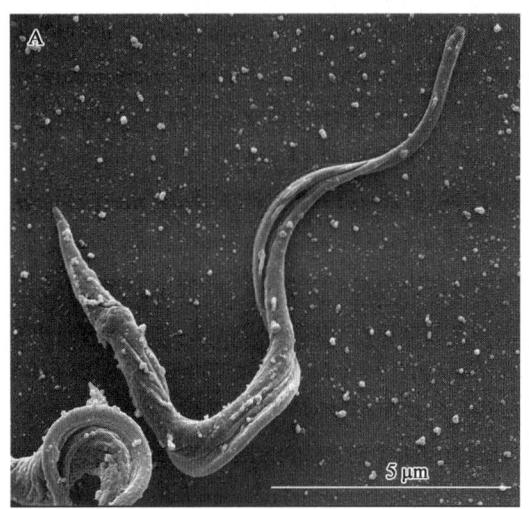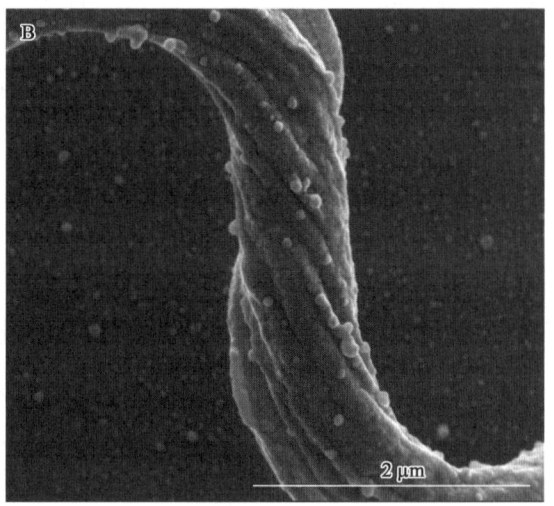

图 8-2 Y 株克氏锥虫锥鞭毛体扫描电镜显示 EV 脱落。在含有 2%葡萄糖的 DMEM 中将锥鞭毛体预孵育,其黏附在含有聚赖氨酸的盖玻片上,如图 8-1 所示进行固定和扫描电镜观察。每个图像中用标尺显示了大小

不同克氏锥虫分离株均可释放 EV,而 YuYu 株比 Y 株分泌物更具感染性,所含的 EV 也比 Y 株更多[41]。对这些 EV 的蛋白质组学分析表明,在这两种不同 EV 中均存在一些 TS/gp85 超家族成员。而这些蛋白最有可能参与虫体黏附到宿主细胞,因此可能由于毒性更强的虫株分泌更多 EV 而导致感染性的差异。此外,这些蛋白家族的一些组分与反式唾液酸酶相呼应,反式唾液酸酶催化唾液酸从宿主分子转移到虫体黏蛋白,并已被证实参与宿主细胞的黏附和侵入,虫体从宿主细胞的细胞质的吞噬溶酶体中逃逸,并从哺乳动物细胞中退出。TS 的存在还可保护寄生虫免受宿主补体和溶解性抗 α-半乳糖抗体的侵害,调控宿主免疫应答和凋亡反应。有研究认为,寄生虫的免疫逃避机制依赖于寄生虫诱导释放宿主细胞源囊泡的能力,这些囊泡通过保护寄生虫免受补体攻击而有助于其免疫逃避,最终使虫体的感染性和存活率增加[43]。

值得注意的是,TS 在种系发育的 2 个主要分支:克氏锥虫 I 和 II 中表达有差异;后者通常与人感染有关,TS 的表达和脱落量更高。这一现象清晰地强调了激活 TS 的重要性,其可能在 EV 中为虫体的一个毒力因子。EV 中存在 TS/gp85 超家族中其他不具有酶活性的相关成员,可能在与宿主细胞的相互作用中发挥重要作用。与 Y 株相比,YuYu 株(毒性更强)释放的 EV 对巨噬细胞的感染性更弱,但在细胞内增殖更强。相比之下,YuYu 株源 EV 比 Y 株源 EV 引起的上皮细胞感染更强[41]。此外,还发现不同克氏锥虫虫株源 EV 也存在质的差异,但目前尚不能将其与感染力/毒力差异联系起来。

除血液中锥鞭毛体释放 EV 外,其他一些发育阶段的虫体也可释放特异性 EV。例如,增殖型克氏锥虫的短鞭毛体不具有感染性,在虫媒的后肠可发育为具有感染性的循环后期锥鞭毛体,表明在其 EV 中有不同的蛋白质组分[44]。这些差异可能源于这些不同发育阶段虫体的代谢和基因表达不同,提示每个 EV 的特殊作用,可能与虫媒的相互作用和(或)虫体感染的起始阶段有关。EV 似乎是由于 MVB 的胞外融合产生外泌体,并直接从细胞膜上出芽形成微泡(microvesicle,MV),也称为胞外体或细胞膜源囊泡。总之,克氏锥虫所有发育阶段均会采取将 EV 作为一种释放虫体主要表面组分的策略,这些组分参与虫体的黏附、侵入、生存和逃避宿主免疫反应。

四、布氏锥虫

布氏锥虫动质体(锥虫属)是昏睡病或非洲锥虫病的病原体,影响撒哈拉以南非洲 36 个国家数百万人和动物的那加那病[45]。布氏锥虫有三个亚种,即感染哺乳动物的布氏锥虫,以及感染人的布氏冈比亚锥虫和布氏罗得西亚锥虫。这些锥虫通过舌蝇(舌蝇属)传播,舌蝇在吸食血液时将锥鞭毛体刺入皮肤组织。被叮咬后,锥鞭毛体先进入淋巴系统,随后进入血液。虫体滞留在血液中,如果不及时治疗,会导致贫血、神经系统紊乱和死亡[45]。布氏锥虫是一种细胞外寄生虫,寄生在哺乳动物血液或舌蝇肠道和虫媒唾液腺中。血液中的锥鞭毛体主要表达表面糖蛋白,围绕虫体周围形成保护膜。该蛋白称为变异表面糖蛋白(variant surface glycoprotein,VSG),由一个多基因家族编码,每次仅表达该家族的一个成员。在布氏锥虫感染的过程中,一旦宿主建立了免疫反应,就会表达另一个 VSG,使虫体逃避宿主免疫防御,导致慢性感染。而在长期感染中,虫体会穿过血脑屏障。

VSG 通过 GPI-锚定黏附在细胞膜上,通过补体替代途径保护虫体免受裂解,并产生抗非特异性抗体[46]。在感染宿主过程中,VSG 和含有 CqG 的锥虫 DNA 分别被 SR-A 和 TLR9 识别,进而促进巨噬细胞和 DC 的活化和促炎细胞因子(TNF-α、IL-6 和 IL-12)的产生。这些锥虫组分以及激活 NK 细胞和 T 细胞而产生的 INF-γ 可诱导激活 I 型巨噬细胞(type 1 macrophages,M1)。这些强烈的 Th1 型反应诱导 NO 的产生,有助于控制布氏锥虫感染。同时在疾病急性期,红细胞摄取增加,可引起贫血[47]。最新研究表明,布氏锥虫 EV 也可促进红细胞被清除,从而导致贫血[48]。

布氏冈比亚锥虫通过从鞭毛袋伸出的纳米管释放 EV。这些 EV 从虫体分泌物和感染大鼠血清中分离获得,直径在 50~100 nm,外泌体大小一致[49]。虫体分泌物中鉴定的蛋白似乎对寄生虫的生存策略有直接作用[49]。例如,经血液释放的布氏罗得西亚锥虫 EV 含血清耐药相关蛋白(serum resistance-associated protein，SRA)，这种蛋白可保护锥虫在人血液中生存。这种蛋白不存在布氏锥虫 EV 中，可能是这种亚种不感染人和一些具有天然免疫因子的灵长类动物的原因之一[48]。研究表明，布氏锥虫源 EV 与红细胞膜融合，传递脂质和 VSG 糖蛋白。红细胞膜的改变造成被肝和脾中的巨噬细胞识别和吞噬，进而导致宿主贫血[48]。一些真核细胞分泌机制(ESCRT 机制)已在布氏锥虫中有相似报道[50]，并表明抑制 Vsp36(一种 ESCRT 成分)会损害 EV 的分泌，但对纳米管源 EV 没有影响[51]。因此，这两种类型的囊泡可能有不同的分泌机制，且在生化上也不同[51]。

布氏锥虫 EV 也与虫体活动力有关，可诱导虫体从受损的细胞和有害的环境中迁移出来。这些 EV 通过昆虫(昆虫体内的布氏锥虫前循环体)被内化，是虫体-虫体间通信的关键组成部分[51]。综上所述，布氏锥虫源 EV 在宿主的细胞与细胞间通信以及宿主与细胞间通信中发挥重要作用，并为开发新的潜在治疗靶点或诊断标志物提供新见解。

五、疟原虫

疟疾是热带和亚热带地区的一种疾病，在 91 个国家均发现有该病(WHO，2017)。据 WHO 报道，全球有 2.19 亿例疟疾病例，43.5 万人死于疟疾。目前，估计有 33 亿人生活在危险地区(WHO，2017 年)(https://www.who.int/malaria/en)。疟疾的病原体为疟原虫，其中三种疟原虫对人体健康具有重大威胁，分别为间日疟原虫、三日疟原虫和恶性疟原虫。人的感染为正在吸食血液的雌性按蚊将子孢子射入真皮层引起。子孢子到达肝脏，侵入肝细胞。在肝细胞内，子孢子发生分裂发育，成千上万的裂殖子释放到血液中。裂殖子侵入红细胞，在血液中开始无性裂体增殖的慢性循环。宿主网织红细胞被间日疟原虫感染。一部分无性繁殖的裂殖子重复裂体增殖，形成配子体，发育为雌雄配子体。蚊子摄取外周循环中的雌雄配子体，在外周循环经历几个循环，并在按蚊中肠中进行增殖，直到产生子孢子，这些子孢子迁移到唾液腺，按蚊吸血时随唾液进入下一个人体内[52]。

疟疾致病机制和防控中包含免疫应答，但反复的疟原虫感染不能形成完全免疫，进而导致流行区人群一生中可多次感染。皮肤感染后，天然免疫反应被触发[53]。一些天然受体被疟原虫 PAMP 激活并参与 DC 的功能，如 T 细胞、B 细胞被激活[54]。然而，寄生虫可通过多种机制逃避免疫反应，包括抑制 DC 的成熟。

研究表明，包括人疟疾和啮齿动物疟疾在内的几种疟原虫病原体，在感染活跃期的人和小鼠血清或血浆可释放 EV[1,2,55]。在小鼠疟疾模型中发现，注射 EV 可控制约氏疟原虫感染网织红细胞[56]。在感染伯氏疟原虫(ANKA 株)的小鼠中，从被约氏疟原虫感染的红细胞分离获得的 EV 通过 TLR 诱导巨噬细胞产生强烈的刺激作用[57]，这些 EV 中含有疟原虫蛋白和 RNA，具有促炎作用，并刺激 TLR 通路。且被约氏疟原虫感染的网织红细胞源外泌体中含有许多宿主和虫体蛋白。研究发现，这些蛋白在感染约氏疟原虫 17X 株的 BALB/c 小鼠中参与调控宿主免疫反应[56]，这些蛋白包括裂殖子表面蛋白 1 和 9 以及与蛋白水解和代谢相关的酶，可诱导强烈的 IgG 反应。此外，在 85% 实验小鼠中，这些外泌体可结合 CpG 寡核苷酸，诱导对致死性感染的保护。在其他研究中，也发现感染恶性疟原虫的红细胞会释放 EV,且这些 EV 也含有宿主和虫体蛋白,在宿主和虫体间的细胞间通信中发挥作用[6]。此外,感染红细胞(infected erythrocytes,iRBC)释放的 EV 可将遗传物质转移到细胞上。从 iRBC 中分离获得的 EV 还可诱导配子体的生成,并对获得这些含有虫体遗传物质的虫体产生抗性。许多研究表明,疟原虫 EV 定位于脑内,可调节宿主免疫系统,引起疟疾的严重临床症状。在脑病变的疟疾患者中,EV 释放增加。此外,血小板 EV 可参与 iRBC 细胞黏附。

EV 被认为是严重脑型疟的生物标志物,与临床表现(如发热)和脑功能障碍(如炎症反应)相关[58]。因此,网织红细胞或红细胞源 EV 可作为疟原虫与宿主细胞间的联络,调控几种疟疾感染的致病机制。更重要的是,网织红细胞源外泌体可作为抗疟疾感染的疫苗平台。

六、刚地弓形虫

弓形虫病是由刚地弓形虫感染引起的一种重要的细胞内原虫,全球近三分之一的人口受感染[59]。大多数感染弓形虫的患者无症状,但免疫功能低下者可致死。原发性感染的孕妇可引起胎儿先天性感染,并导致严重的后遗症或胎儿死亡[60]。

刚地弓形虫在猫科动物小肠中进行有性生殖,在包括人在内的感染动物中进行无性生殖。人的感染是摄入卵囊(在感染的猫粪便中释放)或包囊(在未煮熟的肉中)。在肠腔内,包囊或卵囊释放裂殖子和子孢子侵入细胞,转化为速殖子,到达血管系统或淋巴系统。速殖子几乎可感染所有有核细胞和组织,在急性期可在生物液体中被检测到;在慢性期,速殖子转化为生长缓慢的缓殖子,并持续存在于宿主组织的包囊内[61]。

在健康人中,天然和适应性免疫反应的激活可清除大部分虫体。因为在感染过程中,虫体分泌产物可激活巨噬细胞和 DC。而 TLR 和其他 PAMP 受体的刺激诱导天然免疫反应,产生促炎细胞因子,促进适当的炎性环境,随后招募中性粒细胞、单核细胞和 NK 细胞。然后,适应性免疫细胞(T 淋巴细胞和 B 淋巴细胞)被激活。然而,对速殖子的免疫压力诱导其转化为缓殖子,从而逃避宿主的免疫应答,致疾病进展到慢性阶段[62]。

弓形虫在速殖子和缓殖子的细胞表面表达多种抗原[63]。这些抗原具有多种作用,包括虫体黏附于宿主细胞和虫体在细胞环境中生存[63]。表面抗原(surface antigen,SAG)1 和 SAG2 家族为 GPI 锚定抗原,是最重要的表面抗原之一[64]。此外,刚地弓形虫的分泌抗原可刺激抗体和 T 细胞反应。致密颗粒、微线体和棒状体上的分子为弓形虫进入细胞后的结构,具有高度的免疫原性,除了用于血清学诊断,还可诱导保护性免疫反应[65-67]。

采用蛋白质组学方法可检测弓形虫释放的 EV 中的一些细胞表面抗原和分泌蛋白[68],在这些 EV 中也可检测到小 RNA 和 miRNA[69]。这表明弓形虫 EV 可传递毒力因子和其他有助于宿主-寄生虫相互作用的分子。慢性感染者血清或小鼠血清可识别这些 EV,也证实了免疫原性分子在 EV 中的存在和表达[69]。

体内外研究证实了弓形虫 EV 的免疫作用。弓形虫 EV 可刺激小鼠巨噬细胞高表达 IL-10、iNOS 和 TNF-α[69]。用弓形虫 EV 处理的 RAW 264.7 细胞可诱导 IL-12、TNF-α、IFN-γ 的产生,同时抑制 IL-10 的表达[70]。在体内,与对照组相比,用弓形虫 EV 免疫的小鼠显示出 IgG2a 优于 IgG1,并且 IFN-γ 和 IL-12 的水平较高,表明用 EV 免疫可诱导 Th1 型细胞免疫谱[70]。且与对照组相比,EV 免疫小鼠受到弓形虫致命性感染后,存活时间显著延长,表明 EV 对实验室感染的弓形虫病具有部分保护作用[70]。

感染弓形虫的 DC 和携带弓形虫抗原的脉冲 EV 释放具有免疫调控特性的外泌体,这些 EV 在免疫动物中诱导特异性的 Th1 免疫应答[71]。此外,这些 EV 对弓形虫攻击感染的小鼠产生全身性保护免疫[71]。这种免疫调控作用在感染弓形虫的 THP-1 细胞释放的 EV 实验中也可观察到。EV 可刺激未感染弓形虫的 THP-1 细胞产生 TNF-α[72]。因此,感染弓形虫的免疫细胞释放的 EV 可刺激促炎反应,有助于产生有效的抗弓形虫免疫。更好地了解弓形虫或肝吸虫感染细胞释放的 EV 在免疫和免疫监视中的作用,有助于研发新的抗弓形虫感染策略,以保护孕妇和生活在风险地区的人。

七、十二指肠贾第虫

肠道原虫十二指肠贾第虫,每年可导致全球 2.8 亿例腹泻感染(贾第虫病),其中发展中国家患病率最高[73]。贾第虫感染可表现为无症状到严重的吸收障碍综合征。肠上皮细胞在抵御微生物入侵中发挥重要作用,并表达 PRR,能捕获病原体,建立第一道免疫反应防线。$CD4^+$ Th17 细胞产生 IL-17,诱导肠上皮细胞产生 NO、抗菌肽、趋化因子和转运 IgA[74]。

感染形成的贾第虫包囊是通过污染的食物或水被摄入。当包囊进入体内,接触到酸性 pH 值及囊壁蛋白(cyst wall proteins,CWP)被肠蛋白酶降解后脱囊(释放滋养体)。随后,包囊在肠内释放滋养体(复制形式),并附着在肠上皮细胞上。在包囊形成过程中,滋养体通过胞吞作用释放含有 CWP 的包囊特异性囊泡(encystation-specific vesicle,ESV)[75,76]。这些囊泡的释放与包囊形成有关。一些研究者认为,由于 pH 的变化和胆汁的存在,滋养体中 ESV 增加[77],这可能对贾第虫在宿主感染期间的生存很重要。

富含半胱氨酸的蛋白称为可变表面蛋白(variable surface protein,VSP),覆盖在滋养体表面,并通过不断转换帮助虫体逃避宿主免疫系统[77,79]。其中一些蛋白具有分泌半胱氨酸蛋白酶活性的功能,可作为毒力因子[80-83]。贾第虫分泌一种组织蛋白酶 B 样半胱氨酸蛋白酶,可降解 CXCL8 并减弱中性粒细胞的趋化性[82]。一项蛋白质组学研究发现,寄生虫分泌物中有多种蛋白,其中一些为 EV 释放[84]。贾第虫 EV 大小为 100~250 nm[84]。最近研究表明,贾第虫释放的 EV 有助于贾第虫定植,增加对上皮细胞的黏附,并诱导免疫反应[85]。由于贾第虫没有高尔基复合体和明确的内吞系统,其囊泡运输和生物学功能尚不完全清楚[86]。ESCRT 复合物的亚基在酵母和哺乳动物中参与了内溶酶体分选过程,但似乎这些蛋白不仅在序列上,而且在功能特征上也存在差异[87]。这些研究虽然强调了囊泡在贾第虫病致病中的重要性,然而仍需要更多的研究来阐明 EV 在其感染过程中的作用。

八、总结

本章中,我们从多方面阐述了 EV 如何与一些致病性原虫及宿主相互作用。一些病原微生物分泌膜和胞质作为外泌体和(或)不同类型的 EV,这一认识使我们能更好地理解寄生虫与宿主相互作用的复杂机制。EV 参与多种活动,如组织和细胞侵袭,还直接影响宿主的天然和适应性免疫应答,最终促进寄生虫的生存和传播。因此,EV 的释放在疾病的致病机制中也有很多作用。表 8-1 总结了目前有关寄生虫的生物学特性以及与宿主细胞源 EV 相互作用中主要作用的知识点。此外,EV 也可从感染的细胞中释放出来,其中一些细胞含有寄生虫组分,扩展了这些结构在疾病和愈合过程中的作用。然而,一些重要问题仍未得到解答。例如,不同寄生虫释放 EV 的机制仍需阐明,以及作为预防疾病进程的可能策略尚需更多研究。此外,从寄生虫中分离出的 EV 对免疫预防和治疗具有很强的潜力,尚待进一步探讨,这里主要指被忽略的热带病。

表 8-1 与寄生虫 EV 相关的不同糖蛋白、脂质或核酸及其与宿主-寄生虫的相互作用

寄生虫	分子	对宿主的影响	参考文献
杜氏利什曼原虫 婴儿利什曼原虫 墨西哥利什曼原虫	GP63 LPG HSP	通过改变补体介导的裂解以及促进寄生虫吞噬作用,使虫体实现免疫逃避	[25,88]
克氏锥虫	反式唾液酸酶 Cruzipnai 黏蛋白 GP85 虫体抗原	通过 TLR2,促进虫体与宿主相互作用、侵入,并诱导宿主炎症和天然免疫应答,进而使虫体逃避补体的攻击(携带 TGF-β 的 EV 从单核细胞和淋巴细胞释放),EV 增强通信克氏锥虫和宿主(人)细胞之间的通信,以促进虫体侵入	[1,41-43,89]
刚地弓形虫	小 RNA/微小 RNA	诱导体液和细胞免疫反应	[69]
间日疟原虫 恶性疟原虫 伯氏疟原虫 约氏疟原虫	寄生虫 蛋白质 CSP? ABCA1 转运蛋白	与宿主细胞的相互作用 EV 与发热、脑功能障碍等临床表现相关,提示 EV 在疟疾发病机制中的作用是通过 TLR 调节质膜外层存在磷脂酰丝氨酸(phosphatidylserine,PS)诱导巨噬细胞的有效活化,PS 是 MV 表面的主要成分 在体内调控免疫应答作用 促进 iRBC 之间遗传物质的转换(iRBC 衍生的 EV 和诱导配子体细胞发生)	[2,6,56]
布氏锥虫	VSG 蛋白酶	逃避宿主免疫系统,增加侵入血脑屏障	[48]
十二指肠贾第虫	蛋白	寄生虫在感染过程中适应宿主环境变化的机制	[85]

注:LPG,磷酸酯多糖;VSG,变异表面糖蛋白;CSP,环子孢子蛋白;PS,磷脂酰丝氨酸;MV,微泡;iRBC,感染红细胞;BBB,血脑屏障。

(沈玉娟 译,曹建平 审校)

参考文献

[1] Campos JH, Soares RP, Ribeiro K, Andrade AC, Batista WL, Torrecilhas AC. Extracellular vesicles: role in inflammatory responses and potential uses in vaccination in cancer and infectious diseases. J Immunol Res 2015; 832057. https://doi.org/10.1155/2015/832057.

[2] Marcilla A, Martin-Jaular L, Trelis M, de Menezes-Neto A, Osuna A, Bernal D, Fernandez-Becerra C, Almeida IC, Del Portillo HA. Extracellular vesicles in parasitic diseases. J Extracell Vesicles 2014; 3: 25040.

[3] Torrecilhas AC, Schumacher RI, Alves MJ, Colli W. Vesicles as carriers of virulence factors in parasitic protozoan diseases. Microbes Infect 2012; 14(15): 1465-74. https://doi.org/10.1016/j.micinf.2012.07.008.

[4] Trocoli Torrecilhas AC, Tonelli RR, Pavanelli WR, da Silva JS, Schumacher RI, de Souza W, Silva NCE, de Almeida Abrahamsohn I, Colli W, Manso Alves MJ. *Trypanosoma cruzi*: parasite shed vesicles increase heart parasitism and generate an intense inflammatory response. Microbes Infect 2009; 11(1): 29-39. https://doi.org/10.1016/j.micinf.2008.10.003.

[5] Coakley G, Maizels RM, Buck AH. Exosomes and other extracellular vesicles: the new communicators in parasite infections. Trends Parasitol 2015; 31(10): 477-89. https://doi.org/10.1016/j.pt.2015.06.009.

[6] Regev-Rudzki N, Wilson DW, Carvalho TG, Sisquella X, Coleman BM, Rug M, Bursac D, Angrisano F, Gee M, Hill AF, Baum J, Cowman AF. Cell-cell communication between malaria-infected red blood cells via exosome-kike vesicles. Cell 2013; 153(5): 1120-33. https://doi.org/10.1016/j.cell.2013.04.029.

[7] Alvar J, Vélez ID, Bern C, Herrero M, Desjeux P, Cano J, Jannin J, den Boer M, Leishmaniasis Control Team WHO. Leishmaniasis worldwide and global estimates of its incidence. PLoS ONE 2012; 7(5): e35671. https://doi.org/10.1371/journal.pone.0035671.

[7a] Ross R. Note on the bodies recently described by Leishman and Donovan. Br Med J 1903; 2: 1261-2.

[7b] Ross R. Further notes of Leishman's bodies. Br Med J 1903; 2: 1401.

[8] Lainson R, Ryan L, Shaw JJ. Infective stages of *Leishmania* in the sandfly vector and some observations on the mechanism of transmission. Mem Inst Oswaldo Cruz 1987; 82(3): 421-4.

[9] Chappuis F, Sundar S, Hailu A, Ghalib H, Rijal S, Peeling RW, Alvar J, Boelaert M. Visceral leishmaniasis: what are the needs for diagnosis, treatment and control? Nat Rev Microbiol 2007; 5(11): 873-82. https://doi.org/10.1038/nrmicro1748.

[10] Gurung P, Kanneganti TD. Innate immunity against *Leishmania* infections. Cell Microbiol 2015; 17(9): 1286-94. https://doi.org/10.1111/cmi.12484.

[11] Liu D, Uzonna JE. The early interaction of *Leishmania* with macrophages and dendritic cells and its influence on the host immune response. Front Cell Infect Microbiol 2012; 2: 83. https://doi.org/10.3389/fcimb.2012.00083.

[12] Ueno N, Wilson ME. Receptor-mediated phagocytosis of *Leishmania*: implications for intracellular survival. Trends Parasitol 2012; 28(8): 335-44. https://doi.org/10.1016/j.pt.2012.05.002.

[13] Faria MS, Reis FC, Lima AP. Toll-kike receptors in *Leishmania* infections: guardians or promoters? J Parasitol Res 2012; 2012: 930257. https://doi.org/10.1155/2012/930257.

[14] Gupta AK, Ghosh K, Palit S, Barua J, Das PK, Ukil A. inhibits inflammasome-dependent macrophage activation by exploiting the negative regulatory proteins A20 and UCP2. FASEB J 2017; 31(11): 5087-101. https://doi.org/10.1096/fj.201700407R.

[15] Scott P, Novais FO. Cutaneous leishmaniasis: immune responses in protection and pathogenesis. Nat Rev Immunol 2016; 16: 581-92. https://doi.org/10.1038/nri.2016.72.

[16] Soong L. Subversion and utilization of host innate defense by *Leishmania amazonensis*. Front Immunol 2012; 3: 58. https://doi.org/10.3389/fimmu.2012.00058.

[17] Silveira FT, Lainson R, De Castro Gomes CM, Laurenti MD, Corbett CE. Immunopathogenic competences of *Leishmania* (V.) *braziliensis* and *L.* (*L.*) *amazonensis* in American cutaneous leishmaniasis. Parasite Immunol 2009; 31(8): 423-31. https://doi.org/10.1111/j.1365-3024.2009.01116.x.

[18] Lopez Kostka S, Dinges S, Griewank K, Iwakura Y, Udey MC, von Stebut E. IL-17 promotes progression of cutaneous leishmaniasis in susceptible mice. J Immunol 2009; 182(5): 3039-46. https://doi.org/10.4049/jimmunol.0713598.

[19] Katara GK, Ansari NA, Verma S, Ramesh V, Salotra P. Foxp3 and IL-10 expression correlates with parasite burden in lesional tissues of post kala azar dermal leishmaniasis (PKDL) patients. PLoS Negl Trop Dis 2011; 5(5): e1171. https://doi.org/10.1371/journal.pntd.0001171.

[20] Bhardwaj S, Srivastava N, Sudan R, Saha B. *Leishmania* interferes with host cell signaling to devise a survival strategy. J Biomed Biotechnol 2010; 2010: 109189. https://doi.org/10.1155/2010/109189.

[21] Isnard A, Shio MT, Olivier M. Impact of *Leishmania* metalloprotease GP63 on macrophage signaling. Front Cell Infect Microbiol 2012; 2: 72. https://doi.org/10.3389/fcimb.2012.00072.

[22] Forestier CL, Gao Q, Boons GJ. Leishmania lipophosphoglycan: how to establish structureactivity relationships for this highly complex and multifunctional glycoconjugate? Front Cell Infect Microbiol 2014; 4: 193. https://doi.org/10.3389/fcimb.2014.00193.

[23] Paape D, Aebischer T. Contribution of proteomics of *Leishmania* spp. to the understanding of differentiation, drug resistance mechanisms, vaccine and drug development. J Proteomics 2011; 74(9): 1614-24. https://doi.org/10.1016/j.jprot.2011.05.005.

[24] Paranaiba LF, Pinheiro LJ, Macedo DH, Menezes-Neto A, Torrecilhas AC, Tafuri WL, Soares RP. An overview on *Leishmania* (Mundinia) *enriettii*: biology, immunopathology, LRV and extracellular vesicles during the host-parasite interaction. Parasitology 2017; 1-9. https://doi.org/10.1017/S0031182017001810.

[25] Silverman JM, Clos J, de' Oliveira CC, Shirvani O, Fang Y, Wang C, Foster LJ, Reiner NE. An exosome-based secretion pathway is responsible for protein export from *Leishmania* and communication with macrophages. J Cell Sci 2010; 123(Pt. 6): 842-52. https://doi.org/10.1242/jcs.056465.

[26] Silverman JM, Chan SK, Robinson DP, Dwyer DM, Nandan D, Foster LJ, Reiner NE. Proteomic analysis of the secretome of *Leishmania donovani*. Genome Biol 2008; 9(2): R35. https://doi.org/10.1186/gb-2008-9-2-r35.

[27] Atayde VD, Aslan H, Townsend S, Hassani K, Kamhawi S, Olivier M. Exosome secretion by the parasitic protozoan *Leishmania* within the sand fly midgut. Cell Rep 2015; 13(5): 957-67. https://doi.org/10.1016/j.celrep.2015.09.058.

[28] Silverman JM, Reiner NE. *Leishmania* exosomes deliver preemptive strikes to create an environment permissive for early infection. Front Cell Infect Microbiol 2011; 1: 26. https://doi.org/10.3389/fcimb.2011.00026.

[29] Silverman JM, Clos J, Horakova E, Wang AY, Wiesgigl M, Kelly I, Lynn MA, McMaster WR, Foster LJ, Levings MK, Reiner NE. *Leishmania* exosomes modulate innate and adaptive immune responses through effects on monocytes

and dendritic cells. J Immunol 2010; 185(9): 5011-22. https://doi.org/10.4049/jimmunol.1000541.

[30] Schwab A, Meyering SS, Lepene B, Iordanskiy S, van Hoek ML, Hakami RM, Kashanchi F. Extracellular vesicles from infected cells: potential for direct pathogenesis. Front Microbiol 2015; 6: 1132. https://doi.org/10.3389/fmicb.2015.01132.

[31] Hassani K, Olivier M. Immunomodulatory impact of *Leishmania*-induced macrophage exosomes: a comparative proteomic and functional analysis. PLoS Negl Trop Dis 2013; 7(5): e2185. https://doi.org/10.1371/journal.pntd.0002185.

[32] Cronemberger-Andrade A, Aragão-França L, de Araujo CF, Rocha VJ, Borges-Silva MC, Figueira CP, Figueiras CP, Oliveira PR, de Freitas LA, Veras PS, Pontes-de-Carvalho L. Extracellular vesicles from *Leishmania*-infected macrophages confer an anti-infection cytokine-production profile to naïve macrophages. PLoS Negl Trop Dis 2014; 8(9): e3161. https://doi.org/10.1371/journal.pntd.0003161.

[33] Burleigh BA, Andrews NW. The mechanisms of *Trypanosoma cruzi* invasion of mammalian cells. Annu Rev Microbiol 1995; 49: 175-200. https://doi.org/10.1146/annurev.mi.49.100195.001135.

[34] Burleigh BA, Woolsey AM. Cell signalling and *Trypanosoma cruzi* invasion. Cell Microbiol 2002; 4(11): 701-11.

[35] Sibley LD, Andrews NW. Cell invasion by un-palatable parasites. Traffic 2000; 1(2): 100-6.

[36] Ouaissi A, Ouaissi M. Molecular basis of *Trypanosoma cruzi* and *Leishmania* interaction with their host(s): exploitation of immune and defense mechanisms by the parasite leading to persistence and chronicity, features reminiscent of immune system evasion strategies in cancer diseases. Arch Immunol Ther Exp (Warsz) 2005; 53(2): 102-14.

[37] Almeida IC, Gazzinelli RT. Proinflammatory activity of glycosylphosphatidylinositol anchors derived from *Trypanosoma cruzi*: structural and functional analyses. J Leukoc Biol 2001; 70(4): 467-77.

[38] Almeida IC, Camargo MM, Procópio DO, Silva LS, Mehlert A, Travassos LR, Gazzinelli RT, Ferguson MA. Highly purified glycosylphosphatidylinositols from *Trypanosoma cruzi* are potent proinflammatory agents. EMBO J 2000; 19(7): 1476-85. https://doi.org/10.1093/emboj/19.7.1476.

[39] Colli W. Trans-sialidase: a unique enzyme activity discovered in the protozoan *Trypanosoma cruzi*. FASEB J 1993; 7(13): 1257-64.

[40] Gonçalves MF, Umezawa ES, Katzin AM, de Souza W, Alves MJ, Zingales B, Colli W. *Trypanosoma cruzi*: shedding of surface antigens as membrane vesicles. Exp Parasitol 1991; 72(1): 43-53.

[41] Ribeiro KS, Vasconcellos CI, Soares RP, Mendes MT, Ellis CC, Aguilera-Flores M, de Almeida IC, Schenkman S, Iwai LK, Torrecilhas AC. Proteomic analysis reveals different composition of extracellular vesicles released by two. J Extracell Vesicles 2018; 7(1): 1463779. https://doi.org/10.1080/20013078.2018.1463779.

[42] Nogueira PM, Ribeiro K, Silveira AC, Campos JH, Martins-Filho OA, Bela SR, Campos MA, Pessoa NL, Colli W, Alves MJ, Soares RP, Torrecilhas AC. Vesicles from different *Trypanosoma cruzi* strains trigger differential innate and chronic immune responses. J Extracell Vesicles 2015; 4: 28734.

[43] Cestari I, Ansa-Addo E, Deolindo P, Inal JM, Ramirez MI. *Trypanosoma cruzi* immune evasion mediated by host cell-derived microvesicles. J Immunol 2012; 188(4): 1942-52. https://doi.org/10.4049/jimmunol.1102053.

[44] Bayer-Santos E, Aguilar-Bonavides C, Rodrigues SP, Cordero EM, Marques AF, Varela-Ramirez A, Choi H, Yoshida N, da Silveira JF, Almeida IC. Proteomic analysis of *Trypanosoma cruzi* secretome: characterization of two populations of extracellular vesicles and soluble proteins. J Proteome Res 2013; 12(2): 883-97. https://doi.org/10.1021/pr300947g.

[45] Büscher P, Cecchi G, Jamonneau V, Priotto G. Human African trypanosomiasis. Lancet 2017; 390(10110): 2397-409. https://doi.org/10.1016/S0140-6736(17)31510-6.

[46] Borst P, Ulbert S. Control of VSG gene expression sites. Mol Biochem Parasitol 2001; 114(1): 17-27.

[47] Stijlemans B, Caljon G, Van Den Abbeele J, Van Ginderachter JA, Magez S, De Trez C. Immune evasion strategies of *Trypanosoma brucei* within the mammalian host: progression to pathogenicity. Front Immunol 2016; 7: 233. https://doi.org/10.3389/fimmu.2016.00233.

[48] Szempruch AJ, Sykes SE, Kieft R, Dennison L, Becker AC, Gartrell A, Martin WJ, Nakayasu ES, Almeida IC, Hajduk SL, Harrington JM. Extracellular vesicles from *Trypanosoma brucei* mediate virulence factor transfer and cause host anemia. Cell 2016; 164(1-2): 246-57. https://doi.org/10.1016/j.cell.2015.11.051.

[49] Geiger A, Hirtz C, Becue T, Bellard E, Centeno D, Gargani D, Rossignol M, Cuny G, Peltier JB. Exocytosis and protein secretion in *Trypanosoma*. BMC Microbiol 2010; 10: 20. https://doi.org/10.1186/1471-2180-10-20.

[50] Silverman JS, Muratore KA, Bangs JD. Characterization of the late endosomal ESCRT machinery in *Trypanosoma brucei*. Traffic 2013; 14(10): 1078-90. https://doi.org/10.1111/tra.12094.

[51] Eliaz D, Kannan S, Shaked H, Arvatz G, Tkacz ID, Binder L, Waldman Ben-Asher H, Okalang U, Chikne V, Cohen-Chalamish S, Michaeli S. Exosome secretion affects social motility in *Trypanosoma brucei*. PLoS Pathog 2017; 13(3): e1006245. https://doi.org/10.1371/journal.ppat.1006245.

[52] Cowman AF, Healer J, Marapana D, Marsh K. Malaria: biology and disease. Cell 2016; 167(3): 610-24. https://doi.org/10.1016/j.cell.2016.07.055.

[53] Yamauchi LM, Coppi A, Snounou G, Sinnis P. *Plasmodium* sporozoites trickle out of the injection site. Cell Microbiol 2007; 9(5): 1215-22. https://doi.org/10.1111/j.1462-5822.2006.00861.x.

[54] Good MF, Doolan DL. Malaria vaccine design: immunological considerations. Immunity 2010; 33(4): 555-66. https://doi.org/10.1016/j.immuni.2010.10.005.

[55] Campos FM, Franklin BS, Teixeira-Carvalho A, Filho AL, de Paula SC, Fontes CJ, Brito CF, Carvalho LH. Augmented plasma microparticles during acute *Plasmodium vivax* infection. Malar J 2010; 9: 327. https://doi.org/10.1186/1475-2875-9-327.

[56] Martin-Jaular L, Nakayasu ES, Ferrer M, Almeida IC, Del Portillo HA. Exosomes from *Plasmodium yoelii*-infected reticulocytes protect mice from lethal infections. PLoS ONE 2011; 6(10): e26588. https://doi.org/10.1371/journal.pone.0026588.

[57] Couper KN, Barnes T, Hafalla JC, Combes V, Ryffel B, Secher T, Grau GE, Riley EM, de Souza JB. Parasite-derived plasma microparticles contribute significantly to malaria infection-induced inflammation through potent macrophage stimulation. PLoS Pathog 2010; 6(1): e1000744. https://doi.org/10.1371/journal.ppat.1000744.

[58] Martin-Jaular L, Ferrer M, Calvo M, Rosanas-Urgell A, Kalko S, Graewe S, Soria G, Cortadellas N, Ordi J, Planas A, Burns J, Heussler V, del Portillo HA. Strain-specific spleen remodelling in *Plasmodium yoelii* infections in Balb/c mice facilitates adherence and spleen macrophage-clearance escape. Cell Microbiol 2011; 13(1): 109–22. https://doi.org/10.1111/j.1462-5822.2010.01523.x.

[59] Skorokhod OA, Alessio M, Mordmüller B, Arese P, Schwarzer E. Hemozoin (malarial pigment) inhibits differentiation and maturation of human monocyte-derived dendritic cells: a peroxisome proliferator-activated receptor-gamma-mediated effect. J Immunol 2004; 173(6): 4066–74.

[60] Montoya JG, Remington JS. Management of *Toxoplasma gondii* infection during pregnancy. Clin Infect Dis 2008; 47(4): 554–66. https://doi.org/10.1086/590149.

[61] Saadatnia G, Golkar M. A review on human toxoplasmosis. Scand J Infect Dis 2012; 44(11): 805–14. https://doi.org/10.3109/00365548.2012.693197.

[62] Sasai M, Pradipta A, Yamamoto M. Host immune responses to *Toxoplasma gondii*. Int Immunol 2018; 30(3): 113–9. https://doi.org/10.1093/intimm/dxy004.

[63] Lekutis C, Ferguson DJ, Grigg ME, Camps M, Boothroyd JC. Surface antigens of *Toxoplasma gondii*: variations on a theme. Int J Parasitol 2001; 31(12): 1285–92.

[64] Jung C, Lee CY, Grigg ME. The SRS superfamily of *Toxoplasma* surface proteins. Int J Parasitol 2004; 34(3): 285–96. https://doi.org/10.1016/j.ijpara.2003.12.004.

[65] Carruthers VB. Host cell invasion by the opportunistic pathogen *Toxoplasma gondii*. Acta Trop 2002; 81(2): 111–22.

[66] Denkers EY, Gazzinelli RT. Regulation and function of T-cell-mediated immunity during *Toxoplasma gondii* infection. Clin Microbiol Rev 1998; 11(4): 569–88.

[67] Meira CS, Costa-Silva TA, Vidal JE, Ferreira IM, Hiramoto RM, Pereira-Chioccola VL. Use of the serum reactivity against *Toxoplasma gondii* excreted-secreted antigens in cerebral toxoplasmosis diagnosis in human immunodeficiency virus-infected patients. J Med Microbiol 2008; 57(Pt.7): 845–50. https://doi.org/10.1099/jmm.0.47687-0.

[68] Wowk PF, Zardo ML, Miot HT, Goldenberg S, Carvalho PC, Mörking PA. Proteomic profiling of extracellular vesicles secreted from *Toxoplasma gondii*. Proteomics 2017; 17(15–16): 1600477. https://doi.org/10.1002/pmic.201600477.

[69] Silva VO, Maia MM, Torrecilhas AC, Taniwaki NN, Namiyama GM, Oliveira KC, Ribeiro KS, Toledo MDS, Xander P, Pereira-Chioccola VL. Extracellular vesicles isolated from *Toxoplasma gondii* induce host immune response. Parasite Immunol 2018; 40(9): e12571. https://doi.org/10.1111/pim.12571.

[70] Li Y, Liu Y, Xiu F, Wang J, Cong H, He S, Shi Y, Wang X, Li X, Zhou H. Characterization of exosomes derived from *Toxoplasma gondii* and their functions in modulating immune responses. Int J Nanomedicine 2018; 13: 467–77. https://doi.org/10.2147/IJN.S151110.

[71] Aline F, Bout D, Amigorena S, Roingeard P, Dimier-Poisson I. *Toxoplasma gondii* antigen-pulsed-dendritic cell-derived exosomes induce a protective immune response against *T. gondii* infection. Infect Immun 2004; 72(7): 4127–37. https://doi.org/10.1128/IAI.72.7.4127-4137.2004.

[72] Bhatnagar S, Schorey JS. Exosomes released from infected macrophages contain *Mycobacterium avium* glycopeptidolipids and are proinflammatory. J Biol Chem 2007; 282(35): 25779–89. https://doi.org/10.1074/jbc.M702277200.

[73] Einarsson E, Ma'ayeh S, Svärd SG. An up-date on Giardia and giardiasis. Curr Opin Microbiol 2016; 34: 47–52. https://doi.org/10.1016/j.mib.2016.07.019.

[74] Fink MY, Singer SM. The intersection of immune responses, microbiota, and pathogenesis in giardiasis. Trends Parasitol 2017; 33(11): 901–13. https://doi.org/10.1016/j.pt.2017.08.001.

[75] Benchimol M. The release of secretory vesicle in encysting *Giardia lamblia*. FEMS Microbiol Lett 2004; 235(1): 81–7. https://doi.org/10.1016/j.femsle.2004.04.014.

[76] Gottig N, Elías EV, Quiroga R, Nores MJ, Solari AJ, Touz MC, Luján HD. Active and passive mechanisms drive secretory granule biogenesis during differentiation of the intestinal parasite *Giardia lamblia*. J Biol Chem 2006; 281(26): 18156–66. https://doi.org/10.1074/jbc.M602081200.

[77] Deolindo P, Evans-Osses I, Ramirez MI. Microvesicles and exosomes as vehicles between protozoan and host cell communication. Biochem Soc Trans 2013; 41(1): 252–7. https://doi.org/10.1042/BST20120217.

[78] Papanastasiou P, Hiltpold A, Bommeli C, Köhler P. The release of the variant surface protein of *Giardia* to its soluble isoform is mediated by the selective cleavage of the conserved carboxy-terminal domain. Biochemistry 1996; 35(31): 10143–8. https://doi.org/10.1021/bi960473b.

[79] Prucca CG, Slavin I, Quiroga R, Elías EV, Rivero FD, Saura A, Carranza PG, Luján HD. Antigenic variation in *Giardia lamblia* is regulated by RNA interference. Nature 2008; 456(7223): 750–4. https://doi.org/10.1038/nature07585.

[80] Amat CB, Motta JP, Fekete E, Moreau F, Chadee K, Buret AG. Cysteine protease-dependent mucous disruptions and differential mucin gene expression in giardia duodenalis infection. Am J Pathol 2017; 187(11): 2486–98. https://doi.org/10.1016/j.ajpath.2017.07.009.

[81] Bhargava A, Cotton JA, Dixon BR, Gedamu L, Yates RM, Buret AG. *Giardia duodenalis* surface cysteine proteases induce cleavage of the intestinal epithelial cytoskeletal protein villin via myosin light chain kinase. PLoS One 2015; 10(9): e0136102. https://doi.org/10.1371/journal.pone.0136102.

[82] Cotton JA, Bhargava A, Ferraz JG, Yates RM, Beck PL, Buret AG. *Giardia duodenalis* cathepsin B proteases degrade intestinal epithelial interleukin-8 and attenuate interleukin-8-induced neutrophil chemotaxis. Infect Immun 2014; 82(7): 2772–87. https://doi.org/10.1128/IAI.01771-14.

[83] Ortega-Pierres G, Argüello-García R, Laredo-Cisneros MS, Fonseca-Linán R, Gómez-Mondragón M, Inzunza-Arroyo R, Flores-Benítez D, Raya-Sandino A, Chavez-Munguía B, Ventura-Gallegos JL, Zentella-Dehesa A, Bermúdez-Cruz

RM, González-Mariscal L. Giardipain-1, a protease secreted by *Giardia duodenalis* trophozoites, causes junctional, barrier and apoptotic damage in epithelial cell monolayers. Int J Parasitol 2018; 48(8): 621-39. https://doi.org/10.1016/j.ijpara.2018.01.006.

[84] Ma'ayeh SY, Liu J, Peirasmaki D, Hörnaeus K, Bergström Lind S, Grabherr M, Bergquist J, Svärd SG. Characterization of the *Giardia intestinalis* secretome during interaction with human intestinal epithelial cells: the impact on host cells. PLoS Negl Trop Dis 2017; 11(12): e0006120. https://doi.org/10.1371/journal.pntd.0006120.

[85] Evans-Osses I, Mojoli A, Monguió-Tortajada M, Marcilla A, Aran V, Amorim M, Inal J, Borràs FE, Ramirez MI. Microvesicles released from *Giardia intestinalis* disturb hostpathogen response in vitro. Eur J Cell Biol 2017; 96(2): 131-42. https://doi.org/10.1016/j.ejcb.2017.01.005.

[86] Touz MC, Rivero MR, Miras SL, Bonifacino JS. Lysosomal protein trafficking in *Giardia lamblia*: common and distinct features. Front Biosci (Elite Ed) 2012; 4: 1898-909.

[87] Saha N, Dutta S, Datta SP, Sarkar S. The minimal ESCRT machinery of *Giardia lamblia* has altered inter-subunit interactions within the ESCRT-II and ESCRT-III complexes. Eur J Cell Biol 2018; 97(1): 44-62. https://doi.org/10.1016/j.ejcb.2017.11.004.

[88] Hassani K, Antoniak E, Jardim A, Olivier M. Temperature-induced protein secretion by *Leishmania mexicana* modulates macrophage signalling and function. PLoS One 2011; 6(5): e18724. https://doi.org/10.1371/journal.pone.0018724.

[89] Ramirez MI, de Ruiz RC, Araya JE, Da Silveira JF, Yoshida N. Involvement of the stagespecific 82-kilodalton adhesion molecule of *Trypanosoma cruzi* metacyclic trypomastigotes in host cell invasion. Infect Immun 1993; 61(9): 3636-41.

| 第9章 |

外泌体作为心脑血管疾病的细胞间通信信使
Exosomes as intercellular communication messengers for cardiovascular and cerebrovascular diseases

Antonia Teona Deftu[a,b,#], Beatrice Mihaela Radu[a,b,#], Dragos Cretoiu[c,d], Alexandru Florian Deftu[a,b], Sanda Maria Cretoiu[c], Junjie Xiao[e,f]

[a]*Department of Anatomy, Animal Physiology and Biophysics, Faculty of Biology, University of Bucharest, Bucharest, Romania*, [b]*Life, Environmental and Earth Sciences Division, Research Institute of the University of Bucharest (ICUB), Bucharest, Romania*, [c]*Department of Cell and Molecular Biology and Histology, Carol Davila University of Medicine and Pharmacy, Bucharest, Romania*, [d]*Alessandrescu-Rusescu National Institute of Mother and Child Health, Fetal Medicine Excellence Research Center, Bucharest, Romania*, [e]*Department of Cardiology, The First Affiliated Hospital of Nanjing Medical University, Nanjing, People's Republic of China*, [f]*Cardiac Regeneration and Ageing Lab, Experimental Center of Life Sciences, School of Life Science, Shanghai University, Shanghai, People's Republic of China*

一、概述

细胞分泌蛋白质组被认为包含细胞分泌的所有蛋白质,包括旁分泌物质、外泌体和微泡[1]。目前对细胞释放的囊泡的命名还没有达成共识,正努力以达成共识[2]。目前外泌体、微泡以及凋亡小体被统一命名为EV(由国际EV协会引入的术语),这些EV可以通过负载分子影响附近或远处的细胞[3]。目前有几个公共在线数据库可用,如Vesiclepedia(www.microvesicles.org)、EVpedia(www.evpedia.info)和ExoCarta(www.exocarta.org)[4]。

外泌体在正常和病理条件下介导细胞间通信,它们存在于体液中,如血浆、恶性腹水、尿液、羊水、痰液、精液、母乳、唾液和心包液[5-8]。

外泌体是细胞衍生的小细胞外膜囊泡,直径为50～100 nm,在生理和病理条件下都会主动分泌和释放。通常,外泌体和微泡之间没有明显区别[9]。外泌体起源于细胞质多泡体,其与质膜融合以释放外泌体。微泡,也称为核外颗粒体,是比外泌体更大的囊泡,由质膜直接出芽产生[10]。外泌体在化学成分上也不同于微泡,富含脂质,特别是胆固醇(微泡富含GM1神经节苷脂,外泌体中也有少量存在)和跨膜蛋白——四跨膜蛋白如CD9、CD63和CD81(被视为外泌体标志物)[11]。

外泌体是蛋白质(如细胞因子受体、肿瘤相关抗原、癌蛋白和抗原提呈分子)、编码RNA(mRNA)、非编码RNA(miRNA),甚至DNA的重要负载工具,并确保细胞、组织或器官水平的信息传递[12-16]。凭借小尺寸和外泌体提供的保护,miRNA可以从血清或血浆中蛋白酶和核酸酶降解逃逸[17]。

尽管人们对外泌体在正常条件下的作用知之甚少，但对它们在病理条件下的作用已有广泛研究[18]。外泌体具有细胞的特定基因组和蛋白质组学特征，被认为是检测各种疾病的有效手段[19]。基于外泌体的生物标志物与心血管疾病的预后高度相关[20,21]，并被普遍认为是心血管疾病预防、修复或进展的关键[22]。

在本章中，我们旨在更新心脑血管病理学中外泌体相关的知识。我们回顾了分离和分析外泌体的方法，并对临床实践中心血管疾病中基于外泌体的生物标志物进行了概述。

二、外泌体的产生和释放

外泌体的产生和释放是一个自动调节的过程。因此，在外泌体产生的过程中，产生外泌体的细胞及其局部微环境会影响外泌体的含量，而外泌体的含量决定了向靶细胞发送或释放的信息[23]。在心脑血管系统（图9-1）的生理和病理状态下，确保细胞间通信的外泌体来源于并作用于各种细胞亚型，如心肌细胞、内皮细胞、MSC/基质细胞、红细胞、脑细胞衍生的外泌体等。

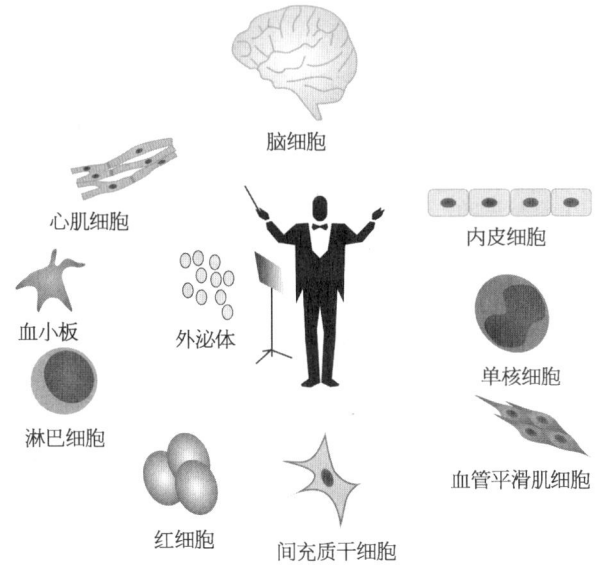

图9-1 外泌体确保心脑血管系统中的细胞间信息传递

研究还表明，不同类型干细胞（包括MSC、造血干细胞、心肌祖细胞、心肌球细胞、诱导多能干细胞）释放的外泌体作用于内皮细胞、心肌细胞、成纤维细胞等类型的细胞，通过增加心脏血管生成，减少氧化应激、炎症和细胞凋亡，发挥心脏保护作用[24]。

（一）心肌细胞来源的外泌体

心肌细胞在生理和病理条件下释放EV（如外泌体或微泡）。一些压力条件，如缺氧、炎症或损伤，会促使心脏细胞分泌EV，这些囊泡（即促进血管生成、抗凋亡、有丝分裂和传递生长因子）有助于心脏再生[25]。

内皮细胞可以摄取心肌细胞衍生的外泌体,这形成了心肌细胞和内皮细胞之间重要的串扰。在心肌细胞-内皮细胞通信系统中,已证实外泌体含有功能性葡萄糖转运蛋白和糖酵解酶,并可以转移至内皮细胞。有趣的是,葡萄糖饥饿可以刺激心肌细胞衍生的外泌体的产生,在这些应激条件下产生的外泌体会诱导内皮细胞生成血管[27]。

不同心脏细胞之间的串扰(如心肌细胞-内皮细胞-干细胞-成纤维细胞-平滑肌细胞)对于维持心脏稳态至关重要。除了心肌细胞和内皮细胞之间的主动交流,心肌细胞衍生的外泌体也可以转移至成纤维细胞[28,29]。

心肌祖细胞还释放外泌体,这些外泌体被内皮细胞吸收,通过激活 ERK/Akt 信号通路刺激内皮细胞迁移和生成血管[30]。

(二) 内皮细胞衍生的外泌体

体内外研究表明,来自内皮祖细胞的外泌体传递 mRNA 并诱导内皮细胞生成血管[31,32]。另一方面,各种细胞产生的外泌体有可能通过传递物质(如 miRNA、蛋白质、脂质、转录因子或信号通路的活化因子)在内皮细胞的信号传导中起更强的生成血管或抗血管生成作用(通过 LDL 受体介导的内吞作用、CD36 依赖的 EV 摄取、氧化应激的诱导)。这是一个动态的过程,外泌体根据局部微环境的变化调整血管生成[23]。

2 型糖尿病患者内皮细胞衍生的微泡水平没有改变[33,34],而代谢综合征患者的循环水平显著增加[35]。

血管并发症、糖尿病或代谢综合征患者的药物治疗可能会增加或减少内皮细胞衍生的微泡水平[36,37]。

心脏内皮细胞(cardiac endothelial cell,CEC)是心脏生理学和病理生理学的重要参与者,与其他内皮细胞(如肾、脑或肺内皮细胞)相比,具有独特的转录组[38]。CEC 衍生的外泌体表达标志物整合素 $\alpha v \beta 6$,并可激活 B 细胞中的 TGF-β[38]。

(三) MSC/基质细胞衍生的外泌体

MSC 是多能干细胞,可以从不同类型的组织(如骨髓、脂肪、肌肉、骨、脑、脾、肝、肺、胸腺和胰腺)中分离出来。MSC 衍生的外泌体具有多种作用,包括组织修复、抗炎、免疫调节和神经保护。有趣的是,MSC 衍生的外泌体比 MSC 本身更稳定。在体内注射时,由于缺乏非整倍性,外泌体比原始细胞更不容易被免疫系统排斥[39]。有研究表明,人 MSC 衍生的外泌体对外周血单核细胞(如 T 淋巴细胞)发挥体外免疫调节作用,可以增加它们的凋亡,但对单核细胞增殖没有任何影响[40]。

与其他细胞亚型(包括成肌细胞、人急性单核细胞白血病细胞或人胚胎肾细胞)相比,MSC 已被证明能够产生更多的外泌体[41]。

(四) 血小板衍生外泌体

已有文献报道血小板可产生外泌体[42]。有趣的是,血小板承载着复杂的转录组,包括大约 9 500 个 mRNA、不同类别的非编码 RNA(如 miRNA)和蛋白质(参与黏附、聚集、颗粒分泌、RNA 转移、mRNA 翻译和免疫调节过程)[43-49]。与其他细胞亚型的外泌体相比,血小板衍生外泌体具有相似的大小、蛋白质标记、CD81 标记与外泌体计数的比率[42,50]。细胞外的钙通过改变血小板糖蛋白 VI、CXCL7 或高迁移率族蛋白 1 的总外泌体含量和每个外泌体的水平,影响血小板衍生外泌体的含量[50]。

在脓毒症患者中,血小板衍生外泌体被证明会导致心肌功能障碍[51]。血小板在血管损伤和血栓形成后的恢复中起重要作用。具体而言,在血管损伤时,血小板与内皮细胞相互作用并释放其负载的物质(如黏附分子,包括血管性血友病因子和纤维蛋白原、生长因子以及炎症和血管生成介质)[52]。在小鼠中,血小板衍生外泌体被证明可以增加蛋白质泛素化并增加 CD36 的蛋白酶体降解,从而有助于抑制动脉粥样硬化-血栓形成过程[53]。此外,血小板衍生外泌体促使内皮细胞凋亡[54]。

(五)白细胞衍生外泌体

白细胞衍生外泌体表达多种与细胞来源相关的蛋白质标志物,如白细胞(CD45)、中性粒细胞(CD15、CD64、CD66b、CD66e)、单核细胞(CD11a、CD14、CD18)和淋巴细胞(CD2、CD3、CD4、CD8、CD19、CD20)[55]。当细胞饥饿或暴露于内毒素、钙离子载体 A23187 的刺激时,单核细胞(即单核细胞系 THP-1)会释放负载标志物的外泌体:Tsg101、负电荷磷脂、CD18、CD14 和活性组织因子(tissue factor,TF)[56]。有趣的是,如果内皮细胞暴露于这些白细胞衍生外泌体,会触发核分裂和凋亡,激活促凝作用[56]。

对白细胞(如 T 细胞、单核细胞、NK 细胞和 B 细胞)及其衍生外泌体之间蛋白质标志物的分析表明,一些细胞表面蛋白质没有转移至 EV,包括 CD3、CD14、CD16 和 CD19[57]。另一方面,其他细胞表面蛋白如 CD9、CD63 和 CD81,可以从白细胞转移至 EV[57]。

(六)红细胞衍生外泌体

红细胞根据其发育阶段释放外泌体和胞外颗粒体,并且红细胞衍生外泌体(erythrocytes-derived exosomes,EDE)仅在骨髓中的红细胞发育期间释放[58]。EDE 在血液中被鉴定,并可以与单核细胞结合,诱导促炎细胞因子(如 TNF-α)的分泌。此外,EDE 促进丝裂原诱导的 $CD4^+$ 和 $CD8^+$ T 细胞增殖[59]。红细胞衍生外泌体诱导的促炎作用(即产生 TNF、IL-6 和 IL-8)受红细胞储存持续时间的影响[60]。需要注意的是,EDE 可能不利于血液储存,从而阻碍输血。其中的机制与红细胞内血红蛋白清除 NO 失调[61]及血管调节异常相关[62]。

红细胞产生囊泡的触发因素有很多,包括胞质中 Ca^{2+} 增加[63]、ATP 耗竭、K^+ 外流增加[64]以及各种细胞内信号级联反应(如 GPCR、PI3K-Akt、Jak-STAT 和 Raf-MEK 通路)[65]。EDE 在各种血液疾病和心血管疾病中也发挥着重要作用。目前已表明 EDE 有助于血液感染性疾病(如疟疾)中的细胞间信号传递[66]。在镰状细胞病患者中,红细胞以棒状和微球形式释放无血影蛋白的含血红蛋白的外泌体,而含有聚合血红蛋白的棒状体最终可能成为微囊泡链[67]。镰状红细胞释放的棒状体显示出凝血改变,这可能是由于磷脂在无血影蛋白膜内的重组[68]。在患有 2 型糖尿病的肥胖患者的血浆中检测到高水平的 CD235a 阳性红细胞衍生微泡,与血浆血红蛋白 A1c 水平没有直接相关性[69]。伴有糖尿病代谢综合征患者的红细胞衍生微泡也显著增加(1/3 的患者)[70]。

(七) 血管平滑肌细胞衍生外泌体

血管平滑肌细胞(vascular smooth muscle cell,VSMC)也产生具有潜在促血管生成活性的外泌体。VSMC 衍生外泌体直径为 60～150 nm,表达蛋白质标志物,如 flotillin-1、CD81 和 Syntenin-1[71]。通过基于液相色谱质谱(nanoLC-MS/MS)的蛋白质组学分析,结果显示人 VSMC 衍生外泌体存在 459 种蛋白质[72]。另一项蛋白质组学研究在 VSMC 衍生外泌体中鉴定了 349 种蛋白质,其中大部分是 ECM 或 ECM 相关蛋白质和细胞黏附分子,这意味着 VSMC 衍生外泌体参与细胞黏附和传递细胞间信号[73]。

VSMC 衍生外泌体在血管病变中发挥重要作用,包括再狭窄、动脉粥样硬化、钙化和凝血[74,75]。在 VSMC 过表达 Krüppel 样因子 5(Krüppel-like factor 5,KLF5)中,VSMC 衍生外泌体将 miR-155 从 VSMC 转移至内皮细胞,从而扰乱血管内皮的完整性并刺激动脉粥样硬化的进展[76]。

(八) 脑细胞衍生外泌体

除了脑外组织,所有脑细胞(即神经元、星形胶质细胞、脑内皮细胞、小胶质细胞、少突胶质细胞等)都可以合成和释放外泌体[77-80]。研究表明,胶质母细胞瘤细胞[81]、脑微血管内皮细胞[82,83]、原代培养的大鼠微胶质细胞[84]、PC12 神经元分化细胞[85]和星形胶质细胞[80]均分泌外泌体。

生理或病理刺激对神经血管单元不同细胞成分的激活决定了外泌体的释放水平。在 HIV 感染中,TLR3 激活的脑微血管内皮细胞的外泌体确保了脑微血管内皮细胞和巨噬细胞之间的信息传递[86]。脑癌的血管生成过程也由 EV 介导,这些囊泡促进了脑微血管内皮细胞和胶质母细胞瘤之间的信息交流[87]。在神经元应激条件下(如氧化应激、缺氧、缺血或低血糖),具有高含量朊病毒蛋白的星形胶质细胞释放的外泌体保证了神经元的存活[88]。在脊髓再生中,在用视黄酸受体 β(retinoic acid receptor β,RARβ)激动剂治疗后,神经元细胞质中的磷酸酶和张力蛋白同源物失活,由外泌体进一步转移至星形胶质细胞,从而促进轴突再生[89]。

在这种情况下,大脑重塑受到外泌体介导的细胞间通信的强烈影响,血管成分起着至关重要的作用。

三、外泌体表征及研究和分析方法

(一) 外泌体大小

一般认为外泌体的直径在 40～100 nm。外泌体的大小因几何(水合或干燥)、流体动力学和体积估计而异。各种方法或细胞亚型被用于表征外泌体,结果表明外泌体大小和形状存在差异[90]。外泌体的大小可以通过多种技术获得,包括原子力显微术、动态光散射、纳米粒子追踪分析、内皮集落形成细胞、扫描电子显微术、透射电子显微术和冷冻断裂透射电子显微术。

外泌体的大小可能也受到干燥方法的影响,如 MSC 衍生外泌体的直径通过纳米粒子追踪分析约为 98 nm,而通过透射电子显微术测量约为 55.5 nm[91]。

分离外泌体的方法也会导致外泌体大小的差异[92-94]。有趣的是,外泌体的数量及其大小分布可能受患者年龄、性别和健康状况的影响[95,96]。

(二) 外泌体分离

外泌体通常与条件培养基和体液(如血液、尿液、唾液、CSF、关节液、母乳、腹水等)分离。尽管已经开发出多种外泌体分离方法,目前还没有可靠的外泌体纯化和分析方案[97]。

外泌体纯化最常用的方法包括差速离心(低速,约 1 500×g)、高速超速离心(>100 000×g)、超滤、溶剂沉淀、微流体技术、免疫亲和分离、密度梯度和尺寸排阻色谱[92,98-102]。

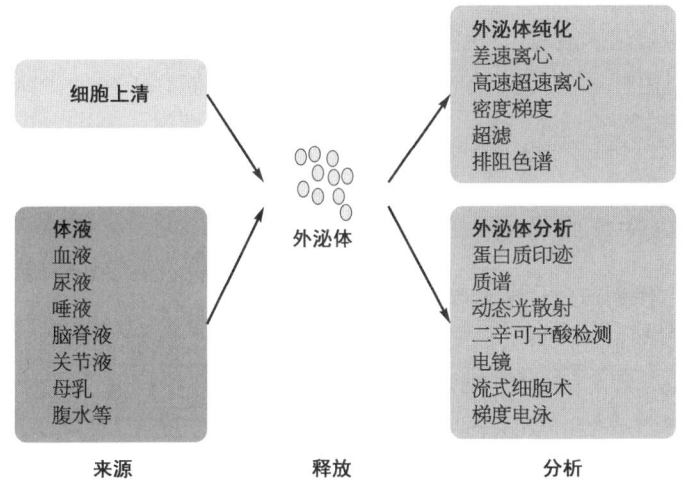

图 9-2 外泌体生物发生和分析概述

由于外泌体标志物和外泌体相关蛋白的富集,与超速离心和密度梯度分离相比,免疫亲和捕获被认为是外泌体分离的最佳方法[92]。

值得注意的是,神经元衍生外泌体的分离具有挑战性。目前已开发出从母体血液中分离胎儿神经元外泌体的方法,可进行神经元标记分析以确定胎儿来源(如 CD81、神经元特异性烯醇化酶、神经丝轻链、L1 细胞黏附分子)或排除胎盘来源(1 型妊娠特异性 β-1-糖蛋白)[50]。最近,已从体内脑组织中分离出外泌体[103]。

由于存在外泌体的体液的可及性和多样性,外泌体分离具有临床相关性。然而,由于缺乏标准化的外泌体分离方案,临床分离外泌体存在困难[104]。临床中 EV 的分离方案应适合所需的输出参数,如 EV 的最终浓度、纯度、亚型分选以及时间/成本效益[102]。

(三) 外泌体分析

已有多种方法可用于外泌体分析,包括蛋白质印迹法、质谱法[105]、动态光散射、二辛可宁酸微量测定法[97]、电子显微镜[106]、流式细胞术[107,108]和梯度电泳[109]。

数十纳米的外泌体尺寸无法通过常规光学显微镜观察到,因此需要电子显微镜来表征其形态[110]。通过透射电子显微镜,塌陷的 EV 呈现出特征性的杯状或甜甜圈形态,而完整的外泌体则是球形的(直径从 30 nm 到 1 μm)[108]。原子力显微镜也是一种用于表征 EV 和外泌体的方法,尤其适用于分析它们的大小和拓扑结构[111]。

由于外泌体富含胆固醇、鞘磷脂、神经节苷脂 GM3 或脂质,外泌体具有脂筏[109]。对于一些外泌体,浮选密度在蔗糖梯度中测量值为 1.10~1.18 g/mL[107]。

心脏外泌体具有特定的蛋白质标志物,包括来自运输机制所需内体分选复合物的蛋白质、四跨膜蛋白(如 CD9、CD63、CD81)和 HSP70[112]。根据来源的不同,白细胞衍生的微粒具有多种标志物[55]。

外泌体的蛋白质含量受细胞来源和外界刺激的影响。蛋白质印迹法证明了心脏外泌体在不同生理或病理条件下保留其负载的蛋白质。此外,质谱分析表明心脏外泌体的蛋白质含量与其他类型的外泌体显著不同,包含细胞溶质、肌节和线粒体蛋白质[105]。

对于红细胞衍生外泌体,它们的检测受红细胞浓缩物储存条件的影响较强。在红细胞浓缩物储存达到特定浓度之前(42~43 天),流式细胞术和动态光散射无法详细说明红细胞衍生外泌体[113]。

四、外泌体与冠状动脉疾病

(一) 外泌体作为冠状动脉疾病的生物标志物

尽管越来越多的证据表明 EV,尤其是外泌体在心血管疾病中的重要性,但它们作为疾病标志物的应用仍受到不同技术障碍的限制(如大多数研究是在体外进行的)。

冠状动脉疾病(coronary artery disease,CAD)是最常见的心脏病类型,是动脉炎症和含胆固醇沉积物(斑块)的结果。斑块形成过程存在由白细胞、红细胞、平滑肌细胞和内皮细胞等产生的 EV[114];而血浆中的 EV 是由血小板产生的,而非平滑肌细胞。结果表明,EV 是内皮细胞功能障碍、血管钙化、不稳定斑块进展和破裂后血栓形成的重要原因[115]。

有多种方法可以评估 CAD、预测死亡风险,如 Killip 分类、加拿大心血管学会心绞痛分级量表、预后生物标志物(包括高敏心肌肌钙蛋白、高敏 C-反应蛋白和肌酸激酶 MB),然而目前并没有金标准。研究表明,在预测心血管疾病方面,PTX3 似乎比 C 反应蛋白更具特异性[116]。最近的研究表明,血浆中的 miRNA 由循环蛋白、脂蛋白以及外泌体转运[117],外泌体可以反映疾病阶段或进展,可确定为有用的生物标志物[118]。几种 miRNA 在冠心病中有变(miR-17、miR-19a、miR-21、miR-92a、miR-126、miR-146a、miR-222 和 miR-223)[119]。

更多的研究指出,miRNA 可以作为心血管疾病预后和治疗的靶点[120]。2017 年,Karakas 等进行了广泛研究,评估了血液中 miRNA 在心血管疾病中的预后价值。他们的研究表明,miR-132、miR-140-3p 和 miR-210 能够可靠地预测心血管死亡。三种 miRNA:miR-223、miR-197 和 miR-126 具有统计学意义,然而,没有一项能预测早期和晚期心血管的意外事件[121]。另一项研究表明,miR-142-3p 和 miR-17-5p 可能用作未来评估 CAD 风险的生物标志物[122]。此外,与健康对照相比,CAD 患者的 miR-126 水平显著下降[119],这表明开发基于 EV 的 miR-126 治疗策略或能治疗 CAD。

(二)冠状动脉疾病康复过程中的外泌体

随着心脏动脉血管不同程度的阻塞,动脉粥样硬化斑块会发生演变,从而导致心肌缺血。严重时斑块会破裂,导致动脉血栓闭塞,产生急性心肌梗死(acute myocardial infarction,AMI)。此时最合适的治疗是尝试对梗死的心肌区域进行再灌注。然而,这伴随着导致额外损伤的缺血再灌注综合征[123]。许多研究人员旨在减少再灌注的影响,以改善受影响心肌区域的活动。这些尝试包括清除由干细胞释放的细胞因子[124]或由心肌中新细胞类型,即端细胞[21,125,126]释放的因子。

这些因子可能通过旁分泌或自分泌下起作用,并且它们可以在外泌体的帮助下运输[127]。Sahoo 等证明 CD34$^+$ 干细胞分泌的外泌体可在体外和体内表现出独立的血管生成活性[128]。MSC 分泌的外泌体在大鼠体内灌注、直接在心肌中灌注或在再灌注前静脉灌注中,则具有心脏保护作用[76,129,130]。有人提出外泌体对 Langendorff 灌注大鼠心脏具有保护作用[131]。

已有提议将外泌体作为细胞疗法的替代方案。例如,由人类心肌球衍生细胞分泌的外泌体通过抑制细胞凋亡、促进心肌细胞增殖及血管生成,具有再生和心脏保护的特性[132]。

五、心肌缺血和梗死中的外泌体

(一)外泌体作为心肌缺血/梗死的生物标志物

众所周知,生物标志物是许多疾病的诊断工具。在心血管内科中,此类生物标志物的发现对于早期诊断梗死前的坏死前阶段具有重要价值[133]。体外实验表明,缺氧的心肌细胞释放的外泌体携带细胞因子 TNF-α 和 HSP60[134,135]。这些发现表明,当细胞处于缺氧状态时,一些标志物可能会在心肌细胞坏死前释放出来,冠状动脉搭桥手术后血浆外泌体含量增加证明了这一观点[136]。有许多研究旨在鉴定 AMI 心肌细胞的特异性 miRNA,一些作者认为 miRNA 的所有变化并非都由心肌细胞产生,因为其他类型的细胞也参与了 AMI,如内皮细胞[137]。最近描述了一组可用于区分 Takotsubo 心肌病(Takotsubo cardiomyopathy,TTC)和 AMI 的 miRNA:miR-1、miR-16、miR-26a 和 miR-133a 可将 TTC 与健康受试者和 ST 段抬高心肌梗死(ST segment elevation myocardial infarction,STEMI)患者区分开来[138]。有研究表明,与健康对照相比,STEMI 患者的心脏特异性 miR-1 和 miR-133a 增加[138]。

外泌体 miRNA-133a 可被视为心肌梗死的生物标志物[139,140]。小鼠中 miR-1、miR-133a、miR-208a 和 miR-499 水平在梗死和邻近梗死心脏区域显著下降[140]。此外,邻近梗死心脏区域对 miR-133a 的捕获有助于抑制心肌肥大[139]。在 AMI 等心脏损伤中,上述心肌细胞产生的 miRNA(miR-1、miR-133a/b、miR-208a 和 miR-499)在血液中的水平显著升高,表明存在心肌损伤[141,142]。这表明未来将 miRNA 作为 AMI 早期诊断的生物学标志物具有潜在价值[143,144]。

(二) 心肌缺血/梗死康复过程的外泌体

1. 参与心肌缺血/梗死后内源性恢复机制的外泌体

几种类型的细胞,包括 MSC、心肌成纤维细胞、心肌祖细胞和造血干细胞释放外泌体,有助于心肌缺血或梗死时的心脏再生。

目前,据报道,MSC 衍生的外泌体及其 miRNA 参与缺血性心脏损伤后的心脏组织再生,其机制包括减少胶原蛋白生成、防止细胞凋亡和增加血管生成[91]。此外,在急性缺血/再灌注损伤的小鼠模型中,心肌祖细胞衍生外泌体通过抑制心肌细胞凋亡来保护缺血心肌[145]。特别是,心肌祖细胞衍生外泌体的 miR-21 显示出通过靶向程序性细胞死亡 4 (programmed cell death 4,PDCD4)基因来抑制心肌细胞的凋亡[146]。有研究表明,在大鼠心脏冠状动脉闭塞后一小时,将人心肌祖细胞衍生的外泌体注射到心脏梗死周围区域时,可抑制心肌细胞凋亡并改善心肌梗死时的心脏功能[147]。

据描述,心肌成纤维细胞在梗死后的心脏修复过程中发挥重要作用。目前的研究表明,心肌梗死与炎症介质产生、基质降解激活以及心肌成纤维细胞增殖和迁移的急性炎症过程有关[148]。在心肌损伤部位,成纤维细胞响应局部炎症介质(如 TGF-β)迁移,并转化为肌成纤维细胞,从而促进修复过程[149]。心肌修复增殖期的特征是心肌成纤维细胞对增殖剂(如成纤维细胞生长因子 2、血小板衍生生长因子、血管紧张素 II、血管升压素、内皮素 I、心肌营养素、类胰蛋白酶和糜蛋白酶)的增殖反应及其向损伤部位的迁移[150-155]。在心肌梗死的恢复过程中,外泌体与复杂的细胞间通信相关,这意味着心肌细胞-内皮细胞-干细胞-成纤维细胞-平滑肌细胞之间存在串扰[156]。

miR-302-367 促进胚胎心肌细胞增殖,因此对其在心肌梗死中的作用进行了研究[157]。心肌梗死后的心肌再生直接受 miR-302-367、miR-17-92、miR-590、miR-199a、miR-17-92 簇、miR-199a-214 簇、miR-34a 和 miR-15 家族的瞬时激活影响[158]。此外,据报道,miR-31a-5p 通过靶向 RhoBTB1 控制出生后心肌细胞的增殖,这表明其可能具有促进患者心肌再生的治疗作用[159]。

2. 用于心肌缺血/梗死后治疗的外泌体

通过体外、离体或体内方法将外泌体递送到损伤部位,测试外泌体在心肌缺血和梗死后心脏恢复中的治疗潜力。此外,已经采用了多种工程方法来封装和递送外泌体。

体外试验表明,与成纤维细胞相比,源自 AC10 心室心肌细胞系的 EV 更容易被内皮细胞吞并,并且心肌细胞-内皮细胞-成纤维细胞之间的旁分泌串扰被认为有助于心脏重塑[160]。

体内实验证明,注射源自 MSC 的外泌体通过 AMPK/mTOR 和 Akt/mTOR 信号通路触发心肌细胞自噬,在缺血/再灌注损伤后的心肌恢复中是有效的[161]。研究证明,MSC 衍生外泌体注射到心肌梗死附近的区域可以通过刺激血管生成和减少炎症反应来发挥局部作用[162]。此外，心肌梗死后 DC 衍生外泌体通过激活 CD4（＋）T 淋巴细胞改善了心脏功能[163]。

有研究将与心脏归巢肽（cardiac homing peptide，CHP；CSTSMLKAC）结合的心脏干细胞外泌体递送到心脏切片或新生大鼠心肌细胞中，并证明了它们在治疗心肌梗死中的功效[164]。此外，与缺血心肌靶向肽（ischemic myocardium-targeting peptide，IMTP）CSTSMLKAC 融合的外泌体富集膜蛋白（Lamp2b）对缺氧损伤的 H9C2 细胞具有抗凋亡作用，而在心肌梗死的小鼠模型中，IMTP-外泌体能够优先靶向缺血心肌并减少缺血区域内的心脏炎症和细胞凋亡[165]。

技术的进步使研究人员能够获得由心肌细胞、平滑肌细胞和人诱导多能干细胞分化而来的内皮细胞改造而成的人心肌贴片，这些贴片已在体外成功测试或移植到小鼠心肌梗死模型中。实验表明，人心肌贴片可释放外泌体，刺激内皮细胞的血管生成活性并发挥心肌细胞保护作用[166]。

六、心力衰竭中的外泌体

（一）外泌体作为心力衰竭的生物标志物

许多 CAD 进展为慢性心力衰竭（heart failure，HF），并且数量逐年增加。HF 管理的一个挑战是如何确定一种可靠的疾病预后方法。HF 的进展由心脏重塑和血管功能障碍的复杂过程决定[167]。外泌体可能是评估患者 HF 进展的有用工具，多项研究报告了它们在调节这种病理状况中的作用[168,169]。

外泌体是一种介导细胞间通信的新型旁分泌调节剂。心肌细胞和心肌成纤维细胞之间的串扰由心肌成纤维细胞衍生的富含 miRNA 的外泌体介导，这一过程导致心肌细胞肥大并形成 HF[170]。

使用外泌体作为生物标志物有一定的优势，但在 HF 患者的风险分层方面仍然存在局限性。评估 HF 程度的经典方法是纽约心脏协会（New York Heart Association，NYHA）功能分类，它仍然可以说是临床中最重要的预后方法，尽管这种评估具有局限性，如将患者归于 Ⅱ 级或 Ⅲ 级仍不太精确。此外，如果评估依赖患者的主观陈述而不是客观条件，结果的准确性可能会受到显著影响[171]。

NYHA Ⅰ 级或更高等级的 HF 患者中内皮细胞衍生外泌体的水平显著增加。分析证明，高外泌体水平与心血管事件概率的显著增加有关[172]。

1. HF 中的外泌体蛋白

研究表明，内皮细胞功能和血管完整性的退化、血管生成失衡和炎症对 HF 的进展至关重要。有研究表明，血管内皮功能障碍与内皮细胞衍生的外泌体水平密切相关[21]。慢性 HF 患者具有高水平的外泌体 $CD144^+/CD31^+/AnnexinV^+$ 和 $CD31^+/AnnexinV^+$ 水平。通过使用 NYHA 功能分级及检测内皮细胞外泌体水平（$CD144^+/CD31^+/AnnexinV^+$ 和 $CD31^+/AnnexinV^+$），可以获得对 HF 患者的良好临床预测[169]。有研究报告了慢性 HF 患者的死亡率与 $CD31^+/$膜联蛋白 V^+ 内皮细胞衍生的凋亡外泌体及单核祖细胞的比率升高之间的相关性[173]。这些外泌体检测被认为是这种高风险病理类型的潜在生物标志物[21]。

欧洲心脏病学会和美国心脏协会/美国心脏病学会推荐利尿钠肽、五聚体蛋白-3、半乳糖蛋白-3和心脏特异性肌钙蛋白作为具有高预测价值的HF生物标志物[174]。

用于慢性HF研究最多的生物标志物之一是B型利尿钠肽,用于评估HF严重程度及诊断病理。然而,一些临床试验报告B型利尿钠肽水平与死亡率或临床结果之间缺乏相关性,因此其预后价值存在争议[175]。

HSP20对小鼠心脏中高血糖的急性和慢性进展均有反应,预测低水平的HSP20会影响糖尿病心肌病的演变和向HF的传播[176]。

含有AT1R的外泌体由心肌细胞在压力超负荷时传递,可能在高血压和HF等环境中调节血压方面发挥重要作用[21]。

SCL8A1参与线粒体和心肌细胞的Ca^{2+}稳态,并与心律失常和HF的发展有关[177]。

Guescini等研究表明,慢性HF患者的血浆外泌体颗粒数和外泌体线粒体DNA(mitochondrial DNA,mtDNA)拷贝数均增加。已有研究发现,星形胶质细胞、胶质母细胞瘤细胞和C2C12细胞衍生的外泌体含有mtDNA[178,179]。

暴露于THP-1细胞或Raji的HF患者和健康对照者的血浆中的外泌体被细胞摄取。随后,被摄取的外泌体诱导IL-1和IL-8的分泌,并增加TLR9-NF-κB途径中蛋白质的表达。炎性细胞因子的增加与mtDNA拷贝数有很大关系,与外泌体mtDNA的来源、患者及对照并不完全相关。氯喹是TLR9的抑制剂,可以阻断TLR9-NF-κB通路并降低该通路中蛋白质的表达。最近一项研究报告表明,THP-1细胞表达TLR2和TLR4,这与外泌体诱导的炎症有关。除TLR2/4通路外,外泌体还可以通过mtDNA激活TLR9-NF-κB通路并导致炎症。在慢性HF患者中,随着血浆外泌体数量的增加,更多的外泌体mtDNA进入目标免疫细胞并通过激活TLR9-NF-κB通路促进细胞因子的分泌,这促进了HF的慢性炎症过程[180]。

经THP-1细胞或Raji处理的HF患者和健康对照者血浆来源的外泌体掺入细胞。随后,内化的外泌体诱导IL-1和IL-8分泌,并增加TLR9-NF-κB途径蛋白的表达。炎性细胞因子含量升高与mtDNA拷贝数密切相关,与外泌体mtDNA来源、患者或对照没有确切关系。TLR9抑制剂氯喹可阻断TLR9-NF-κB通路,降低该通路中蛋白的表达。最近的一项研究报道,THP-1细胞表达TLR2和TLR4与外泌体诱导的炎症有关。除TLR2/4途径外,外泌体还可通过线粒体DNA激活TLR9-NF-κB途径参与炎症反应。在慢性HF患者中,随着血浆外泌体数目的增加,更多的外泌体mtDNA进入靶免疫细胞,通过激活TLR9-NF-κB途径促进细胞因子的分泌,从而参与HF患者的慢性炎症过程。

由于缺乏特异性的诊断生物标志物,围生期心肌病(peripartum cardiomyopathy,PPCM)心力衰竭的死亡风险很高。虽然PPCM的特异性生物标志物尚未被发现,但常规的血常规检查仍有助于PPCM的早期诊断。炎症标志物IL-6、TNF-α、CPR升高,凋亡标志物Fas/Apo-1也升高。脑钠肽(brain natriuretic peptide,BNP)和ProBNP的N末端部分(N-terminal portion of proBNP,pro-NT BNP)是HF的敏感生物标志物,但对PPCM无特异性,高水平pro-NT BNP提示预后较差。此外,特定外泌体相关的miRNA在HF

中受到不同的调控,这表明它们在 HF 的诊断中具有潜在的互补作用。

2. 来源于 HF 的外泌体 miRNA

之前报告表明 miRNA 是人类多种心血管疾病的生物标志物。HF 相关文献中反复出现过许多失调的 miRNA,并证实这些 miRNA 在人类各种疾病和受损的心脏组织中发生了改变。

临床研究表明 HF 时,一种预测靶向红系衍生的核因子 2 相关因子 2(nuclear factor erythroid 2 - related factor 2,Nrf2)的 miRNA - 27a 显著上调,提示 miRNA 可能参与了 HF 发生发展过程中 Nrf2 的异常调节。最近的研究表明,miRNA 可以通过与 RNA 结合蛋白来抵抗核酸酶或包裹在外泌体中来实现主动转运,从而参与信号传递和细胞间通信。富含 miRNA 外泌体介导心肌成纤维细胞和心肌细胞之间的细胞间通信,并参与了 Nrf2/ARE 信号通路失调。研究表明,潜在靶向 Nrf2 mRNA 的 miRNA,在心肌梗死后的心脏中高表达,在心肌成纤维细胞释放的外泌体中大量表达,可能具有与心肌细胞通信的潜力。这种机制可能有助于抑制慢性 HF 中由心肌梗死和氧化应激诱导的细胞间通信信使 Nrf2 的表达。Nrf2 相关的 miRNA 是否参与了心肌梗死和 HF 中 Nrf2 的失调目前尚不清楚。

一些研究表明,基于循环 p53 反应性 miRNA(miRNA - 34a,miRNA - 192 和 miRNA - 194)外泌体,不仅与 HF 的发生高度相关,而且在急性心肌梗死后 HF 患者中显著增加,被视为急性心肌梗死后发生缺血性 HF 的预测因子。有趣的是,这三种 miRNA 在 HF 患者的外泌体组分中含量丰富。上述 miRNA 的敲降可增强阿霉素治疗后的细胞活力,而这些 miRNA 的过度表达可降低细胞存活率,表明这些 miRNA 的水平增加可能导致心脏功能不全。值得注意的是,miR - 34a 和 miR - 194 水平与心肌梗死后左室舒张末期尺寸相关,这表明两者可能有助于预测心肌梗死患者 HF 的发展。

几项研究证明,循环中的 miRNA - 92 与心血管疾病密切相关,且 HF 患者的血清外泌体中 miRNA - 92 的浓度明显高于对照组。NYHA Ⅲ 级和 Ⅳ 级 HF 患者血浆 miRNA 表达水平显著高于 Ⅱ 级 HF 患者和对照组。

据报道,MiRNA - 146a 是一种诊断 PPCM 相关 HF 的应急工具。Halkein 等进行的一项研究表明,急性 PPCM 患者的循环 miRNA - 146a 水平显著升高,在接受 HF 常规治疗后循环外泌体 miRNA - 146a 水平降低,提示 miRN146a 很可能是一种 PPCM 相关急性 HF 的生物标志物。

在不同来源和程度的 HF 中 miR - 1、miR - 21、miR - 24、miR - 29b、miR - 133a、miR - 133b、miR - 199、miR - 208、miR - 214 和 miR - 499 持续受到影响。这组 miRNA 可作为 HF 中 miRNA 介导心脏-骨骼肌通信的初步模板。MiR - 21 在不同程度的 HF 中上调。

需要更多的实验来描述人类心肌细胞源性 EV 的 miRNA 图谱。与心肌组织和 HF 循环中发现的一致,从人类祖细胞培养的心肌细胞强烈表达 miR - 1 和 miR - 499。有趣的是,循环 miR - 1 水平降低与老年患者 HF 的严重程度直接相关。衰老与 HF 衰老之间的相互作用表现在循环 miRNA 的表达上。HF 时在心肌和循环中富集的 miRNA 中,myOmiR(即 miR - 1、miR - 133、miR - 208 和 miR - 499)对发达的骨骼肌有强烈影响。这些 myOmiR 中,miR - 1 和 miR - 133a 在各种心血管疾病的循环中升高,并在心肌梗死后三个月仍然升高。也有报道称,在最晚期 HF 患者中,循环中的 myOMIR(包括 miR-1)上调。可能通过 IGF-1 生长信号轴的抗抑制靶向,抑制 miR-1 和 miR-133a 参与成熟骨骼肌肥大。因此,循环中增加的 miR-1 和 miR-133a 可能促进创伤性心血管事件后骨骼肌萎缩。有趣的是,一旦用左心室辅助装置补偿 HF,心肌中的 myomiR 水平(特别是 miR-1、miR-133a 和 miR-133b)就会降低。

最近发现了一组循环 miRNA,其敏感性足以区分射血分数保留型与降低型慢性 HF,并且循环 miR-221 和 miR-328 水平可以协助循环 B 型利尿钠肽评估 HF。

一些研究已确定了慢性 HF 患者中有类似于急性力竭运动的标志物。例如,一项研究表明,急性运动后不久,血清 miR-21、miR-378 和 miR-940 水平显著升高。

在相对稳定的慢性 HF 患者中,外周血单核细胞中 miR-548 家族成员(如 miR-548c、miR-548i)与对照组相比水平降低,而 miR-22、miR-92b、miR-320 水平似乎升高了。

在小鼠心肌梗死后 HF 模型中,一个研究小组调查了人胚胎干细胞来源的心血管祖细胞(human embryonic stem cell-derived cardiovascular progenitors,hESC-Pg)合成的梗死后外泌体治疗是否能获得与注射 hESC-PG 类似的益处。数据显示,通过介导旁分泌因子刺激细胞分裂和存活,外泌体在改善心脏功能方面与干细胞一样有效。

在动物实验中,在慢性 HF 演变和实验性心室起搏后,观察到犬心室肌和心房肌有不同 miRNA 浓度的变化,包括 cFa-miR-1、cFa-miR-26a、cFa-miR-26b、cFa-miR-29a、cFa-miR-30a、cFa-miR-133a、cFa-miR-133b、cFa-miR-208a 和 cFA-miR-218 的下调,cfa-miR-21 和 cfa-miR-146b 的上调。另一项研究表明,cFamiR-9、cfa-miR-181c、cfa-miR-495 和 cFa-miR-599 的表达与 HF 的发生与发展不同,但也随着年龄的变化而改变。

(二)外泌体与 HF 后的康复

螺内酯和地高辛是治疗 HF 的传统药物。血管紧张素转换酶抑制药(angiotensin converting enzyme inhibitors,ACEI)和 β 受体阻滞剂多年来一直被认为是治疗 HF 的基本药物。尽管它们降低了所有耐受的 HF 患者的死亡率,但也有许多不良反应,如早产、骨畸形、羊水过少、肢体挛缩、宫内发育迟缓、新生儿死亡和肺发育不全。肼屈嗪是一种更好的替代品,通常用来取代 ACEI。扩张性 HF 的治疗方法与目前 PPCM 的治疗方法相似。

研究表明,儿童 HF 的特殊分子模式导致了年龄相关变化的治疗反应,包括磷酸二酯酶治疗的众多效应、肾上腺素能受体系统调节、纤维化基因图谱和 miRNA 表达水平。

NrF2 相关的 miRNA 被认为是慢性 HF 或心肌梗死后状态的潜在治疗靶点。

先前的研究表明,抑制 miRNA-195 后,恢复了正常心脏活动、改善了冠状动脉血流量、增加了 Sirtuin 1 和 B 细胞白血病/淋巴瘤 2 的表达水平,所以降低 miRNA-195 水平可以延缓糖尿病心肌病向完全性 HF 的发生或发展。

欧洲心脏病学会和美国心脏协会/美国心脏病学会已经公布了几项针对 HF 患者的心脏状况诊断和治疗指南。

七、外泌体在心肌肥厚中的作用

（一）外泌体作为心肌肥厚的生物标志物

心肌肥厚由广泛的心脏应激引起，通常与心脏重构有关。应该强调的是，心肌肥厚可能导致 HF。心肌成纤维细胞来源的外泌体含量分析显示，几种 miRNA[如 miR-21_3p（miR-21）]变多，可诱导心肌肥大。此外，蛋白质组分析显示一些 miR-21 靶点，包括 Sorbin、SH3 结构域蛋白 2（SH3 domain-containing protein 2，SORBS2）、PDZ 和 LIM 结构域 5（PDZ and LIM domain 5，PDLIM5）和心肌细胞肥大与沉默 SORBS2 或 PDLIM5 相关。人和动物研究表明，氧化应激是导致心肌肥大的关键因素之一。目前，在 Friedreich 共济失调影响的患者中，有研究表明，氧化应激与心肌肥厚有关，服用艾地苯醌（即辅酶 Q10 的短链类似物）可降低大约 50% 患者的心肌肥厚。此外，异丙肾上腺素诱导 Wistar 大鼠的心肌肥厚与血浆和心肌组织中脂质过氧化物的增加有关，而磷脂对自由基的产生有保护作用。

心肌肥厚的另一个生物标志物是肌浆网钙 ATPase 泵的心脏亚型 Serca2a 的翻译后改变，这种改变可被小泛素样修饰物 1（small ubiquitin-like modifier type 1，SUMO-1）减弱。

在右肾动脉诱导的大鼠心肌肥厚中，结扎证实了含有 HSP90 和 IL-6 的心肌细胞来源外泌体迁移到心肌成纤维细胞，从而有助于心肌成纤维细胞信号转导和转录激活因子 3（signal transducer and activator of transcription 3，STAT-3）信号的双相激活，从而触发胶原合成的增加。

（二）外泌体在心肌肥厚恢复中的作用

从梗死区周围的正常细胞中捕获的外泌体 miRNA-133a 可以减轻由心肌梗死引起的心肌肥厚，刺激氧化应激也可能减轻心肌肥厚。因此，过氧化氢刺激心脏前体细胞产生的氧化应激导致含有高水平 miRNA-21 的外泌体释放，最终阻止了心肌细胞的凋亡。

通过激活血管紧张素Ⅱ1型和2型受体，靶向血管紧张素Ⅱ诱导的心肌成纤维细胞释放外泌体，被认为是治疗心肌肥厚的一种方法。

体外将脂肪细胞来源的外泌体 miR-200a 导入心肌细胞，可诱导心肌细胞肥大，而将反义寡核苷酸导入 miR-200a 可逆转心肌细胞肥大。此外，在体内消融过氧化物酶体增殖物激活受体 γ（proliferator-activated receptor gamma，PPAR-γ）可减少心肌肥厚。

在转基因小鼠中过表达 HSP20 可以减轻链脲佐菌素诱导的心脏功能障碍和肥大。在这些转基因小鼠中，心肌细胞来源的外泌体具有高含量的 HSP20、p-Akt、生存素和超氧化物歧化酶 1，并对体内链脲佐菌素诱导的心脏重塑具有保护作用。

八、外泌体在心律失常中的作用

（一）外泌体作为心律失常的生物标志物

外泌体在心律失常中所起的作用大多是未知的。然而，一些研究表明，富含 miR-1 和

miR-133 的外泌体(通常认为是由冠心病患者或大鼠心肌缺血模型中的心肌细胞分泌)在心律失常中也发挥着重要作用,能够通过钙/钙调蛋白依赖的蛋白激酶Ⅱ信号调节动作电位和心脏传导。

此外,一些外泌体 miR(如 miR-328)被认为具有致心律失常的特性。研究表明,缺血与外泌体 miR-328 上调有关,提示其致心律失常的作用可能与靶向 L 型钙通道有关。应该强调的是,外泌体 miR 以 L 型钙通道的靶向作用在心律失常中是非常重要的,临床和实验证实心房颤动与 L 型钙电流的减少和动作电位时程的缩短有关。

(二)外泌体与心律失常后的恢复

一些研究证实干细胞对心律失常的恢复有积极作用,而另一些研究则证明了干细胞移植会诱发心律失常。将成人 MSC 注入犬左心室心肌使其起搏正常化,6 周内没有异种移植排斥反应。有趣的是,新生大鼠心肌细胞与人骨髓间充质干细胞来源的外泌体孵育并没有增加动作电位时程(action potential duration,APD)。另一方面,植入成人 MSC 时应谨慎,因为它可能诱发心律失常,如减慢传导或降低复极率。一项综合的实验和模拟研究表明,人骨髓间充质干细胞释放的外泌体主要通过旁分泌信号影响人心肌收缩力和导致心律失常,其次是异质细胞偶联。

九、外泌体在脑血管疾病中的作用

(一)外泌体作为脑血管疾病的生物标志物

外泌体含量是确定脑血管疾病中有价值的生物标志物(见表 9-1)。

表 9-1 外泌体作为人类脑血管疾病的生物标志物

脑血管病	外泌体类型	生物标志物
急性缺血性脑卒中	血清外泌体	脑特异性 miR-9 和 miR-124
急性缺氧缺血性脑病	血清外泌体	Synaptopodin
恶性脑肿瘤 多形性胶质母细胞瘤	细胞上清液	缺氧调节蛋白
阿尔茨海默病 额颞痴呆	血浆(星形胶质细胞和神经元衍生的外泌体)	● β位点淀粉样前体蛋白裂解酶 1(β-site amyloid precursor protein-cleaving enzyme 1,BACE-1) ● γ分泌酶 ● 可溶性 Aβ42 ● 可溶性淀粉样前体蛋白 β(soluble amyloid precursor protein β,sAPPβ) ● 可溶性淀粉样前体蛋白 α(soluble amyloid precursor protein α,sAPPα) ● 胶质细胞源性神经营养因子(glial-derived neurotrophic factor,GDNF) ● P-T181-tau ● P-S396-tau

续 表

脑血管病	外泌体类型	生物标志物
帕金森病	红细胞源性外泌体	α - Synuclein
创伤性脑损伤	脑源性细胞外小泡 CSF（脑源性外泌体）	↓ miR - 212 ↑ miR - 212 miR - 21、miR - 146、miR7a 和 miR - 7b 核苷酸结合寡聚化结构域样受体蛋白 - 1、炎症体、αⅡ - 血影蛋白分解产物、GFAP 及其分解产物、泛素羧基末端水解酶 L1

急性缺血性脑卒中患者血清中，脑特异性 miR - 9 和 miR - 124 的外泌体数量增加，与美国国立卫生研究院卒中评分、梗死体积和血清 IL - 6 水平呈正相关，有望成为急性缺血性脑卒中的生物标志物。此外，在急性缺氧缺血性脑病的新生儿血清中，发现神经元外体突触素是一种很有前途的生物标志物，它的水平与短期神经预后相关。

在缺氧相关病理（即脑卒中、心肌梗死、先兆子痫、肿瘤缺氧等）患者中，循环外泌体被认为是与疾病状态相关的生物标志物。

在多形性胶质母细胞瘤患者中，从肿瘤中获得的外泌体提示 U87MG 胶质瘤细胞处于缺氧状态，该外泌体的内容也十分丰富，含有受缺氧调节的 mRNA 和蛋白质如基质金属蛋白酶、IL - 8、PDGF、caveolin 1 和赖氨酰氧化酶。此外，胶质瘤细胞释放的外泌体可以通过调节内皮细胞的活性促进肿瘤的发展。

在阿尔茨海默病患者血浆中，星形胶质细胞来源外泌体的蛋白质含量（如 β 位点淀粉样前体蛋白裂解酶 1、γ 分泌酶、可溶性 Aβ42、可溶性淀粉样前体蛋白 β、可溶性淀粉样前体蛋白 α、胶质源性神经营养因子、P - T181 - tau 和 P - S396 - tau）比神经源性外泌体的含量更高。

帕金森病的发生和发展受到含有 α - synuclein 的红细胞来源外泌体通过血脑屏障的路径影响。

在创伤性脑损伤中，体液特别是血液和 CSF 中的外泌体可以识别出多种生物标志物。脑源性外泌体中的 miRNA 通过表达下调（miR - 212）或上调（miR - 21、miR - 146、miR - 7a 和 miR - 7b）介导创伤性脑损伤。在诱导创伤性脑损伤的大鼠脑中，证实了连接蛋白 43 的磷酸化刺激了脑源性外泌体的释放，并需要激活 ERK 信号。在脊髓损伤或创伤性脑损伤的患者中，核苷酸结合寡聚化结构域样受体蛋白 - 1 炎性小体的成分被确定为 CSF 中外泌体的生物标志物。此外，一项对创伤性脑损伤患者的广泛蛋白质组学研究表明，CSF 中有一些生物标志物，包括 αⅡ- spectrin 分解产物、GFAP 及其分解产物，以及泛素羧基末端水解酶 L1。

（二）外泌体作为大脑中的货物

外泌体对于细胞间的通信是必不可少的，目前认为它们将各种来源（如细胞和体液）的外泌体蛋白和 RNA 转移到脑组织。另一方面，在脑损伤后外泌体的转移也表现为相反的方向。因此，研究表明，脑源性外泌体可以通过血脑屏障（blood-brain barrie，BBB）

(图9-3),并且有证据表明它们存在于外周血或CSF中。体外脑微血管内皮细胞单层研究证实了在卒中样和TNF-α诱导的炎症条件下,外泌体可以通过血脑屏障,而在对照条件下则不能。

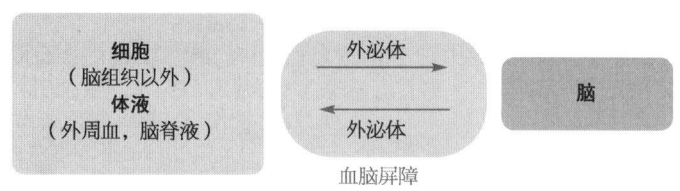

图9-3 外泌体通过血脑屏障

含有miR-132的神经细胞外泌体转移到内皮细胞调节脑血管的完整性。此外,MSC来源的外泌体在体外促进皮层神经元的轴突生长中发挥了积极作用。

有趣的是,在人类早期神经发育过程中,外泌体也充当母体血液的货物。

(三)外泌体在脑血管病治疗中的应用

在几种动物模型中测试了脑卒中后静脉注射MSC释放的外泌体,这可能代表了大脑修复的转化治疗策略。到目前为止,在成年雄性Wistar大鼠受到大脑中动脉闭塞2小时后全身应用MSC衍生的外泌体,可以通过刺激轴突重塑、神经再生和血管生成,改善脑卒中后的功能恢复。

此外,全身应用多能间充质基质细胞或小胶质细胞来源的外泌体可以诱导创伤性脑损伤后的功能恢复(图9-4)。具体地说,将多能间充质基质细胞移植到有创伤性脑损伤的Wistar大鼠后,可改善其感觉运动功能的恢复,促进血管生成和神经再生,并减少炎症。在创伤性脑损伤后的大鼠中,全身应用来自人骨髓间充质干细胞的外泌体,可以增加损伤部位新细胞(即内皮细胞和神经元)的生成,减少神经炎症,改善功能恢复。此外,将来自人脱落乳牙干细胞的外泌体注射到创伤性脑损伤的大鼠模型中,这些外泌体能够通过改变小胶质细胞的极化(即阻止M1小胶质细胞表型和促进M2小胶质细胞表型)来减轻神经炎症,并恢复运动功能。在体外模型中,将小胶质细胞来源的外泌体miR-124-3p转移到神经元,抑制了神经细胞的炎症,促进了创伤性脑损伤小鼠脑提取液中突起的生长。

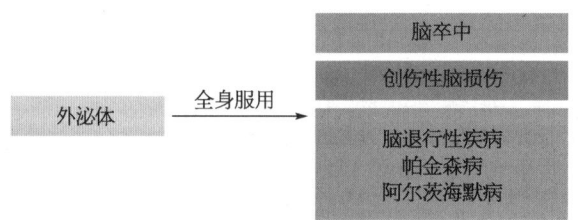

图9-4 外泌体用于脑血管疾病

神经退行性疾病也被认为是脑血管病。对诱发阿尔茨海默病的小鼠活体研究表明,通过腹腔注射中性鞘磷脂酶2抑制剂GW4869阻止外泌体的分泌,可以减少淀粉样斑块的形成。基于外泌体的治疗方法在帕金森病中也很有前景。因此,牙髓干细胞中提取的外泌体被证明可以防止人类多巴胺能神经元的凋亡。负载过氧化氢酶的外泌体在体外被神经元吸收,并能够在诱导帕金森病小鼠鼻内给药时发挥体内神经保护作用。

十、总结

外泌体是未来感兴趣的货运囊泡,因为它们反映了其起源细胞的病理生理状态。供体细胞外泌体含有 RNA 信息,能够影响局部或远距离发现的受体细胞。甚至有研究者假设它们可能携带着能够影响受体细胞的表观遗传调节剂。而且,外泌体可作为心血管疾病进化和进展的生物标志物,但其程度与治疗或再生不同程度心脏损伤的手段相同。外泌体携带的信息对心血管器官可能是保护性的,也可能是破坏性的,这取决于它们起源的细胞。一些转运的 miRNA 免受 RNA 酶和蛋白酶降解,被认为是心血管系统中有吸引力的候选生物标志物,如 AMI 患者中存在的血清 miR-192、miR-194 和 miR-34a。这些生物标志物可以预测来年心室重塑向 HF 的演变。将来,随着一些其他的生物标志物被发现,外泌体作为生物标志物、诊断和预后因子将变得越来越重要。

虽然体外和体内的研究表明,使用干细胞对损伤后的心脏恢复有积极的作用,但应该谨慎考虑在心血管病理中植入干细胞。许多研究表明,这一结果是由旁分泌作用介导的。如今,外泌体被认为是能够运送到特定靶点的天然纳米颗粒。根据它们的来源,如干细胞或心脏祖细胞、体细胞等,外泌体将在心血管系统的修复或再生过程中发挥重要作用。而且,人工设计的外泌体可以通过操纵它们的内容物,治疗缺血性心脏病。

外泌体作为药物递送系统的应用前景非常广阔,但在实际应用之前,还需要进行大量的临床前和临床研究。

(黄宁 译,胡长平 审校)

参考文献

[1] Bruno S, Deregibus MC, Camussi G. The secretome of mesenchymal stromal cells: role of extracellular vesicles in immunomodulation. Immunol Lett 2015; 168(2): 154-8.
[2] Kalra H, Simpson RJ, Ji H, Aikawa E, Altevogt P, Askenase P, et al. Vesiclepedia: a compendium for extracellular vesicles with continuous community annotation. PLoS Biol 2012; 10(12): e1001450.
[3] Camussi G, Deregibus MC, Bruno S, Cantaluppi V, Biancone L. Exosomes/microvesicles as a mechanism of cell-to-cell communication. Kidney Int 2010; 78(9): 838-48.
[4] Yanez-Mo M, Siljander PR, Andreu Z, Zavec AB, Borras FE, Buzas EI, et al. Biological properties of extracellular vesicles and their physiological functions. J Extracell vesicles 2015; 4: 27066.
[5] Keller S, Ridinger J, Rupp AK, Janssen JW, Altevogt P. Body fluid derived exosomes as a novel template for clinical diagnostics. J Transl Med 2011; 9: 86.
[6] Machida T, Tomofuji T, Ekuni D, Maruyama T, Yoneda T, Kawabata Y, et al. MicroRNAs in salivary exosome as potential biomarkers of aging. Int J Mol Sci 2015; 16(9): 21294-309.
[7] Beltrami C, Besnier M, Shantikumar S, Shearn AI, Rajakaruna C, Laftah A, et al. Human pericardial fluid contains exosomes enriched with cardiovascular-expressed microRNAs and promotes therapeutic angiogenesis. Mol ther 2017; 25(3): 679-93.
[8] Barcelo M, Mata A, Bassas L, Larriba S. Exosomal microRNAs in seminal plasma are markers of the origin of azoospermia and can predict the presence of sperm in testicular tissue. Hum Reprod 2018; 33(6): 1087-98.
[9] Evans-Osses I, Reichembach LH, Ramirez MI. Exosomes or microvesicles? Two kinds of extracellular vesicles with different routes to modify protozoan-host cell interaction. Parasitol Res 2015; 114(10): 3567-75.
[10] Cocucci E, Meldolesi J. Ectosomes and exosomes: shedding the confusion between extracellular vesicles. Trends Cell Biol 2015; 25(6): 364-72.
[11] Kalra H, Drummen GP, Mathivanan S. Focus on extracellular vesicles: introducing the next small big thing. Int J Mol Sci 2016; 17(2): 170.

[12] Thery C, Zitvogel L, Amigorena S. Exosomes: composition, biogenesis and function. Nat Rev Immunol 2002; 2(8): 569-79.
[13] Rink J, Ghigo E, Kalaidzidis Y, Zerial M. Rab conversion as a mechanism of progression from early to late endosomes. Cell 2005; 122(5): 735-49.
[14] Balaj L, Lessard R, Dai L, Cho YJ, Pomeroy SL, Breakefield XO, et al. Tumour microvesicles contain retrotransposon elements and amplified oncogene sequences. Nat Commun 2011; 2: 180.
[15] Buzas EI, Gyorgy B, Nagy G, Falus A, Gay S. Emerging role of extracellular vesicles in inflammatory diseases. Nat Rev Rheumatol 2014; 10(6): 356-64.
[16] Abels ER, Breakefield XO. Introduction to extracellular vesicles: biogenesis, rna cargo selection, content, release, and uptake. Cell Mol Neurobiol 2016; 36(3): 301-12.
[17] Henderson MC, Azorsa DO. The genomic and proteomic content of cancer cell-derived exosomes. Front Oncol 2012; 2: 38.
[18] Gangoda L, Boukouris S, Liem M, Kalra H, Mathivanan S. Extracellular vesicles including exosomes are mediators of signal transduction: are they protective or pathogenic? Proteomics 2015; 15(2-3): 260-71.
[19] Raimondo F, Morosi L, Chinello C, Magni F, Pitto M. Advances in membranous vesicle and exosome proteomics improving biological understanding and biomarker discovery. Proteomics 2011; 11(4): 709-20.
[20] Cosme J, Liu PP, Gramolini AO. The cardiovascular exosome: current perspectives and potential. Proteomics 2013; 13 (10-11): 1654-9.
[21] Bei Y, Yu P, Cretoiu D, Cretoiu SM, Xiao J. Exosomes-based biomarkers for the prognosis of cardiovascular diseases. Adv Exp Med Biol 2017; 998: 71-88.
[22] Vanhaverbeke M, Gal D, Holvoet P. Functional role of cardiovascular exosomes in myocardial injury and atherosclerosis. Exosomes in cardiovascular diseases advances in experimental medicine and biology. In: Exosomes in Cardiovascular Diseases. vol. 998. Singapore: Springer; 2017. p.45-58.
[23] Todorova D, Simoncini S, Lacroix R, Sabatier F, Dignat-George F. Extracellular vesicles in angiogenesis. Circ Res 2017; 120(10): 1658-73.
[24] Ailawadi S, Wang X, Gu H, Fan GC. Pathologic function and therapeutic potential of exosomes in cardiovascular disease. Biochim Biophys Acta 2015; 1852(1): 1-11.
[25] Chistiakov DA, Orekhov AN, Bobryshev YV. Cardiac extracellular vesicles in normal and infarcted heart. Int J Mol Sci 2016; 17(1): 63-81.
[26] Garcia NA, Moncayo-Arlandi J, Sepulveda P, Diez-Juan A. Cardiomyocyte exosomes regulate glycolytic flux in endothelium by direct transfer of GLUT transporters and glycolytic enzymes. Cardiovasc Res 2016; 109(3): 397-408.
[27] Garcia NA, Ontoria-Oviedo I, Gonzalez-King H, Diez-Juan A, Sepulveda P. Glucose starvation in cardiomyocytes enhances exosome secretion and promotes angiogenesis in endothelial cells. PLoS One 2015; 10(9): e0138849.
[28] Kakkar R, Lee RT. Intramyocardial fibroblast myocyte communication. Circ Res 2010; 106(1): 47-57.
[29] Cervio E, Barile L, Moccetti T, Vassalli G. Exosomes for intramyocardial intercellular communication. Stem Cells Int 2015; 2015: 482171.
[30] Vrijsen KR, Maring JA, Chamuleau SA, Verhage V, Mol EA, Deddens JC, et al. Exosomes from cardiomyocyte progenitor cells and mesenchymal stem cells stimulate angiogenesis via EMMPRIN. Adv Healthc Mater 2016; 5(19): 2555-65.
[31] Deregibus MC, Cantaluppi V, Calogero R, Lo Iacono M, Tetta C, Biancone L, et al. Endothelial progenitor cell derived microvesicles activate an angiogenic program in endothelial cells by a horizontal transfer of mRNA. Blood 2007; 110(7): 2440-8.
[32] Cantaluppi V, Biancone L, Figliolini F, Beltramo S, Medica D, Deregibus MC, et al. Microvesicles derived from endothelial progenitor cells enhance neoangiogenesis of human pancreatic islets. Cell Transplant 2012; 21(6): 1305-20.
[33] Tsimerman G, Roguin A, Bachar A, Melamed E, Brenner B, Aharon A. Involvement of microparticles in diabetic vascular complications. Thromb Haemost 2011; 106(2): 310-21.
[34] Sabatier F, Darmon P, Hugel B, Combes V, Sanmarco M, Velut JG, et al. Type 1 and type 2 diabetic patients display different patterns of cellular microparticles. Diabetes 2002; 51(9): 2840-5.
[35] Helal O, Defoort C, Robert S, Marin C, Lesavre N, Lopez-Miranda J, et al. Increased levels of microparticles originating from endothelial cells, platelets and erythrocytes in subjects with metabolic syndrome: relationship with oxidative stress. Nutr Metab Cardiovasc Dis 2011; 21(9): 665-71.
[36] Esposito K, Ciotola M, Giugliano D. Pioglitazone reduces endothelial microparticles in the metabolic syndrome. Arterioscler Thromb Vasc Biol 2006; 26(8): 1926.
[37] Mobarrez F, Egberg N, Antovic J, Broijersen A, Jorneskog G, Wallen H. Release of endothelial microparticles in vivo during atorvastatin treatment: a randomized double-blind placebocontrolled study. Thromb Res 2012; 129(1): 95-7.
[38] Lother A, Bergemann S, Deng L, Moser M, Bode C, Hein L. Cardiac endothelial cell transcriptome. Arterioscler Thromb Vasc Biol 2018; 38(3): 566-74.
[39] Yu B, Zhang X, Li X. Exosomes derived from mesenchymal stem cells. Int J Mol Sci 2014; 15(3): 4142-57.
[40] Chen W, Huang Y, Han J, Yu L, Li Y, Lu Z, et al. Immunomodulatory effects of mesenchymal stromal cells-derived exosome. Immunol Res 2016; 64(4): 831-40.
[41] Yeo RW, Lai RC, Zhang B, Tan SS, Yin Y, Teh BJ, et al. Mesenchymal stem cell: an efficient mass producer of exosomes for drug delivery. Adv Drug Deliv Rev 2013; 65(3): 336-41.
[42] Heijnen HF, Schiel AE, Fijnheer R, Geuze HJ, Sixma JJ. Activated platelets release two types of membrane vesicles: microvesicles by surface shedding and exosomes derived from exocytosis of multivesicular bodies and alpha-granules. Blood 1999; 94(11): 3791-9.
[43] Landry P, Plante I, Ouellet DL, Perron MP, Rousseau G, Provost P. Existence of a microRNA pathway in anucleate platelets. Nat Struct Mol Biol 2009; 16(9): 961-6.

[44] Rowley JW, Oler AJ, Tolley ND, Hunter BN, Low EN, Nix DA, et al. Genome-wide RNAseq analysis of human and mouse platelet transcriptomes. Blood 2011; 118(14): e101-11.
[45] Bray PF, McKenzie SE, Edelstein LC, Nagalla S, Delgrosso K, Ertel A, et al. The complex transcriptional landscape of the anucleate human platelet. BMC Genomics 2013; 14: 1.
[46] Schubert S, Weyrich AS, Rowley JW. A tour through the transcriptional landscape of platelets. Blood 2014; 124(4): 493-502.
[47] Rondina MT, Weyrich AS. Regulation of the genetic code in megakaryocytes and platelets. J Thromb Haemost 2015; 13 (Suppl 1): S26-32.
[48] Alhasan AA, Izuogu OG, Al-Balool HH, Steyn JS, Evans A, Colzani M, et al. Circular RNA enrichment in platelets is a signature of transcriptome degradation. Blood 2016; 127(9): e1-11.
[49] Ple H, Landry P, Benham A, Coarfa C, Gunaratne PH, Provost P. The repertoire and features of human platelet microRNAs. PLoS One 2012; 7(12): e50746.
[50] Goetzl L, Darbinian N, Goetzl EJ. Novel window on early human neurodevelopment via fetal exosomes in maternal blood. Ann Clin Transl Neurol 2016; 3(5): 381-5.
[51] Azevedo LC, Janiszewski M, Pontieri V, Pedro Mde A, Bassi E, Tucci PJ, et al. Plateletderived exosomes from septic shock patients induce myocardial dysfunction. Crit Care 2007; 11(6): R120.
[52] Heijnen H, van der Sluijs P. Platelet secretory behaviour: as diverse as the granules ... or not? J Thromb Haemost 2015; 13(12): 2141-51.
[53] Srikanthan S, Li W, Silverstein RL, McIntyre TM. Exosome poly-ubiquitin inhibits platelet activation, downregulates CD36 and inhibits pro-atherothrombotic cellular functions. J Thromb Haemost 2014; 12(11): 1906-17.
[54] Gambim MH, do Carmo Ade O, Marti L, Verissimo-Filho S, Lopes LR, Janiszewski M. Platelet-derived exosomes induce endothelial cell apoptosis through peroxynitrite generation: experimental evidence for a novel mechanism of septic vascular dysfunction. Crit Care 2007; 11(5): R107.
[55] Angelillo-Scherrer A. Leukocyte-derived microparticles in vascular homeostasis. Circ Res 2012; 110(2): 356-69.
[56] Aharon A, Tamari T, Brenner B. Monocyte-derived microparticles and exosomes induce procoagulant and apoptotic effects on endothelial cells. Thromb Haemost 2008; 100(5): 878-85.
[57] Niu C, Wang X, Zhao M, Cai T, Liu P, Li J, et al. Macrophage foam cell-derived extracellular vesicles promote vascular smooth muscle cell migration and adhesion. J Am Heart Assoc 2016; 5(10). pii: e004099.
[58] Kuo WP, Tigges JC, Toxavidis V, Ghiran I. Red blood cells: a source of extracellular vesicles. Methods Mol Biol 2017; 1660: 15-22.
[59] Danesh A, Inglis HC, Jackman RP, Wu S, Deng X, Muench MO, et al. Exosomes from red blood cell units bind to monocytes and induce proinflammatory cytokines, boosting T-cell responses in vitro. Blood 2014; 123(5): 687-96.
[60] Straat M, Boing AN, Tuip-De Boer A, Nieuwland R, Juffermans NP. Extracellular vesicles from red blood cell products induce a strong pro-inflammatory host response, dependent on both numbers and storage duration. Transfus Med Hemother 2016; 43(4): 302-5.
[61] Azarov I, Liu C, Reynolds H, Tsekouras Z, Lee JS, Gladwin MT, et al. Mechanisms of slower nitric oxide uptake by red blood cells and other hemoglobin-containing vesicles. J Biol Chem 2011; 286(38): 33567-79.
[62] Said AS, Doctor A. Influence of red blood cell-derived microparticles upon vasoregulation. Blood transfusion = Trasfusione del sangue 2017; 15(6): 522-34.
[63] Bevers EM, Comfurius P, Dekkers DW, Zwaal RF. Lipid translocation across the plasma membrane of mammalian cells. Biochim Biophys Acta 1999; 1439(3): 317-30.
[64] Burger P, Kostova E, Bloem E, Hilarius-Stokman P, Meijer AB, van den Berg TK, et al. Potassium leakage primes stored erythrocytes for phosphatidylserine exposure and shedding of pro-coagulant vesicles. Br J Haematol 2013; 160(3): 377-86.
[65] Kostova EB, Beuger BM, Klei TR, Halonen P, Lieftink C, Beijersbergen R, et al. Identification of signalling cascades involved in red blood cell shrinkage and vesiculation. Biosci Rep 2015; 35(2). pii: e00187.
[66] Regev-Rudzki N, Wilson DW, Carvalho TG, Sisquella X, Coleman BM, Rug M, et al. Cellcell communication between malaria-infected red blood cells via exosome-kike vesicles. Cell 2013; 153(5): 1120-33.
[67] Allan D, Limbrick AR, Thomas P, Westerman MP. Release of spectrin-free spicules on reoxygenation of sickled erythrocytes. Nature 1982; 295(5850): 612-3.
[68] Westerman MP, Cole ER, Wu K. The effect of spicules obtained from sickle red cells on clotting activity. Br J Haematol 1984; 56(4): 557-62.
[69] Alkhatatbeh MJ, Enjeti AK, Acharya S, Thorne RF, Lincz LF. The origin of circulating CD36 in type 2 diabetes. Nutrition & diabetes 2013; 3: e59.
[70] Agouni A, Lagrue-Lak-Hal AH, Ducluzeau PH, Mostefai HA, Draunet-Busson C, Leftheriotis G, et al. Endothelial dysfunction caused by circulating microparticles from patients with metabolic syndrome. Am J Pathol 2008; 173(4): 1210-9.
[71] Boyer M, Baggett A, Scalia R, Eguchi S, Rizzo V. Characterization of exosomes isolated from cultured vascular endothelial and smooth muscle cells. FASEB J 2017; 31(1_supplement): 837.7-837.7.
[72] Qiu H, Shi S, Wang S, Peng H, Ding SJ, Wang L. Proteomic profiling exosomes from vascular smooth muscle cell. Proteomics Clin Appl 2018; 12(5): e1700097.
[73] Comelli L, Rocchiccioli S, Smirni S, Salvetti A, Signore G, Citti L, et al. Characterization of secreted vesicles from vascular smooth muscle cells. Mol BioSyst 2014; 10(5): 1146-52.
[74] Kapustin AN, Chatrou ML, Drozdov I, Zheng Y, Davidson SM, Soong D, et al. Vascular smooth muscle cell calcification is mediated by regulated exosome secretion. Circ Res 2015; 116(8): 1312-23.
[75] Kapustin AN, Shanahan CM. Emerging roles for vascular smooth muscle cell exosomes in calcification and coagulation. J Physiol 2016; 594(11): 2905-14.

[76] Zheng B, Yin WN, Suzuki T, Zhang XH, Zhang Y, Song LL, et al. Exosome-mediated miR-155 transfer from smooth muscle cells to endothelial cells induces endothelial injury and promotes atherosclerosis. Mol ther 2017; 25(6): 1279-94.

[77] Faure J, Lachenal G, Court M, Hirrlinger J, Chatellard-Causse C, Blot B, et al. Exosomes are released by cultured cortical neurones. Mol Cell Neurosci 2006; 31(4): 642-8.

[78] Fruhbeis C, Frohlich D, Kuo WP, Kramer-Albers EM. Extracellular vesicles as mediators of neuron-glia communication. Front Cell Neurosci 2013; 7: 182.

[79] Zhang ZG, Chopp M. Exosomes in stroke pathogenesis and therapy. J Clin Invest 2016; 126(4): 1190-7.

[80] Goetzl EJ, Mustapic M, Kapogiannis D, Eitan E, Lobach IV, Goetzl L, et al. Cargo proteins of plasma astrocyte-derived exosomes in Alzheimer's disease. FASEB J 2016; 30(11): 3853-9.

[81] Skog J, Wurdinger T, van Rijn S, Meijer DH, Gainche L, Sena-Esteves M, et al. Glioblastoma microvesicles transport RNA and proteins that promote tumour growth and provide diagnostic biomarkers. Nat Cell Biol 2008; 10(12): 1470-6.

[82] Haqqani AS, Delaney CE, Tremblay TL, Sodja C, Sandhu JK, Stanimirovic DB. Method for isolation and molecular characterization of extracellular microvesicles released from brain endothelial cells. Fluids Barriers CNS 2013; 10(1): 4.

[83] Yamamoto S, Niida S, Azuma E, Yanagibashi T, Muramatsu M, Huang TT, et al. Inflammation-induced endothelial cell-derived extracellular vesicles modulate the cellular status of pericytes. Sci Rep 2015; 5: 8505.

[84] Hooper C, Sainz-Fuertes R, Lynham S, Hye A, Killick R, Warley A, et al. Wnt3a induces exosome secretion from primary cultured rat microglia. BMC Neurosci 2012; 13: 144.

[85] Bahrini I, Song JH, Diez D, Hanayama R. Neuronal exosomes facilitate synaptic pruning by up-regulating complement factors in microglia. Sci Rep 2015; 5: 7989.

[86] Sun L, Wang X, Zhou Y, Zhou RH, Ho WZ, Li JL. Exosomes contribute to the transmission of anti-HIV activity from TLR3-activated brain microvascular endothelial cells to macrophages. Antivir Res 2016; 134: 167-71.

[87] Giusti I, Delle Monache S, Di Francesco M, Sanita P, D'Ascenzo S, Gravina GL, et al. From glioblastoma to endothelial cells through extracellular vesicles: messages for angiogenesis. Tumour Biol 2016; 37(9): 12743-53.

[88] Guitart K, Loers G, Buck F, Bork U, Schachner M, Kleene R. Improvement of neuronal cell survival by astrocyte-derived exosomes under hypoxic and ischemic conditions depends on prion protein. Glia 2016; 64(6): 896-910.

[89] Goncalves MB, Malmqvist T, Clarke E, Hubens CJ, Grist J, Hobbs C, et al. Neuronal RARbeta signaling modulates PTEN activity directly in neurons and via exosome transfer in astrocytes to prevent glial scar formation and induce spinal cord regeneration. J Neurosci 2015; 35(47): 15731-45.

[90] Chernyshev VS, Rachamadugu R, Tseng YH, Belnap DM, Jia Y, Branch KJ, et al. Size and shape characterization of hydrated and desiccated exosomes. Anal Bioanal Chem 2015; 407(12): 3285-301.

[91] Ferguson SW, Wang J, Lee CJ, Liu M, Neelamegham S, Canty JM, et al. The microRNA regulatory landscape of MSC-derived exosomes: a systems view. Sci Rep 2018; 8(1): 1419.

[92] Tauro BJ, Greening DW, Mathias RA, Ji H, Mathivanan S, Scott AM, et al. Comparison of ultracentrifugation, density gradient separation, and immunoaffinity capture methods for isolating human colon cancer cell line LIM1863-derived exosomes. Methods 2012; 56(2): 293-304.

[93] Alvarez ML, Khosroheidari M, Kanchi Ravi R, DiStefano JK. Comparison of protein, microRNA, and mRNA yields using different methods of urinary exosome isolation for the discovery of kidney disease biomarkers. Kidney Int 2012; 82(9): 1024-32.

[94] Rekker K, Saare M, Roost AM, Kubo AL, Zarovni N, Chiesi A, et al. Comparison of serum exosome isolation methods for microRNA profiling. Clin Biochem 2014; 47(1-2): 135-8.

[95] Rautou PE, Mackman N. Microvesicles as risk markers for venous thrombosis. Expert Rev Hematol 2013; 6(1): 91-101.

[96] Gustafson CM, Shepherd AJ, Miller VM, Jayachandran M. Age- and sex-specific differences in blood-borne microvesicles from apparently healthy humans. Biol Sex Differ 2015; 6: 10.

[97] Malik ZA, Liu TT, Knowlton AA. Cardiac myocyte exosome isolation. Methods Mol Biol 2016; 1448: 237-48.

[98] Chen C, Skog J, Hsu CH, Lessard RT, Balaj L, Wurdinger T, et al. Microfluidic isolation and transcriptome analysis of serum microvesicles. Lab Chip 2010; 10(4): 505-11.

[99] Szczepanski MJ, Szajnik M, Welsh A, Whiteside TL, Boyiadzis M. Blast-derived microvesicles in sera from patients with acute myeloid leukemia suppress natural killer cell function via membrane-associated transforming growth factor-beta1. Haematologica 2011; 96(9): 1302-9.

[100] Taylor DD, Zacharias W, Gercel-Taylor C. Exosome isolation for proteomic analyses and RNA profiling. Methods Mol Biol 2011; 728: 235-46.

[101] Hong CS, Muller L, Whiteside TL, Boyiadzis M. Plasma exosomes as markers of therapeutic response in patients with acute myeloid leukemia. Front Immunol 2014; 5: 160.

[102] Saenz-Cuesta M, Arbelaiz A, Oregi A, Irizar H, Osorio-Querejeta I, Munoz-Culla M, et al. Methods for extracellular vesicles isolation in a hospital setting. Front Immunol 2015; 6: 50.

[103] Levy E. Exosomes in the diseased brain: first insights from in vivo studies. Front Neurosci 2017; 11: 142.

[104] van der Meel R, Krawczyk-Durka M, van Solinge WW, Schiffelers RM. Toward routine detection of extracellular vesicles in clinical samples. Int J Lab Hematol 2014; 36(3): 244-53.

[105] Malik ZA, Kott KS, Poe AJ, Kuo T, Chen L, Ferrara KW, et al. Cardiac myocyte exosomes: stability, HSP60, and proteomics. Am J Physiol Heart Circ Physiol 2013; 304(7): H954-65.

[106] van Weering JR, Brown E, Sharp TH, Mantell J, Cullen PJ, Verkade P. Intracellular membrane traffic at high resolution. Methods Cell Biol 2010; 96: 619-48.

[107] Admyre C, Johansson SM, Qazi KR, Filen JJ, Lahesmaa R, Norman M, et al. Exosomes with immune modulatory features are present in human breast milk. J Immunol 2007; 179(3): 1969-78.

[108] Arraud N, Linares R, Tan S, Gounou C, Pasquet JM, Mornet S, et al. Extracellular vesicles from blood plasma: determination of their morphology, size, phenotype and concentration. J Thromb Haemost 2014; 12(5): 614-27.

[109] Wubbolts R, Leckie RS, Veenhuizen PT, Schwarzmann G, Mobius W, Hoernschemeyer J, et al. Proteomic and biochemical analyses of human B cell-derived exosomes. Potential implications for their function and multivesicular body formation. J Biol Chem 2003; 278(13): 10963-72.

[110] van der Pol E, Hoekstra AG, Sturk A, Otto C, van Leeuwen TG, Nieuwland R. Optical and non-optical methods for detection and characterization of microparticles and exosomes. J Thromb Haemost 2010; 8(12): 2596-607.

[111] Ashcroft BA, de Sonneville J, Yuana Y, Osanto S, Bertina R, Kuil ME, et al. Determination of the size distribution of blood microparticles directly in plasma using atomic force microscopy and microfluidics. Biomed Microdevices 2012; 14(4): 641-9.

[112] Davidson SM, Takov K, Yellon DM. Exosomes and cardiovascular protection. Cardiovasc Drugs Ther 2017; 31(1): 77-86.

[113] Almizraq RJ, Seghatchian J, Holovati JL, Acker JP. Extracellular vesicle characteristics in stored red blood cell concentrates are influenced by the method of detection. Transfus Apher Sci 2017; 56(2): 254-60.

[114] Leroyer AS, Isobe H, Leseche G, Castier Y, Wassef M, Mallat Z, et al. Cellular origins and thrombogenic activity of microparticles isolated from human atherosclerotic plaques. J Am Coll Cardiol 2007; 49(7): 772-7.

[115] Jansen F, Li Q, Pfeifer A, Werner N. Endothelial- and immune cell-derived extracellular vesicles in the regulation of cardiovascular health and disease. JACC Basic to Transl Sci 2017; 2(6): 790-807.

[116] Yayan J. Emerging families of biomarkers for coronary artery disease: inflammatory mediators. Vasc Health Risk Manag 2013; 9: 435-56.

[117] Kosaka N, Iguchi H, Yoshioka Y, Takeshita F, Matsuki Y, Ochiya T. Secretory mechanisms and intercellular transfer of microRNAs in living cells. J Biol Chem 2010; 285(23): 17442-52.

[118] Cretoiu SM. Circulating microRNAs in cardiovascular diseases: recent progress and challenges. J Hypertens Res 2016; 2(1): 15-8.

[119] Fichtlscherer S, De Rosa S, Fox H, Schwietz T, Fischer A, Liebetrau C, et al. Circulating microRNAs in patients with coronary artery disease. Circ Res 2010; 107(5): 677-84.

[120] Bei Y, Tao L, Cretoiu D, Cretoiu SM, Xiao J. MicroRNAs mediate beneficial effects of exercise in heart. Adv Exp Med Biol 2017; 1000: 261-80.

[121] Karakas M, Schulte C, Appelbaum S, Ojeda F, Lackner KJ, Munzel T, et al. Circulating microRNAs strongly predict cardiovascular death in patients with coronary artery diseaseresults from the large AtheroGene study. Eur Heart J 2017; 38(7): 516-23.

[122] Zhong Z, Hou J, Zhang Q, Zhong W, Li B, Li C, et al. Circulating microRNA expression profiling and bioinformatics analysis of dysregulated microRNAs of patients with coronary artery disease. Medicine 2018; 97(27): e11428.

[123] Hausenloy DJ, Garcia-Dorado D, Botker HE, Davidson SM, Downey J, Engel FB, et al. Novel targets and future strategies for acute cardioprotection: position paper of the european society of cardiology working group on cellular biology of the heart. Cardiovasc Res 2017; 113(6): 564-85.

[124] Davidson SM, Yellon DM. Exosomes and cardioprotection — a critical analysis. Mol Asp Med 2018; 60: 104-14.

[125] Marini M, Ibba-Manneschi L, Manetti M. Cardiac telocyte-derived exosomes and their possible implications in cardiovascular pathophysiology. Adv Exp Med Biol 2017; 998: 237-54.

[126] Cretoiu D, Radu BM, Banciu A, Banciu DD, Cretoiu SM. Telocytes heterogeneity: from cellular morphology to functional evidence. Semin Cell Dev Biol 2017; 64: 26-39.

[127] Yellon DM, Davidson SM. Exosomes: nanoparticles involved in cardioprotection? Circ Res 2014; 114(2): 325-32.

[128] Sahoo S, Klychko E, Thorne T, Misener S, Schultz KM, Millay M, et al. Exosomes from human CD34(+) stem cells mediate their proangiogenic paracrine activity. Circ Res 2011; 109(7): 724-8.

[129] Lai RC, Arslan F, Lee MM, Sze NS, Choo A, Chen TS, et al. Exosome secreted by MSC reduces myocardial ischemia/reperfusion injury. Stem Cell Res 2010; 4(3): 214-22.

[130] Arslan F, Lai RC, Smeets MB, Akeroyd L, Choo A, Aguor EN, et al. Mesenchymal stem cell-derived exosomes increase ATP levels, decrease oxidative stress and activate PI3K/Akt pathway to enhance myocardial viability and prevent adverse remodeling after myocardial ischemia/reperfusion injury. Stem Cell Res 2013; 10(3): 301-12.

[131] Bell R, Beeuwkes R, Botker HE, Davidson S, Downey J, Garcia-Dorado D, et al. Trials, tribulations and speculation! Report from the 7th biennial hatter cardiovascular institute workshop. Basic Res Cardiol 2012; 107(6): 300.

[132] Ibrahim AG, Cheng K, Marban E. Exosomes as critical agents of cardiac regeneration triggered by cell therapy. Stem Cell Rep 2014; 2(5): 606-19.

[133] Xiao J, Cretoiu D, Lei Z, Das S, Li X. Genetic and epigenetic regulation networks: governing from cardiovascular development to remodeling. Biomed Res Int 2017; 2017: 4135956.

[134] Yu X, Deng L, Wang D, Li N, Chen X, Cheng X, et al. Mechanism of TNF-alpha autocrine effects in hypoxic cardiomyocytes: initiated by hypoxia inducible factor 1alpha, presented by exosomes. J Mol Cell Cardiol 2012; 53(6): 848-57.

[135] Gupta S, Knowlton AA. HSP60 trafficking in adult cardiac myocytes: role of the exosomal pathway. Am J Physiol Heart Circ Physiol 2007; 292(6): H3052-6.

[136] Emanueli C, Shearn AI, Laftah A, Fiorentino F, Reeves BC, Beltrami C, et al. Coronary artery-bypass-graft surgery increases the plasma concentration of exosomes carrying a cargo of cardiac MicroRNAs: an example of exosome trafficking out of the human heart with potential for cardiac biomarker discovery. PLoS One 2016; 11(4): e0154274.

[137] Meder B, Keller A, Vogel B, Haas J, Sedaghat-Hamedani F, Kayvanpour E, et al. MicroRNA signatures in total peripheral blood as novel biomarkers for acute myocardial infarction. Basic Res Cardiol 2011; 106(1): 13-23.

[138] Jaguszewski M, Osipova J, Ghadri JR, Napp LC, Widera C, Franke J, et al. A signature of circulating microRNAs differentiates takotsubo cardiomyopathy from acute myocardial infarction. Eur Heart J 2014; 35(15): 999-1006.

[139] Care A, Catalucci D, Felicetti F, Bonci D, Addario A, Gallo P, et al. MicroRNA-133 controls cardiac hypertrophy. Nat Med 2007; 13(5): 613-8.

[140] Kuwabara Y, Ono K, Horie T, Nishi H, Nagao K, Kinoshita M, et al. Increased microRNA-1 and microRNA-133a levels in serum of patients with cardiovascular disease indicate myocardial damage. Circ Cardiovasc Genet 2011; 4(4): 446-54.

[141] Corsten MF, Dennert R, Jochems S, Kuznetsova T, Devaux Y, Hofstra L, et al. Circulating microRNA-208b and MicroRNA-499 reflect myocardial damage in cardiovascular disease. Circ Cardiovasc Genet 2010; 3(6): 499-506.

[142] Oliveira-Carvalho V, Carvalho VO, Bocchi EA. The emerging role of miR-208a in the heart. DNA Cell Biol 2013; 32(1): 8-12.

[143] Cheng C, Wang Q, You W, Chen M, Xia J. MiRNAs as biomarkers of myocardial infarction: a meta-analysis. PLoS One 2014; 9(2): e88566.

[144] Bei Y, Chen T, Banciu DD, Cretoiu D, Xiao J. Circulating exosomes in cardiovascular diseases. Adv Exp Med Biol 2017; 998: 255-69.

[145] Chen L, Wang Y, Pan Y, Zhang L, Shen C, Qin G, et al. Cardiac progenitor-derived exosomes protect ischemic myocardium from acute ischemia/reperfusion injury. Biochem Biophys Res Commun 2013; 431(3): 566-71.

[146] Xiao J, Pan Y, Li XH, Yang XY, Feng YL, Tan HH, et al. Cardiac progenitor cell-derived exosomes prevent cardiomyocytes apoptosis through exosomal miR-21 by targeting PDCD4. Cell Death Dis 2016; 7(6): e2277.

[147] Barile L, Lionetti V, Cervio E, Matteucci M, Gherghiceanu M, Popescu LM, et al. Extracellular vesicles from human cardiac progenitor cells inhibit cardiomyocyte apoptosis and improve cardiac function after myocardial infarction. Cardiovasc Res 2014; 103(4): 530-41.

[148] Chistiakov DA, Orekhov AN, Bobryshev YV. The role of cardiac fibroblasts in post-myocardial heart tissue repair. Exp Mol Pathol 2016; 101(2): 231-40.

[149] Meng XM, Nikolic-Paterson DJ, Lan HY. TGF-beta: the master regulator of fibrosis. Nat Rev Nephrol 2016; 12(6): 325-38.

[150] Booz GW, Baker KM. Molecular signalling mechanisms controlling growth and function of cardiac fibroblasts. Cardiovasc Res 1995; 30(4): 537-43.

[151] Dostal DE, Booz GW, Baker KM. Angiotensin II signalling pathways in cardiac fibroblasts: conventional versus novel mechanisms in mediating cardiac growth and function. Mol Cell Biochem 1996; 157(1-2): 15-21.

[152] Piacentini L, Gray M, Honbo NY, Chentoufi J, Bergman M, Karliner JS. Endothelin-1 stimulates cardiac fibroblast proliferation through activation of protein kinase C. J Mol Cell Cardiol 2000; 32(4): 565-76.

[153] Virag JI, Murry CE. Myofibroblast and endothelial cell proliferation during murine myocardial infarct repair. Am J Pathol 2003; 163(6): 2433-40.

[154] Virag JA, Rolle ML, Reece J, Hardouin S, Feigl EO, Murry CE. Fibroblast growth factor-2 regulates myocardial infarct repair: effects on cell proliferation, scar contraction, and ventricular function. Am J Pathol 2007; 171(5): 1431-40.

[155] Zymek P, Bujak M, Chatila K, Cieslak A, Thakker G, Entman ML, et al. The role of platelet-derived growth factor signaling in healing myocardial infarcts. J Am Coll Cardiol 2006; 48(11): 2315-23.

[156] Yuan MJ, Maghsoudi T, Wang T. Exosomes mediate the intercellular communication after myocardial infarction. Int J Med Sci 2016; 13(2): 113-6.

[157] Tian Y, Liu Y, Wang T, Zhou N, Kong J, Chen L, et al. A microRNA-Hippo pathway that promotes cardiomyocyte proliferation and cardiac regeneration in mice. Sci Transl Med 2015; 7(279): 279ra38.

[158] Wang J, Martin JF. Macro advances in microRNAs and myocardial regeneration. Curr Opin Cardiol 2014; 29(3): 207-13.

[159] Xiao J, Liu H, Cretoiu D, Toader DO, Suciu N, Shi J, et al. miR-31a-5p promotes postnatal cardiomyocyte proliferation by targeting RhoBTB1. Exp Mol Med 2017; 49(10): e386.

[160] Ontoria-Oviedo I, Dorronsoro A, Sanchez R, Ciria M, Gomez-Ferrer M, Buigues M, et al. Extracellular vesicles secreted by hypoxic AC10 cardiomyocytes modulate fibroblast cell motility. Front Cardiovas Med 2018; 5: 152.

[161] Liu L, Jin X, Hu CF, Li R, Zhou Z, Shen CX. Exosomes derived from mesenchymal stem cells rescue myocardial ischaemia/reperfusion injury by inducing cardiomyocyte autophagy via AMPK and Akt pathways. Cell Physiol Biochem 2017; 43(1): 52-68.

[162] Teng X, Chen L, Chen W, Yang J, Yang Z, Shen Z. Mesenchymal stem cell-derived exosomes improve the microenvironment of infarcted myocardium contributing to angiogenesis and anti-inflammation. Cell Physiol Biochem 2015; 37(6): 2415-24.

[163] Liu H, Gao W, Yuan J, Wu C, Yao K, Zhang L, et al. Exosomes derived from dendritic cells improve cardiac function via activation of CD4(+) T lymphocytes after myocardial infarction. J Mol Cell Cardiol 2016; 91: 123-33.

[164] Vandergriff A, Huang K, Shen D, Hu S, Hensley MT, Caranasos TG, et al. Targeting regenerative exosomes to myocardial infarction using cardiac homing peptide. Theranostics 2018; 8(7): 1869-78.

[165] Huang S, Ge X, Yu J, Han Z, Yin Z, Li Y, et al. Increased miR-124-3p in microglial exosomes following traumatic brain injury inhibits neuronal inflammation and contributes to neurite outgrowth via their transfer into neurons. FASEB J 2018; 32(1): 512-28.

[166] Gao L, Gregorich ZR, Zhu W, Mattapally S, Oduk Y, Lou X, et al. Large cardiac muscle patches engineered from human induced-pluripotent stem cell-derived cardiac cells improve recovery from myocardial infarction in swine. Circulation 2018; 137(16): 1712-30.

[167] Shen L, Wang H, Bei Y, Cretoiu D, Cretoiu SM, Xiao J. Formation of new cardiomyocytes in exercise. Adv Exp Med Biol 2017; 999: 91-102.

[168] Waldenström A, Ronquist G. Role of exosomes in myocardial remodeling. Circ Res 2014; 114(2): 315-24.

[169] Berezin AE, Kremzer AA, Samura TA, Martovitskaya YV, Malinovskiy YV, Oleshko SV, et al. Predictive value of apoptotic microparticles to mononuclear progenitor cells ratio in advanced chronic heart failure patients. J Cardiol 2015; 65(5): 403-11.

[170] Bang C, Batkai S, Dangwal S, Gupta SK, Foinquinos A, Holzmann A, et al. Cardiac fibroblast-derived microRNA passenger strand-enriched exosomes mediate cardiomyocyte hypertrophy. J Clin Invest 2014; 124(5): 2136-46.

[171] Raphael C, Briscoe C, Davies J, Ian Whinnett Z, Manisty C, Sutton R, et al. Limitations of the New York Heart Association functional classification system and self-reported walking distances in chronic heart failure. Heart 2007; 93(4): 476-82.

[172] Nozaki T, Sugiyama S, Sugamura K, Ohba K, Matsuzawa Y, Konishi M, et al. Prognostic value of endothelial microparticles in patients with heart failure. Eur J Heart Fail 2010; 12(11): 1223-8.

[173] Berezin AE, Kremzer AA, Martovitskaya YV, Samura TA, Berezina TA. The predictive role of circulating microparticles in patients with chronic heart failure. BBA Clin 2015; 3: 18-24.

[174] Dubin R, Li Y, Ix JH, Shlipak MG, Whooley M, Peralta C. Associations of pentraxin-3 with cardiovascular events, incident heart failure and mortality among persons with coronary heart disease: data from the heart and soul study. Am Heart J 2012; 163: 274-9.

[175] Schneider HG, Lam L, Lokuge A, Krum H, Naughton M, De Villiers SP, et al. B-Type natriuretic peptide testing, clinical outcomes, and health services use in emergency department patients with dyspnea a randomized trial. Ann Intern Med 2009; 150: 365-71.

[176] Salem ESB, Fan GC. Pathological effects of exosomes in mediating diabetic cardiomyopathy. Adv Exp Med Biol 2017; 998: 113-38.

[177] Khananshvili D. The SLC8 gene family of sodium-calcium exchangers (NCX) — structure, function, and regulation in health and disease. Mol Aspects Med 2013; 34: 220-35.

[178] Guescini M, Guidolin D, Luciana V, Casadei L, Gioacchini A, Tibollo P, et al. C2C12 myoblasts release micro-vesicles containing mtDNA and proteins involved in signal transduction. Exp Cell Res 2010; 316: 1977-84.

[179] Guescini M, Genedani S, Stocchi V, Agnati LF. Astrocytes and glioblastoma cells release exosomes carrying mtDNA. J Neural Transm 2010; 117(1): 1-4.

[180] Ye W, Tang X, Yang Z, Liu C, Zhang X, Jin J, et al. Plasma-derived exosomes contribute to inflammation via the TLR9-NF-kappaB pathway in chronic heart failure patients. Mol Immunol 2017; 87: 114-21.

[181] Halkein J, Tabruyn SP, Ricke-Hoch M, Haghikia A, Nguyen NQ, Scherr M, et al. MicroRNA-146a is a therapeutic target and biomarker for peripartum cardiomyopathy. J Clin Invest 2013; 123(5): 2143-54.

[182] Natarelli L, Schober A. MicroRNAs and the response to injury in atherosclerosis. Hamostaseologie 2015; 35(2): 142-50.

[183] Divakaran V, Mann DL. The emerging role of microRNAs in cardiac remodeling and heart failure. Circ Res 2008; 103(10): 1072-83.

[184] Matsumoto S, Sakata Y, Suna S, Nakatani D, Usami M, Hara M, et al. Circulating p53-responsive microRNAs are predictive indicators of heart failure after acute myocardial infarction. Circ Res 2013; 113(3): 322-6.

[185] Wu T, Chen Y, Du Y, Tao J, Zhou Z, Yang Z. Serum exosomal MiR-92b-5p as a potential biomarker for acute heart failure caused by dilated cardiomyopathy. Cell Physiol Biochem 2018; 46(5): 1939-50.

[186] Melman YF, Shah R, Das S. MicroRNAs in heart failure: is the picture becoming less miRky? Circ Heart Fail 2014; 7(1): 203-14.

[187] Matkovich SJ, Van Booven DJ, Youker KA, Torre-Amione G, Diwan A, Eschenbacher WH, et al. Reciprocal regulation of myocardial microRNAs and messenger RNA in human cardiomyopathy and reversal of the microRNA signature by biomechanical support. Circulation 2009; 119(9): 1263-71.

[188] Turchinovich A, Weiz L, Langheinz A, Burwinkel B. Characterization of extracellular circulating microRNA. Nucleic Acids Res 2011; 39(16): 7223-33.

[189] Valadi H, Ekstrom K, Bossios A, Sjostrand M, Lee JJ, Lotvall JO. Exosome-mediated transfer of mRNAs and microRNAs is a novel mechanism of genetic exchange between cells. Nat Cell Biol 2007; 9(6): 654-9.

[190] Tian C, Gao L, Zimmerman MC, Zucker IH. Myocardial infarction-induced microRNA-enriched exosomes contribute to cardiac Nrf2 dysregulation in chronic heart failure. Am J Physiol Heart Circ Physiol 2018; 314(5): H928-39.

[191] O'Neill S, Bohl M, Gregersen S, Hermansen K, O'Driscoll L. Blood-based biomarkers for metabolic syndrome. Trends Endocrinol Metab 2016; 27(6): 363-74.

[192] Evans S, Mann DL. Circulating p53-responsive microRNAs as predictive biomarkers in heart failure after acute myocardial infarction: the long and arduous road from scientific discovery to clinical utility. Circ Res 2013; 113(3): 242-4.

[193] Lindenfeld J, Albert NM, Boehmer JP, Collins SP, Ezekowitz JA, Givertz MM, et al. HFSA 2010 comprehensive heart failure practice guideline. J Card Fail 2010; 16(6): e1-194.

[194] Jansen F, Yang X, Proebsting S, Hoelscher M, Przybilla D, Baumann K, et al. MicroRNA expression in circulating microvesicles predicts cardiovascular events in patients with coronary artery disease. J Am Heart Assoc 2014; 3(6): e001249.

[195] Endo K, Naito Y, Ji X, Nakanishi M, Noguchi T, Goto Y, et al. MicroRNA 210 as a biomarker for congestive heart failure. Biol Pharm Bull 2013; 36(1): 48-54.

[196] Thum T, Galuppo P, Wolf C, Fiedler J, Kneitz S, van Laake LW, et al. MicroRNAs in the human heart: a clue to fetal gene reprogramming in heart failure. Circulation 2007; 116(3): 258-67.

[197] van Rooij E, Sutherland LB, Liu N, Williams AH, McAnally J, Gerard RD, et al. A signature pattern of stress-responsive microRNAs that can evoke cardiac hypertrophy and heart failure. Proc Natl Acad Sci U S A 2006; 103(48): 18255-60.

[198] van Rooij E, Sutherland LB, Thatcher JE, DiMaio JM, Naseem RH, Marshall WS, et al. Dysregulation of microRNAs after myocardial infarction reveals a role of miR-29 in cardiac fibrosis. Proc Natl Acad Sci U S A 2008; 105(35): 13027-32.

[199] Bostjancic E, Zidar N, Stajer D, Glavac D. MicroRNAs miR-1, miR-133a, miR-133b and miR-208 are dysregulated in

human myocardial infarction. Cardiology 2010; 115(3): 163-9.
[200] Satoh M, Minami Y, Takahashi Y, Tabuchi T, Nakamura M. Expression of microRNA-208 is associated with adverse clinical outcomes in human dilated cardiomyopathy. J Card Fail 2010; 16(5): 404-10.
[201] Ikeda S, Kong SW, Lu J, Bisping E, Zhang H, Allen PD, et al. Altered microRNA expression in human heart disease. Physiol Genomics 2007; 31(3): 367-73.
[202] Murach KA, McCarthy JJ. MicroRNAs, heart failure, and aging: potential interactions with skeletal muscle. Heart Fail Rev 2017; 22(2): 209-18.
[203] Goren Y, Kushnir M, Zafrir B, Tabak S, Lewis BS, Amir O. Serum levels of microRNAs in patients with heart failure. Eur J Heart Fail 2012; 14(2): 147-54.
[204] Sygitowicz G, Tomaniak M, Blaszczyk O, Koltowski L, Filipiak KJ, Sitkiewicz D. Circulating microribonucleic acids miR-1, miR-21 and miR-208a in patients with symptomatic heart failure: preliminary results. Arch Cardiovasc Dis 2015; 108(12): 634-42.
[205] van Rooij E, Liu N, Olson EN. MicroRNAs flex their muscles. Trends Genet 2008; 24(4): 159-66.
[206] Zile MR, Mehurg SM, Arroyo JE, Stroud RE, DeSantis SM, Spinale FG. Relationship between the temporal profile of plasma microRNA and left ventricular remodeling in patients after myocardial infarction. Circ Cardiovasc Genet 2011; 4: 614-9.
[207] Akat KM, Moore-McGriff D, Morozov P, Brown M, Gogakos T, Correa Da Rosa J, et al. Comparative RNA-sequencing analysis of myocardial and circulating small RNAs in human heart failure and their utility as biomarkers. Proc Natl Acad Sci U S A 2014; 111(30): 11151-6.
[208] McCarthy JJ, Esser KA. MicroRNA-1 and microRNA-133a expression are decreased during skeletal muscle hypertrophy. J Appl Physiol 2007; 102(1): 306-13.
[209] Elia L, Contu R, Quintavalle M, Varrone F, Chimenti C, Russo MA, et al. Reciprocal regulation of microRNA-1 and insulin-kike growth factor-1 signal transduction cascade in cardiac and skeletal muscle in physiological and pathological conditions. Circulation 2009; 120(23): 2377-85.
[210] Huang MB, Xu H, Xie SJ, Zhou H, Qu LH. Insulin-kike growth factor-1 receptor is regulated by microRNA-133 during skeletal myogenesis. PLoS One 2011; 6(12): e29173.
[211] Schipper ME, van Kuik J, de Jonge N, Dullens HF, de Weger RA. Changes in regulatory microRNA expression in myocardium of heart failure patients on left ventricular assist device support. J Heart Lung Transplant 2008; 27(12): 1282-5.
[212] Watson CJ, Gupta SK, O'Connell E, Thum S, Glezeva N, Fendrich J, et al. MicroRNA signatures differentiate preserved from reduced ejection fraction heart failure. Eur J Heart Fail 2015; 17(4): 405-15.
[213] Xu T, Zhou Q, Che L, Das S, Wang L, Jiang J, et al. Circulating miR-21, miR-378, and miR-940 increase in response to an acute exhaustive exercise in chronic heart failure patients. Oncotarget 2016; 7(11): 12414-25.
[214] Gupta MK, Halley C, Duan Z-H, Lappe J, Viterna J, Jana S, et al. miRNA-548c: a specific signature in circulating PBMCs from dilated cardiomyopathy patients. J Mol Cell Cardiol 2013; 62: 131-41.
[215] Kervadec A, Bellamy V, El Harane N, Arakelian L, Vanneaux V, Cacciapuoti I, et al. Cardiovascular progenitor-derived extracellular vesicles recapitulate the beneficial effects of their parent cells in the treatment of chronic heart failure. J Heart Lung Transplant 2016; 35(6): 795-807.
[216] Chen Y, Wakili R, Xiao J, Wu CT, Luo X, Clauss S, et al. Detailed characterization of microRNA changes in a canine heart failure model: relationship to arrhythmogenic structural remodeling. J Mol Cell Cardiol 2014; 77: 113-24.
[217] Yang VK, Loughran KA, Meola DM, Juhr CM, Thane KE, Davis AM, et al. Circulating exosome microRNA associated with heart failure secondary to myxomatous mitral valve disease in a naturally occurring canine model. J Extracell vesicles 2017; 6(1): 1350088.
[218] Shotan A, Widerhorn J, Hurst A, Elkayam U. Risks of angiotensin-converting enzyme inhibition during pregnancy: experimental and clinical evidence, potential mechanisms, and recommendations for use. Am J Med 1994; 96(5): 451-6.
[219] Modi KA, Illum S, Jariatul K, Caldito G, Reddy PC. Poor outcome of indigent patients with peripartum cardiomyopathy in the United States. Am J Obstet Gynecol 2009; 201(2): 171.e1-5.
[220] Jiang X, Sucharov J, Stauffer BL, Miyamoto SD, Sucharov CC. Exosomes from pediatric dilated cardiomyopathy patients modulate a pathological response in cardiomyocytes. Am J Physiol Heart Circ Physiol 2017; 312(4): H818-26.
[221] Stauffer BL, Russell G, Nunley K, Miyamoto SD, Sucharov CC. miRNA expression in pediatric failing human heart. J Mol Cell Cardiol 2013; 57: 43-6.
[222] Zheng D, Ma J, Yu Y, Li M, Ni R, Wang G, et al. Silencing of miR-195 reduces diabetic cardiomyopathy in C57BL/6 mice. Diabetologia 2015; 58(8): 1949-58.
[223] Hunt SA, Abraham WT, Chin MH, Feldman AM, Francis GS, Ganiats TG, et al. ACC/AHA 2005 guideline update for the diagnosis and management of chronic heart failure in the adult: a report of the American College of Cardiology/American Heart Association task force on practice guidelines (writing committee to update the 2001 guidelines for the evaluation and management of heart failure): developed in collaboration with the American College of Chest Physicians and the international society for heart and lung transplantation: endorsed by the Heart Rhythm Society. Circulation 2005; 112(12): e154-235.
[224] McMurray JJ, Adamopoulos S, Anker SD, Auricchio A, Bohm M, Dickstein K, et al. ESC Guidelines for the diagnosis and treatment of acute and chronic heart failure 2012: the task force for the diagnosis and treatment of acute and chronic heart failure 2012 of the European Society of Cardiology. Developed in collaboration with the Heart Failure Association (HFA) of the ESC. Eur Heart J 2012; 33(14): 1787-847.
[225] Maulik SK, Kumar S. Oxidative stress and cardiac hypertrophy: a review. Toxicol Mech Methods 2012; 22(5): 359-66.

[226] Hausse AO, Aggoun Y, Bonnet D, Sidi D, Munnich A, Rötig A, et al. Idebenone and reduced cardiac hypertrophy in Friedreich's ataxia. Heart 2002; 87(4): 346-9.
[227] Balta N, Dumitru IF, Stoian G, Petec G, Dinischiotu A. Influence of isoproterenol-induced cardiac hypertrophy on oxydative myocardial stress. Rom J Physiol 1995; 32(1-4): 149-54.
[228] Lee A, Jeong D, Mitsuyama S, Oh JG, Liang L, Ikeda Y, et al. The role of SUMO-1 in cardiac oxidative stress and hypertrophy. Antioxid Redox Signal 2014; 21(14): 1986-2001.
[229] Datta R, Bansal T, Rana S, Datta K, Datta Chaudhuri R, Chawla-Sarkar M, et al. Myocytederived Hsp90 modulates collagen upregulation via biphasic activation of STAT-3 in fibroblasts during cardiac hypertrophy. J Mol Cell Biol 2017; 37(6). pii: e00611-16.
[230] Lyu L, Wang H, Li B, Qin Q, Qi L, Nagarkatti M, et al. A critical role of cardiac fibroblastderived exosomes in activating renin angiotensin system in cardiomyocytes. J Mol Cell Cardiol 2015; 89(Pt B): 268-79.
[231] Fang X, Stroud MJ, Ouyang K, Fang L, Zhang J, Dalton ND, et al. Adipocyte-specific loss of PPARgamma attenuates cardiac hypertrophy. JCI insight 2016; 1(16): e89908.
[232] Wang X, Gu H, Huang W, Peng J, Li Y, Yang L, et al. Hsp20-Mediated activation of exosome biogenesis in cardiomyocytes improves cardiac function and angiogenesis in diabetic mice. Diabetes 2016; 65(10): 3111-28.
[233] Belevych AE, Sansom SE, Terentyeva R, Ho H-T, Nishijima Y, Martin MM, et al. MicroRNA-1 and -133 Increase arrhythmogenesis in heart failure by dissociating phosphatase activity from RyR2 complex. PLoS One 2011; 6(12): e28324.
[234] Lu Y, Zhang Y, Wang N, Pan Z, Gao X, Zhang F, et al. MicroRNA-328 contributes to adverse electrical remodeling in atrial fibrillation. Circulation 2010; 122(23): 2378-87.
[235] Neppl RL, Wang D-Z. The myriad essential roles of microRNAs in cardiovascular homeostasis and disease. Genes & diseases 2014; 1(1): 18-39.
[236] Lai LP, Su MJ, Lin JL, Lin FY, Tsai CH, Chen YS, et al. Down-regulation of L-type calcium channel and sarcoplasmic reticular Ca(2+)-ATPase mRNA in human atrial fibrillation without significant change in the mRNA of ryanodine receptor, calsequestrin and phospholamban: an insight into the mechanism of atrial electrical remodeling. J Am Coll Cardiol 1999; 33(5): 1231-7.
[237] Schotten U, Ausma J, Stellbrink C, Sabatschus I, Vogel M, Frechen D, et al. Cellular mechanisms of depressed atrial contractility in patients with chronic atrial fibrillation. Circulation 2001; 103(5): 691-8.
[238] Mancarella S, Yue Y, Karnabi E, Qu Y, El-Sherif N, Boutjdir M. Impaired Ca2+ homeostasis is associated with atrial fibrillation in the alpha1D L-type Ca2+ channel KO mouse. Am J Physiol Heart Circ Physiol 2008; 295(5): H2017-24.
[239] Plotnikov AN, Shlapakova I, Szabolcs MJ, Danilo Jr. P, Lorell BH, Potapova IA, et al. Xenografted adult human mesenchymal stem cells provide a platform for sustained biological pacemaker function in canine heart. Circulation 2007; 116(7): 706-13.
[240] Askar SF, Ramkisoensing AA, Atsma DE, Schalij MJ, de Vries AA, Pijnappels DA. Engraftment patterns of human adult mesenchymal stem cells expose electrotonic and paracrine proarrhythmic mechanisms in myocardial cell cultures. Circ Arrhythm Electrophysiol 2013; 6(2): 380-91.
[241] Mayourian J, Cashman TJ, Ceholski DK, Johnson BV, Sachs D, Kaji DA, et al. Experimental and computational insight into human mesenchymal stem cell paracrine signaling and heterocellular coupling effects on cardiac contractility and arrhythmogenicity. Circ Res 2017; 121(4): 411-23.
[242] Ji Q, Ji Y, Peng J, Zhou X, Chen X, Zhao H, et al. Increased brain-specific MiR-9 and MiR-124 in the serum exosomes of acute ischemic stroke patients. PLoS One 2016; 11(9): e0163645.
[243] Goetzl L, Merabova N, Darbinian N, Martirosyan D, Poletto E, Fugarolas K, et al. Diagnostic potential of neural exosome cargo as biomarkers for acute brain injury. Ann Clin Transl Neurol 2017; 5(1): 4-10.
[244] Kucharzewska P, Christianson HC, Welch JE, Svensson KJ, Fredlund E, Ringner M, et al. Exosomes reflect the hypoxic status of glioma cells and mediate hypoxia-dependent activation of vascular cells during tumor development. Proc Natl Acad Sci U S A 2013; 110(18): 7312-7.
[245] Matsumoto J, Stewart T, Sheng L, Li N, Bullock K, Song N, et al. Transmission of alphasynuclein-containing erythrocyte-derived extracellular vesicles across the blood-brain barrier via adsorptive mediated transcytosis: another mechanism for initiation and progression of Parkinson's disease? Acta Neuropathol Commun 2017; 5(1): 71.
[246] Harrison EB, Hochfelder CG, Lamberty BG, Meays BM, Morsey BM, Kelso ML, et al. Traumatic brain injury increases levels of miR-21 in extracellular vesicles: implications for neuroinflammation. FEBS Open Bio 2016; 6(8): 835-46.
[247] de Rivero Vaccari JP, Brand 3rd F, Adamczak S, Lee SW, Perez-Barcena J, Wang MY, et al. Exosome-mediated inflammasome signaling after central nervous system injury. J Neurochem 2016; 136(Suppl 1): 39-48.
[248] Manek R, Moghieb A, Yang Z, Kumar D, Kobessiy F, Sarkis GA, et al. Protein biomarkers and neuroproteomics characterization of microvesicles/exosomes from human cerebrospinal fluid following traumatic brain injury. Mol Neurobiol 2018; 55(7): 6112-28.
[249] Belting M, Christianson HC. Role of exosomes and microvesicles in hypoxia-associated tumour development and cardiovascular disease. J Intern Med 2015; 278(3): 251-63.
[250] Chen W, Guo Y, Yang W, Chen L, Ren D, Wu C, et al. Phosphorylation of connexin 43 induced by traumatic brain injury promotes exosome release. J Neurophysiol 2018; 119(1): 305-11.
[251] Zhuang X, Xiang X, Grizzle W, Sun D, Zhang S, Axtell RC, et al. Treatment of brain inflammatory diseases by delivering exosome encapsulated anti-inflammatory drugs from the nasal region to the brain. Mol ther 2011; 19(10): 1769-79.
[252] Otero-Ortega L, Laso-Garcia F, Gomez-de Frutos M, Fuentes B, Diekhorst L, Diez-Tejedor E, et al. Role of exosomes as a treatment and potential biomarker for stroke. Transl Stroke Res 2019; 10: 241-49.

[253] Chen CC, Liu L, Ma F, Wong CW, Guo XE, Chacko JV, et al. Elucidation of exosome migration across the blood-brain barrier model in vitro. Cell Mol Bioeng 2016; 9(4): 509-29.

[254] Xu B, Zhang Y, Du XF, Li J, Zi HX, Bu JW, et al. Neurons secrete miR-132-containing exosomes to regulate brain vascular integrity. Cell Res 2017; 27(7): 882-97.

[255] Zhang Y, Chopp M, Liu XS, Katakowski M, Wang X, Tian X, et al. Exosomes derived from mesenchymal stromal cells promote axonal growth of cortical neurons. Mol Neurobiol 2017; 54(4): 2659-73.

[256] Xin H, Li Y, Cui Y, Yang JJ, Zhang ZG, Chopp M. Systemic administration of exosomes released from mesenchymal stromal cells promote functional recovery and neurovascular plasticity after stroke in rats. J Cereb Blood Flow Metab 2013; 33(11): 1711-5.

[257] Zhang Y, Chopp M, Meng Y, Katakowski M, Xin H, Mahmood A, et al. Effect of exosomes derived from multipluripotent mesenchymal stromal cells on functional recovery and neurovascular plasticity in rats after traumatic brain injury. J Neurosurg 2015; 122(4): 856-67.

[258] Li Y, Yang YY, Ren JL, Xu F, Chen FM, Li A. Exosomes secreted by stem cells from human exfoliated deciduous teeth contribute to functional recovery after traumatic brain injury by shifting microglia M1/M2 polarization in rats. Stem Cell Res Ther 2017; 8(1): 198.

[259] Dinkins MB, Dasgupta S, Wang G, Zhu G, Bieberich E. Exosome reduction in vivo is associated with lower amyloid plaque load in the 5XFAD mouse model of Alzheimer's disease. Neurobiol Aging 2014; 35(8): 1792-800.

[260] Jarmalaviciute A, Tunaitis V, Pivoraite U, Venalis A, Pivoriunas A. Exosomes from dental pulp stem cells rescue human dopaminergic neurons from 6-hydroxy-dopamine-induced apoptosis. Cytotherapy 2015; 17(7): 932-9.

[261] Haney MJ, Klyachko NL, Zhao Y, Gupta R, Plotnikova EG, He Z, et al. Exosomes as drug delivery vehicles for Parkinson's disease therapy. J Control Release 2015; 207: 18-30.

第 10 章

皮肤生物学和皮肤病中的外泌体
Exosomes in cutaneous biology and dermatologic disease

Jeffrey D. McBride, Divya Aickara, Evangelos Badiavas

Department of Dermatology and Cutaneous Surgery, University of Miami, Miami, FL, United States

一、角质形成细胞是上层皮肤的主要细胞，分泌外泌体调节黑素细胞产生的色素

外泌体在基础皮肤生物学最基本的方面之一——皮肤色素沉着中发挥着作用。皮肤色素沉着依靠角质形成细胞和黑素细胞间的通信形成。皮肤色素沉着是保护皮肤细胞及其DNA免受紫外线伤害的主要方式。在皮肤的最外层，紫外线辐射激活角质形成细胞与黑素细胞形成的表皮-黑素单元[1]。这种辐射部分以UVA和UVB形式，激活诱导生长因子和细胞外蛋白质分泌的信号传导途径，导致了黑色素这一皮肤中主要色素的产生。细胞分泌的EV（外泌体和微囊泡）可以转运蛋白质、脂质和RNA来调节受体细胞的功能[1]。角质形成细胞分泌的外泌体可通过增加黑素体蛋白的表达和活性来增强黑色素的合成[1]。这些外泌体的功能取决于皮肤光型（皮肤的明暗程度和皮肤通常在日光下晒伤的难易程度），并且受到紫外线B的调节[1]。携带选定miRNA的外泌体针对黑素细胞，并通过改变黑素细胞的基因和蛋白质表达调节皮肤色素沉着（图10-1）[1]。当角质形成细胞和黑素细胞共培养时，MVB（封闭的$CD63^+$-腔内囊泡一定会被挤压成$CD63^+$-外泌体）被重新分配到角质形成细胞与黑素细胞接触的区域[1]。在分泌入细胞外环境后不久，黑素细胞就会吸收角质形成细胞的外泌体[1]。来自光型Ⅴ型皮肤（较深色素的个体）的角质形成细胞中的外泌体显著增加了来自Ⅰ～Ⅱ型/光复杂型或白种人黑素细胞中的黑色素含量[1]。因此，高光型来源的角质形成细胞分泌的外泌体可能具有内在特性和刺激黑色素生成的物质[1]。当使用白种人角质形成细胞的外泌体刺激来自同一供体的黑素细胞时，酪氨酸酶（黑色素产生途径中主要的酶）没有增加。但是，当使用UVB刺激过的角质形成细胞中的外泌体刺激来自同一供体的黑素细胞时，酪氨酸酶和小眼转录因子（黑色素生成的主要调节剂）的表达显著增加，这提示了UVB刺激过的角质形成细胞中的外泌体是白种人产生色素沉着的重要诱因[1]。当UVB诱导的角质形成细胞外泌体应用于体外的人造表皮时也能见到相同的效应[1]。外泌体携带调节色素沉着的miRNA，在暴露于UVB后miRNA的含量会发生改变，特别是miR-3196[1]。此外，发现miR-203这一通过上调TYR蛋白调节黑色素瘤细胞中黑色素生成的关键调节剂在深色皮肤个体的外泌体中高表达[1]。miRNA可能依赖于背景分子，如蛋白质或脂质补充或调节差异表达的角质形成细胞的整体作用[1]。角质形成细胞外泌体的miRNA可能通过miR-3196和MITF依赖性及miR-203和MITF独立性的信号通路对

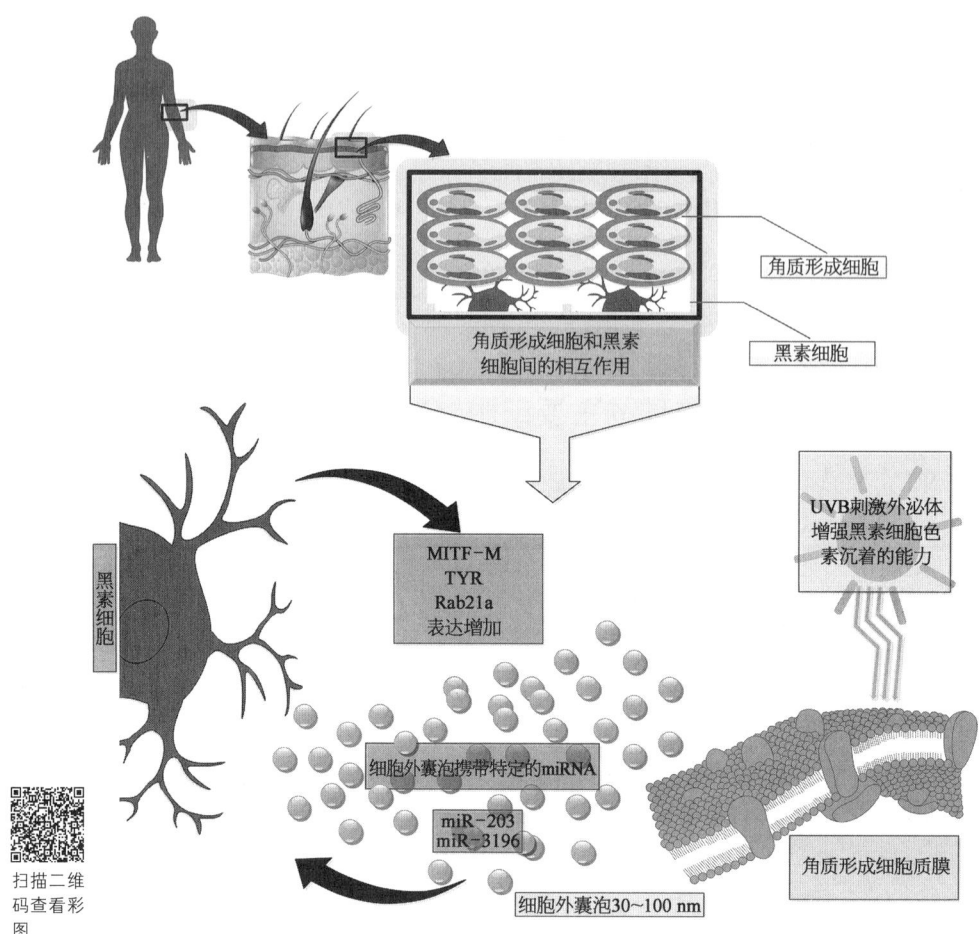

图 10-1 紫外线 B 刺激角质形成细胞分泌外泌体从而刺激黑素细胞产生黑色素。UVB 刺激角质形成细胞产生 miRNA miR-203 和 miR-3196,最终通过上调的 MITF、TRY 和 Rab21a 刺激黑色素生成

黑素细胞的色素沉着进行微调。因此,皮肤色素沉着依靠角质形成细胞间外泌体的传递,环境和遗传因素可能也在外泌体中起作用,最终影响皮肤色素沉着。

紫外线照射通过黑色素从黑素细胞到角质形成细胞的细胞间转移在皮肤中引起色素沉着[2]。Wäster 等显示了用 UVA 照射后的新型细胞反应,导致来源于溶酶体的 EV 从黑素细胞转移到角质形成细胞中[2]。UVA 可能引起细胞质膜损伤,诱导黑素细胞质膜上的 EV 立即发生脱落[2]。这些囊泡中许多都是 CD63 和其他典型的外泌体标志物呈阳性[2]。这些 EV 优先被角质形成细胞内吞[2]。IVA 和 UVB 同样会刺激黑素小体从黑素细胞转移到角质形成细胞,并且依赖功能性的细胞骨架[2]。UVA 引起的黑素细胞质膜损伤可通过钙依赖性溶酶体胞吐作用快速修复[2]。此外,黑素细胞来源的外泌体增强了角质形成细胞的增殖[2]。

一组研究人员发现含有纤维连接蛋白的 EV 能够保护黑素细胞免受紫外线辐射引起的毒性[3]。紫外线照射可激活皮肤黑素细胞分泌黑素小体,防止紫外线引起的损伤[3]。

这表明黑素细胞可以利用自身的 EV 和细胞外基质成分保护彼此免受紫外线的辐射[3]。使用蛋白质组学分析鉴定纤维连接蛋白[3]。有趣的是,黄褐斑患者的皮肤与正常皮肤相比,黑素细胞周围的细胞外空间含有更多的纤维连接蛋白,这与细胞外纤维连接蛋白参与促进黑素细胞甚至病理性存活的模型有关[3]。由于黑素细胞的细胞周期更慢,表达的抗凋亡 Bcl-2 水平更高,非常需要保护其基因组的稳定性,因此迫切需要一种保护黑素细胞免受紫外线引起的基因组损伤的生物学机制[3]。在这项研究中,对 EV 相关蛋白的分析表明,基于膜蛋白间的程度、中间状态、紧密性和径向性,纤维连接蛋白是具有最高集中度的主要组成成分[3]。共焦显微术分析表明 CD81(外泌体标志物)与纤维连接蛋白共定位[3]。

二、角质形成细胞和免疫系统外泌体调节修饰细胞外基质蛋白质的成纤维细胞表达

角质形成细胞分泌与外泌体相关的蛋白质,最终调节蛋白质的表达,如修饰细胞外基质的基质金属蛋白酶。分层蛋白(也称为 14-3-3σ)是一种已知被角质形成细胞"外部化"并刺激成纤维细胞中基质金属蛋白-1 的蛋白质,但是"外部化"的机制在发现其与外泌体相关前是不清楚的[4]。研究发现,分层蛋白(14-3-3σ)从角质形成细胞的纯化外泌体中排出,这些含有分层蛋白的外泌体能够刺激成纤维细胞表达 MMP-1,与 p38/MAPK 途径的激活有关(图 10-2)[4]。这一概念为角质形成细胞利用其外泌体诱导成纤维细胞重塑细胞外基质提供了可能性,这对皮肤稳态很重要,也将可能对理解皮肤病学中纤维化疾病的发病机制很重要。例如,尚不清楚缺少向成纤维细胞转移的角质形成细胞外泌体是否会导致 MMP 产生减少,从而导致体内平衡偏向纤维化。通常在各种器官中,上皮层可能通过这些机制调节下方的结缔组织。此外,免疫系统还会分泌含有 14-3-3 蛋白质的外泌体,调节 MMP-1 的表达(图 10-3)[5]。因此,上皮和免疫系统都能影响主要的真皮细胞和成纤维细胞,以调节 MMP 的表达,从而重塑周围的胶原蛋白。这些概念证明了影响细胞外基质重塑蛋白表达的多细胞间通信途径的复杂性。这些概念还表明上皮或免疫系统的缺陷可能会影响成纤维细胞的状态和真皮中的纤维化。

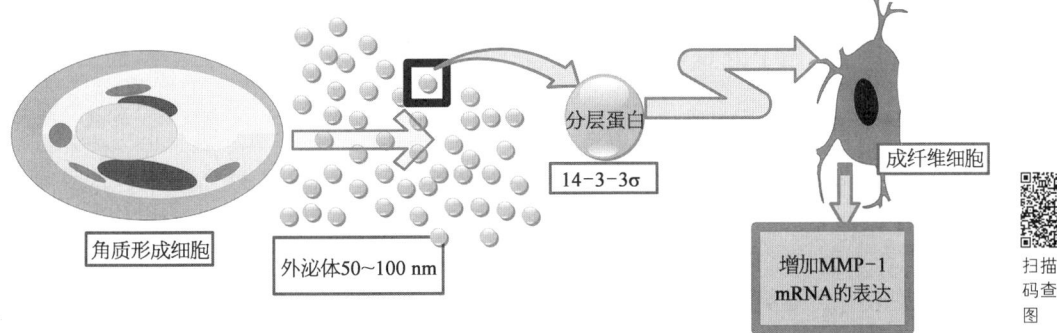

图 10-2 角质形成细胞分泌外泌体相关的分层蛋白增加基质金属蛋白酶的表达。P38/MAPK 途径的激活导致成纤维细胞分泌 MMP-1

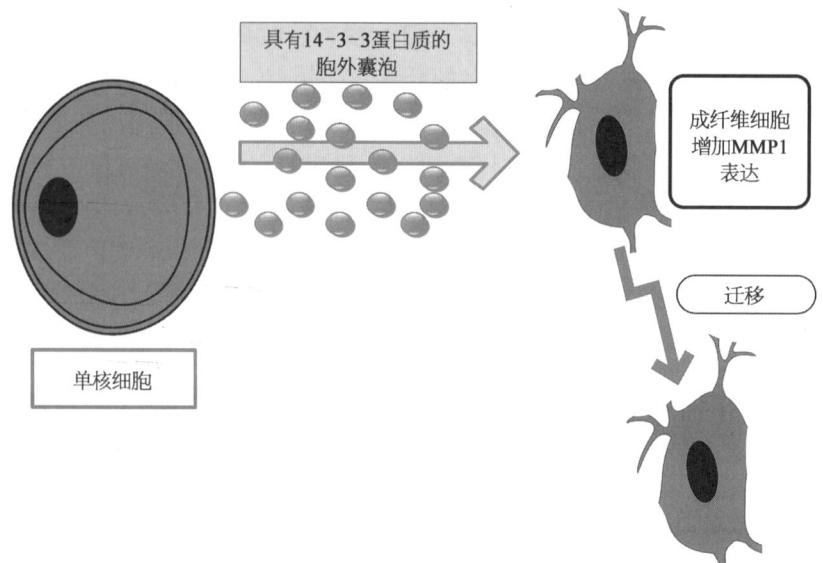

图 10-3 单核细胞分泌具有 14-3-3 蛋白质的外泌体,引起基质金属蛋白酶的表达。成纤维细胞 MMP-1 表达增加促进细胞外基质重塑和成纤维细胞迁移

三、角质形成细胞外泌体可调控免疫系统

上皮与微生物群的相互作用利用外泌体向免疫系统传递信息。皮肤是免疫系统的重要器官,每个细胞具有不同的功能有助于在整体上获得最佳的免疫系统功能。金黄色葡萄球菌是存在于健康皮肤上的常见细菌。在特应性皮炎(湿疹)患者中,金黄色葡萄球菌感染也很常见,这是由于患者的皮肤屏障受损、炎症增加和皮肤水分不足使皮肤更容易感染。皮肤中的外泌体在免疫系统的功能和对感染的反应中起着非常重要的作用。例如,在特应性皮炎和银屑病中,金黄色葡萄球菌的感染和定植会引发炎症,这部分是通过分泌肠毒素 B 引起的。角质形成细胞是表皮的主要细胞类型,约占表皮的 90%。角质形成细胞作为非专业的 APC 促进超抗原诱导的 T 细胞增殖[6]。先前的研究表明,角质形成细胞在与抗原相互作用后有助于 T 细胞增殖[7]。在一个涉及跨孔共培养系统的实验中,人角质形成细胞可以通过外泌体的间接接触诱导 T 细胞增殖[6]。外泌体可以将抗原转移到受体 T 细胞,角质形成细胞外泌体含有 MHC Ⅰ 和 MHC Ⅱ 分子并与 T 细胞相互作用成为抗原提呈的一部分[6]。在干扰素 γ 刺激后,角质形成细胞(先前载有金黄色葡萄球菌肠毒素 B)分泌外泌体诱导 CD4 和 CD8 T 细胞增殖[6]。因此,角质形成细胞利用外泌体使 T 细胞对金黄色葡萄球菌的感染做出反应。外泌体是外部环境与免疫系统反应之间交流系统的重要组成部分。在另一项研究中,鼠角质形成细胞系(MPEK 细胞)在炎性和非炎性条件下都能产生外泌体,并且骨髓 DC 吸收这些外泌体(可能通过直接融合或其他机制进行,有关这些吸收机制的讨论参见本书前面的章节),通过增加 CD40 的表达和细胞因子包括 IL-6、IL-10、IL-12 的产生诱导

成熟表型(图 10-4)[8]。当角质形成细胞暴露于卵清蛋白抗原时,它们将其转移到它们的外泌体中。但有趣的是,这些外泌体不会通过骨髓 DC 引起对 T 细胞的特异性免疫反应[8]。因此,该报道认为角质形成细胞可通过外泌体激活 T 细胞的广泛应答,而与刺激性抗原无关。角质形成细胞来源的外泌体能够影响骨髓 DC 表型和白介素产生,这表明利用外泌体的角质形成细胞和 DC 间的交互作用激活免疫系统很重要[8]。

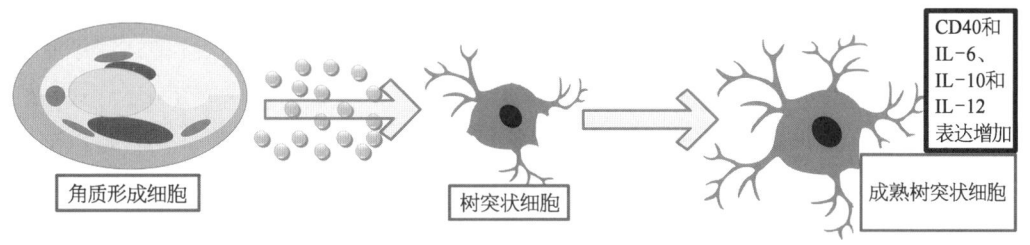

图 10-4　角质形成细胞分泌能刺激成熟 DC 发育的外泌体。角质形成细胞外泌体通过成熟 DC 诱导 CD40 和 IL-6、IL-10 和 IL-12 表达增加

四、真皮成纤维细胞,特别是真皮乳头细胞,分泌外泌体刺激毛囊生长的阶段称为生长期

毛囊密度对于皮肤细菌的稳态、温度调节、性信号甚至人的修饰和自尊非常重要。研究发现,由真皮乳头细胞分泌的外泌体在毛囊发育中也很重要。真皮乳头细胞在调节毛囊的生长、形成和循环周期中起着关键作用[9]。假设真皮乳头通过旁分泌机制,部分通过外泌体调节毛囊生长[9]。在这项研究中,毛囊在生长周期的不同阶段被注射了来自真皮乳头细胞的外泌体,这些外泌体表达 CD9、CD63 和 TSG101[9]。然后评估外泌体对外根鞘细胞增殖、迁移和细胞周期状态的影响[9]。真皮乳头细胞来源的外泌体加速了小鼠毛囊从静止期(休止阶段)到生长期(卵泡生长阶段)和退行期(卵泡破裂阶段)[9]。外泌体上调毛囊中的 β-联蛋白和 Shh 水平并增加外根鞘的增殖和迁移[9]。因此,很可能是真皮乳头中的外泌体激活 Wnt/β-联蛋白信号通路和 sonic hedgehog 途径来刺激发育中的毛囊[9]。因此,来自成纤维细胞的外泌体刺激毛囊生长对皮肤稳态至关重要。

五、纤维化疾病使成纤维细胞外泌体表达失调

系统性硬化是一种慢性、自身免疫性疾病,以皮肤和内脏器官组织纤维化为特征。一项研究尝试确定外泌体在系统性硬化中可能的作用并阐明外泌体对伤口愈合的影响[10]。与正常受试者的成纤维细胞相比,系统性硬化患者的真皮成纤维细胞中外泌体的常见标志物(CD9、CD63 和 CD81)增加[10]。系统性硬化患者成纤维细胞中的外泌体刺激正常成纤维细胞中Ⅰ型胶原的产生[10]。这表明系统性硬化患者的外泌体含量(特别是 mRNA)发生了改变[10]。有趣的是,系统性硬化患者血清中的外泌体水平显著下降[10]。作者假设系统性硬化的血管异常可能导致外泌体下降[10]。系统性硬化患者血清中外泌体的减少可能使胶原蛋白下调、溃疡和凹陷性瘢痕可能性升高,从而导致伤口愈合延迟[10]。关于外泌体在如系统

性硬化等纤维化疾病中的调节作用仍知之甚少。然而,成纤维细胞外泌体的释放对如系统性硬化等结缔组织疾病的状态可能至关重要。

六、含有磷脂酶活性的肥大细胞刺激朗格汉斯细胞将脂质抗原提呈给T细胞

银屑病被认为是一种慢性炎症性皮肤疾病,但也可能累及其他器官,并与辅助性T细胞17反应有关[11]。它与多种细胞的浸润有关,包括$CD4^+$和CD^+ T细胞、嗜中性粒细胞、NK细胞、肥大细胞、先天淋巴细胞和单核细胞/巨噬细胞[11]。肽链型抗原的作用尚不明确,有研究者假设非肽链型抗原如脂质可能在银屑病的发病机制中发挥作用。此外,肥大细胞及其促炎细胞因子的活化和脱颗粒可能促进皮肤银屑病的病理[11]。朗格汉斯细胞是皮肤中的APC,并在银屑病的皮损中高表达CD1a,CD1a可向T细胞提呈脂质抗原(如脂肪酸、蜡酯和鲨烯)[11]。在银屑病中,干扰素-α诱导肥大细胞释放外泌体将磷脂酶A2(一种产生脂质抗原并与脂质特异性T细胞炎性皮肤反应有关的酶)转移到表达CD1a的细胞中(图10-5)[11]。银屑病患者皮肤皮损部位外泌体反应的CD1a反应性T细胞比外周血和非皮损部位的比例更高[11]。这些外泌体导致脂质抗原向T细胞提呈增加,诱导IL-17a和IL-22产生[11]。在外泌体中发现磷脂酶A2的活性解释了肥大细胞如何促进脂质抗原的生成,将其最终由朗格汉斯细胞提呈给T细胞,在此之前,这一点一直无法解释[11]。因此,该模型表明肥大细胞外泌体在银屑病的发病机制中处于上游[11]。

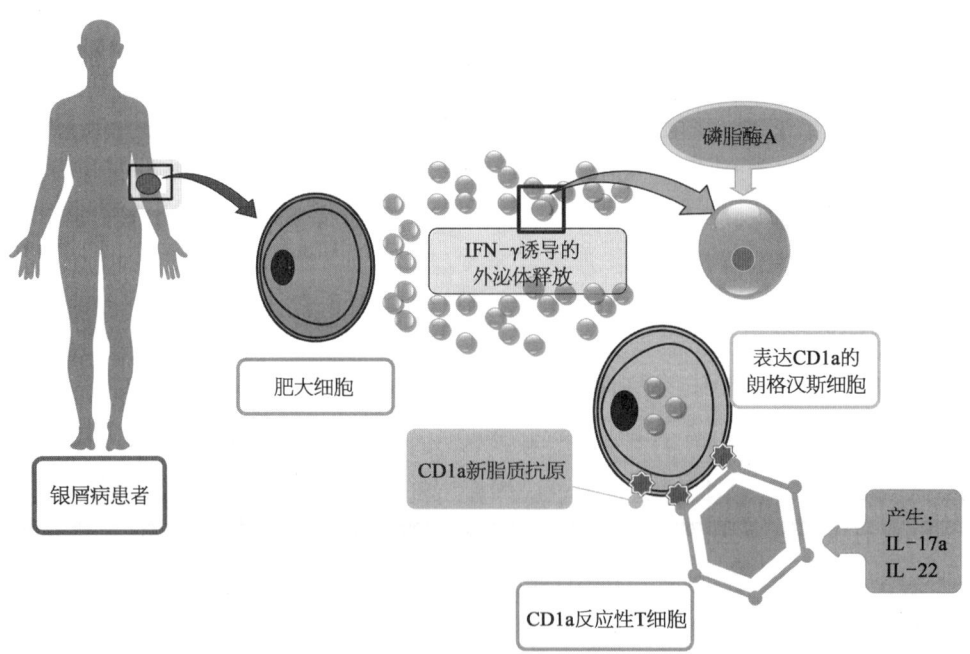

图10-5 银屑病中携带磷脂酶A活性外泌体的表达促进脂质抗原表达至T细胞。通过肥大细胞释放IFN-γ诱导的携带磷脂酶的外泌体刺激CD1a-朗格汉斯细胞向T细胞提呈新脂质抗原,T细胞表达IL-17和IL-22促进银屑病的发病机制

七、大疱性类天疱疮患者体液中的外泌体增强病原性炎症

大疱性类天疱疮是一种自身免疫性水疱病,其 B 细胞产生的抗体针对基底膜半桥粒抗原 BP180 和 BP230,从而导致表皮下水疱的形成。水疱内的液体含有大量的炎症细胞,包括嗜酸性粒细胞、嗜中性粒细胞及 $CD9^+$、$CD63^+$ 和 $CD81^+$ 外泌体[12]。这些水疱液体中的外泌体最可能来自浸润的粒细胞。外泌体被原代角质形成细胞内化,诱导促炎细胞因子和趋化因子的表达并激活 ERK1/2 和 STAT3 信号通路,形成一个促炎放大环(图 10-6)[12]。在水疱液体外泌体的质谱分析中,与对照外泌体相比,免疫和炎性分子如 s100-A8、基质金属蛋白酶 1、HSP 和 HLA Ⅱ类组织相容性抗原发生富集[12]。中性粒细胞标志物如 MPO 和嗜酸性粒细胞生物标志物如嗜酸性粒细胞过氧化物酶和嗜酸性粒细胞阳离子蛋白存在于水疱液体外泌体中,而在对照外泌体中不存在[12]。总体而言,大疱性类天疱疮水疱液体中外泌体的蛋白质组学特征表明它们可能促进或至少反映了大疱性类天疱疮的炎症机制[12]。总之,水疱性疾病中的外泌体有助于病原性炎症的持续。

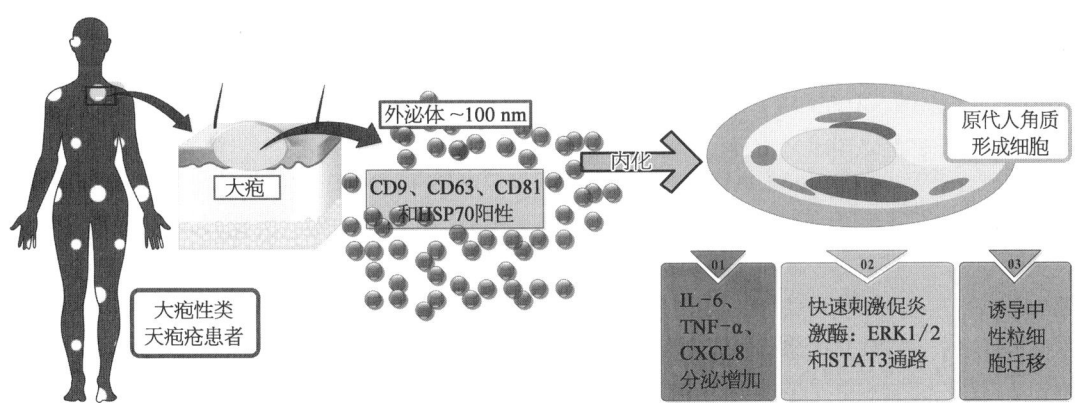

图 10-6 大疱性类天疱疮中角质形成细胞吸收水疱液体外泌体,进一步促进促炎活性。CD9、CD63、CD81 和 HSP70+外泌体被角质形成细胞内化并导致 IL-6,TNF-α 和 CXCL8 分泌增加,刺激促炎激酶、ERK1/2 和 STAT3 通路,诱导中性粒细胞迁移

八、皮肤修复

干细胞外泌体刺激皮肤修复

尽管皮肤外伤和破裂很常见,但是许多皮肤伤口难以愈合。当它们愈合时,会留下瘢痕损害皮肤外观或功能。加速愈合的常规方法包括皮肤移植、应用特殊的生物材料或敷料、应用生长因子、基因疗法甚至是激光治疗。单独注射生长因子可能导致细胞外液中的蛋白酶降解。皮肤修复的目标包括缩短愈合时间和减少瘢痕。人们一直关注外泌体作为再生工具,因为它们可以保护生长因子免于降解,并帮助将蛋白质从一个细胞转运到另一个细胞。外泌体在皮肤伤口愈合中的作用一直是积极探索的领域,因为它们被认为具有高度稳定性和低免疫原性。此外,外泌体回到组织损伤部位的能力对皮肤潜在的修复至关重要。就制药潜力而言,外泌体的剂量和浓度可能更易实现标准化[13]。在皮肤病学中,外泌体被认为

是皮肤伤口愈合有希望的潜在再生工具。

越来越多的证据表明 MSC 有益于皮肤的修复和再生。骨髓来源的间充质干细胞(BM-MSC)剂量依赖性地增强了来自正常供体和慢性伤口患者成纤维细胞的增殖和迁移[14]。BM-MSC 外泌体激活成纤维细胞中的多个信号通路包括 Akt、ERK 和 STAT3 介导的途径,并诱导许多生长因子表达包括肝细胞生长因子、胰岛素样生长因子-1、神经生长因子和基质衍生生长因子-1[14]。此外,发现 BM-MSC 含有活化转录因子(STAT3)[14]并帮助促进疏水/脂化糖蛋白生长因子(如 Wnt3a)[15]和基底膜蛋白(如胶原Ⅶ)[16]的运输。BM-MSC 外泌体对 Wnt3a 的转移可以刺激成纤维细胞增殖、迁移和内皮血管生成[15]。BM-MSC EV 介导的Ⅶ型胶原蛋白和 COL7A mRNA 的转移刺激隐性营养不良型大疱性表皮松解症(recessive dystrophic epidermolysis bullosa,RDEB)的成纤维细胞(缺少Ⅶ型胶原产生)增殖并诱导它们制造新的Ⅶ型胶原蛋白[16]。当用 BM-MSC EV 处理细胞,然后洗涤并使其在无血清培养基中分泌新蛋白时,培养基中的Ⅶ型胶原发生剂量依赖性积累,这表明 BM-MSC EV 可以在 RDEB 的成纤维细胞中诱导Ⅶ型胶原产生(图 10-7)[16]。成纤维细胞导致的瘢痕形成过多在瘢痕的预防和治疗中是重要的治疗目标[17]。在鼠全层皮肤伤口模型中,脐带源性的 MSC 在很大程度上依靠外泌体及其微 RNA 的含量(特别是 miR-21、miR-23a、miR-125b 和 miR-145),通过抑制 TGF-β2/SMAD2 途径从而减少瘢痕形成和成肌纤维细胞累积[17]。

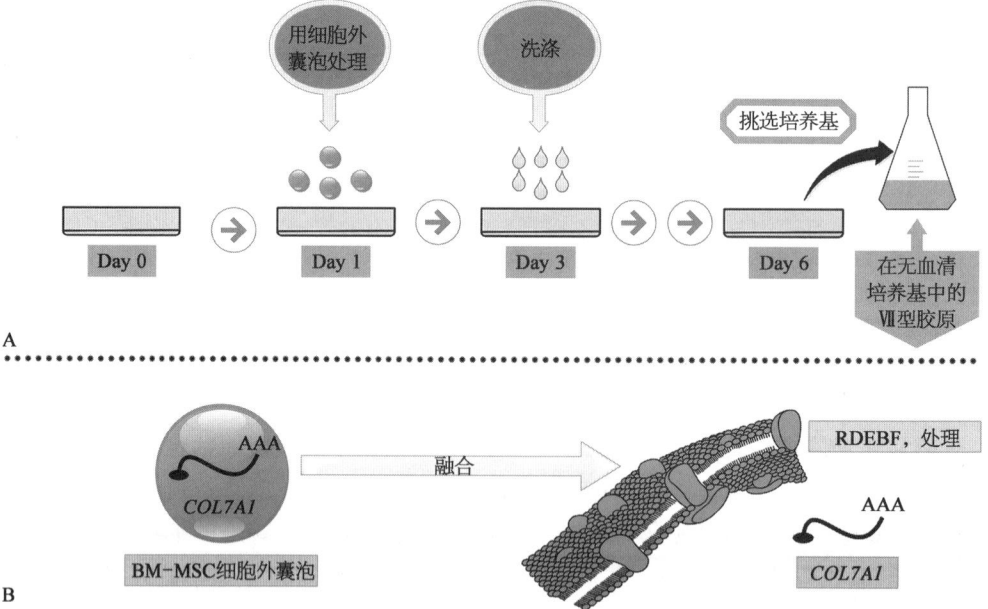

图 10-7 骨髓源性的间充质干细胞 EV 诱导隐性营养不良型大疱性表皮松解症患者的成纤维细胞产生Ⅶ型胶原。A. 在第 1 天处理 RDEB 成纤维细胞 48 小时后进行彻底清洗,第 6 天在无血清培养基中可检测到Ⅶ型胶原的产生。B. 在 BM-MSC EV 中检测到 COL7A1 mRNA;当这些囊泡与 RDEB 成纤维细胞融合时,可以将 mRNA 内化到细胞中,使其可用于生产新的Ⅶ型胶原蛋白

来自人脂肪 MSC 的外泌体(AD-MSC 外泌体)也显示通过成纤维细胞重编程来加速皮肤伤口愈合[13]。由于脂肪组织是一种活跃的内分泌器官,它支持皮肤正常的生理状态、提供营养和支持并含有干细胞和生长因子,因此人们一直关注利用脂肪组织促进皮肤再生的潜力[13]。在处理 AD-MSC 外泌体后,成纤维细胞以剂量依赖性的方式被刺激进行增殖、迁移和产生Ⅰ型、Ⅲ型胶原和弹性蛋白[13]。各种基因的表达也得到增强:N-钙黏着蛋白、周期蛋白-1、PCNA 和Ⅰ型、Ⅲ型胶原[13]。在体内,AD-MSC 适应伤口环境并分泌外泌体,在伤口愈合的早期阶段,组织学证据表明伤口中Ⅰ型和Ⅲ型胶原增加[13]。有趣的是,在急性伤口愈合的后期,AD-MSC 外泌体反而似乎会抑制胶原表达以减少瘢痕形成。人脐带 MSC 分泌的外泌体可以诱导 Wnt/β-连环蛋白信号传导加速皮肤修复[18]。然而,在高细胞密度环境中,通过 14-3-3σ 蛋白,脐带外泌体以 YAP 磷酸化作用抑制 Wnt/β-连环蛋白,最终减弱 Wnt 信号,这可能有助于在重塑阶段减少伤口修复时的瘢痕形成[18]。

血管生成指从原有的血管中形成新的血管芽和血管,这是皮肤伤口愈合的重要过程。血管生成需要内皮细胞与周围环境的合作使内皮细胞增殖、迁移、侵袭、发芽和三维组织构建从而形成新血管[19]。AD-MSC 成为血管生成过程中内皮细胞候选的内源性调节剂,因为它们被认为通过旁分泌机制为新血管生成创造主要的环境[19,20]。BM-MSC 外泌体和 AD-MSC 外泌体都可被内皮细胞(HUVEC)吸收,并且无论在体内还是体外环境都可促进血管生成[14,19]。在 AD-MSC 外泌体中,miR-125a 发生富集并抑制血管生成抑制剂 delta-like4(DLL4)的表达,通过靶向其 3′非翻译区促进血管内皮尖端细胞的形成[19]。总之,外泌体,特别是来自干细胞的外泌体诱导了复杂的程序使其在各种模型中改善皮肤修复。

九、与外泌体相关的细胞间黏附分子如恶性细胞分泌的桥粒黏蛋白能调节细胞外环境促进肿瘤进展

有趣的是,细胞间黏附分子的一些成分显示出调节某些类型皮肤癌的外泌体表达。越来越多的证据表明,分泌到体液中的癌源性 EV 可以在调节肿瘤微环境、发病机制和肿瘤转移中发挥重要作用[21]。鳞状细胞癌(squamous cell carcinoma, SCC)来源的 EV 富含桥粒黏蛋白 2(Dsg2)的 C-末端片段[21]。当 Dsg2 过表达时,SCC 的细胞会增加 EV 的释放[21]。当成纤维细胞与表达 Dsg2-绿荧光蛋白(green fluorescent protein, GFP)的 SCC 细胞共培养时,可在成纤维细胞内部检测到 GFP[21]。Dsg2 增强 EV 的丝裂原活性从而促进成纤维细胞的生长[21]。SCC EV 激活 Erk1/2 和 Akt 信号传导并刺激成纤维细胞增殖[21]。在头颈部鳞状细胞癌中,Dsg2 高度上调,鳞状细胞癌患者血清中的 EV 显示其富含 Dsg2 C-末端片段和生长因子如表皮生长因子[21]。在鳞状细胞肿瘤细胞中,Dsg2 下调陷窝蛋白-1 的水平表明 Dsg2 可能增强陷窝蛋白-1 的内吞作用[21]。

十、外泌体对恶性黑色素瘤的发病机制起重要作用

外泌体已显示出其在黑色素瘤细胞发病机制中的重要作用。CD147 最初被认为是免疫球蛋白超家族中的一种细胞表面蛋白,在各种肿瘤细胞表面高度表达并且是黑色素瘤细胞

表面的一种恶性肿瘤标志物[22]。恶性细胞上表达的 CD147 能通过刺激成纤维细胞产生基质金属蛋白酶，诱导肿瘤细胞侵袭并促进血管生成[22]。黑色素瘤 EV 表面存在断裂的 CD147 片段[22]。基质金属蛋白酶是一类降解细胞外基质不同成分的酶家族，许多研究表明它们在细胞外环境的重塑中起重要作用[22]。研究发现恶性黑色素瘤细胞能无须直接接触刺激成纤维细胞中 MMP 的产生，这提示外泌体可能参与了向成纤维细胞转运刺激因子（如 CD147 通过细胞外泌体）[22]。黑色素瘤是一种具有高度侵袭性的肿瘤，在美国占男性和女性肿瘤比例的 4%，约占 80% 的皮肤癌相关死亡[23]。miRNA 是一类有 22～25 个核苷酸的 RNA，可调节转录后的基因表达[23]。目前缺少一种非侵入性的筛查工具来识别易患黑色素瘤的患者，而血液作为生物标志物标本有几个关键的优势，即采样和处理比皮肤更简单，或作为一种极端的方法对所有高危患者进行全身 PET-CT 扫描来寻找转移性黑色素瘤。与未受影响的对照组相比，在临床上受影响的家族性黑色素瘤患者（携带 CDKN2A/p16 基因）的血浆源性外泌体 miRNA 中，相比没有转移性黑色素瘤的患者，转移性黑色素瘤的患者的 miR-17、miR-19a、miR-21、miR-126 和 miR-149 明显更高[23]。这些 miRNA 参与调控核激素受体、细胞间黏附分子、酪氨酸激酶受体、淋巴细胞转录因子、p63 表达、锌指蛋白和肿瘤坏死因子受体超家族成员等[23]。转移性黑色素瘤患者中差异表达的 miRNA 可用作预测性生物标志物监测发作、缓解、复发和治疗反应[23]。外泌体 miRNA 出色的稳定性使其成为监测各种肿瘤疾病进展的理想候选[23]。

尽管转移性肿瘤可以产生在远程微环境中适应转移前环境的外泌体从而促进转移，但也有证据表明黑色素瘤转移前会分泌抑制转移的外泌体[24]。这些抗转移的外泌体通过单核细胞亚群的扩张刺激先天免疫反应，这些单核细胞在骨髓中被称为 Ly6C^{low} 巡逻单核细胞[24]。这些单核细胞反而能够通过募集 NK 细胞和巨噬细胞从转移前环境中清除肿瘤细胞[24]。非常有趣的是，这些事件的发生依赖于外泌体外表面上的 Nr4a1 转录因子和色素上皮衍生因子（pigment epithelium-derived factor，PEDF）的诱导[24]。从原发性黑色素瘤患者（无转移）中分离出的外泌体具有抑制肺转移的能力。因此，黑色素瘤细胞的外泌体最初可能通过刺激骨髓和免疫系统间接抑制转移，在潜在的转移部位增强监视和肿瘤细胞的清除率[24]。

十一、外泌体的循环信号存在于转移性鳞状细胞癌，特别是在隐性营养不良型大疱性表皮松解症患者中

鳞状细胞癌利用外泌体促进肿瘤的进展。TGF-β 的信号转导促进肿瘤生长和纤维化，但根据情况也能成为肿瘤抑制因子或启动子[25]。口腔部 SCC 常有 TGF-βⅡ型受体功能突变的缺失[25]。在 SCC 研究的前沿领域，TGF-β 活性的异质性可以影响耐药性[25]。口腔 SCC 源性成纤维细胞中的外泌体含有 TGF-βⅡ型受体[25]。SCC 的 TGF-βⅡ型受体的转移使缺少该受体的角质形成细胞对 TGF-β 具有反应性，这提示肿瘤细胞与非肿瘤细胞间的基质通信能改变对 TGF-β 信号转导的敏感性[25]。RDEB 患者在 COL7A1 中携带功能丧失的突变，而这对于维持皮肤和黏膜的基底膜非常重要。由于创伤、炎症、感染和尝试伤口愈合的持续和重复循环，RDEB 患者容易发展为浸润性和侵袭性 SCC。假设这些 SCC 肿

瘤在循环中释放含有可检测特征的外泌体,这些外泌体可能就标志着浸润性 SCC 的存在[26]。转移到内部组织的肿瘤在每次临床就诊时不容易检测或筛选出。一个研究小组调查了使用 SCC 源性的 EV 作为"液体活检"检测肿瘤标志物基因 Ct-SLCO1B3 的可行性,该基因编码有机阴离子转运多肽超家族的成员,这一成员通常在肝脏中表达,但有报道指出其在 RDEB-SCC 中会过表达[26]。在 7 种不同的 RDEB-SCC 细胞系的 EV 中可检测到 Ct-SLCO1B3,但在正常人的角质形成细胞或 RDEB 患者角质形成细胞的外泌体中无法被检测到[26]。

十二、黑色素瘤患者血液循环中的外泌体标志转移和预后恶化

越来越多的证据表明外泌体能调节肿瘤转移,皮肤肿瘤源性的外泌体也不例外。肿瘤源性的外泌体正在成为肿瘤发生的介质。高度转移性黑色素瘤来源的外泌体通过激活骨髓祖细胞中的酪氨酸激酶 MET 增加原发性黑色素瘤的转移性行为[27]。黑色素瘤源性的外泌体在转移前部位引起血管渗漏并重编程骨髓祖细胞来支持致病性血管形成[27]。转移性黑色素瘤患者骨髓祖细胞中 MET 升高和外泌体中 MET 表达减少使恶性黑色素瘤环境中骨髓祖细胞的促转移行为减少[27]。在同样的研究中,Peinado 等发现了一个同时具有预后和治疗潜力的外泌体特异性黑色素瘤标志物,包含 TYRP2、VLA-4、HSP70、HSP90 亚型和 MET 癌蛋白及许多与细胞外基质重塑和炎症相关的基因[27]。与控制组或 I 期疾病相比,III 期和 IV 期黑色素瘤血液循环外泌体中 MET 含量更高[27]。在 IV 期黑色素瘤患者中,如果每毫升血浆中分离出的循环外泌体的蛋白质总量大于 50 μg/mL(与少于 50 μg/mL 相比),患者的累积生存概率会显著降低,前组中所有患者都在 11 个月内死亡(后组 28 个月后存活率超过 50%)。因此,恶性黑色素瘤患者循环中的外泌体含量,无论是外泌体中的总蛋白还是特定的基因产物都有助于预测生存[27]。

十三、总结

人们开始认识到外泌体在皮肤病学中的作用对于理解皮肤的基础生物学过程至关重要。此外,外泌体在特应性皮炎、大疱性类天疱疮、银屑病和皮肤癌的发病机制中起关键作用。干细胞外泌体可以作为治疗方法刺激皮肤修复和再生。根据迄今为止的发现,外泌体研究将有益于皮肤病学领域,可以开发更佳的生物标志物用于疾病检测和预后及治疗工具以管理皮肤疾病。

(庄昊俊 译,邓辉 审校)

参考文献

[1] Lo Cicero A, et al. Exosomes released by keratinocytes modulate melanocyte pigmentation. Nat Commun 2015; 6: 7506.
[2] Waster P, et al. Extracellular vesicles are transferred from melanocytes to keratinocytes after UVA irradiation. Sci Rep 2016; 6: 27890.
[3] Bin BH, et al. Fibronectin-containing extracellular vesicles protect melanocytes against ultraviolet radiation-induced cytotoxicity. J Invest Dermatol 2016; 136(5): 957-66.
[4] Chavez-Munoz C, et al. Primary human keratinocytes externalize stratifin protein via exosomes. J Cell Biochem 2008; 104(6): 2165-73.
[5] Medina A, Ghahary A. Transdifferentiated circulating monocytes release exosomes containing 14-3-3 proteins with

matrix metalloproteinase-1 stimulating effect for dermal fibroblasts. Wound Repair Regen 2010; 18(2): 245-53.
[6] Cai XW, et al. A novel noncontact communication between human keratinocytes and T cells: exosomes derived from keratinocytes support superantigen-induced proliferation of resting T cells. Mol Med Rep 2017; 16(5): 7032-8.
[7] Nickoloff BJ, et al. Accessory cell function of keratinocytes for superantigens. Dependence on lymphocyte function-associated antigen-1/intercellular adhesion molecule-1 interaction. J Immunol 1993; 150(6): 2148-59.
[8] Kotzerke K, et al. Immunostimulatory activity of murine keratinocyte-derived exosomes. Exp Dermatol 2013; 22(10): 650-5.
[9] Zhou L, et al. Regulation of hair follicle development by exosomes derived from dermal papilla cells. Biochem Biophys Res Commun 2018; 500(2): 325-32.
[10] Nakamura K, et al. Altered expression of CD63 and exosomes in scleroderma dermal fibroblasts. J Dermatol Sci 2016; 84(1): 30-9.
[11] Cheung KL, et al. Psoriatic T cells recognize neolipid antigens generated by mast cell phospholipase delivered by exosomes and presented by CD1a. J Exp Med 2016; 213(11): 2399-412.
[12] Fang H, et al. Proinflammatory role of blister fluid-derived exosomes in bullous pemphigoid. J Pathol 2018; 245(1): 114-25.
[13] Hu L, et al. Exosomes derived from human adipose mensenchymal stem cells accelerates cutaneous wound healing via optimizing the characteristics of fibroblasts. Sci Rep 2016; 6: 32993.
[14] Shabbir A, et al. Mesenchymal stem cell exosomes induce proliferation and migration of normal and chronic wound fibroblasts, and enhance angiogenesis in vitro. Stem Cells Dev 2015; 24(14): 1635-47.
[15] McBride JD, et al. Bone marrow mesenchymal stem cell-derived CD63(+) exosomes transport Wnt3a exteriorly and enhance dermal fibroblast proliferation, migration, and angiogenesis in vitro. Stem Cells Dev 2017; 26(19): 1384-98.
[16] McBride JD, et al. Dual mechanism of type VII collagen transfer by bone marrow mesenchymal stem cell extracellular vesicles to recessive dystrophic epidermolysis bullosa fibroblasts. Biochimie 2018; 155: 50-8.
[17] Fang S, et al. Umbilical cord-derived mesenchymal stem cell-derived exosomal microRNAs suppress myofibroblast differentiation by inhibiting the transforming growth factor-beta/SMAD2 pathway during wound healing. Stem Cells Transl Med 2016; 5(10): 1425-39.
[18] Zhang B, et al. HucMSC exosome-delivered 14-3-3zeta orchestrates self-control of the Wnt response via modulation of YAP during cutaneous regeneration. Stem Cells 2016; 34(10): 2485-500.
[19] Liang X, et al. Exosomes secreted by mesenchymal stem cells promote endothelial cell angiogenesis by transferring miR-125a. J Cell Sci 2016; 129(11): 2182-9.
[20] Bronckaers A, et al. Mesenchymal stem/stromal cells as a pharmacological and therapeutic approach to accelerate angiogenesis. Pharmacol Ther 2014; 143(2): 181-96.
[21] Overmiller AM, et al. Desmoglein 2 modulates extracellular vesicle release from squamous cell carcinoma keratinocytes. FASEB J 2017; 31(8): 3412-24.
[22] Hatanaka M, et al. Cleaved CD147 shed from the surface of malignant melanoma cells activates MMP2 produced by fibroblasts. Anticancer Res 2014; 34(12): 7091-6.
[23] Pfeffer SR, et al. Detection of exosomal miRNAs in the plasma of melanoma patients. J Clin Med 2015; 4(12): 2012-27.
[24] Plebanek MP, et al. Pre-metastatic cancer exosomes induce immune surveillance by patrolling monocytes at the metastatic niche. Nat Commun 2017; 8(1): 1319.
[25] Languino LR, et al. Exosome-mediated transfer from the tumor microenvironment increases TGFbeta signaling in squamous cell carcinoma. Am J Transl Res 2016; 8(5): 2432-7.
[26] Sun Y, et al. Extracellular vesicles as biomarkers for the detection of a tumor marker gene in epidermolysis bullosa-associated squamous cell carcinoma. J Invest Dermatol 2018; 138(5): 1197-200.
[27] Peinado H, et al. Melanoma exosomes educate bone marrow progenitor cells toward a prometastatic phenotype through MET. Nat Med 2012; 18(6): 883-91.

第 11 章

泌尿系统中的外泌体
Exosomes in nephrology

Robert W. Hunter, James W. Dear, and Matthew A. Bailey

University/BHF Centre for Cardiovascular Science, Queen's Medical Research Institute, University of Edinburgh, Edinburgh, United Kingdom

一、概述

（一）目的

本章旨在提供泌尿系统外泌体的最新研究进展。我们将回顾外泌体在正常生理和疾病中的作用。我们将首先考虑尿液外泌体，这是肾脏和尿路相关的临床和实验研究外泌体材料的主要来源。我们将讨论尿液外泌体作为肾脏疾病生物标志物的潜力，回顾外泌体通过介导肾脏细胞间的信号传导发挥重要生理（和病理生理）功能的证据。最后，我们将分析基于外泌体的治疗方案在治疗泌尿系统疾病中的潜力。

（二）肾脏和尿路中的外泌体：特殊性

出于多种原因，肾脏和尿路可被视为外泌体信号通路的"特例"。第一，尿液中提供了易于获取且用之不竭的器官特异性外泌体，为研究人员和临床医师提供了大量的生物资源。第二，尿路内排列着空间分离的不同细胞类型，这促成了尿液中混合外泌体的形成。这是一个可以研究细胞特异性外泌体信号的理想系统，而且尿液的流动为我们研究外泌体信号的定向（沿着尿路从近端到远端）提供了条件。第三，肾小球滤过屏障和肾小管-间质-血管界面的复杂显微解剖结构为我们提供了探讨外泌体在身体组织中传播机制的体系。

这些特征都是研究者和临床医师面临的机遇与挑战，我们将在本章中详细阐述。

（三）命名

与其他领域一样，许多关于肾脏外泌体的文献也存在着命名混乱的问题。特别是在 21 世纪早期进行的研究中，EV 亚群要么没有命名，要么是形形色色的非标准定义。因此，"胞外囊泡（extracellular vesicle）""外泌体（exosome）""微囊泡（microvesicle）""微粒子（microparticle）""纳米囊泡（nanovesicle）"等术语被用来指代具有不同特征的囊泡群。研究者甚至创造了一些如"前列腺体（prostasomes）"的术语来指代尿路特有的囊泡。在本章中，我们将遵循最新关于命名法的共识声明[1,2]，即 EV 根据其生物成因进行分类。因此，我们将"外泌体"一词限定为那些具备与来自内吞途径的起泡事件相匹配物质的囊泡（直径 30～100 nm 并且高表达如 CD63、CD81、flotillin-1 和 Tsg101 等标志物）[3,4]。我们将使用

"微泡"一词来指那些可能起源于质膜处起泡事件的颗粒(直径 100~1 000 nm)。当讨论定义模糊的 EV 时,我们将笼统地称之为 EV。

二、尿液外泌体

(一) 外泌体的提取方法

肾脏和尿路细胞将外泌体释放到尿液中,这一现象最先由 Knepper 实验室[5]发现。这为我们提供了充足的生物原材料,非常有助于进行肾脏病学中外泌体的相关研究。然而,从尿液中提取外泌体需要一些特殊方法。

1. 尿蛋白干预尿液外泌体的提取

尿蛋白可以与尿液外泌体相互作用并干扰外泌体的分离。尿调节素(又称 Tamm-Horsfall 蛋白)是尿液最丰富的尿蛋白,它与透明带蛋白在结构上相关,在低温(−4℃)及尿液 pH 和离子强度改变时沉淀[6,7]。沉淀形成细长的绳索状聚合物细丝,细丝在电子显微镜下可见[6,8]。在差速离心方案中,外泌体可能会被尿调节素形成的网状结构捕获并丢失在低速颗粒中。可以通过使用还原剂(如二硫苏糖醇)破坏尿调节素形成的聚合物[6,7,9]或在 D_2O 蔗糖梯度上进行等密度离心来避免外泌体丢失[8]。

在病理性蛋白尿的情况下,如肾病综合征,尿蛋白的混杂干扰作用将进一步增强。如使用标准的超速离心法,大量蛋白质如白蛋白和 α1-抗胰蛋白酶将与外泌体共纯化。在一定程度上,这一问题可以通过尺寸排除色谱分离外泌体和游离蛋白组分[10]或使用 D_2O 蔗糖梯度上进行等密度离心来解决[11]。分离外泌体方法的细微变化可能会对最终样品的组成产生影响。例如,使用密度梯度超速离心法可产生富含水通道蛋白-2、多囊蛋白-1、多囊蛋白-2 或足细胞素的外泌体亚群[8]。这些蛋白在不同的肾单位节段中表达,因此这些外泌体组分很可能来自不同的肾单位节段。例如,足细胞素富集的提取物具有与肾小球相同的分子标记[11]。

2. 外泌体在尿液标本中的标准化问题

研究人员或临床医师在处理尿液外泌体时面临的另一个挑战是使结果标准化。在生理与病理的不同情况,尿流速率变化很大,因此利用外泌体浓度衡量结果缺少价值(如每毫升样品中外泌体颗粒的数量或外泌体蛋白的微克数)。肾小管液或尿液的流速改变可能对外泌体释放或被尿路细胞吸收的速率有影响(据我们所知,这还有待严格的测试)。因此,测量排泄率,即单位时间内尿中排出的外泌体数量,可能也是不太可行的。

为了解决这个问题,不同的研究者尝试了不同的方法,多数人使用尿肌酐浓度来标化外泌体浓度,临床上广泛使用其不定时对尿液样本中的蛋白质和其他溶质的排泄进行标化。另一种替代方法是使用尿调节素浓度进行标化,这种蛋白通常会与 EV 一起被分离出来,并且尿调节素的丰度与健康志愿者尿液中典型 EV 标记物的丰度高度相关[6]。然而,尿调节素的排泄率在不同的个体之间存在显著差异,因此,当需要对不同受试者的尿液外泌体产物进行标准化化比较时,这种方法是不完善的。总尿蛋白也可用于标化外泌体浓度,但不适用于病理性蛋白尿患者。

3. 尿液外泌体的提取方法

除了有干扰作用的尿蛋白,尿液与其他生物液体相比,唯一需要特别注意的是其样本量可能很大(通常是 10～100 mL)。差速离心法仍然被许多人认为是从尿液中制备外泌体的金标准,但过滤、沉淀、免疫亲和捕获或尺寸排除色谱的方法成为更适合大输入量的替代方法[13-15]。在对这些替代方案的比较中,一种改进的沉淀方案中外泌体和 RNA 的产量最高[13]。

(二) 尿液外泌体的细胞源性与分子结构特点

尿液中外泌体的分子载体与其他生物液体中外泌体的分子载体相似,包括脂质、蛋白质和核酸,尤其富含非编码 RNA。同时,尿液外泌体具备复杂的表面糖基化[16]。

尿中外泌体蛋白的浓度约为 2 μg/mL,约占尿总蛋白的 3%[17]。尿液外泌体蛋白组(以及磷蛋白组)富含顶膜蛋白[9],这与外泌体的生物成因相关:即尿道内膜细胞从顶面直接释放 EV 进入尿腔。然而,细胞质和核蛋白如转录因子也被检测到[18]。

尿液外泌体中的核酸主要包括易受 DNA 感染的 DNA(可能包覆在囊泡外)和耐 RNA 酶的 RNA(可能被保护在囊泡内)[19]。在健康人类受试者的 RNA 测序数据中,几乎 90% 的读码与核糖体 RNA 对齐,其余约 60% 与非编码 RNA 序列对齐[20]。mRNA 序列在肾单位、肾集合系统和下尿路特异性表达的转录本中富集[19,20]。

(三) 肾脏细胞对外泌体的摄取

沿尿路排列的细胞将外泌体释放到尿液中,但这些细胞也能通过尿路和血管间隙吸收外泌体。此外,肾细胞摄取外泌体(或至少是外泌体中的某个亚群)似乎是选择性并受生理调节。

1. 摄取外泌体的分子基础

关于肾脏细胞对外泌体的摄取,目前大量研究集中在肾小管上皮细胞方面。外泌体可以穿过顶端或基底外侧的细胞膜[21],根尖纤毛也可能在促进外泌体摄取方面发挥作用:一些外泌体会与肾小管(IMCD)细胞和胆道上皮细胞[8]上的初级纤毛发生物理作用。

荧光型外泌体(来源于表达 CD63-GFP 的肾小管细胞)的细胞摄取被非荧光型外泌体竞争性抑制,这证明 EV 的摄取是通过饱和途径发生的[22]。

无论体外还是体内,外泌体的胰蛋白酶化使其无法被肾细胞吸收[23],这表明外泌体的吸收依赖于其表面蛋白的表达。一些研究者已经定义了对 EV 摄取很重要的特定表面蛋白(对于特定细胞和特定 EV)。例如,阻断 CD29 或 CD44 可抑制肾小管细胞对 MSC 源性外泌体的摄取[23,24]。作为 CD44 的内源性配体,透明质酸在肾间质和肾小管基底膜上表达[25,26]。阻断 CD36 可抑制足细胞源性外泌体与肾小管上皮细胞的相互作用[27]。

在某种程度上,细胞对外泌体的摄取是选择性的,这与外泌体的起源有关。小鼠远端肾小管上皮细胞吸收人近端肾小管上皮细胞源性外泌体而非小鼠肾小球旁细胞源性 EV 外泌体[21]。

这些结果证明,外泌体的吸收依赖于细胞表面蛋白质与外泌体之间的独特互动(图 11-1)。这一观点逐渐得到广泛认可,即外泌体选择地与受体细胞通过特定受体-配体相互作用,然后通过活跃的内吞作用完成内化[28]。

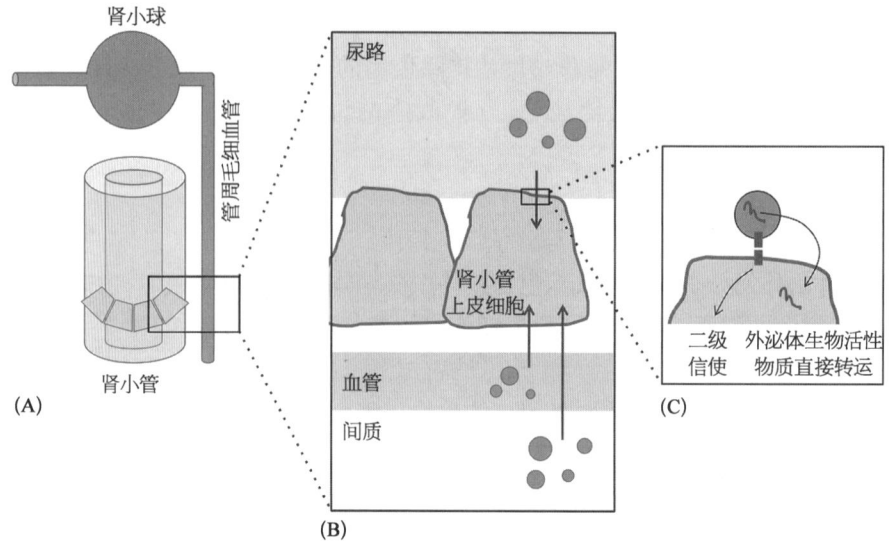

图 11-1 肾小管内的外泌体信号传导模型。(A 和 B)理论上,外泌体可以通过多种途径进入尿路。它们可以由尿路内壁的细胞释放,也可以通过肾小球滤过屏障或肾小管从血管或间质进入。这些路径均有实验结果支持(见正文)。(C)与其他系统一样,外泌体通过与特定的细胞表面分子相互作用进入肾脏细胞。它们可以通过转运生物活性物质(核酸/蛋白质/脂质)或刺激细胞表面受体激活第二信使级联作用来影响靶细胞功能

2. 外泌体摄取与释放的生理调节

集合管细胞对外泌体的摄取受到血管升压素和内皮素-1的调节,这两种物质都是集合管细胞功能的生理调节因子[21,29]。由于所有的尿液外泌体都必须经过集合管,尿液的外泌体成分可能会随着抗利尿激素信号活性变化而有所不同(如水合状态)。为了支持这一假说,在一名中立性尿崩性糖尿病患者中,使用血管升压素治疗后,其表达足细胞和近端小管标志物的外泌体的尿排泄下降[21]。至于其他(非抗利尿激素应答的)肾脏细胞中外泌体摄取的生理调节因子,目前尚未被广泛研究。

3. 外泌体在体内可转运至肾脏细胞

来自远端器官的外泌体是否可以进入尿液仍存在争议,有待最终解决。一方面,EV的大小和电荷分布决定了它们不能穿越肾小球和肾小管基底膜[30,31]。与此相一致的是,健康受试者尿液外泌体中检测到的绝大多数RNA和蛋白分子来自肾脏和尿路[9,19]。

另一方面,有证据表明,至少在肾损伤的情况下,循环中的外泌体(或外泌体活性物质)会被肾细胞吸收。将荧光标记的外泌体注射到小鼠体循环后,可以在肾小管细胞中检测到荧光标记[21,23,32]。同样地,在大肠埃希菌相关溶血性尿毒症综合征患者和小鼠的肾细胞中检测到血细胞来源的EV标志物[33]。然而,在一些研究中,仅在急性肾损伤的情况下可观察到这一现象,而在健康对照中缺少相关发现[23,32]。

值得注意的是,也有证据表明完整的外泌体可以从血管间隙进入肾细胞和尿液。通过纳米追踪分析检测到了注射进循环系统的荧光标记外泌体[21]。而在注射游离染料的情况下,研究者没能在尿液中检测到尿荧光信号。而用洗涤剂处理尿液后,荧光信号大大降低。

三、外泌体用作生物标志物

（一）作为生物标志物的两方面应用

外泌体具有作为生物标志物的潜力，其分子载体可以用于推断起源细胞的分子状态。蛋白组学、转录组学和脂质组学已被用于识别尿液外泌体中的分子生物标志物。外泌体作为生物标记物的潜力可能会在以下两个方面被广泛应用：一是作为机械性生物标志物，帮助了解人类疾病或动物模型中特定细胞类型的功能；二是作为临床生物标志物，帮助诊断肾脏或其他泌尿系统疾病。

（二）反应肾小管功能的机械标志物

1. 水的运输

尿液外泌体中管状转运蛋白的丰度已被证明与多种环境下体内转运活性有关。事实上，这一现象的首次证明早于研究者对尿路外泌体的普遍认识，即升压素增加了中枢性尿崩症患者尿水通道蛋白2（aquaporin，AQP2）的排泄[34]。已知，大多数尿中AQP2是通过外泌体排泄出来的[35]，而在尿液外泌体中AQP2的表达与体内加压素信号活性之间的相关性已经被多次证明[29,36]。

2. 钠的运输

肾小管钠转运体的转运活性与它们在顶端细胞膜中的丰度相关，并受转录后修饰（如磷酸化）的调控。因此，在尿液EV中管状钠转运体的丰度和（或）磷酸化状态与它们在体内的转运活性相关，而这在罕见的孟德尔疾病中得到了验证。Gitelman和Gordon综合征分别导致噻嗪敏感的NaCl共转运体NCC活性不足和过度活跃。在Gitelman综合征中，尿液外泌体中NCC蛋白的丰度明显降低[37,38]；而在Gordon综合征中，NCC蛋白的丰度升高[39]。在Ⅰ型Bartter综合征中也观察到类似现象，这是由呋塞米敏感的Na-K-Cl共转运体NKCC2突变引起[9,37]。

但在生理条件下，尿中钠转运蛋白的丰度是否与肾脏中的表达相关？这已经在动物模型和人类身上进行了测试，Esteva-Font等发现，在饮食钠含量的干扰下，大鼠的NCC和NKCC2确实存在这种相关性[40]。然而，在饮食摄入钠的变化足以改变钠排泄的情况下，他们并没有观察到高血压受试者的尿液外泌体中NCC和NKCC2表达的变化。其他研究小组发现，原发性醛固酮增多症患者尿液外泌体中NCC和磷酸化NCC表达增加，这种疾病预计会增加其在肾小管的表达[41]。类似地，肾移植患者的环孢素治疗（已知通过其对WNK-SPAK信号通路的影响增加NCC表达）增加了尿液外泌体中NCC和NKCC2的丰度[42]。噻嗪类利尿剂（NCC抑制剂）的治疗增加了尿液外泌体中NCC的丰度和磷酸化，并且在使用噻嗪类药物出现血压反应的患者中，这种作用更大[43]。这与在啮齿类动物上的研究一致，即慢性噻嗪类药物的摄入导致NCC表达增加。

同样地，肾移植患者尿液外泌体中NCC的丰度和磷酸化受到钙调磷酸酶抑制剂和血压对噻嗪类药物敏感的影响[44]。

尿液外泌体中NCC的表达在人类和啮齿动物中表现出日变化[45,46]，这与已知的啮齿类动物肾脏表达的日变化一致。但有趣的是,很多其他外泌体蛋白也观察到了日变化[45]。

3. 酸碱运输

与观察到的水和钠转运蛋白的作用类似,尿液外泌体中酸碱转运蛋白的丰度随着酸碱稳态的变化而变化。在酸中毒中,液泡 ATP 酶 B1 亚单位的排泄(在分泌酸的闰细胞上表达)增加,而 pendrin 的排泄(在分泌碱的细胞上表达)减少[47,48];在碱中毒中则恰恰相反。

4. 肾小管的相关介绍

一些研究小组试图对尿液外泌体中的一组转运蛋白进行定量分析,以获得肾小管不同段转运活性的"概况"。这种方法曾被用于研究美国皮肤利什曼病患者尿液浓缩和酸化缺陷的机制。外泌体转运蛋白的表达若向一个方向改变且能够代表肾脏的表达,则将提供一个机制上的解释。尿浓缩缺陷患者往往具有较低的 AQP2 和(可能是补偿性的)较高的 NKCC2 表达;尿酸化缺陷患者常常有较高的 NHE3、液泡 ATP 酶和潘蛋白表达[49]。

接受内皮素激动剂治疗的健康受试者游离水清除率增高。对尿液外泌体蛋白的分析表明,这发生在 NKCC2 和 AQP2 排泄增加的情况下。这表明水尿症是由 Henle 循环中钠转运增加引起的(而不是由收集管中 AQP2 活性降低引起的)。与之一致的是,肾清除参数也表明循环中的钠吸收增加[50]。

在噻嗪类药物引起的低钠血症患者中,与血钠正常的对照组相比,NCC 和 AQP2 的尿液外泌体丰度分别减少和增加[51]。如果这些变化指标能代表肾脏中的转运蛋白/通道活性,那便可以解释低钠血症发生的原因,因为它们有利于钠的排出和水分的保留。此外,这些差异在噻嗪类药物停用几个月后仍然存在,表明这种变化可能在噻嗪类药物暴露之前就存在,因此有可能被用作预测噻嗪类药物诱发低钠血症的生物标志物。

(三)反应肾脏疾病的生物标志物

尿液外泌体在协助诊断罕见的单基因疾病上有巨大潜力(如上文所述)。然而,鉴于泌尿上皮细胞携带的核酸、蛋白质、脂质和其他大分子的多样性,许多研究人员采用系统生物学的方法,试图发现复杂的尿液外泌体活性物质中编码的临床信号。

与全尿或尿中可溶性物质相比,外泌体作为生物标志物储库具有几个潜在优势。首先,外泌体富含某些特殊分子(如膜结合蛋白、非编码 RNA)。RNA 甚至可以在囊泡核心内得到保护,免受核酸酶降解。此外,通过寻找与来源细胞相关的标记物的共表达,有可能用于评估某种特定细胞类型中某特定生物标志物的丰度,从而获得比全尿更高的信噪比。

1. 采用外泌体丰度作为细胞损伤的生物标志物

一种假设是,外泌体的数量或理化性质可以提供其起源细胞状态的相关信息。举一个简单的例子,如果在细胞损伤时外泌体释放的速率增加,那么在尿液中检测到的外泌体数量可能与细胞损伤相关。而这一假设在糖尿病肾病和先兆子痫中有一定的证据支持。在这两种情况下,足细胞来源的尿液外泌体的丰度都有所增加,且都观测到了肾小球损伤[52-54]。在这种方法中,一个分子标记可被用来定义一种起源细胞,如足细胞的足细胞素或肾素。

更复杂的方法是使用一种以上分子标志物的共表达来定义来自细胞亚群的外泌体。例如,肾移植后几天,共表达肾小球或近端肾小管标记物的 $CD133^+$ 尿液外泌体(即来源于祖细胞)增加。这表明祖细胞可能有助于移植后肾小球和肾小管的修复[55,56]。

2. 外泌体活性物质作为疾病生物标志物

同时,外泌体的分子内容物可以提供疾病状态的信息。转录组学、蛋白质组学和脂质组学方法发现了各种肾脏疾病的潜在生物标志物,如急性肾小管损伤、肾小球疾病和移植排斥方面(表11-1),目前已有大量相关报道[72,56]。比如,一项队列研究比较了15名慢性肾脏病(chronic kidney disease,CKD)(混合病因)患者与10名健康对照组的尿液外泌体,结果显示15名CKD患者的尿液外泌体中显示了30种非编码RNA存在差异表达[66]。这是一项鼓舞人心的结果,但在更集中的疾病群体中进行更大规模的研究是否会发现RNA"信号",从而帮助做出可靠且有益于临床的决策,仍有待进一步研究。

类似于"机械性生物标志物"的研究,动物研究在探索特定"损伤"生物标志物在尿液外泌体中的丰度与其在肾脏中的表达丰度之间的相关性至关重要。例如,对来自足细胞损伤模型的尿液外泌体转录组的分析显示胱抑素C在损伤中受到不同程度的调节。在体内足细胞和小管细胞的mRNA和蛋白表达也反映了这种差异表达[73]。

表11-1 已在患者中检测的尿液外泌体生物标志物

细胞来源	生物标志物	疾病	参考文献
肾小球疾病和糖尿病肾病			
足细胞	外泌体数量	糖尿病肾病(1型)	[54]
?	miRNA	糖尿病肾病(1型)	[57]
?	外泌体大小、密度即蛋白组学	糖尿病肾病(2型)	[58]
?	钙调素	糖尿病肾病	[59]
足细胞	WT-1	祖细胞损伤/FSGS	[60]
?	蛋白组学	IgAN和TBMN	[61]
足细胞	ADAM10	肾小球疾病	[62]
?	miRNA	SLE和狼疮肾炎	[63]
足细胞	外泌体数量	先兆子痫	[53]
肾小管疾病、AKI、CKD、高血压			
?	胎球蛋白A	AKI	[64]
肾小管上皮细胞	护骨素	CKD	[65]
肾小管上皮细胞	ncRNA	CKD	[66]
足细胞		肾血管性高血压	[67]
?	蛋白组学	原发性高血压	[68]
肾小管上皮细胞	NCC、AQP2、PGT	噻嗪类药物引起的低钠	[51]
肾移植			
progenitor	CD133	移植物功能	[55]
?	NGAL	延迟移植物功能	[69]
?	蛋白组学	排异反应/肾小管损伤	[70]
?	蛋白组学	急性排异反应	[71]

四、外泌体在肾脏与尿路中的生物学作用

与其他身体系统一样,越来越多的研究支持外泌体在肾脏和尿路中发挥功能性作用的假说,外泌体不仅仅是细胞废物。宽泛地讲,它们可能通过与受体细胞表面受体相互作用或通过将有功能的蛋白质、脂质或核酸转运到受体细胞来发挥生物学功能。关于外泌体改变肾细胞功能的报道很多(表 11-2 及图 11-2),其中大多数描述了对肾小管上皮细胞的影响,因此我们的讨论集中在这些细胞上。

(一)外泌体信号通路调节小管间质细胞

1. EV 外泌体信号通路调控管状细胞转运功能

最初的一篇报道描述了加压素刺激集合管细胞释放的外泌体如何促进加压素受体阴性的集合管细胞进行水运输[29]。使用后叶升压素治疗后,外泌体中的 APQ2 丰度增加,而"外泌体标志物"flotillin-1 和 Tsg101 的丰度保持不变。我们后来了解到,尿液外泌体中含有功能性 AQP2 水通道[98]。因此,这一效应可能与功能性 AQP2 通道的转移有关,但还有待进一步验证。

也有研究检测了离体肾小管细胞近端到远端的信号传递。由多巴胺激动剂刺激的近端小管细胞产生的外泌体降低了受体远端小管细胞中活性氧的产生[22]。造成这种效应的机制尚不明确,但研究人员使用荧光 CD63 和 CD9 标记证明,外泌体被受体细胞内化,且在一些细胞中,荧光标记显示外泌体进入细胞后定位于多泡体。Jella 等也检测了外泌体从近端肾单位向远端肾单位传递信号的可能性。他们发现,来自近端肾小管细胞的外泌体降低了远端肾小管细胞中上皮性钠通道 ENaC 的活性,从顶端释放的外泌体比基底外侧细胞表面释放的外泌体作用更强[91]。研究者发现了一种涉及 GAPDH 蛋白转移的机制,即外泌体表达出具有催化活性的 GAPDH,外泌体中 GAPDH 的药理抑制作用消除了它们对 ENaC 的刺激作用,免疫共免疫沉淀实验表明远端小管细胞中 ENaC 亚基和 GAPDH 之间存在物理上的相互作用。

Fiona Karet 的研究小组进行了更广泛的检测,即验证尿液外泌体将调节型 microRNA 转移到肾小管细胞的一般假设。利用小 RNA 测序,他们发现健康志愿者的尿液外泌体富含靶向膜转运体及其调节因子的 miRNA。在体外实验培养的细胞上,尿液外泌体能够调节远端和近端小管细胞中溶质转运体的表达[86],这表明 miRNA 可能是形成外泌体生物功能活性物质中的关键成分,在靶向肾小管细胞中发挥功能性作用。

表 11-2 外泌体在肾脏中的功能性通信

起源细胞	受体细胞	转运物质	功能	实验研究	参考文献
起源于干细胞且能起到保护作用的外泌体					
MSC	肾小管上皮细胞	RMA	增强急性肾损伤时的细胞修复功能;抗凋亡作用	体内与体外实验;RNAse 作用性阴性对照	[23]

续 表

起源细胞	受体细胞	转运物质	功 能	实验研究	参考文献
MSC	?	?	肾损伤时起保护作用（5/6肾切除情况）	体内试验；所用于注射MSC相当	[74]
MSC	?	?	肾损伤时起保护作用（氧化应激通路）	体内与体外实验（缺血再灌注损伤模型）	[75]
MSC	肾小管上皮细胞	miRNA	急性肾损伤时起保护作用	体外实验；使用放线菌素D推断miRNA的转移	[24]
MSC	肾小管上皮细胞	肝细胞生长因子mRNA	肾小管损伤时的保护作用	体内与体外实验；使用RNAse验证其作用依赖于RNA	[76]
MSC	肾小管上皮细胞(HK2)	miR	抑制TGF-β诱导的EMT；修复UUO引发的肾损伤	体内与体外实验	[77]
MSC	肾小管上皮细胞	miRNA	急性肾损伤时起保护作用	体内实验；敲低Drosha做阴性对照	[78]
MSC	肾小管上皮细胞(NRK52E)	miRNA (let7c)	纤维化时起保护作用	体内与体外实验；采用Cy-3标记pre-miRNA来检测其转运情况	[79]
	肾小管上皮细胞	miRNA/mRNA	急性肾损伤时起保护作用&促进肾小管上皮细胞增殖	体内与体外实验	[80]
MSC	肾小管上皮细胞&巨噬细胞	IL-10	减轻肾脏炎症反应	体内实验；代谢综合征和肾动脉狭窄的猪模型	[81]
MSCs & HLSC	系膜细胞	miR-222	高糖损伤时起保护作用	体外实验	[82]
BMDC	成纤维细胞	miR	移植肾小管间质纤维化(tPA信号通路)	体内与体外试验；证明外泌体中的miR-144在肾纤维化时靶向tPA的3'UTR	[83]
EPC	肾小管上皮细胞	miRNA	急性肾损伤时起保护作用	体内实验；使用RNase、敲低Dicer基因及miR抑制剂做阴性对照	[84]
EPC	系膜细胞	miRNA	肾小球系膜损伤时起保护作用(Thy1.1肾炎)	体内与体外试验；使用RNAse验证其作用依赖于RNA	[85]
肾小管上皮细胞间的信号传递					
?（可能取自全尿）	肾小管上皮细胞	miRNA	溶质运输途径表达水平发生改变	体外试验	[86]
肾小管上皮细胞	肾小管上皮细胞	AQP2蛋白	转变水运输能力	体外试验	[29]
肾小管上皮细胞	肾小管上皮细胞	?	增强急性肾损伤时的细胞修复功能	体外试验	[87]

续 表

起源细胞	受体细胞	转运物质	功 能	实验研究	参考文献
肾小管上皮细胞	肾小管上皮细胞	miRNA	下调 miRNA 靶基因的表达	体内与体外试验；使用外源性 miRNA 做阳性对照	[21]
肾小管上皮细胞	肾小管上皮细胞	?	转变多巴胺信号通路的激活	荧光标记 CD9 与 CD63 检测其转运	[22]
肾小管上皮细胞	肾小管上皮细胞	HIF-1α	抑制凋亡	体外实验	[88]
全肾/HK-2	?	?	缺氧诱导产生的外泌体可以在缺血再灌注损伤时保护肾脏	体内与体外试验	[89]
肾小管上皮细胞	肾小管上皮细胞	?	移植损伤修复	体外试验；检测外泌体对 EGFR 通路的影响	[90]
肾小管上皮细胞（近端）	肾小管上皮细胞（远端）	GAPDH	ENaC 活动	体外试验	[91]
肾小管上皮细胞	肾小管上皮细胞	ATF3（转录因子）	肾损伤时起保护作用（MCP-1 通路）	体内与体外试验	[92]
其他肾成分间的信号通路					
HUVEC/单核细胞	足细胞	?	TNF-α 诱导的促炎表型转变	体外试验	[93]
足细胞	肾小管上皮细胞	无（表观相互作用）	前纤维化信号通路	体外试验；通过阻断 CD36 证明其表观的相互作用	[27]
肾小球系膜细胞	足细胞	TGF-β1	高糖诱导的损伤转变	体外试验	[94]
白细胞	肾小球内皮细胞和 HEK	激肽 B1 受体	血管炎中的激肽信号	以患者为研究对象的体内与体外试验	[95]
肾小管上皮细胞	MSC	miRNA	诱导产生 MET	体外试验；使用 miR 替代物做阳性对照	[96]
肾小管上皮细胞	巨噬细胞	CCL2 mRNA	诱导对蛋白尿的炎症反应	体内与体外实验；构建 GFP-CCL2 证明 mRNA 转移至巨噬细胞	[97]

注：AQP2，水通道蛋白 2；BMDC，骨髓源细胞；EPC，血管内皮祖细胞；HLSC，人肝脏干细胞；HUVEC，人脐静脉内皮细胞；MET，间质-上皮细胞转化；miRNA，microRNA；MSC，间充质干细胞；UUO，单侧输尿管阻断。

2. 干细胞源外泌体使肾小管细胞对肾损伤产生抵抗性

在 21 世纪初，许多研究团队探讨了干细胞疗法改善器官损伤的潜力。他们发现干细胞可以防止器官损伤（包括肾脏损伤），但是这种作用并不是由注入的干细胞移植和增殖介导的。

干细胞迁移到损伤部位，并产生旁分泌因子影响该部位的细胞[99]。研究发现，来自 MSC 的 EV 足以解释 MSC 为什么会在肾损伤模型中起到保护作用[23,74]。

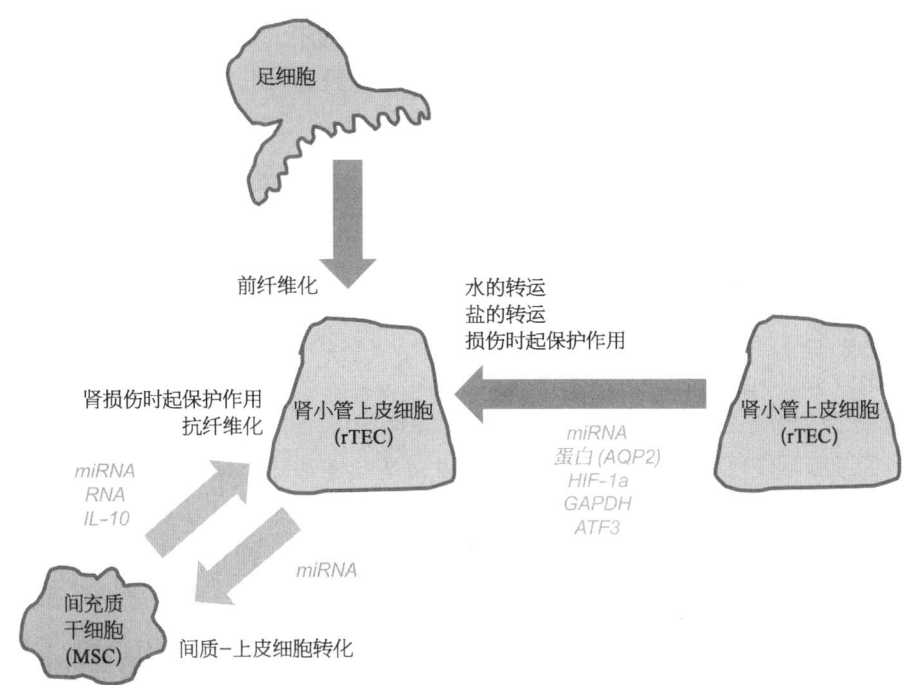

图 11-2 外泌体起到向肾小管上皮细胞发出信号的功能作用。多项研究表明,外泌体对肾小管上皮细胞具有功能性作用。总结如图,详见表 11-2

Camussi 研究团队发表了大量论文来检测干细胞来源外泌体促进肾脏修复的能力[23,24,78,84,96]。当将来自 MSC 或内皮祖细胞(endothelial progenitor cell, EPC)的外泌体注射到小鼠的体循环中时,均能保护小鼠免受肾脏损伤[23,78,84]。比较外泌体(100 000 g 颗粒)或微囊泡(10 000 g 颗粒)这两种生物制剂,似乎只有外泌体发挥这种治疗效果[80]。这种治疗效果取决于能将关键的 RNA 种类转移到肾小管细胞。miRNA 是最有力的证据。EV 中富含 miRNA,当 miRNA 被一般(Dicer 或 Drosha 敲除)或特异性(antagomirs)敲除时,这种保护作用就会消失[78,84]。

其他研究小组也发现了相似现象。Wang 等发现 MSC 过表达 miRNA-let7c 对体内肾损伤具有保护作用。在体外,他们发现 MSC 通过外泌体将荧光标记的 miRNA 转移到肾小管细胞,这些外泌体减弱了肾小管细胞中 TGF-β 信号的促纤维化作用[79]。Dominguez 等研究证明,在大鼠模型中,来自肾小管上皮细胞的外泌体能够加速肾脏损伤后的恢复[87];而从缺氧肾小管细胞中获得外泌体的效果更强,可以将之理解为缺血预处理的一种形式。

综上所述,这一系列研究支持两个关键结论:干细胞源性外泌体可以对肾小管细胞进行再编辑,保护它们免受损伤,而外泌体携带的 RNA 在介导这一效应方面至关重要。因此,核糖核酸是直接还是间接在靶细胞中发挥作用,即外泌体传递到靶细胞的 mRNA 分子是否会被翻译成蛋白质?递送的 miRNA 分子是否进入 RNA 诱导沉默复合体(RNA-induced silencing complex, RISC)并抑制靶 mRNA 的表达?这些问题尚无明确回答,但现有的证据支持外泌体发挥直接作用。在体外,骨髓 MSC 衍生的外泌体被肾小管细胞内化,减轻了 ATP 耗竭的损害效应[24]。外泌体疗法改变了靶细胞内 miRNA 的表达。使用放线菌素D抑制转录的实验表明,外泌体的一些作用是由其携带的微小核糖核酸直接转移介导的,而其他效应受到外泌体介导的靶细胞微小核糖核酸转录变化影响。也有证据表明内源性干细胞释放的外泌体携带的miRNA可以直接沉默靶基因表达。红细胞生成素在小鼠输尿管梗阻模型中对肾损伤有保护作用。机制很有趣:促红细胞生成素刺激骨髓细胞释放含miR-144的外泌体,miR-144靶向成纤维细胞中组织纤溶酶原激活剂的3´UTR。同时,miR-144拮抗剂可以阻断这种作用[83]。

miRNA靶标预测和基因本体分析已被用于预测可能由MSC源性外泌体RNA内容物调节的关键细胞过程,包括调节细胞增殖、凋亡、脂肪酸代谢、炎症、基质受体相互作用、细胞黏附和细胞骨架组织等途径[24,78,80]。

3. 由肾小管细胞传递至其他组分的外泌体信号

肾小管细胞不仅仅是外泌体信号的靶点,也是功能性外泌体的来源。这种信号在疾病状态中可能发挥重要作用。暴露于白蛋白的肾小管细胞释放能够在巨噬细胞中诱导促炎状态的外泌体。这些外泌体富含编码趋化因子CCL2的mRNA,而使用GFP-CCL2融合基因构建体的实验表明,外泌体携带的基因直接传递至巨噬细胞[97]。这一途径可能会导致蛋白尿时常见的肾小管间质炎症。肾小管细胞源外泌体也显示出诱导部分MSC向上皮细胞转化的能力,这可能是通过转移miRNA实现的[96]。

4. 外泌体通过细胞表面受体向肾小管细胞传递信号

RNA的转移介导了外泌体的许多功能效应,但这并不排除其他机制也在发挥作用。足细胞源性微泡在体外肾小管细胞中诱导细胞内促纤维化信号通路,但这种诱导作用随着表面受体CD36的阻断被完全抑制[27]。这表明表面受体对外泌体的内化至关重要,或者外泌体通过结合靶细胞表面受体以及激活细胞内二级信使级联反应发挥作用。

(二)外泌体介导的与泌尿系统病原体的相互作用

外泌体与同物种的受体细胞发生相互作用,但也有证据表明在尿路感染的情况下存在跨物种相互作用。宿主来源的尿液外泌体富含固有免疫系统的蛋白,包括抗菌肽。它们在体外表现出抗菌功能,能够溶解常见的泌尿系统病原体,如大肠埃希菌[100]。同时,病原体源性外泌体可以被宿主的尿路上皮细胞内化,从而影响宿主细胞的功能。性传播的寄生虫,如阴道毛滴虫,释放的外泌体会被尿路上皮细胞内化,进而增加寄生虫与受体细胞的结合[101]。而在其他身体系统中,外泌体介导的病原体和宿主之间的相互作用也有文献进行了描述[102]。

五、外泌体疗法的潜在应用

由于外泌体在动物疾病模型中能够发挥功能性作用,研究者热衷于探索外泌体疗法用于治疗人类肾脏疾病的潜能。与传统的小分子药物和细胞疗法相比,外泌体在理论上具备诸多优势。它们可以通过传递复杂的多效性信号(如miRNA的混合)调控靶细胞中的多种通路,而且外泌体具有稳定的表型,但细胞疗法却保留了恶变的潜力[103]。在肾脏和尿道之外,涉及原理验证的相关研究表明,携带小非编码RNA活性物质及经过人工培养的外泌体能够靶向肿瘤细胞并提高小鼠肿瘤模型的存活率[104]。

然而，想要开发安全有效的外泌体疗法仍需克服一些困难，尤其是需要发展和充分理解最基础的外泌体生物学机制。我们进一步研究外泌体发挥生物学功能的机制，以及它们是如何选择性地靶向特定细胞。

肾小管是外泌体疗法的一个重要靶点。如上文所述，系统递送的外泌体会进入肾小管细胞，甚至能够优先转运到肾小管损伤部位。在啮齿动物模型上进行的相关原理验证研究表明，以这种方式输入外泌体可以在急性肾损伤的情况下起保护作用。肾小管细胞的病变是许多临床重要疾病的基础，包括各种形式的急性肾损伤和CKD[105-107]。然而，这种改善了结局的干预手段可能涉及协调细胞生理的多种复杂改变，如促进上皮细胞向间充质细胞转化[108]。由于外泌体能够递送多种活性物质，因此可以作为实现多种生理变化的理想手段。

外泌体可以以一种开创性的方式在临床上发挥有益作用。例如，促红细胞生成素可以促进骨髓细胞释放大量外泌体，从而可能实现对内源性外泌体释放的控制[83]，或者使用外泌体作为辅助治疗手段，以增强对常规药物的反应。例如，膀胱肿瘤细胞释放的微泡能够通过增加递送进入细胞核的药物来增强小鼠膀胱癌模型中的化疗效果[109]。

六、总结

肾脏和尿道中的外泌体与其他人体系统有颇多相似。我们逐步了解了控制外泌体释放和摄取的机制以及决定外泌体所含生物活性物质的因素（图11-1）。外泌体可以改变靶细胞功能，这可能是通过RNA、蛋白质和脂质等多种生物活性物质的递送实现的，其中miRNA可能起到关键作用。初步研究表明，外泌体有成为生物标志物和治疗药物的潜力，但目前尚未应用至临床实践中。

然而，肾和尿道中的外泌体也具有一些明显的特点。采用尿液作为外泌体的材料来源，我们仍需面对许多特殊的挑战和机遇。尿液的流动为我们提供了研究沿肾单位从近端到远端定向外泌体信号的条件。同时，外泌体能够通过循环系统进入泌尿器官，这为我们提供了详细探讨外泌体运输机制的模型器官——肾。

肾小管细胞从尿道和血管中吸收外泌体，而这一过程在一定程度上必然受生理调节（图11-1）。细胞对外泌体的摄取是饱和的，依赖于细胞表面受体，并受已知的肾小管细胞分泌的激素调控。肾小管细胞对外泌体的内化诱导产生细胞功能改变。肾小管细胞（在相同或远端的肾单位阶段）之间由外泌体介导的信号可以影响靶细胞的转运功能。同时，从干细胞传递至肾小管细胞的信号传递影响细胞的存活、增殖和对损伤的易感性（图11-2）。

目前，对外泌体的研究还处于起步阶段，仍有大量的问题亟须解答。本章末，我们在框11-1中列出了一些肾脏外泌体领域的亟须解决的问题。

框11-1　肾脏与尿路外泌体有待解决的相关问题

外泌体释放、摄取和运输的基本机制

- 外泌体的摄取是否具备特异性（包括外泌体和靶细胞的类型）？如果具备，这种特异性由何种机制解释？

- 外泌体释放的生理调节因子有哪些,这些因子在不同类型肾细胞中有区别吗?
- 不同类型肾细胞中外泌体摄取的生理调节因子是什么?外泌体如何从血管转运至泌尿系统?在肾小球或肾小管基底膜结构完整性受损的病理状态下,情况是否有所不同?

外泌体信号传导的机制

- 蛋白质和 RNA 等活性物质转运在肾脏外泌体信号通路的生物学功能中起到多大作用?
- 细胞表面外泌体的相互作用在外泌体信号通路的生物学功能中起到多大作用?

临床应用

- 如使用尿液外泌体作为生物标志物,最佳采样方法是什么(如何优化外泌体活性物质的获取成本、时间和稳定性)?
- 使用尿液外泌体作为生物标志物的潜在效用是否会在大型临床研究中得到证实?
- 外源性肠道外泌体如何用于肾脏疾病的治疗?
- 我们如何调节内源性外泌体信号以提高肾脏疾病的治疗效果?

(张光远　姚弛　译,王锋　审校)

参考文献

[1] Lötvall J, Hill AF, Hochberg F, Buzás EI, Di Vizio D, Gardiner C, Gho YS, Kurochkin IV, Mathivanan S, Quesenberry P, Sahoo S, Tahara H, Wauben MH, Witwer KW, Théry C. Minimal experimental requirements for definition of extracellular vesicles and their functions: a position statement from the International Society for Extracellular Vesicles. J Extracell Vesicles 2014; 3: 26913.

[2] Witwer KW, Buzás EI, Bemis LT, Bora A, Lässer C, Lötvall J, Nolte-'t Hoen EN, Piper MG, Sivaraman S, Skog J, Théry C, Wauben MH, Hochberg F. Standardization of sample collection, isolation and analysis methods in extracellular vesicle research. J Extracell Vesicles 2013; 2. https://doi.org/10.3402/jev.v2i0.20360.

[3] Erdbrugger U, Le TH. Extracellular vesicles in renal diseases: more than novel biomarkers? J Am Soc Nephrol 2015. https://doi.org/10.1681/ASN.2015010074.

[4] van Niel G, D'Angelo G, Raposo G. Shedding light on the cell biology of extracellular vesicles. Nat Rev Mol Cell Biol 2018; 19: 213-28. https://doi.org/10.1038/nrm.2017.125.

[5] Pisitkun T, Shen R-F, Knepper MA. Identification and proteomic profiling of exosomes in human urine. Proc Natl Acad Sci U S A 2004; 101: 13368-73. https://doi.org/10.1073/pnas.0403453101.

[6] Fernández-Llama P, Khositseth S, Gonzales PA, Star RA, Pisitkun T, Knepper MA. Tamm-Horsfall protein and urinary exosome isolation. Kidney Int 2010; 77: 736-42.

[7] Gonzales PA, Zhou H, Pisitkun T, Wang NS, Star RA, Knepper MA, Yuen PST. Isolation and purification of exosomes in urine. In: Rai AJ, editor. The urinary proteome. Totowa, NJ: Humana Press; 2010. p.89-99.

[8] Hogan MC, Manganelli L, Woollard JR, Masyuk AI, Masyuk TV, Tammachote R, Huang BQ, Leontovich AA, Beito TG, Madden BJ, Charlesworth MC, Torres VE, LaRusso NF, Harris PC, Ward CJ. Characterization of PKD protein-positive exosome-kike vesicles. J Am Soc Nephrol 2009; 20: 278-88. https://doi.org/10.1681/ASN.2008060564.

[9] Gonzales PA, Pisitkun T, Hoffert JD, Tchapyjnikov D, Star RA, Kleta R, Wang NS, Knepper MA. Large-scale proteomics and phosphoproteomics of urinary exosomes. J Am Soc Nephrol 2009; 20: 363-79. https://doi.org/10.1681/ASN.2008040406.

[10] Rood IM, Deegens JKJ, Merchant ML, Tamboer WPM, Wilkey DW, Wetzels JFM, Klein JB. Comparison of three methods for isolation of urinary microvesicles to identify biomarkers of nephrotic syndrome. Kidney Int 2010; 78: 810-6. https://doi.org/10.1038/ki.2010.262.

[11] Hogan MC, Johnson KL, Zenka RM, Charlesworth MC, Madden BJ, Mahoney DW, Oberg AL, Huang BQ, Leontovich AA, Nesbitt LL, et al. Subfractionation, characterization, and in-depth proteomic analysis of glomerular membrane vesicles in human urine. Kidney Int 2014; 85: 1225-37.

[12] Troyanov S, Delmas-Frenette C, Bollée G, Youhanna S, Bruat V, Awadalla P, Devuyst O, Madore F. Clinical,

genetic, and urinary factors associated with uromodulin excretion. Clin J Am Soc Nephrol 2016; 11: 62‑9. https://doi.org/10.2215/CJN.04770415.

[13] Alvarez ML, Khosroheidari M, Kanchi Ravi R, DiStefano JK. Comparison of protein, microRNA, and mRNA yields using different methods of urinary exosome isolation for the discovery of kidney disease biomarkers. Kidney Int 2012; 82: 1024‑32. https://doi.org/10.1038/ki.2012.256.

[14] Prunotto M, Farina A, Lane L, Pernin A, Schifferli J, Hochstrasser DF, Lescuyer P, Moll S. Proteomic analysis of podocyte exosome-enriched fraction from normal human urine. J Proteomics 2013; 82: 193‑229. https://doi.org/10.1016/j.jprot.2013.01.012.

[15] Vergauwen G, Dhondt B, Van Deun J, De Smedt E, Berx G, Timmerman E, Gevaert K, Miinalainen I, Cocquyt V, Braems G, Van den Broecke R, Denys H, De Wever O, Hendrix A. Confounding factors of ultrafiltration and protein analysis in extracellular vesicle research. Sci Rep 2017; 7: 2704. https://doi.org/10.1038/s41598-017-02599-y.

[16] Gerlach JQ, Krüger A, Gallogly S, Hanley SA, Hogan MC, Ward CJ, Joshi L, Griffin MD. Surface glycosylation profiles of urine extracellular vesicles. PLoS ONE 2013; 8: e74801. https://doi.org/10.1371/journal.pone.0074801.

[17] Zhou H, Yuen PS, Pisitkun T, Gonzales PA, Yasuda H, Dear JW, Gross P, Knepper MA, Star RA. Collection, storage, preservation, and normalization of human urinary exosomes for biomarker discovery. Kidney Int 2006; 69: 1471‑6.

[18] Zhou H, Cheruvanky A, Hu X, Matsumoto T, Hiramatsu N, Cho ME, Berger A, Leelahavanichkul A, Doi K, Chawla LS, et al. Urinary exosomal transcription factors, a new class of biomarkers for renal disease. Kidney Int 2008; 74: 613‑21.

[19] Miranda KC, Bond DT, McKee M, Skog J, Paunescu TG, Da Silva N, Brown D, Russo LM. Nucleic acids within urinary exosomes/microvesicles are potential biomarkers for renal disease. Kidney Int 2010; 78: 191‑9.

[20] Miranda KC, Bond DT, Levin JZ, Adiconis X, Sivachenko A, Russ C, Brown D, Nusbaum C, Russo LM. Massively parallel sequencing of human urinary exosome/microvesicle RNA reveals a predominance of non-coding RNA. PLoS ONE 2014; 9: e96094. https://doi.org/10.1371/journal.pone.0096094.

[21] Oosthuyzen W, Scullion KM, Ivy JR, Morrison EE, Hunter RW, Starkey Lewis PJ, O'Duibhir E, Street JM, Caporali A, Gregory CD, Forbes SJ, Webb DJ, Bailey MA, Dear JW. Vasopressin regulates extracellular vesicle uptake by kidney collecting duct cells. J Am Soc Nephrol 2016. https://doi.org/10.1681/ASN.2015050568.

[22] Gildea JJ, Seaton JE, Victor KG, Reyes CM, Bigler Wang D, Pettigrew AC, Courtner CE, Shah N, Tran HT, Van Sciver RE, Carlson JM, Felder RA. Exosomal transfer from human renal proximal tubule cells to distal tubule and collecting duct cells. Clin Biochem 2014; 47: 89‑94. https://doi.org/10.1016/j.clinbiochem.2014.06.018.

[23] Bruno S, Grange C, Deregibus MC, Calogero RA, Saviozzi S, Collino F, Morando L, Busca A, Falda M, Bussolati B, Tetta C, Camussi G. Mesenchymal stem cell-derived microvesicles protect against acute tubular injury. J Am Soc Nephrol 2009; 20: 1053‑67. https://doi.org/10.1681/ASN.2008070798.

[24] Lindoso RS, Collino F, Bruno S, Araujo DS, Sant'Anna JF, Tetta C, Provero P, Quesenberry PJ, Vieyra A, Einicker-Lamas M, Camussi G. Extracellular vesicles released from mesenchymal stromal cells modulate miRNA in renal tubular cells and inhibit ATP depletion injury. Stem Cells Dev 2014; 23: 1809‑19. https://doi.org/10.1089/scd.2013.0618.

[25] Hansell P, Göransson V, Odlind C, Gerdin B, Hällgren R. Hyaluronan content in the kidney in different states of body hydration. Kidney Int 2000; 58: 2061‑8. https://doi.org/10.1111/j.1523-1755.2000.00378.x.

[26] Herrera MB, Bussolati B, Bruno S, Morando L, Mauriello-Romanazzi G, Sanavio F, Stamenkovic I, Biancone L, Camussi G. Exogenous mesenchymal stem cells localize to the kidney by means of CD44 following acute tubular injury. Kidney Int 2007; 72: 430‑41. https://doi.org/10.1038/sj.ki.5002334.

[27] Munkonda MN, Akbari S, Landry C, Sun S, Xiao F, Turner M, Holterman CE, Nasrallah R, Hébert RL, Kennedy CRJ, Burger D. Podocyte-derived microparticles promote proximal tubule fibrotic signaling via p38 MAPK and CD36. J Extracell Vesicles 2018; 7: 1432206. https://doi.org/10.1080/20013078.2018.1432206.

[28] French KC, Antonyak MA, Cerione RA. Extracellular vesicle docking at the cellular port: extracellular vesicle binding and uptake. Semin Cell Dev Biol 2017; 67: 48‑55. https://doi.org/10.1016/j.semcdb.2017.01.002.

[29] Street JM, Birkhoff W, Menzies RI, Webb DJ, Bailey MA, Dear JW. Exosomal transmission of functional aquaporin 2 in kidney cortical collecting duct cells: exosome signalling in collecting duct. J Physiol 2011; 589: 6119‑27. https://doi.org/10.1113/jphysiol.2011.220277.

[30] Deregibus MC, Figliolini F, D'Antico S, Manzini PM, Pasquino C, De Lena M, Tetta C, Brizzi MF, Camussi G. Charge-based precipitation of extracellular vesicles. Int J Mol Med 2016; 38: 1359‑66. https://doi.org/10.3892/ijmm.2016.2759.

[31] Lawrence MG, Altenburg MK, Sanford R, Willett JD, Bleasdale B, Ballou B, Wilder J, Li F, Miner JH, Berg UB, Smithies O. Permeation of macromolecules into the renal glomerular basement membrane and capture by the tubules. Proc Natl Acad Sci U S A 2017; 114: 2958‑63. https://doi.org/10.1073/pnas.1616457114.

[32] Grange C, Tapparo M, Bruno S, Chatterjee D, Quesenberry PJ, Tetta C, Camussi G. Biodistribution of mesenchymal stem cell-derived extracellular vesicles in a model of acute kidney injury monitored by optical imaging. Int J Mol Med 2014; 33: 1055‑63. https://doi.org/10.3892/ijmm.2014.1663.

[33] Ståhl A, Arvidsson I, Johansson KE, Chromek M, Rebetz J, Loos S, Kristoffersson AC, Békássy ZD, Mörgelin M, Karpman D. A novel mechanism of bacterial toxin transfer within host blood cell-derived microvesicles. PLoS Pathog 2015; 11: e1004619. https://doi.org/10.1371/journal.ppat.1004619.

[34] Kanno K, Sasaki S, Hirata Y, Ishikawa S, Fushimi K, Nakanishi S, Bichet DG, Marumo F. Urinary excretion of aquaporin-2 in patients with diabetes insipidus. N Engl J Med 1995; 332: 1540‑5.

[35] Wen H, Frøkiær J, Kwon T-H, Nielsen S. Urinary excretion of aquaporin-2 in rat is mediated by a vasopressin-dependent apical pathway. J Am Soc Nephrol 1999; 10: 1416‑29.

[36] Higashijima Y, Sonoda H, Takahashi S, Kondo H, Shigemura K, Ikeda M. Excretion of urinary exosomal AQP2 in rats is regulated by vasopressin and urinary pH. Am J Physiol Renal Physiol 2013; 305: F1412‑21. https://doi.org/10.

1152/ajprenal. 00249. 2013.
[37] Corbetta S, Raimondo F, Tedeschi S, Syrèn M-L, Rebora P, Savoia A, Baldi L, Bettinelli A, Pitto M. Urinary exosomes in the diagnosis of Gitelman and Bartter syndromes. Nephrol Dial Transplant Off Publ Eur Dial Transpl Assoc—Eur Ren Assoc 2015; 30: 621 – 30. https://doi.org/10.1093/ndt/gfu362.
[38] Joo KW, Lee JW, Jang HR, Heo NJ, Jeon US, Oh YK, Lim CS, Na KY, Kim J, Cheong HI, Han JS. Reduced urinary excretion of thiazide-sensitive Na-Cl cotransporter in Gitelman syndrome: preliminary data. Am J Kidney Dis 2007; 50: 765 – 73. https://doi.org/10.1053/j. ajkd.2007.07.022.
[39] Mayan H, Attar-Herzberg D, Shaharabany M, Holtzman EJ, Farfel Z. Increased urinary Na-Cl cotransporter protein in familial hyperkalaemia and hypertension. Nephrol Dial Transplant 2008; 23: 492 – 6. https://doi.org/10.1093/ndt/gfm641.
[40] Esteva-Font C, Wang X, Ars E, Guillén-Gómez E, Sans L, González Saavedra I, Torres F, Torra R, Masilamani S, Ballarín JA, Fernández-Llama P. Are sodium transporters in urinary exosomes reliable markers of tubular sodium reabsorption in hypertensive patients? Nephron Physiol 2010; 114. https://doi.org/10.1159/000274468. p 25 – p 34.
[41] van der Lubbe N, Jansen PM, Salih M, Fenton RA, van den Meiracker AH, Danser AJ, Zietse R, Hoorn EJ. The phosphorylated sodium chloride cotransporter in urinary exosomes is superior to prostasin as a marker for aldosteronism. Hypertension 2012; 60: 741 – 8.
[42] Esteva-Font C, Guillén-Gómez E, Diaz JM, Guirado L, Facundo C, Ars E, Ballarin JA, Fernández-Llama P. Renal sodium transporters are increased in urinary exosomes of cyclosporine-treated kidney transplant patients. Am J Nephrol 2014; 39: 528 – 35. https://doi.org/10.1159/000362905.
[43] Pathare G, Tutakhel OAZ, van der Wel MC, Shelton LM, Deinum J, Lenders JWM, Hoenderop JGJ, Bindels RJM. Hydrochlorothiazide treatment increases the abundance of the NaCl cotransporter in urinary extracellular vesicles of essential hypertensive patients. Am J Physiol Renal Physiol 2017; 312: F1063 – 72. https://doi.org/10.1152/ajprenal.00644.2016.
[44] Tutakhel OAZ, Moes AD, Valdez-Flores MA, Kortenoeven MLA, Vrie MvD, Jeleń S, Fenton RA, Zietse R, Hoenderop JGJ, Hoorn EJ, Hilbrands L, Bindels RJM. NaCl cotransporter abundance in urinary vesicles is increased by calcineurin inhibitors and predicts thiazide sensitivity. PLoS ONE 2017; 12: e0176220. https://doi.org/10.1371/journal.pone.0176220.
[45] Castagna A, Pizzolo F, Chiecchi L, Morandini F, Channavajjhala SK, Guarini P, Salvagno G, Olivieri O. Circadian exosomal expression of renal thiazide-sensitive NaCl cotransporter (NCC) and prostasin in healthy individuals. Proteomics Clin Appl 2015; 9: 623 – 9. https://doi.org/10.1002/prca.201400198.
[46] Ivy JR, Oosthuyzen W, Peltz TS, Howarth AR, Hunter RW, Dhaun N, Al-Dujaili EAS, Webb DJ, Dear JW, Flatman PW, Bailey MA. Glucocorticoids induce nondipping blood pressure by activating the thiazide-sensitive cotransporter. Hypertension 2016; 67: 1029 – 37. https://doi.org/10.1161/HYPERTENSIONAHA.115.06977.
[47] Pathare G, Dhayat N, Mohebbi N, Wagner CA, Cheval L, Neuhaus TJ, Fuster DG. Acute regulated expression of pendrin in human urinary exosomes. Pflugers Arch 2018; 470: 427 – 38. https://doi.org/10.1007/s00424-017-2049-0.
[48] Pathare G, Dhayat NA, Mohebbi N, Wagner CA, Bobulescu IA, Moe OW, Fuster DG. Changes in V-ATPase subunits of human urinary exosomes reflect the renal response to acute acid/alkali loading and the defects in distal renal tubular acidosis. Kidney Int 2018; 93: 871 – 80. https://doi.org/10.1016/j.kint.2017.10.018.
[49] Oliveira RA, Diniz LF, Teotônio LO, Lima CG, Mota RM, Martins A, Sanches TR, Seguro AC, Andrade L, Silva GB, et al. Renal tubular dysfunction in patients with American cutaneous leishmaniasis. Kidney Int 2011; 80: 1099 – 106.
[50] Hunter RW, Moorhouse R, Farrah TE, MacIntyre IM, Asai T, Gallacher PJ, Kerr D, Melville V, Czopek A, Morrison EE, Ivy JR, Dear JW, Bailey MA, Goddard J, Webb DJ, Dhaun N. First-in-man demonstration of direct endothelin-mediated natriuresis and diuresis. Hypertension 2017; 70(1): 192 – 200. https://doi.org/10.1161/HYPERTENSIONAHA.116.08832.
[51] Channavajjhala SK, Bramley R, Peltz T, Oosthuyzen W, Jia W, Kinnear S, Sampson B, Martin N, Hall IP, Bailey MA, Dear JW, Glover M. Urinary extracellular vesicle protein profiling and endogenous lithium clearance support excessive renal sodium wasting and water reabsorption in thiazide-induced hyponatremia. Kidney Int Rep 2018; 4(1): 139 – 47. https://doi.org/10.1016/j.ekir.2018.09.011.
[52] Burger D, Thibodeau J-F, Holterman CE, Burns KD, Touyz RM, Kennedy CRJ. Urinary podocyte microparticles identify prealbuminuric diabetic glomerular injury. J Am Soc Nephrol 2014; 25: 1401 – 7. https://doi.org/10.1681/ASN.2013070763.
[53] Gilani SI, Anderson UD, Jayachandran M, Weissgerber TL, Zand L, White WM, Milic N, Suarez MLG, Vallapureddy RR, Nääv Å, Erlandsson L, Lieske JC, Grande JP, Nath KA, Hansson SR, Garovic VD. Urinary extracellular vesicles of podocyte origin and renal injury in preeclampsia. J Am Soc Nephrol 2017; 28: 3363 – 72. https://doi.org/10.1681/ASN.2016111202.
[54] Lytvyn Y, Xiao F, Kennedy CRJ, Perkins BA, Reich HN, Scholey JW, Cherney DZ, Burger D. Assessment of urinary microparticles in normotensive patients with type 1 diabetes. Diabetologia 2017; 60: 581 – 4. https://doi.org/10.1007/s00125-016-4190-2.
[55] Dimuccio V, Ranghino A, Praticò Barbato L, Fop F, Biancone L, Camussi G, Bussolati B. Urinary CD133 + extracellular vesicles are decreased in kidney transplanted patients with slow graft function and vascular damage. PLoS ONE 2014; 9: e104490. https://doi.org/10.1371/journal.pone.0104490.
[56] Ranghino A, Dimuccio V, Papadimitriou E, Bussolati B. Extracellular vesicles in the urine: markers and mediators of tissue damage and regeneration. Clin Kidney J 2015; 8: 23 – 30. https://doi.org/10.1093/ckj/sfu136.
[57] Xie Y, Jia Y, Cuihua X, Hu F, Xue M, Xue Y. Urinary exosomal microRNA profiling in incipient type 2 diabetic kidney disease. J Diabetes Res 2017; 2017: 6978984. https://doi.org/10.1155/2017/6978984.
[58] Kamińska A, Platt M, Kasprzyk J, Kuśnierz-Cabala B, Gala-Błądzińska A, Woźnicka O, Jany BR, Krok F,

[59] Piekoszewski W, Kuźniewski M, Stępień EŁ. Urinary extracellular vesicles: potential biomarkers of renal function in diabetic patients. J Diabetes Res 2016; 2016: 5741518. https://doi.org/10.1155/2016/5741518.

[60] Zubiri I, Posada-Ayala M, Benito-Martin A, Maroto AS, Martin-Lorenzo M, Cannata-Ortiz P, de la Cuesta F, Gonzalez-Calero L, Barderas MG, Fernandez-Fernandez B, Ortiz A, Vivanco F, Alvarez-Llamas G. Kidney tissue proteomics reveals regucalcin downregulation in response to diabetic nephropathy with reflection in urinary exosomes. Transl Res 2015; 166: 474-484.e4. https://doi.org/10.1016/j.trsl.2015.05.007.

[61] Zhou H, Kajiyama H, Tsuji T, Hu X, Leelahavanichkul A, Vento S, Frank R, Kopp JB, Trachtman H, Star RA, Yuen PST. Urinary exosomal Wilms' tumor-1 as a potential biomarker for podocyte injury. Am J Physiol Renal Physiol 2013; 305: F553-9. https://doi.org/10.1152/ajprenal.00056.2013.

[62] Moon P-G, Lee J-E, You S, Kim T-K, Cho J-H, Kim I-S, Kwon T-H, Kim C-D, Park S-H, Hwang D, Kim Y-L, Baek M-C. Proteomic analysis of urinary exosomes from patients of early IgA nephropathy and thin basement membrane nephropathy. Proteomics 2011; 11: 2459-75. https://doi.org/10.1002/pmic.201000443.

[63] Gutwein P, Schramme A, Abdel-Bakky MS, Doberstein K, Hauser IA, Ludwig A, Altevogt P, Gauer S, Hillmann A, Weide T, Jespersen C, Eberhardt W, Pfeilschifter J. ADAM10 is expressed in human podocytes and found in urinary vesicles of patients with glomerular kidney diseases. J Biomed Sci 2010; 17: 3. https://doi.org/10.1186/1423-0127-17-3.

[64] Perez-Hernandez J, Forner MJ, Pinto C, Chaves FJ, Cortes R, Redon J. Increased urinary exosomal microRNAs in patients with systemic lupus erythematosus. PLoS ONE 2015; 10: e0138618. https://doi.org/10.1371/journal.pone.0138618.

[65] Zhou H, Pisitkun T, Aponte A, Yuen PST, Hoffert JD, Yasuda H, Hu X, Chawla L, Shen RF, Knepper MA, Star RA. Exosomal Fetuin-A identified by proteomics: a novel urinary biomarker for detecting acute kidney injury. Kidney Int 2006; 70: 1847-57. https://doi.org/10.1038/sj.ki.5001874.

[66] Benito-Martin A, Ucero AC, Zubiri I, Posada-Ayala M, Fernandez-Fernandez B, Cannata-Ortiz P, Sanchez-Nino MD, Ruiz-Ortega M, Egido J, Alvarez-Llamas G, Ortiz A. Osteoprotegerin in exosome-kike vesicles from human cultured tubular cells and urine. PLoS ONE 2013; 8: e72387. https://doi.org/10.1371/journal.pone.0072387.

[67] Khurana R, Ranches G, Schafferer S, Lukasser M, Rudnicki M, Mayer G, Hüttenhofer A. Identification of urinary exosomal noncoding RNAs as novel biomarkers in chronic kidney disease. RNA 2017; 23: 142-52. https://doi.org/10.1261/rna.058834.116.

[68] Kwon SH, Woollard JR, Saad A, Garovic VD, Zand L, Jordan KL, Textor SC, Lerman LO. Elevated urinary podocyte-derived extracellular microvesicles in renovascular hypertensive patients. Nephrol Dial Transplant 2017; 32: 800-7. https://doi.org/10.1093/ndt/gfw077.

[69] Damkjaer M, Jensen PH, Schwämmle V, Sprenger RR, Jacobsen IA, Jensen ON, Bie P. Selective renal vasoconstriction, exaggerated natriuresis and excretion rates of exosomic proteins in essential hypertension. Acta Physiol (Oxf) 2014; 212: 106-18. https://doi.org/10.1111/apha.12345.

[70] Alvarez S, Suazo C, Boltansky A, Ursu M, Carvajal D, Innocenti G, Vukusich A, Hurtado M, Villanueva S, Carreño JE, Rogelio A, Irarrazabal CE. Urinary exosomes as a source of kidney dysfunction biomarker in renal transplantation. Transplant Proc 2013; 45: 3719-23. https://doi.org/10.1016/j.transproceed.2013.08.079.

[71] Pisitkun T, Gandolfo MT, Das S, Knepper MA, Bagnasco SM. Application of systems biology principles to protein biomarker discovery: urinary exosomal proteome in renal transplantation. Proteomics Clin Appl 2012; 6: 268-78. https://doi.org/10.1002/prca.201100108.

[72] Sigdel TK, Ng YW, Lee S, Nicora CD, Qian W-J, Smith RD, Camp DG, Sarwal MM. Perturbations in the urinary exosome in transplant rejection. Front Med 2015; 1. https://doi.org/10.3389/fmed.2014.00057.

[73] Merchant ML, Rood IM, Deegens JKJ, Klein JB. Isolation and characterization of urinary extracellular vesicles: implications for biomarker discovery. Nat Rev Nephrol 2017; 13: 731-49. https://doi.org/10.1038/nrneph.2017.148.

[74] Spanu S, van Roeyen CRC, Denecke B, Floege J, Mühlfeld AS. Urinary exosomes: a novel means to non-invasively assess changes in renal gene and protein expression. PLoS ONE 2014; 9: e109631. https://doi.org/10.1371/journal.pone.0109631.

[75] He J, Wang Y, Sun S, Yu M, Wang C, Pei X, Zhu B, Wu J, Zhao W. Bone marrow stem cells-derived microvesicles protect against renal injury in the mouse remnant kidney model. Nephrology (Carlton) 2012; 17: 493-500. https://doi.org/10.1111/j.1440-1797.2012.01589.x.

[76] Zhang G, Zou X, Miao S, Chen J, Du T, Zhong L, Ju G, Liu G, Zhu Y. The anti-oxidative role of micro-vesicles derived from human Wharton-Jelly mesenchymal stromal cells through NOX2/gp91(phox) suppression in alleviating renal ischemia-reperfusion injury in rats. PLoS ONE 2014; 9: e92129. https://doi.org/10.1371/journal.pone.0092129.

[77] Ju G, Cheng J, Zhong L, Wu S, Zou X, Zhang G, Gu D, Miao S, Zhu Y, Sun J, Du T. Microvesicles derived from human umbilical cord mesenchymal stem cells facilitate tubular epithelial cell dedifferentiation and growth via hepatocyte growth factor induction. PLoS One 2015; 10: e0121534. https://doi.org/10.1371/journal.pone.0121534.

[78] He J, Wang Y, Lu X, Zhu B, Pei X, Wu J, Zhao W. Micro-vesicles derived from bone marrow stem cells protect the kidney both in vivo and in vitro by microRNA-dependent repairing. Nephrology (Carlton) 2015; 20: 591-600. https://doi.org/10.1111/nep.12490.

[79] Collino F, Bruno S, Incarnato D, Dettori D, Neri F, Provero P, Pomatto M, Oliviero S, Tetta C, Quesenberry PJ, Camussi G. AKI recovery induced by mesenchymal stromal cellderived extracellular vesicles carrying microRNAs. J Am Soc Nephrol 2015; 26: 2349-60. https://doi.org/10.1681/ASN.2014070710.

[80] Wang B, Yao K, Huuskes BM, Shen H-H, Zhuang J, Godson C, Brennan EP, Wilkinson-Berka JL, Wise AF, Ricardo SD. Mesenchymal stem cells deliver exogenous microRNA-ket7c via exosomes to attenuate renal fibrosis. Mol Ther 2016; 24: 1290-301. https://doi.org/10.1038/mt.2016.90.

[81] Bruno S, Tapparo M, Collino F, Chiabotto G, Deregibus MC, Soares Lindoso R, Neri F, Kholia S, Giunti S, Wen S, Quesenberry P, Camussi G. Renal regenerative potential of different extracellular vesicle populations derived from bone marrow mesenchymal stromal cells. Tissue Eng Part A 2017; 23: 1262-73. https://doi.org/10.1089/ten.TEA.

2017.0069.

[81] Eirin A, Zhu X-Y, Puranik AS, Tang H, McGurren KA, van Wijnen AJ, Lerman A, Lerman LO. Mesenchymal stem cell-derived extracellular vesicles attenuate kidney inflammation. Kidney Int 2017; 92: 114–24. https://doi.org/10.1016/j.kint.2016.12.023.

[82] Gallo S, Gili M, Lombardo G, Rossetti A, Rosso A, Dentelli P, Togliatto G, Deregibus MC, Taverna D, Camussi G, Brizzi MF. Stem cell-derived, microRNA-carrying extracellular vesicles: a novel approach to interfering with mesangial cell collagen production in a hyperglycaemic setting. PLoS One 2016; 11: e0162417. https://doi.org/10.1371/journal.pone.0162417.

[83] Zhou Y, Fang L, Yu Y, Niu J, Jiang L, Cao H, Sun Q, Zen K, Dai C, Yang J. Erythropoietin protects the tubular basement membrane by promoting the bone marrow to release extracellular vesicles containing tPA-targeting miR-144. Am J Physiol Renal Physiol 2016; 310: F27–40. https://doi.org/10.1152/ajprenal.00303.2015.

[84] Cantaluppi V, Gatti S, Medica D, Figliolini F, Bruno S, Deregibus MC, Sordi A, Biancone L, Tetta C, Camussi G. Microvesicles derived from endothelial progenitor cells protect the kidney from ischemia-reperfusion injury by microRNA-dependent reprogramming of resident renal cells. Kidney Int 2012; 82: 412–27. https://doi.org/10.1038/ki.2012.105.

[85] Cantaluppi V, Medica D, Mannari C, Stiaccini G, Figliolini F, Dellepiane S, Quercia AD, Migliori M, Panichi V, Giovannini L, Bruno S, Tetta C, Biancone L, Camussi G. Endothelial progenitor cell-derived extracellular vesicles protect from complement-mediated mesangial injury in experimental anti-Thy1.1 glomerulonephritis. Nephrol Dial Transplant Off Publ Eur Dial Transpl Assoc — Eur Ren Assoc 2015; 30: 410–22. https://doi.org/10.1093/ndt/gfu364.

[86] Gracia T, Wang X, Su Y, Norgett EE, Williams TL, Moreno P, Micklem G, Karet Frankl FE. Urinary exosomes contain microRNAs capable of paracrine modulation of tubular transporters in kidney. Sci Rep 2017; 7: 40601. https://doi.org/10.1038/srep40601.

[87] Dominguez JH, Liu Y, Gao H, Dominguez JM, Xie D, Kelly KJ. Renal tubular cell-derived extracellular vesicles accelerate the recovery of established renal ischemia reperfusion injury. J Am Soc Nephrol 2017; 28: 3533–44. https://doi.org/10.1681/ASN.2016121278.

[88] Zhang W, Zhou X, Yao Q, Liu Y, Zhang H, Dong Z. HIF-1-mediated production of exosomes during hypoxia is protective in renal tubular cells. Am J Physiol Renal Physiol 2017; 313: F906–13. https://doi.org/10.1152/ajprenal.00178.2017.

[89] Zhang G, Yang Y, Huang Y, Zhang L, Ling Z, Zhu Y, Wang F, Zou X, Chen M. Hypoxia-induced extracellular vesicles mediate protection of remote ischemic preconditioning for renal ischemia-reperfusion injury. Biomed Pharmacother 2017; 90: 473–8. https://doi.org/10.1016/j.biopha.2017.03.096.

[90] Zhou X, Zhang W, Yao Q, Zhang H, Dong G, Zhang M, Liu Y, Chen J-K, Dong Z. Exosome production and its regulation of EGFR during wound healing in renal tubular cells. Am J Physiol Renal Physiol 2017; 312: F963–70. https://doi.org/10.1152/ajprenal.00078.2017.

[91] Jella KK, Yu L, Yue Q, Friedman D, Duke BJ, Alli AA. Exosomal GAPDH from proximal tubule cells regulate ENaC activity. PLoS One 2016; 11: e0165763. https://doi.org/10.1371/journal.pone.0165763.

[92] Chen H-H, Lai P-F, Lan Y-F, Cheng C-F, Zhong W-B, Lin Y-F, Chen T-W, Lin H. Exosomal ATF3 RNA attenuates pro-inflammatory gene MCP-1 transcription in renal ischemia-reperfusion. J Cell Physiol 2014; 229: 1202–11. https://doi.org/10.1002/jcp.24554.

[93] Eyre J, Burton JO, Saleem MA, Mathieson PW, Topham PS, Brunskill NJ. Monocyte- and endothelial-derived microparticles induce an inflammatory phenotype in human podocytes. Nephron Exp Nephrol 2011; 119: e58–66. https://doi.org/10.1159/000329575.

[94] Wang Y-Y, Tang L-Q, Wei W. Berberine attenuates podocytes injury caused by exosomes derived from high glucose-induced mesangial cells through TGFβ1-PI3K/AKT pathway. Eur J Pharmacol 2018; 824: 185–92. https://doi.org/10.1016/j.ejphar.2018.01.034.

[95] Kahn R, Mossberg M, Ståhl A-L, Johansson K, Lopatko Lindman I, Heijl C, Segelmark M, Mörgelin M, Leeb-Lundberg LMF, Karpman D. Microvesicle transfer of kinin B1-receptors is a novel inflammatory mechanism in vasculitis. Kidney Int 2017; 91: 96–105. https://doi.org/10.1016/j.kint.2016.09.023.

[96] Chiabotto G, Bruno S, Collino F, Camussi G. Mesenchymal stromal cells epithelial transition induced by renal tubular cells-derived extracellular vesicles. PLoS ONE 2016; 11: e0159163. https://doi.org/10.1371/journal.pone.0159163.

[97] Lv L-L, Feng Y, Wen Y, Wu W-J, Ni H-F, Li Z-L, Zhou L-T, Wang B, Zhang J-D, Crowley SD, Liu B-C. Exosomal CCL2 from tubular epithelial cells is critical for albumin-induced tubulointerstitial inflammation. J Am Soc Nephrol 2018; 29: 919–35. https://doi.org/10.1681/ASN.2017050523.

[98] Miyazawa Y, Mikami S, Yamamoto K, Sakai M, Saito T, Yamamoto T, Ishibashi K, Sasaki S. AQP2 in human urine is predominantly localized to exosomes with preserved water channel activities. Clin Exp Nephrol 2018; 22: 782–8. https://doi.org/10.1007/s10157-018-1538-6.

[99] Torres Crigna A, Daniele C, Gamez C, Medina Balbuena S, Pastene DO, Nardozi D, Brenna C, Yard B, Gretz N, Bieback K. Stem/stromal cells for treatment of kidney injuries with focus on preclinical models. Front Med 2018; 5. https://doi.org/10.3389/fmed.2018.00179.

[100] Hiemstra TF, Charles PD, Gracia T, Hester SS, Gatto L, Al-Lamki R, Floto RA, Su Y, Skepper JN, Lilley KS, Karet Frankl FE. Human urinary exosomes as innate immune effectors. J Am Soc Nephrol 2014; 25: 2017–27. https://doi.org/10.1681/ASN.2013101066.

[101] Twu O, de Miguel N, Lustig G, Stevens GC, Vashisht AA, Wohlschlegel JA, Johnson PJ. Trichomonas vaginalis exosomes deliver cargo to host cells and mediate host: parasite interactions. PLoS Pathog 2013; 9: e1003482. https://doi.org/10.1371/journal.ppat.1003482.

[102] Coakley G, Maizels RM, Buck AH. Exosomes and other extracellular vesicles: the new communicators in parasite infections. Trends Parasitol 2015; 31: 477–89. https://doi.org/10.1016/j.pt.2015.06.009.

[103] Robbins PD, Dorronsoro A, Booker CN. Regulation of chronic inflammatory and immune processes by extracellular vesicles. J Clin Invest 2016; 126: 1173-80. https://doi.org/10.1172/JCI81131.

[104] Kamerkar S, LeBleu VS, Sugimoto H, Yang S, Ruivo CF, Melo SA, Lee JJ, Kalluri R. Exosomes facilitate therapeutic targeting of oncogenic KRAS in pancreatic cancer. Nature 2017; 546: 498-503. https://doi.org/10.1038/nature22341.

[105] Chevalier RL. The proximal tubule is the primary target of injury and progression of kidney disease: role of the glomerulotubular junction. Am J Physiol Renal Physiol 2016; 311: F145-61. https://doi.org/10.1152/ajprenal.00164.2016.

[106] Ferenbach DA, Bonventre JV. Mechanisms of maladaptive repair after AKI leading to accelerated kidney ageing and CKD. Nat Rev Nephrol 2015; 11: 264-76. https://doi.org/10.1038/nrneph.2015.3.

[107] Kramann R, Kusaba T, Humphreys BD. Who regenerates the kidney tubule? Nephrol Dial Transplant 2015; 30: 903-10. https://doi.org/10.1093/ndt/gfu281.

[108] Lovisa S, LeBleu VS, Tampe B, Sugimoto H, Vadnagara K, Carstens JL, Wu C-C, Hagos Y, Burckhardt BC, Pentcheva-Hoang T, Nischal H, Allison JP, Zeisberg M, Kalluri R. Epithelial-to-mesenchymal transition induces cell cycle arrest and parenchymal damage in renal fibrosis. Nat Med 2015; 21: 998-1009. https://doi.org/10.1038/nm.3902.

[109] Jin X, Ma J, Liang X, Tang K, Liu Y, Yin X, Zhang Y, Zhang H, Xu P, Chen D, Zhang T, Lu J, Hu Z, Qin X, Zeng X, Li L, Huang B. Pre-instillation of tumor microparticles enhances intravesical chemotherapy of nonmuscle-invasive bladder cancer through a lysosomal pathway. Biomaterials 2017; 113: 93-104. https://doi.org/10.1016/j.biomaterials.2016.10.036.

第12章

神经退行性疾病中的胞外囊泡
Extracellular vesicles in neurodegenerative disorders

Imre Mäger[a], Eduard Willms[a], Scott Bonner[a], Andrew F. Hill[b], Matthew J. A. Wood[a]

[a]University of Oxford, Department of Paediatrics, Oxford, United Kingdom, [b]La Trobe University, La Trobe Institute for Molecular Science, Melbourne, VIC, Australia

一、概述

在中枢神经系统（central nervous system，CNS）中，EV 是信号和通信网络的重要组成部分，这有助于确保大脑的正常生理功能。与其他细胞间信号传感器相比（如神经递质、神经营养因子、激素和细胞因子），在相同的脂质双层包裹中，EV 含有大量不同的信号分子。在其生物发生期间，EV 充满了生物活性蛋白（受体和配体）、脂质和遗传物质（编码和非编码RNA），在本书的其他章节中对此有详细的讨论和全面的回顾[1,2]。

有多种因素决定分泌型 EV 的内容，从而决定其潜在的生物学功能（图 12-1）。首要的是，尽管与母细胞相比，许多物质在 EV 内都特别富集，但 EV 在一定程度上反映了它们的起源细胞。当然，这并不奇怪，因为细胞只能将特定细胞类型本身的物质装入 EV 内。但是，根据细胞状态和应激条件，不仅在基因表达谱中，而且在细胞器的细胞内转运中，以及在不同生物过程（如泛素-蛋白酶体系统、自噬和蛋白质翻译后修饰）的激活/失活中，都可能有巨大的变化。后者反过来可以通过 EV 分泌途径的变化影响 EV 的组成（如膜出芽与通过内溶酶体系统的分泌，通过胚胎干细胞依赖途径与神经酰胺依赖途径的分泌等）。最近的研究非常清楚地表明，由一种细胞类型分泌的 EV 的异质性水平可能非常大[1,3,4]，并且许多不同的 EV 亚群可以仅基于 EV 的流体力学大小来定义[3,5-7]，包括被称为外泌颗粒的无膜小颗粒[4]，而功能多样性可以存在于这些大小定义的 EV 亚群中[5,8-10]。这意味着由于压力或其他细胞外刺激，通过在不同的分泌模式之间切换，分泌型 EV 的总组成可能会发生很大变化。

应该强调的是，CNS 中 EV 的细胞间通信网络与其他信号转导分子的网络同时发挥作用。因此，最终的通信网络可能非常复杂，尤其是因为它涉及许多不同的细胞类型，包括旁分泌和自分泌信号（图 12-2）。然而，研究整个多因素 EV-中介的通信网络是非常具有挑战性的，许多当前的工作试图解决这种复杂性。

关于 EV 介导 CNS 信号网络重要性的大多数证据可能来自对不同疾病的研究。在一系列神经退行性疾病中（如阿尔茨海默病、帕金森病、多发性硬化、肌萎缩侧索硬化和朊病毒病），EV 已经被证明或建议可以调节病理的不同方面，本章将重点介绍这些疾病（图 12-3）。

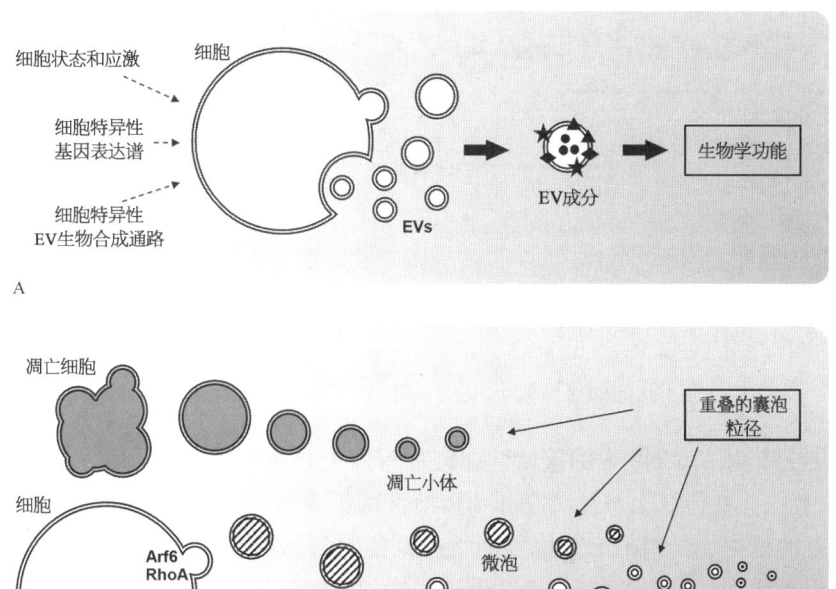

图 12-1　A. EV 的生物学功能由 EV 组成决定，而 EV 组成又受其产生的细胞类型、细胞状态和应激环境的特异性基因表达谱以及被激活的细胞特异性 EV 亚型生物发生途径的影响。B. 一个特定的细胞可以分泌许多具有不同生物发生途径的不同 EV 亚群。虽然微泡是由细胞膜直接向外出芽产生，但外泌体的释放与多泡体和溶酶体内途径的其他成分的转运有关。此外，还存在几个外泌体亚群，通常由它们的流体动力学直径区别。然而，仅根据大小区分 EV 亚群是一项困难的任务，因为不同囊泡类型之间可能有相当大的重叠

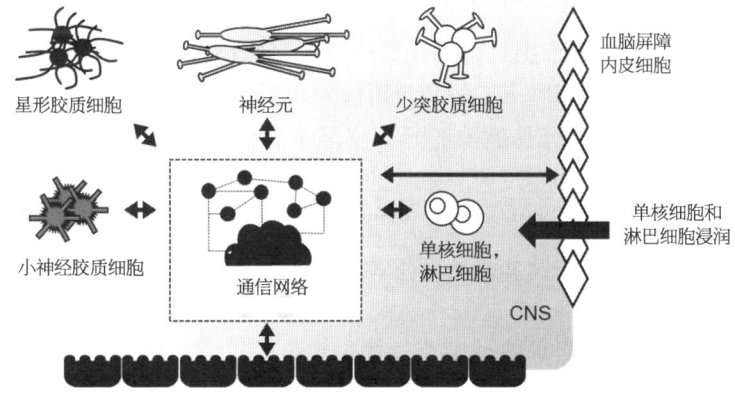

图 12-2　EV 由 CNS 的多种细胞类型分泌，包括常驻细胞（如星形胶质细胞、神经元、少突胶质细胞和小胶质细胞）、血脑屏障和血 CSF 屏障细胞（即脑微血管内皮细胞和脉络丛上皮细胞），以及疾病中浸润的单核细胞和淋巴细胞。多种来源的 EV 能够以旁分泌和自分泌的方式发挥作用，从而形成一个复杂的通信网络，各个细胞成分之间具有多种相互作用，在许多病理条件下可能会解除调节

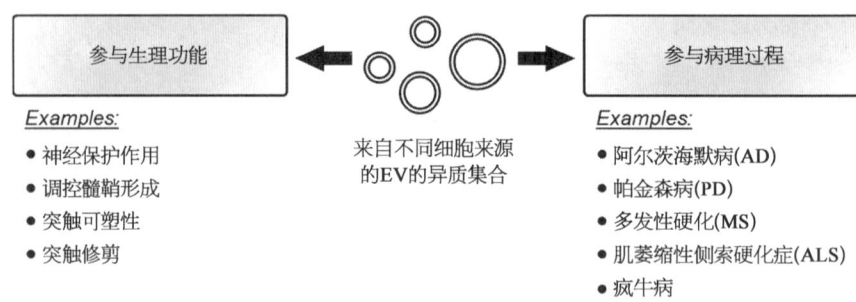

图12-3 几乎所有CNS细胞类型的EV都参与了一系列神经退行性疾病的病理过程。另一方面,EV也是系统的重要组成部分,保证中枢神经生理功能的正常运作。在不同的疾病模型中,这些特性已被尝试开发EV来促进CNS修复

EV在维持健康的CNS中的重要性在某种程度上是难以研究的,部分原因是现在已经证明EV含有一些在传统上被认为是作为可溶性因子或形态形成因子分泌的载物分子。然而,越来越多的证据也强调了EV信号网络在维持正常生理过程中的重要性。在下面的章节中,我们将更详细地讨论EV在CNS生理和病理中的作用。

二、胞外囊泡介导健康的中枢神经系统维护

关于EV参与CNS生理学的大量证据来自对神经元细胞的研究。神经元来源的EV本身和由许多不同类型胶质细胞分泌的EV均可调节或支持神经元的功能。例如,少突胶质细胞,一种参与轴突髓鞘形成的胶质细胞,以Ca^{2+}依赖的方式分泌EV,这是由神经递质谷氨酸[11]触发的。因此,神经元活性导致少突胶质细胞EV的分泌增加,从而通过超氧化物歧化酶、过氧化氢酶[12]或其他酶的转移,增加神经元[11]的代谢活性,从而在氧化应激和饥饿条件下对神经元提供保护。少突胶质细胞EV除具有神经保护作用外,还可增加神经元放电速率,调节细胞信号通路和基因表达,影响正常神经元生理[12]。

然而,应该强调的是,神经元并不是唯一可以与少突胶质细胞EV相互作用的细胞类型。例如,一组选定的小胶质细胞可以内化和降解少突胶质细胞EV[13],这可能表明可用于调节神经元功能的少突胶质细胞EV的数量可能取决于小胶质细胞的活性。此外,为使EV介导的信号网络进一步复杂化,其他神经元分泌因子反而可以抑制少突胶质细胞EV的生成[14],这与上文解释的谷氨酸[14]反应中EV的分泌增加相反。这种抑制性细胞通信途径似乎与少突胶质细胞通过分泌自抑制性EV产生髓鞘的自动调节作用有关[14],而不是神经元对应激的保护作用。神经保护性和髓鞘产生调节性少突胶质细胞EV之间的确切差异仍有待确定。

虽然小胶质细胞可以清除其他细胞分泌的EV,但同时也可以分泌自己的EV,这对靶细胞产生功能上的影响。例如,一群含内源性大麻素的小胶质细胞能抑制γ-氨基丁酸(γ-aminobutyric acid,GABA)能神经元的突触前传递[14]。另一方面,小胶质细胞响应ATP分泌的EV可以增加神经元细胞的兴奋性活性,包括通过调节鞘脂代谢增加谷氨酸的胞吐作用[15,16]。值得注意的是,由于鞘脂代谢途径也参与EV的分泌,因此阐明EV介导的小胶质细胞-神经元如何相互作用进入囊泡介导的CNS细胞通信网络的其他部分,如上文讨论

的针对应激条件的保护,将是重要的。

除了髓鞘形成、抗应激和神经元活动的调节,CNS 的 EV 还参与突触可塑性的调节。调节突触可塑性的能力主要归因于神经元分泌的 EV。在它们的生物发生过程中,神经元 EV 装载了多种与可塑性直接相关的货物分子,如 Arc 蛋白[17,18]、AMPA 受体[19]、Wnt 家族信号蛋白[20-24]、ephrins[25]、音猬因子(sonic hedgehog,SHH)[26,27]和 Syt4[28]。虽然后一种 EV 结合分子是分泌的,主要通过突触和神经肌肉接头起作用,以支持它们在神经元可塑性中的功能,但当与小胶质细胞相互作用时,其他神经元 EV 成分似乎反而会触发突触消除(即突触修剪)。这一过程似乎与小胶质细胞吞噬神经突起的活性增加有关,可能以补体成分 C3 依赖的方式[29]。但是,这种信号分子在突触间的传递和(或)呈现促进了可塑性相关的分子和表型效应,需要进行更多的工作来更好地理解 EV 在整个生物体水平上调节突触可塑性的作用,如在调节记忆、学习和其他顶级过程中。

上面的例子只代表了在维持 CNS 正常生理方面 EV 可能发挥了一定的作用。如前所述,EV 通信是复杂的,因为它取决于所涉及细胞类型的整体状态和激活状态(图 12-1 和图 12-2)。因此,在病理条件下(图 12-3),当产生 EV 的细胞有缺陷、过度激活或以其他方式调节不当时,EV 在 CNS 中的许多功能被更清楚地揭示。这些功能将在下文中讨论,重点是 EV 在与 CNS 病理中的参与。

三、神经退行性疾病中的胞外囊泡

(一)阿尔茨海默病

阿尔茨海默病(Alzheimer's disease,AD)是最常见的痴呆症,严重影响记忆和其他智力[30]。确切的病理生理学和疾病的原因还没有完全了解,但许多机制已经得到了彻底的研究和描述[31]。AD 的许多方面与 β-淀粉样(amyloid beta,Aβ)肽从其前体淀粉样前体蛋白(amyloid precursor protein,APP)产生的增加有关,而 Aβ 肽的产生又与其他几个基因如 APP、PSEN1 和 PSEN2 的突变有关。Aβ 水平的增加积聚在细胞外斑块中,其存在与 AD 病理相关。AD 的另一个标志是稳定细胞骨架/微管的 tau 蛋白的过度磷酸化,特别是在神经元细胞中。过度磷酸化的 tau 蛋白通过一种很大程度上未知的机制聚集成神经原纤维缠结。这两种事件都与神经元丢失增加、神经炎症、氧化应激以及小胶质细胞和星形胶质细胞活化有关。

对 EV 参与 AD 致病性的理解通过逐步发现已经成熟[30,31]。在疾病中关于 EV 潜在作用的最初迹象与发现 Aβ42 肽,即与 AD 相关的 Aβ 肽的同工型,在疾病的 MVB 中积累有关[32,33]。由于 MVB 是外泌体(EV 的一种类型)的生物发生位点,这意味着至少有一种 EV 亚型与形成斑块的 Aβ42 肽有关。后者在随后的研究中得到证实,其中 EV 的标志物 Flotillin-1[34]和 Alix[35]被发现分别在 AD 小鼠和患者的大脑中与 Aβ 共同定位。为了支持后面的观察,有报道称抑制一种对外泌体生物发生重要的酶,即中性鞘磷脂酶 2(nSmase2),可减少小鼠模型的疾病病理[36]。尽管 nSmase2 参与了许多细胞过程,即到目前为止 nSmase2 并不仅仅参与外泌体分泌途径,但这一证据可能被认为是间接的。然而,有报道称星形细胞来源的 EV 可刺激 Aβ42 肽聚集,同时抑制小胶质细胞清除 Aβ42[36],这有力地支持了 EV 网络参与 AD 病理。后者的作用依赖于神经酰胺[37],但这是否与 EV 中存在的神经酰胺或神经酰胺阳性囊泡中的其他 EV 成分直接相关,还需要进一步澄清。

有趣的是,EV 本身似乎参与了 APP 蛋白的致病过程[38]。EV 制剂中存在几种 APP 处理酶,如 BACE1 和其他分泌酶、PSEN1、PSEN2 和 ADAM10。APP 裂解时,在 EV 中可以发现 APP 碳端片段的水平以及裂解产物(包括 Aβ 多肽)[39]。

因此,有许多机制可以导致细胞外环境中 Aβ42 的产生和聚集增加,包括 EV 介导的 Aβ 的分泌、加工和聚集诱导。星形胶质细胞衍生的 EV 可以加速 Aβ 聚集,导致小胶质细胞清除和 Aβ 降解的损害[36]。同时,细胞外高水平的 Aβ 与星形胶质细胞的自身凋亡增加有关,这也导致这些细胞分泌促凋亡 EV[40]。过量 Aβ 的存在也触发小胶质细胞分泌神经毒性 EV,然而,这可能与前纤维 Aβ 有关,而不是预先形成的聚集体[41]。与星形胶质细胞 EV 诱导的 Aβ 聚集体相反,这些小胶质细胞来源的 EV 可以在一定程度上溶解 Aβ 聚集体,可能通过与小胶质细胞 EV 脂质的相互作用[41]。值得注意的是,在 AD 中小胶质细胞分泌神经毒性 EV 不仅与 Aβ 的扩散有关,还与其他蛋白质有关,如磷酸化 Tau 蛋白[38,42-45]。据报道,小胶质细胞不是降解磷酸化的 Tau,而是将这种蛋白质包装到 EV 中,从细胞中排出,并在受体细胞中诱导细胞毒性效应[42]。

上述观察进一步强调了在疾病条件下 EV 相互作用网络的复杂性,其中某些类型的 EV 可能具有保护性,而其他类型的 EV 可能具有致病性,这取决于它们的组成。例如,nSmase2 依赖性分泌含有神经酰胺的 EV 的复杂性就说明了这一点。尽管上述证据表明,通过抑制 nSmase2 活性来抑制 EV 的分泌可能是一种有趣的治疗干预策略[36,41],但其他证据则指向相反的方向。例如,至少在某些条件下促进神经元分泌 nSmase2 依赖性 EV 可能是保护性的,因为它有助于消除 Aβ 的神经毒性,与小胶质细胞接触以清除毒性肽[46,47],并中和 Aβ 诱导的突触可塑性缺陷[48]。为什么神经元型 EV 与星形细胞型和小胶质型 EV 在这方面表现不同仍有待解决,然而,有一种假说认为这可能与神经元 EV 上存在特定的鞘糖脂或细胞型朊蛋白(cellular prion protein,PrP^C)[30,49-51] 或特定的酶,如胰岛素降解酶(insulin-degrading enzyme,IDE)[52-54] 有关。

综上所述,关于 EV 参与 AD 的发现有些矛盾,EV 在 AD 病理中的累积效应不仅取决于给定细胞类型的 EV 的亚型特异性分泌,还取决于 CNS 中不同细胞类型分泌的 EV 的平衡和化学计量。

(二)帕金森病

帕金森病(Parkinson disease,PD)是另一种常见的神经退行性疾病。PD 中受影响的细胞主要是大脑黑质区的多巴胺能神经元,其退化导致 PD 的典型运动症状,如静止性震颤、运动迟缓和姿势不稳定[55]。这种病理的主要原因是 α-突触核蛋白(α-syn),它在神经元的突触前区表达,但其他基因也与 PD 相关(如 DJ-1、PINK1、LRRK2)[56]。尽管并不清楚 α-突触的所有功能,但已经确定在 PD(以及其他突触核蛋白病)中,α-突触错误折叠、细胞间传播和聚集到被称为 Lewy 体的结构是潜在病理学的关键特征。新出现的证据表明,EV 参与了这些过程[2,31]。

EV在聚集的α-syn传播中的作用被认为与朊病毒蛋白的传播有些相似[57-60]，如本章下文所述。虽然α-syn在CNS来源的EV中可明显检测到，但它不一定是α-syn的主要分泌途径[57]。很大一部分α-syn是独立于囊泡分泌的，但与EV相关的较小部分蛋白质似乎在病理学中更重要[51,61-63]。有人认为，α-syn的分泌可能与调节该蛋白胞质浓度的需要有关；未能做到这一点可能与基因变异体和α-syn突变形式错误折叠/聚集的可能性增加有关[56,64]。某些基因如ATP13A2，似乎对调节α-syn的胞质水平很重要，有证据表明，该基因在神经元中的高表达与神经元的高存活率和α-syn EV 分泌的增加有关[65-68]。

然而，当有毒形式的α-syn从细胞中排出时，含有这种蛋白质的EV被其他神经元细胞吸收时会变成具有神经毒性[51,61-63,69]。重要的是，据报道，EV相关的α-突触比可溶性α-突触低聚物更具神经毒性[59,62]。这种神经毒性可以被其他细胞抵消，如星形胶质细胞和小胶质细胞，它们可以清除细胞外α-syn并降低神经毒性α-syn聚集体的细胞外浓度[70]。然而，尽管从细胞外环境中清除α-syn似乎是减少神经毒性的好策略，但它实际上可能导致胶质细胞中α-syn内含物的形成、小胶质细胞过度激活、促炎信号通路的诱导以及氧化还原酶过氧化氢酶、超氧化物歧化酶和其他抗氧化剂的减少[70-74]。通过分泌EV，这些炎症细胞至细胞的信号通路被放大，如通过从小胶质细胞诱导含TNF的EV，这可以在受体细胞（包括神经元）中启动凋亡过程[75]。

导致α-syn扩散的另一个因素与PD伴随的溶酶体功能障碍有关，溶酶体加工缺陷可增加α-syn阳性EV的比例[63]。PD患者分泌的含α-syn的EV的变化非常显著，不仅在患者的CSF中，而且在血浆中均可检测到其水平升高[76,77]。这一观察不仅对开发PD的敏感生物标志物很重要，而且为额外的潜在疾病病理机制，特别是病理的传播提供了额外的信息。

如上所述，通过EV摄取α-syn的可能性大于可溶性α-syn寡聚体，而且可溶性α-syn寡聚体的聚集在EV浓度增加的情况下得到增强，包括从PD患者CSF中分离的EV[59,60,76]。这似乎表明，类似于在AD中观察到的情况，如上所述，EV似乎在PD中起作用，通过神经元、星形胶质细胞和小胶质细胞之间以正反馈调节的方式传递有毒蛋白质作为信号网络。然而，与AD病例类似，PD患者的EV组成似乎表明至少有一群EV可能确实具有神经保护作用[78]。

（三）多发性硬化

多发性硬化（multiple sclerosis，MS）是最常见的获得性脱髓鞘疾病，影响CNS。本病以原发性脱髓鞘的局灶性斑块和脑及脊髓灰质和白质的弥漫性神经变性为特征[79]。疾病发展的风险与免疫调节相关的遗传因素[80]，以及环境因素如EB病毒感染[81]有关。然而，对MS的最终发病机制尚未完全了解。迄今为止，已经证实以髓鞘蛋白为目标的自反应性$CD4^+$ T细胞是MS发病机制的关键组成部分。此外，外周血T辅助性$CD4^+$细胞激活也被观察到可导致促炎、自反应、Th1和Th17 T细胞亚群的产生[82]。此外，B细胞和单核/巨噬细胞也被证明在MS病变中活跃。B细胞和$CD8^+$ T细胞构成了MS病变中脑浸润细胞的很大一部分，尽管迄今为止还没有明确的效应细胞和靶抗原[83]。

与其他多种神经退行性疾病一样,有强有力的证据支持免疫调节性 EV 参与 MS 的病理。例如,MS 患者 CSF 中分泌型 EV 总数明显高于健康人[84,85],表明该疾病中 EV 体内平衡失衡。有几种细胞类型,包括 CNS 浸润的病理相关细胞,可导致 EV 浓度增加,从而触发特定的功能效应。

在 MS 中,分泌促炎性 EV 的细胞类型之一是小胶质细胞。当外源性小胶质细胞病毒被注射到患有实验性自身免疫性脑脊髓炎(experimental autoimmune encephalomyelitis,EAE)小鼠的大脑中时,该实验在动物中模拟 MS,会夸大疾病症状[84]。同时,EV 分泌受损的 aSmase 缺乏小鼠对 EAE 更有抵抗力[84]。然而,必须注意的是,aSmase 缺乏也可以减少小胶质细胞以外的其他细胞类型的 EV 分泌,并且 aSmase 也参与 EV 分泌以外的细胞过程。

脑内皮源性 EV 的参与似乎也与 MS 的发病机制高度相关。在某些条件下,内皮 EV 可以激活单核细胞[86],以及 $CD4^+$ 和 $CD8^+$ T 淋巴细胞[87]。这通过多种机制发生,如 ICAM-1 受体的转移(对于单核细胞),以及 CD40、CD275、MHC II、β2-微球蛋白和 CCL5 表达的诱导(对于 T 细胞)。这可能导致单核细胞[86]和 T 细胞[88,89]的黏附和跨内皮迁移增加。除了增加跨内皮 EV 的迁移,内皮细胞也能引起血脑屏障的直接破坏[90,91]。然而,后者并不仅限于内皮型 EV。血脑屏障的破坏可由如来源于 MS 患者血小板的内皮 EV 触发[90,91],以及白细胞、小胶质细胞和星形胶质细胞通过触发含有金属蛋白酶和半胱天冬酶 1 的内皮 EV 对促炎细胞因子刺激的反应而触发[92,93]。累积起来,这些数据强烈地表明外泌体通过炎症信号的传播以及淋巴细胞和髓细胞通过血脑屏障的转移参与了 MS 发病机制和疾病进展。

然而,在 MS 中,类似于在 AD 和 PD 中观察到的情况(见上文),并非所有的 EV 都具有致病性。有证据表明,含有特定物质的 EV 具有保护效益。例如,来自谷氨酸激活的少突胶质细胞的 EV 通过髓鞘蛋白和 RNA 的转移支持髓鞘形成[11,12],来自干扰素 γ 刺激的树突细胞的 EV 促进少突胶质祖细胞生长,增加髓鞘形成,降低氧化应激和促进髓鞘再形成[94]。除了支持髓鞘形成,少突胶质细胞 EV 增加了神经元对压力的抵抗力,并增强了它们的存活和生存能力,这可能对髓鞘形成有积极的影响[12]。因此,EV 在这种能力中的作用可能不仅仅局限于健康个体髓鞘的发育,还包括 MS 和其他脱髓鞘疾病中受损髓鞘的再生。

除了在 MS 发病机制和治疗干预方面的意义,EV 及其载体已经显示出其是该疾病生物标志物的一个有希望的来源。目前 MS 的诊断是一个复杂的过程,其基于临床表现和 MRI 成像的结果。这种复杂的诊断程序需要彻底地寻找更简单、更快、更可靠的诊断方法,并用于预后和治疗性生物标志物[95]。因此,在过去的十年中,许多研究小组致力于鉴定 MS 的生物标志物,特别是轻(NF-L)和重(NF-H)神经丝蛋白、星形胶质细胞衍生的几丁质酶 3-like 1 (astrocyte derived chitinase 3-like 1, CHI3L1)和胶质纤维酸性蛋白(glial fibrillar acidic protein,GFAP)[96-99]。

然而,传统的生物标志物研究的成功率有限[100]。因此,重点已经转移到将 EV 作为 MS 的生物标志物来源,这显示了一些重要的前景。例如,MS 患者 CSF 中髓系细胞来源的 EV 水平与 MS 患者的 MRI 病变相关[84]。同样,血浆中 $CD61^+$、$CD45^+$ 和 $CD14^+$ EV 的数量似乎与疾病的严重程度相关[85]。目前的成功不仅限于来自骨髓细胞的 EV。由于 EV 从

CNS流出,在患者血清中发现部分含髓磷脂蛋白的少突胶质EV可能也是一种预测性生物标志物[101]。在MS患者和对照组之间,循环EV的miRNA似乎也存在差异[102]。然而,在很大程度上尚不清楚是哪些细胞导致了这种差异。虽然大多数研究关注患者与对照组之间生物标志物的差异,但也有一些报道指出一些潜在的生物标志物的正常化,而不是其他的对MS治疗的反应[103-105]。

应该强调的是,在MS中,类似于在AD和PD中观察到的,有关EV参与疾病病理的证据是明确的。此外,来自不同细胞的EV似乎在病理生理和疾病进展中具有特定的功能,这可能与细胞特异性的EV含量有关,甚至可能与特定细胞在病理条件下分泌的EV亚型有关。这些研究也揭示了考虑所有EV类型和亚群体的整个通信网络的重要性,特别是考虑到某些EV可以起到保护和缓解疾病的作用。

(四) 肌萎缩侧索硬化

肌萎缩侧索硬化(amyotrophic lateral sclerosis,ALS)是一种致命的、进行性的神经退行性疾病,由于皮质、脑干和脊髓中运动神经元的退化,导致肌肉无力和瘫痪,并最终死亡。ALS的发病率为(2~3)/10万,患病率为(6~7)/10万,是欧洲最常见的运动神经元疾病[106,107]。通常情况下,患者死亡率为症状出现后2~5年,然而,一些患者由于呼吸障碍而存活时间较短,一些患者由于进展缓慢而存活超过30年[108,109]。

由TARDBP编码的细胞核DNA结合蛋白TAR DNA结合蛋白43(TDP-43)的细胞质内含物阳性是ALS最典型的神经病理学特征[110,111],几乎所有的ALS患者,包括家族性ALS患者,都可以看到TDP-43阳性的包涵体[112]。内含物包含高度磷酸化的泛素化聚集体,主要由TDP-43的碳末端片段组成。TARDBP突变几乎只在C末端发现,然而这些突变占ALS病例的<1%[113]。在TDP-43阳性内含物不可见的ALS病例中(<3%),聚集体由突变基因产生的蛋白质组成,最常见的是超氧化物歧化酶1(superoxide dismutase 1,SOD1),或在罕见情况下融合在肉瘤中(fused in sarcoma,FUS)[114,115]。

当来自ALS患者大脑的不溶性TDP-43被引入表达TDP-43的人类神经母细胞瘤细胞时,TDP-43阳性内含物形成,表明模板聚集发生[116]。SOD1的模板聚集也以类似的方式被观察到[117]。SOD1聚集体由邻近细胞分泌和内吞,在那里它们引发正常细胞质突变SOD1的聚集体,从而繁殖ALS。当聚集的SOD1种子被去除后,聚集仍然存在,这表明新形成的聚集物能够持续繁殖ALS[118]。

EV在ALS的参与尚不清楚,但有证据表明,它们确实通过聚集物的传播在疾病传播中发挥作用,类似于在其他神经退行性疾病,如AD、PD和朊病毒疾病中观察到的情况。从用于培养表达TDP-43的神经母细胞瘤细胞的条件培养基中分离出的EV显示TDP-43富集。此外,在ALS患者CSF分离的EV中也检测到TDP-43。这些发现共同支持了通过EV运输聚集物作为ALS繁殖手段的假设[116,119]。此外,也有证据表明SOD1通过ALS细胞模型的外泌体传播[118,120]。

尽管EV是一种很有吸引力的生物标志物来源,但目前还没有用于检测ALS的生物标志物。对14例ALS患者血清样本的分析表明,循环EV的miRNA特征可能是一个可能的生物标志物[121]。然而,需要更多的工作来确定循环 EV 的哪个亚群负责这一观察,以及这些 EV miRNA 候选生物标志物的功能是什么。此外,一项病例研究报道,与健康对照组相比,一名 ALS 患者 CSF 中白细胞来源的 EV 增加[122],并且在一名 ALS 患者群体 CSF 中分离出的 EV 中检测到 TDP-43[119],尽管这些发现相对不确定。

至于 EV 对 ALS 的治疗益处,已有一些证据表明源自脂肪来源多能干细胞(adipose derived multipotent stem cell,ASC)的外泌体发挥神经保护作用。在一种以转染 SOD1 突变的 NSC-34 运动神经元样细胞为基础的 ALS 体外模型中观察到,ASC-EV 在一定程度上作为病理损伤响应了 H_2O_2 增加 ALS 运动神经元的存活[123]。G93A ALS 小鼠体外模型中,ASC 衍生的 EV 也可以减少神经元细胞中 SOD-1 的聚集增加,并恢复原代神经元中的线粒体功能[124]。然而,正如这两项研究的情况一样,到目前为止,这些证据还没有在体内得到复制。

尽管有一些证据表明 EV 参与了 ALS 的发病机制,基于 EV 的 ALS 生物标志物的早期成功尝试强调了这一点,但迄今为止,关于 CNS 中自然发生的 EV 信号网络是否可以作为疾病保护机制的一部分提供神经保护的信息要少得多。然而,鉴于与其他神经退行性疾病的相似性,未来可能会有更多关于这些问题的信息。

(五)朊病毒病(传染性海绵状脑病)

朊病毒病,在技术上被称为传染性海绵状脑病(transmissible spongiform encephalopathy,TSE),是一组影响大脑和神经系统的进行性神经退行性疾病。朊病毒病导致神经功能受损,导致记忆和人格改变,运动、平衡和协调出现问题,最终导致死亡[125]。宿主编码的细胞朊病毒蛋白(PrP^C)的错误折叠亚型(PrP^{Sc})被认为是朊病毒病发病机制的核心。PrP^{Sc} 的错误折叠、聚集和积累导致神经元变性和随后的死亡,最终导致成簇的充满液体的空腔,使脑组织呈现海绵状外观(因此得名海绵状)。

朊病毒病与其他神经退行性疾病的不同之处在于它们在物种内部以及偶尔在物种之间传播的能力(即朊病毒病是可传播的)。牛海绵状脑病(bovine spongiform encephalopathy,BSE)突出了这一特征的危险和潜在的破坏性影响。从 20 世纪 80 年代末到 20 世纪 90 年代,疯牛病危机主要发生在英国,但也发生在欧洲其他地区[126]。不幸的是,朊病毒不会被烹饪或热处理破坏,这意味着 PrP^{Sc} 可以通过食用受污染的肉制品传播给人类。牛被认为是通过动物饲料感染的,这些饲料中含有患羊瘙痒病(一种影响羊的朊病毒病)的羊的加工残余物/骨粉[127]。令人不安的是,牛也被认为是通过喂养其他被感染的牛的遗骸而被感染,这些遗骸被加工成骨粉。这场危机导致了 200 例人类变异型克雅病(variant Creutzfeldt-Jakob disease,vCJD)。克雅病是最著名的人类朊病毒病。德国神经学家 Hans Gerhard Creutzfeldt 和 Alfons Maria Jakob 在 20 世纪 20 年代首次描述了这种疾病,这种疾病与 BSE 暴露无关,在全球范围内的发病率约为每年百万分之一[128,129]。

然而,除了克雅病,还存在其他朊病毒病,并且很可能会发现更多。例如,α-syn 蛋白在 PD 中的朊病毒样扩散在上面相应的章节中讨论过,而其他一些已知的朊病毒病非常罕见,如库鲁病和致命的家族性失眠。库鲁病是一种非常罕见的朊病毒病,在巴布亚新几内亚独立国的福尔人中很常见。这种疾病通过葬礼或仪式性的内食行为在前部落成员中传播[130]。致命性家族性失眠是一种罕见的遗传性睡眠障碍，以进行性失眠导致痴呆和死亡为特征。它是一种遗传性朊病毒病，与朊病毒蛋白基因突变有关，在极其罕见的情况下会偶发[131]。

朊病毒病可以通过 PRNP 基因突变的遗传偶尔发生[如家族性克雅病和格斯特曼-施特劳斯勒尔-沙因克尔综合征（Gerstmann-Straussler-Scheinker syndrome）]，或者可以通过预先存在的朊病毒的传播获得（如 vCJD 和库鲁病）。朊病毒一词由"蛋白质感染性粒子"演变而来，从这个名字可以看出，朊病毒疾病病理的核心是一种蛋白质。生理上发生的 PrP^C（C 表示细胞）参与许多不同的过程，如神经元分化、突触功能和铜稳态[132]。正如上文在 AD 部分讨论的，PrP^C 甚至可以在神经退行性疾病中起到神经保护作用。然而，PrP 的错误折叠变体（PrP^{Sc}）与朊病毒病密切相关。

PrP^C 的二级蛋白质结构主要由 α 螺旋组成，可被蛋白质降解蛋白酶溶解和消化。PrP^C 转化为毒性 PrP^{Sc}（Sc 用于羊瘙痒病）导致蛋白质二级结构的改变。二级结构以 β 片为主，这使得它不溶于水，并且高度抵抗蛋白酶的消化。PrP^{Sc} 可以促进 PrP^C 的错误折叠，并诱导 PrP^C 在邻近细胞中的错误折叠。这种正反馈循环导致了疾病的进展和传播。

已发现朊病毒蛋白与外泌体有关，携带 PrP^{Sc} 的 EV 可传播朊病毒感染[132]。PrP^{Sc} 特异性地存在于质膜中的脂筏中，在那里它们通过所谓的 GPI 锚与脂筏相连。含有趋化因子调节蛋白的富含脂筏的 EV，而趋化因子锚定已被成功用作将分子束缚在 EV 表面的方法[133]。研究表明，抑制和刺激 EV 生物发生途径会影响 PrP^{Sc} 在细胞间的传递[134-136]。这些发现支持 EV 在 PrP^{Sc} 传播中的作用。

替代机制，如细胞间直接接触和隧道纳米管已被提议在感染性朊病毒蛋白的细胞间转移中发挥作用[137,138]。然而，PrP^C 错误折叠成 PrP^{Sc} 似乎是在多细胞体中 PrP^{Sc} 的存在下触发的[139]，多细胞体是 EV 生物发生的组成部分，这在本书的其他章节中有详细讨论。PrP^{Sc} 感染细胞分泌的 EV 的形态发生显著变化，进一步支持了多泡体和 EV 参与朊病毒病的传播[140]。作为一个正反馈回路，这可以导致 EV 分泌 PrP^{Sc}，再摄取，以及随后一轮 PrP^{Sc} 接种[132,140-142]。值得注意的是，这些观察还表明，除了神经毒性，PrP^{Sc} 还可以通过改变 EV 的组成调节朊病毒蛋白错误折叠的反应。

可见，EV 不仅参与了神经毒性朊病毒蛋白在 CNS 中的传播，而且参与了整个机体的传播，因为在从血液中提取的 EV 上发现了 PrP^{Sc}[143,144]。对与 PrP^{Sc} 分泌相关的 EV 生物学的彻底研究，有助于阐明血液循环中发现的含 PrP^{Sc} 的 EV 是朊病毒病传播病理学的一部分还是疾病存在的指示性迹象，这可以作为朊病毒病的早期生物标志物[132]。

四、总结

EV 是多方面的、复杂的细胞间信号实体。在神经退行性疾病中，这反映在它们的双重作用上，在某些情况下，它们既作为疾病介质，也在某些情况下具有神经保护作用。这可能取决于 EV 来源的细胞类型和 EV 组成的疾病特异性变化。研究这些影响并不简单，因为 EV 在成分和性能上是高度不均一的。此外，不同细胞来源的 EV 是复杂细胞通信网络的一部分，该网络与其他细胞信号分子如细胞因子、神经递质、亲神经因子和激素一起发挥作用。

这意味着 EV 的功能可能不仅取决于其承载成分,还取决于接收信号的细胞的状态。这两种因素在神经退行性疾病中都可能发生显著改变。然而,在神经退行性疾病中开发 EV 和 EV 亚组分的特性在疾病生物标志物研究中显示出前景,并有助于设计这些疾病的新治疗策略。

(崔国红 译,国东海 审校)

参考文献

[1] Andaloussi SEL, Mäger I, Breakefield XO, Wood MJA. Extracellular vesicles: biology and emerging therapeutic opportunities. Nat Rev Drug Discov 2013; 12: 347 - 57.
[2] Thompson AG, et al. Extracellular vesicles in neurodegenerative disease — pathogenesis to biomarkers. Nat Rev Neurol 2016; 12: 346 - 57.
[3] Mathieu M, Martin-Jaular L, Lavieu G, Théry C. Specificities of secretion and uptake of exosomes and other extracellular vesicles for cell-to-cell communication. Nat Cell Biol 2019; 21: 9 - 17.
[4] Zhang H, et al. Identification of distinct nanoparticles and subsets of extracellular vesicles by asymmetric flow field-flow fractionation. Nat Cell Biol 2018; 20: 332 - 43.
[5] Tkach M, Kowal J, Théry C. Why the need and how to approach the functional diversity of extracellular vesicles. Philos Trans R Soc Lond B Biol Sci 2018; 373: 20160479.
[6] Willms E, et al. Cells release subpopulations of exosomes with distinct molecular and biological properties. Sci Rep 2016; 6: 22519.
[7] Willms E, Cabañas C, Mäger I, Wood MJA, Vader P. Extracellular vesicle heterogeneity: subpopulations, isolation techniques, and diverse functions in cancer progression. Front Immunol 2018; 9: 738.
[8] Lai RC, Lim SK. Membrane lipids define small extracellular vesicle subtypes secreted by mesenchymal stromal cells. J Lipid Res 2019; 60. https://doi.org/10.1194/jlr.R087411.
[9] Timmers L, et al. Human mesenchymal stem cell-conditioned medium improves cardiac function following myocardial infarction. Stem Cell Res 2011; 6: 206 - 14.
[10] Lai RC, et al. MSC secretes at least 3 EV types each with a unique permutation of membrane lipid, protein and RNA. J Extracell Vesicles 2016; 1: 1 - 12.
[11] Frühbeis C, et al. Neurotransmitter-triggered transfer of exosomes mediates oligodendrocyte - neuron communication. PLoS Biol 2013; 11: e1001604.
[12] Frohlich D, et al. Multifaceted effects of oligodendroglial exosomes on neurons: impact on neuronal firing rate, signal transduction and gene regulation. Philos Trans R Soc Lond B Biol Sci 2014; 369: 20130510.
[13] Fitzner D, et al. Selective transfer of exosomes from oligodendrocytes to microglia by macropinocytosis. J Cell Sci 2011; 124: 447 - 58.
[14] Bakhti M, Winter C, Simons M. Inhibition of myelin membrane sheath formation by oligodendrocyte-derived exosome-kike vesicles. J Biol Chem 2011; 286: 787 - 96.
[15] Riganti L, et al. Sphingosine-1-phosphate (S1P) impacts presynaptic functions by regulating synapsin I localization in the presynaptic compartment. J Neurosci 2016; 36: 4624 - 34.
[16] Antonucci F, et al. Microvesicles released from microglia stimulate synaptic activity via enhanced sphingolipid metabolism. EMBO J 2012; 31: 1231 - 40.
[17] Pastuzyn ED, et al. The neuronal gene Arc encodes a repurposed retrotransposon Gag protein that mediates intercellular RNA transfer. Cell 2018; 172: 275 - 288.e18.
[18] Ashley J, et al. Retrovirus-kike Gag protein Arc1 binds RNA and traffics across synaptic boutons. Cell 2018; 172: 262 - 274.e11.
[19] Lachenal G, et al. Release of exosomes from differentiated neurons and its regulation by synaptic glutamatergic activity. Mol Cell Neurosci 2011; 46: 409 - 18.
[20] Korkut C, et al. Trans-synaptic transmission of vesicular Wnt signals through Evi/Wntless. Cell 2009; 139: 393 - 404.
[21] Holm MM, Kaiser J, Schwab ME. Extracellular vesicles: multimodal envoys in neural maintenance and repair. Trends Neurosci 2018; 41: 360 - 72.
[22] Koles K, et al. Mechanism of evenness interrupted (Evi)-exosome release at synaptic boutons. J Biol Chem 2012; 287: 16820 - 34.
[23] Beckett K, et al. Drosophila S2 cells secrete wingless on exosome-kike vesicles but the wingless gradient forms independently of exosomes. Traffic 2013; 14: 82 - 96.
[24] Gross JC, Chaudhary V, Bartscherer K, Boutros M. Active Wnt proteins are secreted on exosomes. Nat Cell Biol 2012; 14: 1036 - 45.
[25] Gong J, Körner R, Gaitanos L, Klein R. Exosomes mediate cell contact - independent ephrin-Eph signaling during axon guidance. J Cell Biol 2016; 214: 35 - 44.
[26] Vyas N, et al. Vertebrate hedgehog is secreted on two types of extracellular vesicles with different signaling properties. Sci Rep 2015; 4: 7357.
[27] Matusek T, et al. The ESCRT machinery regulates the secretion and long-range activity of hedgehog. Nature 2014; 516: 99 - 103.
[28] Korkut C, et al. Regulation of postsynaptic retrograde signaling by presynaptic exosome release. Neuron 2013; 77:

1039-46.
[29] Bahrini I, Song J, Diez D, Hanayama R. Neuronal exosomes facilitate synaptic pruning by up-regulating complement factors in microglia. Sci Rep 2015; 5: 7989.
[30] Malm T, Loppi S, Kanninen KM. Exosomes in Alzheimer's disease. Neurochem Int 2016; 97: 193-9.
[31] Vella L, Hill A, Cheng L. Focus on extracellular vesicles: exosomes and their role in protein trafficking and biomarker potential in Alzheimer's and Parkinson's disease. Int J Mol Sci 2016; 17: 173.
[32] Takahashi RH, et al. Intraneuronal Alzheimer Aβ42 accumulates in multivesicular bodies and is associated with synaptic pathology. Am J Pathol 2002; 161: 1869-79.
[33] Verbeek MM, Otte-Höller I, Fransen JAM, de Waal RMW. Accumulation of the amyloid-β precursor protein in multivesicular body-kike organelles. J Histochem Cytochem 2002; 50: 681-90.
[34] Langui D, et al. Subcellular topography of neuronal Aβ peptide in APPxPS1 transgenic mice. Am J Pathol 2004; 165: 1465-77.
[35] Rajendran L, et al. Alzheimer's disease beta-amyloid peptides are released in association with exosomes. Proc Natl Acad Sci U S A 2006; 103: 11172-7.
[36] Dinkins MB, Dasgupta S, Wang G, Zhu G, Bieberich E. Exosome reduction in vivo is associated with lower amyloid plaque load in the 5XFAD mouse model of Alzheimer's disease. Neurobiol Aging 2014; 35: 1792-800.
[37] Dinkins MB, et al. The 5XFAD mouse model of Alzheimer's disease exhibits an age-dependent increase in anti-ceramide IgG and exogenous administration of ceramide further increases anti-ceramide titers and amyloid plaque burden. J Alzheimers Dis 2015; 46: 55-61.
[38] Perez-Gonzalez R, Gauthier SA, Kumar A, Levy E. The exosome secretory pathway transports amyloid precursor protein carboxyl-terminal fragments from the cell into the brain extracellular space. J Biol Chem 2012; 287: 43108-15.
[39] Sharples RA, et al. Inhibition of γ-secretase causes increased secretion of amyloid precursor protein C-terminal fragments in association with exosomes. FASEB J 2008; 22: 1469-78.
[40] Wang G, et al. Astrocytes secrete exosomes enriched with proapoptotic ceramide and prostate apoptosis response 4 (PAR-4): potential mechanism of apoptosis induction in Alzheimer disease (AD). J Biol Chem 2012; 287: 21384-95.
[41] Joshi P, et al. Microglia convert aggregated amyloid-β into neurotoxic forms through the shedding of microvesicles. Cell Death Differ 2014; 21: 582-93.
[42] Asai H, et al. Depletion of microglia and inhibition of exosome synthesis halt tau propagation. Nat Neurosci 2015; 18: 1584-93.
[43] Simon D, Garcia-Garcia E, Royo F, Manuel Falcon-Perez J, Avila J. Proteostasis of tau. Tau overexpression results in its secretion via membrane vesicles. FEBS Lett 2012; 586: 47-54.
[44] Saman S, et al. Exosome-associated tau is secreted in tauopathy models and is selectively phosphorylated in cerebrospinal fluid in early Alzheimer disease. J Biol Chem 2012; 287: 3842-9.
[45] Fiandaca MS, et al. Identification of preclinical Alzheimer's disease by a profile of pathogenic proteins in neurally derived blood exosomes: a case-control study. Alzheimers Dement 2015; 11: 600-607.e1.
[46] Yuyama K, Sun H, Mitsutake S, Igarashi Y. Sphingolipid-modulated exosome secretion promotes clearance of amyloid-β by microglia. J Biol Chem 2012; 287: 10977-89.
[47] Yuyama K, et al. Decreased amyloid-β pathologies by intracerebral loading of glycosphingolipid-enriched exosomes in Alzheimer model mice. J Biol Chem 2014; 289: 24488-98.
[48] An K, et al. Exosomes neutralize synaptic-plasticity-disrupting activity of Aβ assemblies in vivo. Mol Brain 2013; 6: 47.
[49] Falker C, et al. Exosomal cellular prion protein drives fibrillization of amyloid beta and counteracts amyloid beta-mediated neurotoxicity. J Neurochem 2016; 137: 88-100.
[50] Chiasserini D, et al. Proteomic analysis of cerebrospinal fluid extracellular vesicles: a comprehensive dataset. J Proteomics 2014; 106: 191-204.
[51] Bellingham SA, Guo BB, Coleman BM, Hill AF. Exosomes: vehicles for the transfer of toxic proteins associated with neurodegenerative diseases? Front Physiol 2012; 3. https://doi.org/10.3389/fphys.2012.00124.
[52] Tamboli IY, et al. Statins promote the degradation of extracellular amyloid β-peptide by microglia via stimulation of exosome-associated insulin-degrading enzyme (IDE) secretion. J Biol Chem 2010; 285: 37405-14.
[53] Bulloj A, Leal MC, Xu H, Castano EM, Morelli L. Insulin-degrading enzyme sorting in exosomes: a secretory pathway for a key brain amyloid-beta degrading protease. J Alzheimers Dis 2010; 19: 79-95.
[54] Sanderson RD, Bandari SK, Vlodavsky I. Proteases and glycosidases on the surface of exosomes: newly discovered mechanisms for extracellular remodeling. Matrix Biol 2017. https://doi.org/10.1016/j.matbio.2017.10.007.
[55] Olanow CW, Stern MB, Sethi K. The scientific and clinical basis for the treatment of Parkinson disease (2009). Neurology 2009; 72: S1-136.
[56] Chistiakov DA, Chistiakov AA. α-Synuclein-carrying extracellular vesicles in Parkinson's disease: deadly transmitters. Acta Neurol Belg 2017; 117: 43-51.
[57] Lee H-J. Intravesicular localization and exocytosis of -synuclein and its aggregates. J Neurosci 2005; 25: 6016-24.
[58] Lee H-J, Suk J-E, Bae E-J, Lee S-J. Clearance and deposition of extracellular α-synuclein aggregates in microglia. Biochem Biophys Res Commun 2008; 372: 423-8.
[59] Danzer KM, et al. Exosomal cell-to-cell transmission of alpha synuclein oligomers. Mol Neurodegener 2012; 7: 42.
[60] Gray M, et al. Acceleration of α-synuclein aggregation by exosomes. J Biol Chem 2015; 290: 2969-82.
[61] Desplats P, et al. Inclusion formation and neuronal cell death through neuron-to-neuron transmission of -synuclein. Proc Natl Acad Sci U S A 2009; 106: 13010-5.
[62] Emmanouilidou E, et al. Cell-produced -synuclein is secreted in a calcium-dependent manner by exosomes and impacts neuronal survival. J Neurosci 2010; 30: 6838-51.
[63] Alvarez-Erviti L, et al. Lysosomal dysfunction increases exosome-mediated alpha-synuclein release and transmission. Neurobiol Dis 2011; 42: 360-7.

[64] Ali SF, Binienda ZK, Imam SZ. Molecular aspects of dopaminergic neurodegeneration: gene-environment interaction in parkin dysfunction. Int J Environ Res Public Health 2011; 8: 4702–13.
[65] Gitler AD, et al. α-Synuclein is part of a diverse and highly conserved interaction network that includes PARK9 and manganese toxicity. Nat Genet 2009; 41: 308–15.
[66] Kong SMY, et al. Parkinson's disease-kinked human PARK9/ATP13A2 maintains zinc homeostasis and promotes α-Synuclein externalization via exosomes. Hum Mol Genet 2014; 23: 2816–33.
[67] Ramonet D, et al. PARK9-associated ATP13A2 localizes to intracellular acidic vesicles and regulates cation homeostasis and neuronal integrity. Hum Mol Genet 2012; 21: 1725–43.
[68] Ramirez A, et al. Hereditary parkinsonism with dementia is caused by mutations in ATP13A2, encoding a lysosomal type 5 P-type ATPase. Nat Genet 2006; 38: 1184–91.
[69] Hansen C, et al. α-Synuclein propagates from mouse brain to grafted dopaminergic neurons and seeds aggregation in cultured human cells. J Clin Invest 2011; 121: 715–25.
[70] Lee H-J, et al. Direct transfer of α-synuclein from neuron to astroglia causes inflammatory responses in synucleinopathies. J Biol Chem 2010; 285: 9262–72.
[71] Halliday GM, Stevens CH. Glia: initiators and progressors of pathology in Parkinson's disease. Mov Disord 2011; 26: 6–17.
[72] Vekrellis K, Xilouri M, Emmanouilidou E, Rideout HJ, Stefanis L. Pathological roles of α-synuclein in neurological disorders. Lancet Neurol 2011; 10: 1015–25.
[73] Alvarez-Erviti L, Couch Y, Richardson J, Cooper JM, Wood MJA. Alpha-synuclein release by neurons activates the inflammatory response in a microglial cell line. Neurosci Res 2011; 69: 337–42.
[74] Uttara B, Singh A, Zamboni P, Mahajan R. Oxidative stress and neurodegenerative diseases: a review of upstream and downstream antioxidant therapeutic options. Curr Neuropharmacol 2009; 7: 65–74.
[75] Chang C, et al. Exosomes of BV-2 cells induced by alpha-synuclein: important mediator of neurodegeneration in PD. Neurosci Lett 2013; 548: 190–5.
[76] Stuendl A, et al. Induction of α-synuclein aggregate formation by CSF exosomes from patients with Parkinson's disease and dementia with Lewy bodies. Brain 2016; 139: 481–94.
[77] Shi M, et al. Plasma exosomal α-synuclein is likely CNS-derived and increased in Parkinson's disease. Acta Neuropathol 2014; 128: 639–50.
[78] Tomlinson PR, et al. Identification of distinct circulating exosomes in Parkinson's disease. Ann Clin Transl Neurol 2015; 2: 353–61.
[79] Lemus HN, Warrington AE, Rodriguez M. Multiple sclerosis: mechanisms of disease and strategies for myelin and axonal repair. Neurol Clin 2018; 36: 1–11.
[80] Ascherio A, Munger KL. Environmental risk factors for multiple sclerosis. Part I: the role of infection. Ann Neurol 2007; 61: 288–99.
[81] Hohlfeld R, Wekerle H. Autoimmune concepts of multiple sclerosis as a basis for selective immunotherapy: from pipe dreams to (therapeutic) pipelines. Proc Natl Acad Sci U S A 2004; 101: 14599–606.
[82] Sospedra M, Martin R. Immunology of multiple sclerosis. Annu Rev Immunol 2005; 23: 683–747.
[83] Hohlfeld R, Dornmair K, Meinl E, Wekerle H. The search for the target antigens of multiple sclerosis, part 2: CD8+ T cells, B cells, and antibodies in the focus of reverse-translational research. Lancet Neurol 2016; 15: 317–31.
[84] Verderio C, et al. Myeloid microvesicles are a marker and therapeutic target for neuroinflammation. Ann Neurol 2012; 72: 610–24.
[85] Sáenz-Cuesta M, et al. Circulating microparticles reflect treatment effects and clinical status in multiple sclerosis. Biomark Med 2014; 8: 653–61.
[86] Jy W, et al. Endothelial microparticles (EMP) bind and activate monocytes: elevated EMPmonocyte conjugates in multiple sclerosis. Front Biosci 2004; 9: 3137–44.
[87] Wheway J, Latham SL, Combes V, Grau GER. Endothelial microparticles interact with and support the proliferation of T cells. J Immunol 2014; 193: 3378–87.
[88] Barry OP, Praticò D, Savani RC, FitzGerald GA. Modulation of monocyte-endothelial cell interactions by platelet microparticles. J Clin Invest 1998; 102: 136–44.
[89] Quandt J, Dorovini-Zis K. The beta chemokines CCL4 and CCL5 enhance adhesion of specific CD4+ T cell subsets to human brain endothelial cells. J Neuropathol Exp Neurol 2004; 63: 350–62.
[90] Marcos-Ramiro B, et al. Microparticles in multiple sclerosis and clinically isolated syndrome: effect on endothelial barrier function. BMC Neurosci 2014. https://doi.org/10.1186/1471-2202-15-110.
[91] Alexander JS, et al. Blood circulating microparticle species in relapsing-remitting and secondary progressive multiple sclerosis. A case-control, cross sectional study with conventional MRI and advanced iron content imaging outcomes. J Neurol Sci 2015; 355: 84–9.
[92] Hakulinen J, Sankkila L, Sugiyama N, Lehti K, Keski-Oja J. Secretion of active membrane type 1 matrix metalloproteinase (MMP-14) into extracellular space in microvesicular exosomes. J Cell Biochem 2008; 105: 1211–8.
[93] Sarkar A, Mitra S, Mehta S, Raices R, Wewers MD. Monocyte derived microvesicles deliver a cell death message via encapsulated caspase-1. PLoS ONE 2009; 4: e7140.
[94] Pusic AD, Pusic KM, Clayton BLL, Kraig RP. IFNγ-stimulated dendritic cell exosomes as a potential therapeutic for remyelination. J Neuroimmunol 2014; 266: 12–23.
[95] Palmer AJ, Colman S, O'Leary B, Taylor BV, Simmons RD. The economic impact of multiple sclerosis in Australia in 2010. Mult Scler 2013; 19: 1640–6.
[96] Lee JY, Taghian K, Petratos S. Axonal degeneration in multiple sclerosis: can we predict and prevent permanent disability? Acta Neuropathol Commun 2014; 2: 97.
[97] Comabella M, et al. Cerebrospinal fluid chitinase 3-kike 1 levels are associated with conversion to multiple sclerosis.

Brain 2010; 133: 1082-93.
[98] Borràs E, et al. Protein-based classifier to predict conversion from clinically isolated syndrome to multiple sclerosis. Mol Cell Proteomics 2016; 15: 318-28.
[99] Axelsson M, et al. Glial fibrillary acidic protein: a potential biomarker for progression in multiple sclerosis. J Neurol 2011; 258: 882-8.
[100] Trentini A, et al. N-acetylaspartate and neurofilaments as biomarkers of axonal damage in patients with progressive forms of multiple sclerosis. J Neurol 2014; 261: 2338-43.
[101] Galazka G, Mycko MP, Selmaj I, Raine CS, Selmaj KW. Multiple sclerosis: serum-derived exosomes express myelin proteins. Mult Scler 2018; 24: 449-58.
[102] Selmaj I, et al. Global exosome transcriptome profiling reveals biomarkers for multiple sclerosis. Ann Neurol 2017; 81: 703-17.
[103] Jimenez JJ, et al. Elevated endothelial microparticle—monocyte complexes induced by multiple sclerosis plasma and the inhibitory effects of interferon-β1b on release of endothelial microparticles, formation and transendothelial migration of monocyte-endothelial microparticle. Mult Scler J 2005; 11: 310-5.
[104] Lowery-Nordberg M, et al. The effects of high dose interferon-β1a on plasma microparticles: correlation with MRI parameters. J Neuroinflammation 2011; 8: 43.
[105] Dawson G, Qin J. Gilenya (FTY720) inhibits acid sphingomyelinase by a mechanism similar to tricyclic antidepressants. Biochem Biophys Res Commun 2011; 404: 321-3.
[106] Mandrioli J, Faglioni P, Merelli E, Sola P. The epidemiology of ALS in Modena, Italy. Neurology 2003; 60: 683-9.
[107] Chio A, et al. Epidemiology of ALS in Italy: a 10-year prospective population-based study. Neurology 2009; 72: 725-31.
[108] Stambler N, Charatan M, Cedarbaum JM. Prognostic indicators of survival in ALS. Neurology 1998; 50: 66-72.
[109] de Carvalho M, et al. Motor neuron disease presenting with respiratory failure. J Neurol Sci 1996; 139: 117-22.
[110] Arai T, et al. TDP-43 is a component of ubiquitin-positive tau-negative inclusions in frontotemporal lobar degeneration and amyotrophic lateral sclerosis. Biochem Biophys Res Commun 2006; 351: 602-11.
[111] Neumann M, et al. Ubiquitinated TDP-43 in frontotemporal lobar degeneration and amyotrophic lateral sclerosis. Science 2006; 314: 130-3.
[112] Mackenzie IRA, Frick P, Neumann M. The neuropathology associated with repeat expansions in the C9ORF72 gene. Acta Neuropathol 2014; 127: 347-57.
[113] Rutherford NJ, et al. Novel mutations in TARDBP(TDP-43) in patients with familial amyotrophic lateral sclerosis. PLoS Genet 2008; 4: e1000193.
[114] Shibata N, et al. Intense superoxide dismutase-1 immunoreactivity in intracytoplasmic hyaline inclusions of familial amyotrophic lateral sclerosis with posterior column involvement. J Neuropathol Exp Neurol 1996; 55: 481-90.
[115] Deng HX, et al. FUS-immunoreactive inclusions are a common feature in sporadic and non-SOD1 familial amyotrophic lateral sclerosis. Ann Neurol 2010; 67: 739-48.
[116] Nonaka T, et al. Prion-kike properties of pathological TDP-43 aggregates from diseased brains. Cell Rep 2013; 4: 124-34.
[117] Chia R, et al. Superoxide dismutase 1 and tgSOD1G93A mouse spinal cord seed fibrils, suggesting a propagative cell death mechanism in amyotrophic lateral sclerosis. PLoS ONE 2010; 5: e10627.
[118] Münch C, O'Brien J, Bertolotti A. Prion-kike propagation of mutant superoxide dismutase-1 misfolding in neuronal cells. Proc Natl Acad Sci U S A 2011; 108: 3548-53.
[119] Feneberg E, et al. Limited role of free TDP-43 as a diagnostic tool in neurodegenerative diseases. Amyotroph Lateral Scler Frontotemporal Degener 2014; 15: 351-6.
[120] Gomes C, Keller S, Altevogt P, Costa J. Evidence for secretion of Cu, Zn superoxide dismutase via exosomes from a cell model of amyotrophic lateral sclerosis. Neurosci Lett 2007; 428: 43-6.
[121] Saucier D, et al. Identification of a circulating miRNA signature in extracellular vesicles collected from amyotrophic lateral sclerosis patients. Brain Res 2018; 1708: 100-8.
[122] Zachau AC, et al. Leukocyte-derived microparticles and scanning electron microscopic structures in two fractions of fresh cerebrospinal fluid in amyotrophic lateral sclerosis: a case report. J Med Case Reports 2012; 6: 274.
[123] Bonafede R, et al. Exosome derived from murine adipose-derived stromal cells: neuroprotective effect on in vitro model of amyotrophic lateral sclerosis. Exp Cell Res 2016; 340: 150-8.
[124] Lee M, et al. Adipose-derived stem cell exosomes alleviate pathology of amyotrophic lateral sclerosis in vitro. Biochem Biophys Res Commun 2016; 479: 434-9.
[125] Scheckel C, Aguzzi A. Prions, prionoids and protein misfolding disorders. Nat Rev Genet 2018; 19: 405-18.
[126] Ducrot C, Arnold M, de Koeijer A, Heim D, Calavas D. Review on the epidemiology and dynamics of BSE epidemics. Vet Res 2008; 39: 15.
[127] Greig JR. Scrapie in sheep. J Comp Pathol 1950; 60: 263-6.
[128] Richardson EP, Masters CL. The nosology of Creutzfeldt-Jakob disease and conditions related to the accumulation of PrPCJD in the nervous system. Brain Pathol 1995; 5: 33-41.
[129] Creutzfeldt HG. Über eine eigenartige herdförmige erkrankung des zentralnervensystems (Vorläufige mitteilung). Zeitschrift für die gesamte Neurol und Psychiatre 1920; 57: 1-18.
[130] Gajdusek DC, Zigas V. Degenerative disease of the central nervous system in New Guinea: the endemic occurrence of kuru in the native population. N Engl J Med 1957; 257: 974-8.
[131] Llorens F, Zarranz J-J, Fischer A, Zerr I, Ferrer I. Fatal familial insomnia: clinical aspects and molecular alterations. Curr Neurol Neurosci Rep 2017; 17: 30.
[132] Cheng L, Zhao W, Hill AF. Exosomes and their role in the intercellular trafficking of normal and disease associated prion proteins. Mol Aspects Med 2018; 60: 62-8.

[133] Kooijmans SAA, et al. Display of GPI-anchored anti-EGFR nanobodies on extracellular vesicles promotes tumour cell targeting. J Extracell Vesicles 2016; 5: 31053.
[134] Guo BB, Bellingham SA, Hill AF. The neutral sphingomyelinase pathway regulates packaging of the prion protein into exosomes. J Biol Chem 2015; 290: 3455-67.
[135] Guo BB, Bellingham SA, Hill AF. Stimulating the release of exosomes increases the intercellular transfer of prions. J Biol Chem 2016; 291: 5128-37.
[136] Vilette D, et al. Efficient inhibition of infectious prions multiplication and release by targeting the exosomal pathway. Cell Mol Life Sci 2015; 72: 4409-27.
[137] Gousset K, et al. Prions hijack tunnelling nanotubes for intercellular spread. Nat Cell Biol 2009; 11: 328-36.
[138] Kanu N, et al. Transfer of scrapie prion infectivity by cell contact in culture. Curr Biol 2002; 12: 523-30.
[139] Yim Y-I, et al. The multivesicular body is the major internal site of prion conversion. J Cell Sci 2015; 128: 1434-43.
[140] Coleman BM, Hanssen E, Lawson VA, Hill AF. Prion-infected cells regulate the release of exosomes with distinct ultrastructural features. FASEB J 2012; 26: 4160-73.
[141] Vella LJ, et al. Packaging of prions into exosomes is associated with a novel pathway of PrP processing. J Pathol 2007; 211: 582-90.
[142] Bellingham SA, Coleman BM, Hill AF. Small RNA deep sequencing reveals a distinct miRNA signature released in exosomes from prion-infected neuronal cells. Nucleic Acids Res 2012; 40: 10937-49. https://doi.org/10.1093/nar/gks832.
[143] Saá P, et al. First demonstration of transmissible spongiform encephalopathy-associated prion protein (PrPTSE) in extracellular vesicles from plasma of mice infected with mouse-adapted variant Creutzfeldt-Jakob disease by in vitro amplification. J Biol Chem 2014; 289: 29247-60.
[144] Cervenakova L, et al. Are prions transported by plasma exosomes? Transfus Apher Sci 2016; 55: 70-83.

| 第 13 章 |

纤维化疾病中的胞外囊泡：
纤维化诊断和治疗的新应用

Extracellular vesicles in fibrotic diseases: New applications for fibrosis diagnosis and treatment

Tsukasa Kadota[a,b], Nobuyoshi Kosaka[a], Yu Fujita[a,b],
Jun Araya[b], Kazuyoshi Kuwano[b], Takahiro Ochiya[a,c]

[a]Division of Molecular and Cellular Medicine, National Cancer Center Research Institute, Tokyo, Japan,
[b]Division of Respiratory Diseases, Department of Internal Medicine, The Jikei University School of Medicine, Tokyo, Japan, [c]Institute of Medical Science, Tokyo Medical University, Tokyo, Japan

一、概述

纤维化通常表现为 ECM 成分的形成和积聚，导致组织和器官的重塑。如此广泛的组织重塑会导致器官衰竭，并可能导致死亡。据估计，在美国，纤维性疾病导致的死亡高达 45%。虽然这一估计包括动脉粥样硬化，但纤维化疾病具有多种高死亡率和较少见的疾病，如特发性肺纤维化（idiopathic pulmonary fibrosis，IPF）、肝硬化、心脏纤维化、系统性硬化和肾纤维化。因此，我们现在认识到，纤维形成是一个广泛的细胞和分子机制引起的重要疾病过程。然而，目前的纤维化治疗策略数量有限，疗效不佳。这些事实强调了对纤维化发病机制和潜在治疗方法进一步理解的必要性。

EV 包括各种各样的小膜泡，大小从 50 纳米到几微米不等，几乎所有类型的细胞都会释放 EV 到细胞外环境中。根据 EV 的大小、生物起源和分泌机制，EV 通常被归类为外泌体、微泡和凋亡小体。外泌体是由内质体膜向内和反向萌发产生的，并通过 MVB 与质膜的融合释放到细胞外液中。微泡比外泌体大，正常情况下或对刺激做出反应时通过脱落或出芽从质膜产生。凋亡小体直径只有几微米，在细胞凋亡过程中通过滤泡从质膜上释放出来。虽然这些囊泡的起源已经确定，但目前的方法无法区分这些不同类型的 EV。因此，在本文中，我们将 EV 作为细胞外液中所有类型囊泡的通用术语。近年来，EV 通过蛋白质、mRNA 和 miRNA 等内容物的转移，在包括纤维形成在内的多种生物学和病理过程中被鉴定为细胞间通信的调节介质。此外，有大量证据表明 EV 有可能被用作病理状态的生物标志物或治疗药物。因此，研究 EV 在纤维化疾病中的作用，不仅有助于我们进一步了解其发病机制，而且为纤维化疾病的诊断和治疗提供新的临床应用方向。在本文中，我们概述了对组织损伤和修复如何导致纤维化的理解。本文还对 EV 与肝、肺、心等纤维化疾病的关系进行了综述。此外，我们提出了基于 EV 的生物标志物和治疗纤维化疾病的方法。

二、纤维化机制

在许多慢性疾病或损伤中都存在着共同的纤维化发生机制。事实上，在不同的组织和器官中，与纤维化相关的信号通路和介导因子是相似的。例如，Makarev等揭示了肺纤维化和肝纤维化之间的一些共同途径，如TGF-β、IL-6和整合素连接激酶信号。一些抗纤维化药物，如吡非尼酮对不同组织和器官的纤维化也有效。此外，不同组织和器官中的纤维化疾病可以相互作用。例如，随着年龄的增长，心脏和肾脏同时发生纤维化，这是由于利尿钠肽系统（natriuretic peptide system，NPS）、肾素-血管紧张素-醛固酮系统（renin-angiotensin-aldosterone system，RAAS）和TGF-β1通路之间的失衡。因此，揭示多器官纤维化共同的核心分子机制对于了解纤维化疾病的发病机制至关重要。

纤维化发生已被认为是组织损伤后伤口愈合过程的一部分。纤维化是在所有器官中通过肌成纤维细胞增殖和ECM沉积以快速修复损伤。当损伤自然消退时，纤维化反应通常受到限制，细胞外基质蛋白发生再吸收，从而促进器官修复。另一方面，当慢性或反复损伤发生时，效应细胞的持续激活会导致过度活跃的伤口愈合和正常再生过程的丧失。结果，ECM的过度和无序沉积最终损害了器官的结构和功能。

伤口愈合过程有复杂的调控机制，包括多种细胞类型和分子系统的相互作用。在大多数慢性纤维化疾病中，炎症可能是纤维生成的初始步骤（图13-1A）。上皮细胞和内皮细胞的各种应激性损伤导致多种炎症介质（如细胞因子、趋化因子和其他因子）的产生，导致多种炎症细胞（如巨噬细胞和中性粒细胞）的刺激和损伤。这些炎症细胞通过促纤维化介质，包括血小板源性生长因子（platelet-derived growth factor，PDGF）、TGF-β1和IL-13引起间充质细胞（如成纤维细胞）的激活，尤其是TGF-β1在诱导前体细胞向肌成纤维细胞分化中起重要作用。另一种纤维化的方式是没有炎症细胞浸润的上皮驱动的纤维化反应，以IPF为代表（图13-1B）。在IPF的发病机制中，受损和异常激活的肺上皮细胞诱导间充质细胞的迁移并分化为肌成纤维细胞，而这一过程在没有原发性免疫致病成分的情况下发生。在炎症和非炎症机制中，肌成纤维细胞迅速产生多种细胞外基质，在修复过程中维持损伤组织的完整性，并以自分泌和旁分泌的方式进一步增加细胞因子、趋化因子、生长因子和其他因子的产生，进一步触发和促进纤维化。

三、胞外囊泡在器官纤维化发病机制中的作用

纤维化的生物活性可溶性介质包括趋化因子（CCL2、MCP-1、MIP-1β）、细胞因子（TGF-β1、PDGF、IL-1β、IL-6、IL-13、IL-2、IL-33和TNF-α）、VEGF、PDGF、过氧化物酶体增殖物激活受体（proliferator-activated receptor，PPAR）、半胱天冬酶，以及RRAS的成分（ANG Ⅱ）。此外，非肽介质，如活性氧介质和脂质介质已被确定为纤维化的关键因素。近年来，EV已成为纤维形成的新调节因子。在本节中，我们回顾了越来越多的证据表明EV参与了几个器官包括肝、肺和心脏的纤维化过程（表13-1）。

（一）EV 与肝纤维化

肝纤维化是病毒性肝炎、酗酒、非酒精性脂肪肝等慢性肝病的常见转归，可导致肝硬化和肝功能衰竭。肝星状细胞（hepatic stellate cell，HSC）的激活是肝纤维化的关键事件，因为这些细胞在损伤后成为肝细胞外基质的主要来源。肝损伤后，HSC 失去脂滴，迁移到损伤部位，获得肌纤维母细胞分化，分泌过多的细胞外基质蛋白。

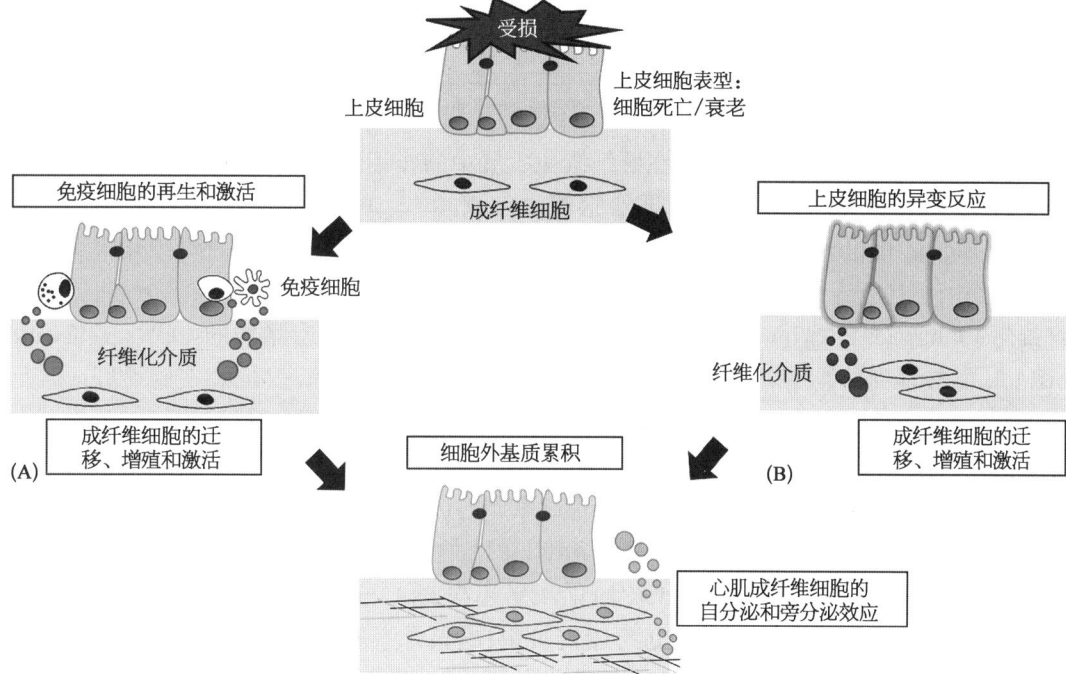

图 13-1　纤维化进展的示意图。多种损伤性刺激导致上皮细胞损伤，导致细胞死亡，包括细胞凋亡和（或）细胞衰老。在大多数情况下，(A) 受损的上皮细胞招募并激活包括巨噬细胞和淋巴细胞在内的各种免疫细胞，而巨噬细胞和淋巴细胞反过来又释放促纤维化介质。这种反应导致组织肌成纤维细胞的扩张、募集和（或）激活，这是以器官纤维化为特征的病理性 ECM 的主要来源。相反，非炎性上皮驱动的纤维化反应是发展纤维化的另一种方式，表现为 IPF(B)。受损的上皮细胞产生各种介质，导致成纤维细胞活化和细胞外基质堆积，这在没有主要免疫致病成分的情况下也可以发生。一旦纤维化反应建立，激活的成纤维细胞对其微环境细胞（如上皮细胞和免疫细胞）具有自分泌和旁分泌作用

表 13-1　EV 参与器官纤维化的病理变化

器官	来源	受体细胞	介质	效应	参考文献
肝	肝星状细胞	肝星状细胞，肝细胞	miR-214	CCN2 抑制	[20]
肝	肝星状细胞	肝星状细胞	Twist1	CCN2 抑制	[21]
肝	肝星状细胞	肝星状细胞	CCN,CCNmRNA	—	[22]
肝	内皮细胞	肝星状细胞	鞘磷脂酶 1	肝星状细胞迁移	[23]
肺	—	肺成纤维细胞	Wint5	成纤维细胞增殖	[24]

续 表

器官	来源	受体细胞	介质	效应	参考文献
肺	内皮细胞	肺成纤维细胞	—	成纤维细胞的迁移能力	[25]
心	成纤维细胞	心肌细胞	miR-23-3p	心肌肥厚的发展	[26]
心	心肌细胞	成纤维细胞	HSP90	心肌纤维化的发展	[27]
心	心脏成纤维细胞	心肌细胞	miRNA	Nrf2 调节异常	[28]

注：CCN：富含半胱氨酸-61/结缔组织生长因子/肾母细胞瘤。Nrf2：核因子红细胞2相关因子2。

到目前为止，有一些关于 EV 在肝纤维化发展中的作用的报道。CCN2 是富含半胱氨酸蛋白 61/结缔组织生长因子/肾母细胞瘤过度表达（cysteine-rich-61/connective tissue growth factor/nephroblastoma-overexpressed，CCN）家族的成员，在各种纤维化疾病中起着关键作用。在肝纤维化中，CCN2 在活化的 HSC 中表达增加，直接促进丝分裂、趋化和纤维化。Charrier 等描述，HSC 衍生的 EV 在 HSC 激活期间含有增加的 CCN2 或 CCN2 mRNA，并转移到其他静止或激活的 HSC 中。Chen 等证明，miR-214 在实验性肝纤维化或 HSC 激活过程中直接调节 CCN2 的表达，并通过 EV 从 HSC 转移到邻近的 HSC 或肝细胞。同一组还报道了 twist 相关蛋白 1（Twist1）的独特功能，Twist1 是 CCN2 依赖性纤维形成中 DNA 结合转录因子的基本螺旋-环-螺旋家族的成员。HSC 衍生的 EV 含有高水平的 Twist1，在 HSC 激活过程中，Twist1 驱动 miR-214 的表达，并通过 EV 转移导致受体 HSC 细胞中 CCN2 的表达。除了调节 HSC 活化，EV 还与 HSC 迁移有关。Wang 等证明，内皮细胞衍生 EV 中的鞘氨醇激酶 1 通过纤维连接蛋白-整合素依赖性 EV 黏附和动力依赖性 EV 内化调节 HSC 信号和迁移[23]。在肝硬化中，血管生成有助于肝硬化期间的血管重塑。Witek 等发现活化的 HSC 和反应性胆管细胞将含 Hedgehog 配体的 EV 转移到肝窦内皮细胞（sinusoidal endothelial cell，SEC），导致肝脏 SEC 活化标志物增加。因此，这些 EV 可能促进肝硬化时的血管重塑。

（二）EV 与肺纤维化

IPF 是最常见的肺纤维化疾病，是一种慢性的、进行性的、不可逆的和致命的肺部疾病，其特征是弥漫性肺泡上皮细胞损伤和结构重塑。IPF 通常对糖皮质激素等抗炎治疗无效。尽管病因尚不清楚，但肺泡上皮细胞和成纤维细胞的异常活化是 IPF 发病机制中最为公认的理论之一。

目前，EV 在 IPF 发病机制中的作用研究较少。Martin-Medina 等发现，IPF 患者支气管肺泡灌洗液中 EV 分泌的 WNT5A 增加，促进肺成纤维细胞增殖。Bacha 等发现，在严重 IPF 患者中，从血浆中分离出的循环内皮细胞微粒水平显著升高，这刺激了肺成纤维细胞的迁移能力。此外，我们还发现香烟烟雾提取物诱导的人支气管上皮细胞衍生 EV 通过 EV miR-210 的自噬调节促进肺成纤维细胞的肌成纤维细胞分化。因为香烟烟雾是 IPF 的重要危险因素，EV 诱导的肌成纤维细胞分化可能参与了 IPF 的发病机制。此外，我们最近的研究表明，IPF 患者肺成纤维细胞来源的 EV 增加了肺上皮细胞线粒体活性氧（mitochondrial reactive oxygen species，mtROS）和相关的线粒体损伤，导致 mtROS 介导的 DNA 损伤反应激活和随后的上皮细胞衰老。从机制上讲，EV 中显著上调的 miR-23b-3p 和 miR-494-3p 负责抑制 SIRT3，导致 EV 诱导的肺上皮细胞表型。衰老的细胞不仅损害再生，还损害生物活性分子的分泌，这对于 IPF 纤维化的发生和发展至关重要。这些结果提示 EV 在 IPF 发病机制中起着重要的调节作用（Kadota 等未发表的数据）。

（三）EV 与心肌纤维化和肥大

心肌纤维化是由大多数心肌疾病引起的病理性心肌重塑所致。在心脏，心脏成纤维细胞是最丰富的细胞类型，是细胞外基质产生的中央调节器。心肌成纤维细胞也通过旁分泌因子，如 TGF-β 和成纤维细胞生长因子（fibroblast growth factor 2，FGF-2）与心肌细胞进行交流。此外，与其他器官不同，心脏的再生能力非常有限。因此，张力性瘢痕对于防止心肌梗死和其他损伤后的破裂是必要的。这种代偿机制引起心室扩张、心肌细胞肥大等病理改变，最终导致心力衰竭的发生。

考虑到 EV 在心肌纤维化和肥大病理发生中的作用，Bang 等证明心肌成纤维细胞衍生的 EV 中的 miR-21-3p 转移到心肌细胞，通过下调 Sorbin 和 SH3 结构域 2（Sorbin and SH3 domain containing 2，SORBS2）或 PDZ 和 LIM 结构域 5（PDZ and LIM domain 5，PDLIM5）诱导心肌肥大，两者都被称为心肌结构和功能的调节器。另一方面，Datta 等揭示了 HSP90 介导的分泌型或 EV 型心肌细胞 IL-6 调节机制，其中 IL-6 通过在心肌纤维化发展过程中成纤维细胞中 STAT-3 信号的双相激活来改变纤维化反应。此外，Tian 等鉴定了心脏成纤维细胞和心肌细胞之间 EV 相关的 miRNA 介导的通信，导致核因子红细胞 2 相关因子 2（nuclear factor erythroid 2-related factor 2，Nrf2）/抗氧化响应元件（antioxidant response element，ARE）信号通路的失调，并可能导致心脏纤维化。Nrf2 是这些区域的主要调节因子。此外，许多 Nrf2 调节的酶参与了心脏病的发病机制，并与氧化应激介导的心脏重塑和心力衰竭有关。这些结果表明，EV 介导的心肌细胞和成纤维细胞之间的相互作用与心肌纤维化有关。

此外，还研究了心肌细胞源性 EV 在运动心脏修复中的作用。在 2 型糖尿病小鼠模型中，运动组细胞外空间、血管壁和心肌细胞周围区域的心肌细胞衍生 EV 水平增加，miR-29b 和 miR-455 上调。有趣的是，EV 中的 miRNA 通过抑制 MMP-9（ECM 降解的决定因素）而减弱纤维化和心肌细胞解偶联，提示 miRNA 参与心肌细胞源性 EV 在心肌纤维化发病机制中的作用。

四、胞外囊泡在纤维性疾病诊断中的作用

死亡风险随着纤维化阶段的增加呈指数增加，非酒精性脂肪肝、肺纤维化和慢性肾脏疾病都证明了这一点。因此，及早准确地检测器官纤维化的存在和程度具有潜在的益处。诊断和分期器官纤维化的金标准是组织学，通常是在细针活检或手术获得的样本上进行。然而，组织学评估器官纤维化有几个局限性：获取组织学具有侵袭性、重复活检困难和缺乏对

纤维化分布的代表性。因此，许多其他的方法，如影像学、机械和功能测试以及液体活检，已经被提出并被用于无创性地评估器官纤维化的阶段。

最近，由于几个原因，EV 已被确定为新的疾病生物标志物。首先，EV 反映其亲代细胞的生理状态和微环境，大多数细胞分泌含有特定蛋白质、核酸和脂质的 EV。其次，在血液和其他体液中发现了 EV。第三，EV 在细胞外环境中非常稳定，因为它们的磷脂双层。到目前为止，许多肠道病毒衍生的蛋白和 miRNA 已经被研究为各种疾病的潜在的、有用的生物标志物。在这一部分中，我们将回顾 EV 在肝和肺纤维化中的生物标志物。

（一）以 EV 为基础的生物标志物在肝纤维化中的作用

几项研究证明了基于 EV 的生物标志物在肝纤维化程度和存在方面的潜在效用。Morattini 等研究发现，EV 中的全长可溶性受体类型酪氨酸蛋白磷酸酶 γ（soluble receptortype tyrosineprotein phosphatase γ，sPTPRG）亚型已被确认为人和小鼠血浆中肝损伤的生物标志物。PTPRG 属于一个酶家族，它能从细胞内特定靶点的磷酸酪氨酸残基中去除磷酸基团，并在杂合性缺失、高甲基化和点突变的情况下发挥肿瘤抑制基因的作用。高谷丙转氨酶（alanine aminotransferase，ALT）或低 ALT 升高的血浆 sPTPRG 水平与肝损伤呈正相关。在另一项研究中，与健康人和康复者相比，慢性丙型肝炎（chronic hepatitis C，CHC）患者血清中可溶性 CD81 升高。EV 相关的可溶性 CD81 水平也与血浆 ALT 水平和严重形式的肝纤维化相关。此外，Lambrecht 等研究了早期 HBV 和 HCV 肝纤维化患者循环中 EV 相关 miRNA 的表达谱，提示这些 EV 相关 miRNA 有可能作为早期肝纤维化的标志物。此外，Kornek 等研究发现，血清中免疫细胞微粒，如 CD4$^+$ 和 CD8$^+$ T 细胞以及不变自然杀伤 T 细胞和巨噬细胞/单核细胞（CD14$^+$）具有评估 CHC 和非酒精性脂肪肝（nonalcoholic fatty liver，NAFL）或非酒精性脂肪性肝炎（nonalcoholic steatohepatitis，NASH）患者组织学分级、严重程度和病理分期的潜力。

（二）以 EV 为基础的生物标志物在肺纤维化中的作用

有几项关于使用 EVS 的肺间质纤维化生物标志物的研究。Makiguchi 等的结果显示，IPF 患者 EV 中 miR-21 的水平高于健康对照组。Njock 等的研究还发现，IPF 患者痰中 EV 中 miR-142-3p 水平与 IPF 严重程度呈负相关，这是通过一氧化碳/肺泡容积的肺弥散能力进行评估。这些结果表明，循环中的 EV 有可能成为诊断和疾病严重程度的潜在生物标志物。

表 13-2 EV 参与器官纤维化的病理变化

疾病	体液	介质	对照组	参考文献
肝损伤	血清，血浆	sPTPRG	无肝者	[48]
丙型肝炎		可溶性 CD81	健康者	[49]
乙肝和丙肝		miRNA	健康者	[50]

续 表

疾 病	体 液	介 质	对照组	参考文献
CHC	血清,血浆	CD4$^+$微粒	健康者	[51]
NAFL/NAFH	血清,血浆	CD4$^+$微粒	健康者	[51]
IPF	血浆	miR-21-5p	健康者	[52]
IPF	唾液	miR-142-3p	健康者	[53]

(三)目前 EV 分析在疾病诊断中的局限性

尽管使用 EV 作为生物标志物有很多优点,但目前仍有一些挑战限制了它们的临床适用性。首先,需要新的分离和富集 EV 的方法来分析数以千计的临床样本。目前,分离肠道病毒最常用的方法是超速离心法。然而,超速离心法分离 EV 需要昂贵的设备、耗时长,且需要大量的样品。虽然依赖于肠道病毒表面标志物的替代方法正在研究中,如微流控芯片、磁珠和流式细胞术[54],但这些方法在临床实践中的诊断性能仍不清楚。其次,目前的隔离技术使得区分不同的 EV 亚群变得困难。EV 主要是通过超速离心按大小分离的。然而,研究表明,当按大小分开时,EV 家族是异质性的。第三,EV 的生物发生机制还有待阐明。因此,需要进一步研究以合理的价格分离高纯度 EV 用于疾病生物标志物分析的技术。

五、胞外囊泡作为纤维化治疗的新应用

(一)器官纤维化的可逆性

传统上,纤维化被认为是一个不可逆转的过程,是伤口无序愈合的末期,因此难以治疗。然而,现在越来越多的证据表明,纤维化在很大限度上是可逆的,即使在后期也是如此。在动物模型中,肝纤维化是可逆的,在大多数情况下,在去掉诱导性致纤维化因素后,器官结构完全或接近完全恢复。例如,在一个公认的博莱霉素诱导的小鼠肺纤维化模型中,气管内给药 3~4 周后,组织结构恢复的自发纤维化消退可以发生。与纤维化诱因明确的动物模型不同,人类纤维性疾病往往是多因素的,纤维化消退的程度似乎取决于器官的分解能力和纤维化疾病的机制。人体器官纤维化解决的最令人信服的证据是在肝脏观察到的。众所周知,肝炎感染引起的肝硬化在抗病毒治疗后表现出明显的消退。相比之下,心脏和肺脏的再生能力非常有限。尽管如此,心脏纤维化患者的左心室射血功能和 IPF 患者的用力肺活量等器官功能的恢复已被证实是通过可能的抗纤维化干预来实现的。

就纤维化疾病的最佳治疗策略而言,根除损伤的根本原因可能是解决纤维化的最有效方法,如肝硬化的抗病毒治疗。当病因不明或无法对损伤的根本原因进行有效治疗时,应考虑针对纤维化的治疗。然而,尽管许多干预措施的目的都是消除纤维化,但很少有干预措施显示出对纤维化患者的疗效。因此,需要新的治疗方法来克服纤维化疾病。

(二)EV 在纤维化治疗中的新应用

EV 因其作为再生或免疫调节剂来源或作为药物输送载体的潜在应用而备受关注。使

用以 EV 为基础的治疗有几个优点。首先，EV 的免疫原性和毒性都很低，在组织和循环中都是稳定的。EV，特别是外泌体，已经在几个临床试验中被用于抗肿瘤疫苗。在肺癌中，使用 DC 来源的 EVe（dendritic cell-derived EVe，DeX）进行的Ⅰ期和Ⅱ期临床试验已经完成。虽然在Ⅱ期研究中，22 名非小细胞肺癌患者中有一人出现了 3 级肝毒性，但地塞米松治疗是可行的，且耐受性良好。其次，EV 可以被靶细胞选择性地、快速地摄取，靶细胞可能针对特定类型的细胞或组织。第三，它们具有特性，如脂质双层结构、纳米尺寸以及血液循环和组织的稳定性。在这一部分中，我们总结了 EV 在逆转纤维化的治疗应用中的效用。

（三）MSC 来源的 EV

由干细胞分泌的 EV 自然携带着来自干细胞的各种分子。在实验模型和临床试验中，有各种类型干细胞来源的 EV 被研究用于纤维化，如胚胎干细胞、诱导的多能干细胞以及多能/单能成人干细胞系，如 MSC。尤其是骨髓间充质干细胞已经得到了广泛的研究，并被认为是一种很有前途的治疗方法，特别是在纤维化疾病领域。

骨髓间充质干细胞是一种多能干细胞，在特定的培养条件下具有自我更新和分化为间充质细胞系的能力，如骨、软骨、肌肉和脂肪。归巢和迁移是 MSC 的其他独特功能。此外，由于分泌各种细胞因子和可溶性因子，它们可以协调组织修复、免疫调节、抗炎和/或免疫抑制。目前，临床前和临床试验表明，骨髓间充质干细胞能够改善各种疾病的预后，如心血管疾病、脑卒中、脊髓损伤、肾损伤、肺损伤和移植物抗宿主病（graft-versus-host disease，GvHD）。重要的是，36 项临床试验的荟萃分析没有反映出任何与骨髓间充质干细胞注射相关的严重并发症。

大量研究表明，MSC 来源的 EV（MSC-derived EV，MSC-EV）可能是 MSC 的替代品。此外，使用 MSC 衍生的 EV 允许将生物活性分子输送到受损器官，而不需要注射异种细胞。因此，到目前为止，已经有许多研究调查了 MSC-EV 在纤维化治疗中的应用。

在肝纤维化方面，Li 等研究发现，来源于人脐带 MSC 的 EV 通过抑制 TGF-β1/Smad 信号通路和抑制肝细胞上皮-间充质转化，在体内减轻了 CCl4 诱导的肝损伤。另一项研究表明，来自绒毛膜板来源的 MSC 的 EV 相关 miR-125b 抑制了 Hedgehog 信号的激活，从而促进了肝纤维化的减轻。此外，已有研究表明，从脂肪组织来源的 MSC 中释放的 EV 可抑制人原代 HSC 的增殖和激活。这些结果提示，EV 通过运送 MSC 中有效的 EV 货物而具有抗纤维化作用。

在肺纤维化方面，Shentu 等研究表明，人骨髓间充质干细胞来源的 EV 可以阻断转化生长因子 β1 诱导的肌成纤维细胞分化。人骨髓间充质干细胞来源的 EV 被成纤维细胞摄取，并可能利用 Thy-1-整合素相互作用依赖的途径促进 EV 的细胞间通信。细胞表面蛋白 Thy-1 是一种 GPI 锚定的糖蛋白，在 MSC 细胞表面高度表达，并与整合素相互作用。BM-MSC 来源的 EV 富含几种 miRNA，包括 miR-630，它针对的是在 IPF 成纤维细胞中上调的促纤维化基因。

在心脏，MSC 来源的 EV 通过各种机制介导心脏组织修复，如调节受损组织环境、诱导血管生成，促进增殖和防止凋亡。此外，心肌梗死后应用 MSC 来源的 EV 可促进心肌修复。

此外，Ma 等的结果显示，Akt 过表达的人脐带 MSC 的 EV 通过激活 PDGFD，促进心脏再生和血管生成。

（四）体液衍生 EV

从体液中分离出的 EV 也被证明在纤维化模型中有治疗效果。例如，来自健康人的血清 EV 可以治疗肝纤维化，因为它们有能力减轻肝星状细胞的激活，减轻肝细胞的损伤和炎症。EV 治疗改善了 CCL4 损伤或硫乙酸损伤的纤维化小鼠模型的肝功能，减少了肝细胞凋亡，抑制了受损肝脏的炎症反应，减少了肝脏或循环中促炎症细胞因子的释放，减少了炎症浸润，并降低了循环中谷草转氨酶/谷丙转氨酶的水平。另一项研究表明，从大鼠血浆中分离出的 EV 具有保护心脏免受缺血再灌注损伤的能力。这种作用是由 EV 上的 HSP70 介导的，刺激 TLR4 信号转导，导致 ERK1/2、p38MAPK 激活，进而导致心肌细胞 HSP27 磷酸化。此外，Beltrami 等研究发现，从人类心包液中提取的 EV 在小鼠肢体缺血模型中显示出促进体内治疗性血管生成的能力，这表明它们在心血管保护和修复方面的重要性。他们从机制上暗示，EV 将功能性的 let-7b-5p 转移到内皮细胞，从而降低其 TGFBR1 的表达，并诱导其促血管生成能力。总体而言，尽管其潜在的机制还不完全清楚，但来自健康人的体液来源的 EV 对纤维化疾病患者是有益的。

（五）基于 EV 治疗目前的局限性

基于 EV 的纤维化疾病治疗还有几个剩余的挑战。首先，应该制订标准化的、有质量控制的 EV 分离方案。选择合适的分离方法可获得纯度和效价可重复的、高质量的、均一的 EV。其次，由于 EV 的生产效率较低，需要有效的、大规模的生产 EV 以保证临床应用。第三，迫切需要对 EV 进行更严格的描述，以更好地探索囊泡的生物发生，并将 EV 应用于临床环境。第四，重要的是建立合适的临床前体内模型，以确定 EV 的剂量、生物分布、毒性和免疫原性。特别是，需要对 EV 进行活体成像，以可视化 EV 在体内的动力学，并量化 EV 递送到目标受损组织。

六、总结和展望

最近的证据表明纤维化在某些情况下是可逆的。消除潜在的有害刺激应该是解决纤维化的最有效的策略。在不可能治疗纤维化的情况下，抑制参与纤维化发展的有害介质似乎是一种很有前景的方法。EV 在生理和病理过程中都是细胞间通信的重要调节因子。本文描述的研究结果证实了 EV 在纤维化疾病的发病机制中起着关键作用。因此，抑制有害的 EV 可能是治疗纤维化疾病的潜在选择。此外，越来越多的证据表明，从干细胞或健康体液中提取的 EV 对纤维化疾病具有治疗作用。尽管 EV 的临床应用仍然存在重大挑战，但 EV 的进一步研究和开发可能会在未来帮助患者进行纤维化管理和治疗。

致谢

本章得到了 Practical Research for Innovative Cancer Control（17ck0106366h001） from Japan Agency for Medical Research and Development（AMED）的支持。

（高晨珊　张雅楠　译，侯磊　审校）

参考文献

[1] Wynn TA. Fibrotic disease and the T(H)1/T(H)2 paradigm. Nat Rev Immunol 2004; 4: 583-94.
[2] Robbins PD, Morelli AE. Regulation of immune responses by extracellular vesicles. Nat Rev Immunol 2014; 14: 195-208.
[3] Colombo M, Raposo G, Théry C. Biogenesis, secretion, and intercellular interactions of exosomes and other extracellular vesicles. Annu Rev Cell Dev Biol 2014; 30: 255-89.
[4] Witwer KW, et al. Standardization of sample collection, isolation and analysis methods in extracellular vesicle research. J Extracell Vesicles 2013; 2: 20360.
[5] Théry C, et al. Minimal information for studies of extracellular vesicles 2018 (MISEV2018): a position statement of the international society for extracellular vesicles and update of the MISEV2014 guidelines. J Extracell Vesicles 2018; 7: 1535750.
[6] Raposo G, Stoorvogel W. Extracellular vesicles: exosomes, microvesicles, and friends. J Cell Biol 2013; 200: 373-83.
[7] Kosaka N, et al. Secretory mechanisms and intercellular transfer of microRNAs in living cells. J Biol Chem 2010; 285: 17442-52.
[8] Makarev E, et al. Common pathway signature in lung and liver fibrosis. Cell Cycle 2016; 15: 1667-73.
[9] Azuma A, et al. Double-blind, placebo-controlled trial of pirfenidone in patients with idiopathic pulmonary fibrosis. Am J Respir Crit Care Med 2005; 171: 1040-7.
[10] Khanna D, et al. An open-kabel, phase II study of the safety and tolerability of pirfenidone in patients with scleroderma-associated interstitial lung disease: the LOTUSS trial. J Rheumatol 2016; 43: 1672-9.
[11] Sangaralingham SJ, et al. Cardiorenal fibrosis and dysfunction in aging: Imbalance in mediators and regulators of collagen. Peptides 2016; 76: 108-14.
[12] Gurtner GC, Werner S, Barrandon Y, Longaker MT. Wound repair and regeneration. Nature 2008; 453: 314-21.
[13] Wynn TA. Cellular and molecular mechanisms of fibrosis. J Pathol 2008; 214: 199-210.
[14] Rockey DC, Bell PD, Hill JA. Fibrosis — a common pathway to organ injury and failure. N Engl J Med 2015; 372: 1138-49.
[15] Kisseleva T, Brenner DA. Fibrogenesis of parenchymal organs. Proc Am Thorac Soc 2008; 5: 338-42.
[16] Wynn TA, Vannella KM. Macrophages in tissue repair, regeneration, and fibrosis. Immunity 2016; 44: 450-62.
[17] King TE, Pardo A, Selman M. Idiopathic pulmonary fibrosis. The Lancet 2011; 378: 1949-61.
[18] Kendall RT, Feghali-Bostwick CA. Fibroblasts in fibrosis: novel roles and mediators. Front Pharmacol 2014; 5: 123.
[19] Weiskirchen R, Weiskirchen S, Tacke F. Organ and tissue fibrosis: molecular signals, cellular mechanisms and translational implications. Mol Aspects Med 2018; 65: 2-15. https://doi.org/10.1016/j.mam.2018.06.003.
[20] Chen L, et al. Epigenetic regulation of connective tissue growth factor by MicroRNA-214 delivery in exosomes from mouse or human hepatic stellate cells. Hepatology 2014; 59: 1118-29.
[21] Chen L, Chen R, Kemper S, Charrier A, Brigstock DR. Suppression of fibrogenic signaling in hepatic stellate cells by Twist1-dependent microRNA-214 expression: role of exosomes in horizontal transfer of Twist1. Am J Physiol Gastrointest Liver Physiol 2015; 309: G491-9.
[22] Charrier A, et al. Exosomes mediate intercellular transfer of pro-fibrogenic connective tissue growth factor (CCN2) between hepatic stellate cells, the principal fibrotic cells in the liver. Surgery 2014; 156: 548-55.
[23] Wang R, et al. Exosome adherence and internalization by hepatic stellate cells triggers sphingosine 1-phosphate-dependent migration. J Biol Chem 2015; 290: 30684-96.
[24] Martin-Medina A, et al. Increased extracellular vesicles mediate WNT-5A signaling in idiopathic pulmonary fibrosis. Am J Respir Crit Care Med 2018; 198. https://doi.org/10.1164/rccm.201708-1580OC.
[25] Bacha NC, et al. Endothelial microparticles are associated to pathogenesis of idiopathic pulmonary fibrosis. Stem Cell Rev 2018; 14: 223-35.
[26] Travers JG, Kamal FA, Robbins J, Yutzey KE, Blaxall BC. Cardiac fibrosis: the fibroblast awakens. Circ Res 2016; 118: 1021-40.
[27] Bang C, et al. Cardiac fibroblast-derived microRNA passenger strand-enriched exosomes mediate cardiomyocyte hypertrophy. J Clin Investig 2014; 124: 2136-46.
[28] Datta R, et al. Myocyte-derived Hsp90 modulates collagen upregulation via biphasic activation of STAT-3 in fibroblasts during cardiac hypertrophy. Mol Cell Biol 2017; 37: 552-625.
[29] Hernandez-Gea V, Friedman SL. Pathogenesis of liver fibrosis. Annu Rev Pathol Mech Dis 2011; 6: 425-56.
[30] Gressner OA, Gressner AM. Connective tissue growth factor: a fibrogenic master switch in fibrotic liver diseases. Liver Int 2008; 28: 1065-79.
[31] Witek RP, et al. Liver cell-derived microparticles activate hedgehog signaling and alter gene expression in hepatic endothelial cells. Gastroenterology 2009; **136**: 320-330.e2.
[32] Gross TJ, Hunninghake GW. Idiopathic pulmonary fibrosis. N Engl J Med 2001; 345: 517-25.
[33] Selman M, Pardo A. Revealing the pathogenic and aging-related mechanisms of the enigmatic idiopathic pulmonary fibrosis. An integral model. Am J Respir Crit Care Med 2014; 189: 1161-72.
[34] Fujita Y, et al. Suppression of autophagy by extracellular vesicles promotes myofibroblast differentiation in COPD pathogenesis. J Extracell Vesicles 2015; 4: 28388.
[35] Kadota T, et al. Emerging role of extracellular vesicles as a senescence-associated secretory phenotype: Insights into the

[36] Kakkar R, Lee RT. Intramyocardial fibroblast myocyte communication. Circ Res 2010; 106: 47-57.
[37] Takeda N, et al. Cardiac fibroblasts are essential for the adaptive response of the murine heart to pressure overload. J Clin Investig 2010; 120: 254-65.
[38] Tian C, Gao L, Zimmerman MC, Zucker IH. Myocardial infarction-induced microRNAenriched exosomes contribute to cardiac Nrf2 dysregulation in chronic heart failure. Am J Physiol Heart Circ Physiol 2018; 314: H928-39.
[39] Ashrafian H, et al. Fumarate is cardioprotective via activation of the Nrf2 antioxidant pathway. Cell Metab 2012; 15: 361-71.
[40] Chaturvedi P, Kalani A, Medina I, Familtseva A, Tyagi SC. Cardiosome mediated regulation of MMP9 in diabetic heart; role of mir29b and mir455 in exercise. J Cell Mol Med 2015; 19: 2153-61.
[41] Dulai PS, et al. Increased risk of mortality by fibrosis stage in nonalcoholic fatty liver disease: systematic review and meta-analysis. Hepatology 2017; 65: 1557-65.
[42] Ley B, Collard HR, King TE. Clinical course and prediction of survival in idiopathic pulmonary fibrosis. Am J Respir Crit Care Med 2011; 183: 431-40.
[43] Tonelli M, et al. Chronic kidney disease and mortality risk: a systematic review. J Am Soc Nephrol 2006; 17: 2034-47.
[44] de Jong OG, et al. Cellular stress conditions are reflected in the protein and RNA content of endothelial cell-derived exosomes. J Extracell Vesicles 2012; 1: 18396.
[45] Beninson LA, Fleshner M. Exosomes: an emerging factor in stress-induced immunomodulation. Semin Immunol 2014; 26: 394-401.
[46] Kadota T, Yoshioka Y, Fujita Y, Kuwano K, Ochiya T. Extracellular vesicles in lung cancerfrom bench to bedside. Semin Cell Dev Biol 2017; 67: 39-47.
[47] Fujita Y, Yoshioka Y, Ochiya T. Extracellular vesicle transfer of cancer pathogenic components. Cancer Sci 2016; 107: 385-90.
[48] Moratti E, Vezzalini M, Tomasello L, Giavarina D, Sorio C. Identification of protein tyrosine phosphatase receptor gamma extracellular domain (sPTPRG) as a natural soluble protein in plasma. PLoS ONE 2015; 10: e0119110.
[49] Welker M-W, et al. Soluble serum CD81 is elevated in patients with chronic hepatitis C and correlates with alanine aminotransferase serum activity. PLoS ONE 2012; 7: e30796.
[50] Lambrecht J, et al. Circulating ECV-associated miRNAs as potential clinical biomarkers in early stage HBV and HCV induced liver fibrosis. Front Pharmacol 2017; 8: 56.
[51] Kornek M, et al. Circulating microparticles as disease-specific biomarkers of severity of inflammation in patients with hepatitis C or nonalcoholic steatohepatitis. Gastroenterology 2012; 143: 448-58.
[52] Makiguchi T, et al. Serum extracellular vesicular miR-21-5p is a predictor of the prognosis in idiopathic pulmonary fibrosis. Respir Res 2016; 17: 110.
[53] Njock M-S, et al. Sputum exosomes: promising biomarkers for idiopathic pulmonary fibrosis. Thorax 2018; 74: 309-312. https://doi.org/10.1136/thoraxjnl-2018-211897.
[54] Xu R, Greening DW, Zhu H-J, Takahashi N, Simpson RJ. Extracellular vesicle isolation and characterization: toward clinical application. J Clin Investig 2016; 126: 1152-62.
[55] Bobrie A, Colombo M, Krumeich S, Raposo G, Théry C. Diverse subpopulations of vesicles secreted by different intracellular mechanisms are present in exosome preparations obtained by differential ultracentrifugation. J Extracell Vesicles 2012; 1: 18397.
[56] Jun J-I, Lau LF. Resolution of organ fibrosis. J Clin Investig 2018; 128: 97-107.
[57] Hecker L, et al. Reversal of persistent fibrosis in aging by targeting Nox4-Nrf2 redox imbalance. Sci Transl Med 2014; 6: 231ra47.
[58] Marcellin P, et al. Regression of cirrhosis during treatment with tenofovir disoproxil fumarate for chronic hepatitis B: a 5-year open-kabel follow-up study. Lancet 2013; 381: 468-75.
[59] Karimi-Shah BA, Chowdhury BA. Forced vital capacity in idiopathic pulmonary fibrosis— FDA review of pirfenidone and nintedanib. N Engl J Med 2015; 372: 1189-91.
[60] Morse MA, et al. A phase I study of dexosome immunotherapy in patients with advanced nonsmall cell lung cancer. J Transl Med 2005; 3: 9.
[61] Besse B, et al. Dendritic cell-derived exosomes as maintenance immunotherapy after first line chemotherapy in NSCLC. OncoImmunology 2016; 5: e1071008.
[62] Hoshino A, et al. Tumour exosome integrins determine organotropic metastasis. Nature 2015; 527: 329-35.
[63] Lener T, et al. Applying extracellular vesicles based therapeutics in clinical trials—an ISEV position paper. J Extracell Vesicles 2015; 4: 30087.
[64] Khan M, et al. Embryonic stem cell-derived exosomes promote endogenous repair mechanisms and enhance cardiac function following myocardial infarction. Circ Res 2015; 117: 52-64.
[65] Hu G-W, et al. Exosomes secreted by human-induced pluripotent stem cell-derived mesenchymal stem cells attenuate limb ischemia by promoting angiogenesis in mice. Stem Cell Res Ther 2015; 6: 10.
[66] Fujita Y, Kadota T, Araya J, Ochiya T, Kuwano K. Clinical application of mesenchymal stem cell-derived extracellular vesicle-based therapeutics for inflammatory lung diseases. J Clin Med 2018; 7: 355.
[67] Nardi NB, da Silva Meirelles L. Mesenchymal stem cells: isolation, in vitro expansion and characterization. In: Handbook of experimental pharmacology. 2008. p.249-82. https://doi.org/10.1007/978-3-540-77855-4_11.
[68] Salem HK, Thiemermann C. Mesenchymal stromal cells: current understanding and clinical status. Stem Cells 2010; 28: 585-96.
[69] Lalu MM, et al. Safety of cell therapy with mesenchymal stromal cells (SafeCell): a systematic review and meta-analysis of clinical trials. PLoS ONE 2012; 7: e47559.
[70] Li T, et al. Exosomes derived from human umbilical cord mesenchymal stem cells alleviate liver fibrosis. Stem Cells Dev

2013; 22: 845-54.
- [71] Hyun J, Wang S, Kim J, Kim GJ, Jung Y. MicroRNA125b-mediated Hedgehog signaling influences liver regeneration by chorionic plate-derived mesenchymal stem cells. Sci Rep 2015; 5: 14135.
- [72] Shentu T-P, et al. Thy-1 dependent uptake of mesenchymal stem cell-derived extracellular vesicles blocks myofibroblastic differentiation. Sci Rep 2017; 7: 18052.
- [73] Lai RC, et al. Exosome secreted by MSC reduces myocardial ischemia/reperfusion injury. Stem Cell Res 2010; 4: 214-22.
- [74] Barile L, et al. Extracellular vesicles from human cardiac progenitor cells inhibit cardiomyocyte apoptosis and improve cardiac function after myocardial infarction. Cardiovasc Res 2014; 103: 530-41.
- [75] Zhang Z, et al. Pretreatment of cardiac stem cells with exosomes derived from mesenchymal stem Cells enhances myocardial repair. J Am Heart Assoc 2016; 5: e002856.
- [76] Ma J, et al. Exosomes derived from Akt-modified human umbilical cord mesenchymal stem cells improve cardiac regeneration and promote angiogenesis via activating platelet-derived growth factor D. Stem Cells Transl Med 2017; 6: 51-9.
- [77] Chen L, et al. Therapeutic effects of serum extracellular vesicles in liver fibrosis. J Extracell Vesicles 2018; 7: 1461505.
- [78] Vicencio JM, et al. Plasma exosomes protect the myocardium from ischemia-reperfusion injury. J Am Coll Cardiol 2015; 65: 1525-36.
- [79] Beltrami C, et al. Human pericardial fluid contains exosomes enriched with cardiovascularexpressed MicroRNAs and promotes therapeutic angiogenesis. Mol Ther 2017; 25: 679-93.
- [80] Adamiak M, Sahoo S. Exosomes in myocardial repair: advances and challenges in the development of next-generation therapeutics. Mol Ther 2018; 26: 1635-43.

第 14 章

炎症疾病中外泌体介导的免疫细胞信号交流机制

Mechanisms of exosome-mediated immune cell crosstalk in inflammation and disease

Todd W. Costantini, Raul Coimbra, Brian P. Eliceiri

Division of Trauma, Surgical Critical Care, Burns and Acute Care Surgery, Department of Surgery, University of California San Diego, San Diego, CA, United States

一、在免疫细胞相互作用过程中外泌体的转运参与炎症反应

健康组织中的组织修复和再生一直被认为是一种多细胞类型的协调反应,这种协调反应直到最近才被认为是由细胞间的直接相互作用和分泌因子的释放所介导的[1-5]。20世纪80年代发现的外泌体是多囊泡胞内体(multi-vesicular endosome,MVE)的产物,其腔内囊泡(现在称为外泌体)是从成熟的血网织红细胞表面释放出来的[6-8],这使得人们认识到外泌体是细胞间交流的普遍机制,这种机制在炎症中起着至关重要的作用[9-12]。近年来外泌体的研究聚焦在其生物发生机制、远距离介导细胞信号的生物活性、有效载荷的表征、外泌体生物标志物以及外泌体治疗上。此外,鼠与人的遗传学,以及外泌体分析技术的进步已经将一类EV从一类构成型的分泌囊泡转变为公认的在细胞生物学、免疫学和炎症调节的生物活性介质。例如,外泌体作为细胞间通信的媒介,已经成为专业APC调节免疫反应的重要机制[13-19],包括DC在内的APC通过经典直接细胞相互作用以及两种不同型APC表面表达的外泌体,来呈现MHC Ⅰ和MHC Ⅱ与肽的复合体。首先共刺激表达在APC表面的调节分子和同在表面的外泌体,这包括MHC Ⅰ/Ⅱ、B7-1、B7-2和其他调节DC与受体细胞对接的分子[9,20-22],即一种被称为变装的机制。其次,APC能摄入外泌体从而导致细胞因子表达发生改变,进而影响共刺激分子的表达和提呈给T细胞的APC源性外泌体的释放。尽管APC在激活幼稚T细胞方面比外泌体更有效,但根据对肿瘤模型[23-28]、感染[29]、耐受性[30]、免疫豁免[31]和关节炎[32,33]的研究,分离的外泌体上存在的抗原可以介导免疫刺激或免疫抑制。

免疫调节细胞因子能够重新编码外泌体释放的生物活性。从而证明了外泌体的可塑性和他们能够远距离调节炎症信号的潜能,特别在原发肿瘤和损伤模型中,局部组织介导的前哨淋巴结的免疫监视反应[9]。巨噬细胞衍生的外泌体转移至T细胞,随后激活了淋巴细胞的扩张和分化,被称为"免疫突触"[29,34,35],从而证明了外泌体增强免疫反应的能力[4,5,20]。肿瘤源性外泌体[10,36,37]调节免疫反应包括控制耐受性和免疫原性[32,38-41],其通过直接提呈

肿瘤源性抗原如 CEA、melan-A、间皮素和细胞调节分子,如 FasL、RAIL、CD154/CD40L 和 PD-L1[31,42-44]。

既然外泌体能够同时介导免疫刺激性和免疫抑制活动,那么细胞源性的表征、释放的机制、有效载荷和效应细胞是区分外泌体在健康基线与疾病模型中生物学相关性的重要考虑因素。例如,伴随细菌性和病毒性感染,从感染巨噬细胞中分离出来的外泌体在小鼠 APC 和 T 细胞的存在下提供保护,这表明外泌体在急性模型中调节免疫反应[45-48]。反之,肿瘤源性外泌体介导免疫抑制通过阻断效应细胞中的分化和细胞因子释放,并可能提呈 PD-L1 和 CD40,两者被熟知能够抑制 T 细胞反应。相反,肿瘤源性外泌体介导肿瘤微环境中的 APC 上免疫抑制和循环中的二级反应。肿瘤源性外泌体的全身反应包括骨髓源性前体细胞的重编码[26],而外泌体表面上特定整合素的存在则定义了肿瘤源性外泌体的向性,可以在局部微环境和二级站点中指导其归巢和生物学活性[28]。尽管本综述没有对这一方面进行全面总结,但在感染和肿瘤方面的外泌体研究已经建立起了外泌体在免疫调节的中心地位,并通过开发肿瘤源性外泌体影响特定免疫反应介导免疫监视的能力,为诊断手段与治疗方式的发展提供了基础。

二、外泌体生物发生和分泌途径与健康和疾病的相关性

外泌体在许多生物系统中介导细胞间串扰信号传导,这种信号在疾病中受到干扰,并导致不同的外泌体特征。尽管本领域的研究人员通常认为外泌体是释放它的细胞质膜表面上蛋白质的"快照",但它们代表了其来源细胞中更为复杂的物质。实际上,存在于 MVE 与质膜融合释放的外泌体表面的蛋白质也可能具有细胞内来源。为了确定外泌体的生物发生以及健康和疾病对该机制的影响,一项对将胞内囊泡分选到溶酶体或 MVE 的内体囊泡运输机制的生物化学概述表明,存在特定的细胞介体融合以及从质膜释放之前"编辑"囊泡有效载荷的过程。外泌体生物发生的调控已鉴定出与分泌和内吞途径相关的蛋白质,如负责运输的 ESCRT、脂质和四跨膜蛋白。各种体外筛选和功能研究已将 ESCRT 分为 ESCRT-0(如 Hrs、STAM)、ESCRT-Ⅰ(如 TSG101)、ESCRT-Ⅱ 和 ESCRT-Ⅲ(如 CHMP4C)。鞘磷脂酶(nSMase2)和神经酰胺的产生对外泌体的生物发生而言也是必不可少的,而 Rab 和相关活化蛋白(即 Rab GTPase 活化蛋白,RabGAP)[49-53]与外泌体释放的分泌步骤有关。由于 Rab 是 GTPase 超家族的一部分,因此 Rab 的利用可能是针对特定细胞类型的。体外筛选已确定 Rab 27 介导了 50% 的外泌体分泌,这与 Rab27a 和 Rab27b 的双敲除小鼠一致,且具有这些 Rab 所介导的调节性 RabGAP 的活性。这些研究表明,外泌体的生物发生和分泌涉及并行机制,特定的 MHCⅠ/Ⅱ、四跨膜蛋白和整联蛋白进入分泌外泌体的细胞内分选还需要其他途径。

microRNA 负载由特定的 RNA 结合蛋白调节,当通过蛋白质折叠和包装机制将其与蛋白一起加载到外泌体中时,它们开始提供对外泌体负载复杂性的了解。在特定 miRNA 的包装中,虽然每个外泌体的绝对浓度较低,但涉及特定 RNA 结合蛋白,这些蛋白可能有助于在源细胞中进行包装,在外泌体中稳定,并且可能并入受体细胞的 RNA 处理途径中,从而允许细胞之间 miRNA 的信号交流[54]。主要通过免疫印迹、免疫金电子显微镜抗体染

色和蛋白质组学定义的蛋白质有效载荷表明,外泌体蛋白质多种多样,包括介导抗原提呈(MHCⅠ、MHCⅡ)、黏附(四连蛋白和整联蛋白)、膜运输(Annexins、Rabs、Arfs、clathrin)、ESCRT蛋白(Alix、Tsg101)、热休克响应(HSP70、HSP90)、细胞骨架(肌动蛋白、cofilin、微管蛋白)、酶(激酶、搪瓷酶)、信号转导(14-3-3、syntenin)和脂筏(flotilins)[55]。

国际胞外囊泡学会(International Society for Extracellular Vesicle,ISEV)建立了报告标准,其中Exocarta(www.exocarta.org)是外泌体有效载荷的数据库,提供了详尽的数据库,详细描述了外泌体的蛋白质、核酸和脂质组成。尽管分离方法和质量控制因外泌体分离和有效载荷的特性而异,但很明显,外泌体的数量和含量可以受多种因素和疾病过程的调节。因此,基于外泌体的细胞内起源、外泌体的组成性释放的贡献以及由于质膜被夹入细胞外空间(即微囊泡)而导致的小囊泡的存在,在特定疾病条件下以细胞类型的特定方式进行外泌体的检测将是未来研究的重点。

复杂器官系统(如大脑)的单细胞转录组学已鉴定出特定细胞类型的不同基因表达谱。这一方法极大地促进了人们对激酶、转录因子和转运蛋白的细胞型特异性表达显著增加的基因超家族的理解。进一步研究发现,调节外泌体释放的机制可能是具有细胞类型特异性的,并受到了疾病状态调节。因此,体内机制研究的挑战将是特定途径的定义以及生物标志物研究,在易于获取的组织和体液(如血浆、尿液、唾液和CSF)中检测更复杂的外泌体特征。

三、疾病中体内释放外泌体的机制

对具有生物有效载荷的外泌体释放机制理解的进步,为研究疾病模型中的外泌体提供了分子学基础,并让人看到其在治疗和诊断方面不可忽视的潜力。着眼于对免疫系统具有生物学活性的外泌体,此篇回顾了:① 外泌体和肿瘤学以及 ② 外泌体在非中枢神经系统损伤和炎症中的最新发现。最新免疫检查点抑制剂治疗的进展彻底改变了肿瘤学领域,它确立了靶向免疫系统激活/重新激活宿主适应性免疫细胞群以识别和减轻肿瘤负担的核心重要性。Paget的"种子和土壤"假说提出,肿瘤微环境将提供重要的因素来支持肿瘤的生长和转移,这取决于异常ECM蛋白、生长因子/趋化因子、免疫细胞以及最近的外泌体的局部积累。在抑制免疫反应的同时,携带促肿瘤恶性有效载荷的肿瘤微环境中所积累的外泌体的不良后果,也将为检测循环血浆中作为生物标志物的外泌体提供了可能性。在将肿瘤视为无法治愈的伤口的概观下,肿瘤相关外泌体的作用机制可为急、慢性损伤和炎症模型提供可验证的假设。

四、肿瘤学中的外泌体和免疫检查点抑制

已知外泌体可介导特定的肿瘤诱导的免疫反应[11,56,57],这可能与个体对免疫检查点抑制剂的反应有关,并可能指导个体化治疗计划的制订。我们在后续部分中详细介绍的最新进展中利用了外泌体概况的多重分析[58,59]和单个外泌体颗粒分析来定义特定的表面目标(即VFC)[60,61]。可以根据其在免疫细胞信号传导和串扰中的已知功能和丰度来选择与APC调节和T细胞活化相关的靶标[11,62,63]。可以使用市售仪器和适当的质量保证(quality assurance,QA)和质量控制(quality control,QC)标准[64-66],仅对一小部分外周血进行外泌

体分析和血浆中目标表位的定量分析。在实验性肿瘤模型中已确定外泌体是激活T细胞的抗原提呈的重要"非典型"机制之一[67-69]。尽管有几项研究将血浆外泌体与肿瘤进展相关联[70-73],从而确定了它们的临床相关性,但还没有公开发表的研究分析外泌体作为免疫检查点抑制剂治疗效果的衡量标准。由于现在存在用于快速评估外泌体大小和数量的定量方法,然后通过表面轮廓分析来评估外泌体的来源和复杂性,因此存在一种针对特定表位进行EV分析的策略,该策略与具有自适应性的那些表位的临床相关性非常吻合的免疫细胞信号传导。然而,这些分析策略在分层患者人群中的广泛实施具有转化潜力,尽管已与现有的分子和临床标准进行交叉比较,但在实验模型中进一步研究外泌体的生物活性支持了分析人类肿瘤中外泌体的目标。在外泌体分析中,生物活性样品的冷冻和储存比细胞更实用,血浆是从健康志愿者和肿瘤患者中取样的理想选择,进一步提高了临床转化的效率。

五、外泌体在创伤与缺血/再灌注损伤中的作用

创伤性损伤所致的出血性休克(traumatic injury causing hemorrhagic shock,T/HS)会导致组织损伤,其中缺血/再灌注会触发一系列炎症反应,从而导致系统性炎症反应综合征(systemic inflammatory response syndrome,SIRS)[74]。尽管此反应是最初对损伤的反应所必需的,并且在大多数患者康复后会缓解,但不受控制的SIRS可能导致远处器官损伤,如急性肺损伤和多器官功能衰竭[75]。尽管对T/HS损伤后多器官功能衰竭的病理生理机制尚不清楚,但外泌体从受伤的肠上皮、免疫细胞、肠神经系统和脉管系统向肠系膜淋巴(mesenteric lymph,ML)输送生物活性免疫调节因子的生物活性是调节SIRS的一个重要组成部分。我们推测,ML外泌体可调节ML和肠系膜淋巴结(mesenteric lymph node,MLN)的免疫细胞活化,并且当它们扩散到体循环中时,会诱发继发性器官损伤。这些外泌体的炎症相关功能有效载荷包括miRNA、蛋白质和脂质,可用于定义免疫信号传导,作为生物标志物或治疗性外泌体。先前我们已经证明ML中的APC激活MLN中的T细胞,并且最近对外泌体的分析表明显示,如MHCⅡ的外泌体表面的免疫相关抗原决定簇可以用作区分假性与ML损伤的标志物。ML中外泌体的核酸和蛋白质组学分析表明,外泌体在损伤后具有独特的miRNA和蛋白质有效负载,这是进一步研究外泌体作为治疗靶点和诊断方法的机会(即"治疗学")。例如,可以通过加载特定的调节性miRNA来改造外泌体,以重新引入肠系膜淋巴管或受伤动物的外周循环来减轻炎症。通过大量调节肠道内稳态的神经免疫调节网络,我们已经探索了肠壁炎症的神经调节的可能性,这种调节可以通过外泌体谱的变化来检测。在这个例子中,迷走神经是肠道和其他器官上消炎性副交感神经输入的明确介体,在电刺激迷走神经后,我们观察到了创伤和缺血性损伤后的保护作用,如改善了肠道上皮的完整性、降低了免疫细胞激活,并确定ML中外泌体蛋白质有效载荷的变化。这些研究为探究ML外泌体在肺等次要器官中的全身作用提供了科学前提。外泌体通过ML进入胸导管从而进入体循环,可以在肺中鉴定出荧光标记的外泌体,并伴有肺损伤标志物的增加[76]。这些观察结果与肿瘤学和免疫学领域的研究一致,在这些领域中,通过淋巴结传播肿瘤、感染或炎症相关的外泌体与疾病进展和远距离传播细胞间信号传递的能力有关[77,78]。

例如，已知 ML 包含炎症介质[79]，并且多项研究表明：ML 导管的结扎可减轻肺部炎症，并且休克后 ML 注入幼稚动物的循环中可再现肺损伤表型[80,81]。我们在动物模型中对外泌体的研究表明，外泌体与 ML 中炎症介质的作用相似，其使用的是成熟的实验方法，与人类创伤和局部缺血的休克和复苏阶段的病理生理学一致。

六、外泌体与炎症性肠病

包括克罗恩病和溃疡性结肠炎在内的炎症性肠病（inflammatory bowel disease，IBD）是一种慢性免疫介导的胃肠道疾病，困扰着超过 150 万美国人，其特点是缓解和复发[82,83]。IBD 通常还与免疫细胞的活化、炎症因子的募集和肠系膜淋巴管系统的扩张有关[84,85]。而 ML 在 IBD 进展中的作用至今仍然未知。我们的研究小组[13,76,86-90]已经确定了外泌体介导 ML 中的促炎生物活性，并提出神经免疫轴通过 ML 调节肠道炎症。释放到肠系膜淋巴系统的外泌体穿过胸导管进入锁骨下静脉并进入全身循环[91]。我们已经证明，ML 中的促炎生物活性是由外泌体介导的。因此，肠损伤后释放的 ML 外泌体对巨噬细胞具有促炎作用，并抑制 DC 的活化。从肿瘤、上皮细胞和免疫细胞释放的外泌体介导细胞间信号传导，因此我们提出肠道壁来源的外泌体调节 IBD 中的炎症。激活的免疫细胞刺激调节先天性和适应性免疫[92]神经元回路的能力导致了数次肠损伤研究，其中迷走神经的刺激通过增强屏障完整性和减少炎症保护肠壁。综上所述，我们之前的研究表明迷走神经刺激可减轻肠道炎症[93-95]，降低 ML 的毒性，并减少周围组织炎症和随后的远处器官损伤[13,76,87-90]。以 ML 外泌体为重点，确定特定外泌体负载的功能相关性非常重要，如通过调节靶细胞中的信号转导通路来介导细胞间通信的 miRNA。肠内免疫细胞的神经调节是否会改变 IBD 和其他慢性疾病中 ML 外泌体的表型是一个悬而未决的问题，我们建议通过分析引流 ML 中的外泌体概况和生物学活性来监测肠道免疫和系统性炎症反应的神经控制。

七、外泌体与伤口愈合

伤口愈合和组织修复领域的临床观察、实验结果和法则认为，损伤的修复包括止血、炎症、血管形成和上皮形成四个主要阶段。我们认为，外泌体所携带能够反映损伤阶段的蛋白质和核酸有效负荷可以影响外泌体的外形、有效载荷和生物活性[13,76,97]。组织修复反应的协调阶段与反应失调形成对比，这种失调定义了与肥胖、糖尿病、衰老、感染和烧伤后瘢痕形成有关的慢性伤口[98,99]。我们认为外泌体在介导慢性伤口免疫反应中的作用可能与肿瘤微环境中外泌体的生物学特性相似。相反，在健康组织中观察到外泌体介导的炎症可能为外泌体蛋白质和核酸提供了模板，从而促进亲修复性外泌体生物学和组织损伤的修复。我们将外泌体生物发生的特定介体的生化活性与具有有效载荷外泌体的群体释放联系在一起，并且通过关注 RabGAP 的生化活性来调节促炎性巨噬细胞与亲性修复性巨噬细胞之间平衡的生物学活性。我们已经建立了基于合成聚乙烯醇（polyvinylalcohol，PVA）海绵的皮下植入物模型用于体内生产外泌体，其中释放外泌体的细胞（即供体细胞）可以通过局部基因传递来靶向，以测试特定外泌体生物发生的介体生物化学活性。尽管迄今为止，大多数定义外泌体生物发生的遗传学研究都使用培养的细胞系，但靶向慢病毒基因递送的 PVA 植入物能够收集募集的白细胞和释放到条件培养基中的外泌体，称为伤口液，因为 PVA 模型是一种无菌炎症和伤口巨噬细胞募集的模型。因此，PVA 模型可用作生成更高密度的 CD9[+]、CD63[+] 和 CD81[+] 外泌体的体内 3D 支架，而通常不受用于体外生长细胞的细胞培养瓶和小牛血清的限制[100]。PVA 也可以用 ECM 蛋白包被，以修饰募集的白细胞的微环境，从而释放外泌体。然后，可以使用 ECM 相关整联蛋白的蛋白质表位分析来预测伤口床中外泌体亚群的向性，并提供许多未开发的机会来设计外泌体的向性，并验证其在体内的生理相关性[28]。

八、外泌体与糖尿病

慢性疾病，如糖尿病是伤口愈合、创伤和感染等并发症的显著危险因素。糖尿病创面、肝脏和脂肪组织的促炎状态以促炎细胞因子如 TNF-α 和胰岛素抵抗为特征。最近的研究表明，脂肪组织巨噬细胞来源的外泌体被释放到血液循环中，其中包含的 miRNA 能够介导胰岛素抵抗。含 miRNA 的外泌体能够介导细胞的胰岛素活性和系统胰岛素敏感度，从而识别 PPARγ 作为治疗靶点。循环的无细胞核酸分析（包括 miRNA）一直是患者样品和动物模型中广泛研究的主题，但是这些研究的一个混杂因素是 miRNA 经常不重叠。Dicer 是一种调节 miRNA 加工酶的基因，使用特定组织 Dicer 敲除的小鼠可用于定义特定 miRNA 的功能要求，这是一种遗传工具，可以完善与疾病过程中功能相关的 miRNA 的子集[101]。

九、外泌体释放的物种特异性机制的潜力

物种进化中的基因重复和重排已成为基本发展过程的重要介体，这些基因被称为人类特异性或独特人类基因（uniquely human gene，UHG）。在神经科学中，特定的 UHG 已从调控神经元形成的基因家族如 Notch（即 Notch2NL）和其他 RabGTPase 超家族（即 ARHGAP11b）进化而来，这些家族调节皮质折叠的形成。在外泌体生物发生领域，RabGTPase 激活蛋白家族的成员（即 TBC1D3）调节生长因子信号转导、巨噬细胞胞吞作用（已知增强抗原的摄取和提呈过程）以及外泌体生物发生。有趣的是，TBC1D3 也与皮质折叠的形成有关，这一活动突显了进一步研究 UHG 在神经科学中的重要性。在外泌体及其形成和释放的调控中，针对 Rab 和 RabGAP 进行了广泛的研究，特别是根据它们各自超家族的大小。研究外泌体形成遗传介质的总体障碍决定了它们的功能要求。迄今为止，大多数研究都使用了酵母和脊椎动物细胞系，但敲除小鼠靶向特定的外泌体生物发生却进展缓慢。此外，迄今为止已确定了大多数基因家族成员的相关性，如 Rab 或 RabGAP。结合序列相关的家族的某些成员实际上可能调控不相关的途径的可能性，以及家族成员在不同细胞类型或发育中的不同时间表达的可能性。我们已经考虑了调节外泌体生物发生的基因的物种特异性表达可能还需要在进化和免疫系统选择压力的背景下进行解释。我们最近提出，免疫系统，特别是适应性免疫系统，可能是 UHG 出现的热点。像在神经发育中一样，炎症反应是对感染和损伤的主要防御反应，很明显，人类和啮齿动物模型中免疫细胞组成的根本差异可能会使实验研究转化为临床研究。我们认为，随着越来越全面的筛选鉴定出新型

的和已知的外泌体生物发生和分泌的调节因子,将需要考虑体外和体内模型的相关性,尤其是外泌体调节基因的物种和细胞类型特异性功能。

十、外泌体和技术驱动的进步

使用各种技术从条件培养基或生物体液中分离外泌体,这些技术包括分步离心、随后的过滤、超速离心或磁珠富集。这些对于在动物模型或人类中部署临床样品的分析测定至关重要。例如,尽管分离方法和质量控制方法的差异限制了绝对比较,但是光散射方法,如纳米颗粒跟踪分析(nanoparticle tracking analysis, NTA)为根据大小分层的外泌体提供了标准化的定量技术。但是,NTA 并没有解决外泌体的有效载荷和多样性,只是大小上的差异。此外,在本领域中,关于囊泡的来源存在争议,因为囊泡是由细胞内 MVE 产生的 EV,而微囊泡则是在质膜上的。尽管微囊泡被定义为从其他来源释放,但质膜,30～150 nm 范围内的小微囊泡可能会被混淆解释。基于磁珠的外泌体特定亚群富集,已经使人们更加了解外泌体的复杂性,可以将其用于分析健康和疾病中的外泌体,但是,这些技术需要大量的 miRNA 或蛋白质组学样本。

解决生物液中外泌体复杂性的技术是囊泡流式细胞术(vesicle flow cytometry, VFC),该技术使用基于荧光膜染料的优化流式细胞术分析程序。VFC 对于分析临床样本的外泌体特别重要,因为它解决了外泌体临床研究领域中对患者血浆样本分析必不可少的三个障碍。有限地采用 VFC 技术的障碍是单个外泌体上表面表位的异质性,通常不对患者血浆样品中的外泌体进行分析。VFC 工作流程通过在脂质双层中掺入荧光的敏感亲脂性荧光染料(即 di-8-ANEPPS)[102],最大限度地减少了由第一步分析的丰度和亲和力而产生的特异性抗体的偏差,从而可重复地检测外泌体根据样品上膜染料的荧光触发,与大小和抗体特异性无关。为了解决可用的已验证的 VFC 抗体的局限性,可以使用多重分析来筛选外泌体表面的水平。一个重要的提示是,不同表位的抗体亲和力范围很大,因此除非进行了适当的校准技术,否则限制了交叉解释。现在存在定量方法的组合,用于快速评估外泌体的大小、数量、外形、有效载荷和生物活性,可以根据患者队列和相匹配的志愿者血液来提供液体活检,以确定外泌体在健康和疾病方面的病理生理作用。

十一、总结

外泌体在介导健康和人类疾病的细胞间通信和免疫反应中的重要性日益得到认可。了解外泌体加工和释放的调控以及外泌体表面和内部携带的物质对于更好地了解外泌体生物学至关重要。结合改进的技术以通过研究其加工和释放的分子更好地表征外泌体的子集,外泌体可能会成为未来重要的诊断和治疗靶点。

(黄晶焕 译,李晓林 审校)

参考文献

[1] Lopez-Verrilli MA, Court FA. Exosomes: mediators of communication in eukaryotes. Biol Res 2013; 46(1): 5-11. https://doi.org/10.4067/S0716-97602013000100001. 23760408.
[2] Raposo G, Stoorvogel W. Extracellular vesicles: exosomes, microvesicles, and friends. J Cell Biol 2013; 200(4): 373-

383. Epub 2013/02/20, https://doi.org/10.1083/jcb.20121113823420871. PMCID 3575529.

[3] Yanez-Mo M, Siljander PR, Andreu Z, Zavec AB, Borras FE, Buzas EI, Buzas K, Casal E, Cappello F, Carvalho J, Colas E, Cordeiro-da Silva A, Fais S, Falcon-Perez JM, Ghobrial IM, Giebel B, Gimona M, Graner M, Gursel I, Gursel M, Heegaard NH, Hendrix A, Kierulf P, Kokubun K, Kosanovic M, Kralj-Iglic V, Kramer-Albers EM, Laitinen S, Lasser C, Lener T, Ligeti E, Line A, Lipps G, Llorente A, Lotvall J, Mancek-Keber M, Marcilla A, Mittelbrunn M, Nazarenko I, Nolte-t Hoen EN, Nyman TA, O'Driscoll L, Olivan M, Oliveira C, Pallinger E, Del Portillo HA, Reventos J, Rigau M, Rohde E, Sammar M, Sanchez-Madrid F, Santarem N, Schallmoser K, Ostenfeld MS, Stoorvogel W, Stukelj R, Van der Grein SG, Vasconcelos MH, Wauben MH, De Wever O. Biological properties of extracellular vesicles and their physiological functions. J Extracell Vesicles 2015; 4: 27066. https://doi.org/10.3402/jev.v4.27066. 25979354. PMCID: PMC4433489.

[4] Gutierrez-Vazquez C, Villarroya-Beltri C, Mittelbrunn M, Sanchez-Madrid F. Transfer of extracellular vesicles during immune cell-cell interactions. Immunol Rev 2013; 251(1): 125 – 142. https://doi.org/10.1111/imr.12013. 23278745. PMCID: PMC3740495.

[5] Mittelbrunn M, Gutierrez-Vazquez C, Villarroya-Beltri C, Gonzalez S, Sanchez-Cabo F, Gonzalez MA, Bernad A, Sanchez-Madrid F. Unidirectional transfer of microRNA-loaded exosomes from T cells to antigen-presenting cells. Nat Commun 2011; 2: 282. https://doi.org/10.1038/ncomms1285. 21505438. PMCID: PMC3104548.

[6] Harding CV, Heuser JE, Stahl PD. Exosomes: looking back three decades and into the future. J Cell Biol 2013; 200(4): 367 – 71. https://doi.org/10.1083/jcb.201212113. 23420870. PMCID 3575527.

[7] Harding C, Heuser J, Stahl P. Receptor-mediated endocytosis of transferrin and recycling of the transferrin receptor in rat reticulocytes. J Cell Biol 1983; 97(2): 329 – 39. 6309857. PMCID: PMC2112509.

[8] Pan BT, Johnstone RM. Fate of the transferrin receptor during maturation of sheep reticulocytes in vitro: selective externalization of the receptor. Cell 1983; 33(3): 967 – 78, 6307529.

[9] Bianco NR, Kim SH, Morelli AE, Robbins PD. Modulation of the immune response using dendritic cell-derived exosomes. Methods Mol Biol 2007; 380: 443 – 55. https://doi.org/10.1007/978-1-59745-395-0_28. 17876111.

[10] Hao S, Bai O, Yuan J, Qureshi M, Xiang J. Dendritic Cell-Derived Exosomes Stimulate Stronger CD8(+) CTL Responses and Antitumor Immunity than Tumor Cell-Derived Exosomes. Cell Mol Immunol 2006; 3(3): 205 – 11. PubMed PMID; WOS: 000208926200006.

[11] Pitt JM, Charrier M, Viaud S, Andre F, Besse B, Chaput N, Zitvogel L. Dendritic cell-derived exosomes as immunotherapies in the fight against cancer. J Immunol 2014; 193(3): 1006 – 11. https://doi.org/10.4049/jimmunol.1400703. 25049431.

[12] Quah BJ, O'Neill HC. The immunogenicity of dendritic cell-derived exosomes. Blood Cells Mol Dis 2005; 35(2): 94 – 110. Epub 2005/06/25 https://doi.org/10.1016/j.bcmd.2005.05.00215975838.

[13] Kojima M, Gimenes-Junior JA, Langness S, Morishita K, Lavoie-Gagne O, Eliceiri B, Costantini TW, Coimbra R. Exosomes, not protein or lipids, in mesenteric lymph activate inflammation: unlocking the mystery of post-shock multiple organ failure. J Trauma Acute Care Surg 2017; 82(1): 42 – 50. https://doi.org/10.1097/TA.0000000000001296. 27779585.

[14] Lee H, Zhang D, Zhu Z, Dela Cruz CS, Jin Y. Epithelial cell-derived microvesicles activate macrophages and promote inflammation via microvesicle-containing microRNAs. Sci Rep 2016; 6: 35250. https://doi.org/10.1038/srep35250. 27731391. PMCID: PMC5059671.

[15] Li D, Liu J, Guo B, Liang C, Dang L, Lu C, He X, Cheung HY, Xu L, Lu C, He B, Liu B, Shaikh AB, Li F, Wang L, Yang Z, Au DW, Peng S, Zhang Z, Zhang BT, Pan X, Qian A, Shang P, Xiao L, Jiang B, Wong CK, Xu J, Bian Z, Liang Z, Guo DA, Zhu H, Tan W, Lu A, Zhang G. Osteoclast-derived exosomal miR-214-3p inhibits osteoblastic bone formation. Nat Commun 2016; 7: 10872. https://doi.org/10.1038/ncomms10872. 26947250. PMCID: PMC4786676.

[16] Shenoda BB, Ajit SK. Modulation of Immune Responses by Exosomes Derived from Antigen-Presenting Cells. Clin Med Insights Pathol 2016; 9(Suppl 1): 1 – 8. https://doi.org/10.4137/CPath.S39925. 27660518. PMCID: PMC5024790.

[17] Garzetti L, Menon R, Finardi A, Bergami A, Sica A, Martino G, Comi G, Verderio C, Farina C, Furlan R. Activated macrophages release microvesicles containing polarized M1 or M2 mRNAs. J Leukoc Biol 2014; 95(5): 817 – 25. https://doi.org/10.1189/jlb.0913485. 24379213.

[18] Truman J-P, Al Gadban MM, Smith KJ, Jenkins RW, Mayroo N, Virella G, Lopes-Virella MF, Bielawska A, Hannun YA, Hammad SM. Differential regulation of acid sphingomyelinase in macrophages stimulated with oxidized low-density lipoprotein (LDL) and oxidized LDL immune complexes: role in phagocytosis and cytokine release. Immunology 2012; 136(1): 30 – 45. https://doi.org/10.1111/j.1365-2567.2012.03552.x. PubMed PMID; WOS: 000302399200005.

[19] Zhang Y, Liu D, Chen X, Li J, Li L, Bian Z, Sun F, Lu J, Yin Y, Cai X, Sun Q, Wang K, Ba Y, Wang Q, Wang D, Yang J, Liu P, Xu T, Yan Q, Zhang J, Zen K, Zhang C-Y. Secreted monocytic miR-150 enhances targeted endothelial cell migration. Mol Cell 2010; 39(1): 133 – 44. https://doi.org/10.1016/j.molcel.2010.06.010. PubMed PMID; WOS: 000280139200014.

[20] Mittelbrunn M, Vicente-Manzanares M, Sanchez-Madrid F. Organizing polarized delivery of exosomes at synapses. Traffic 2015; 16(4): 327 – 37. https://doi.org/10.1111/tra.12258. PubMed PMID 25614958.

[21] Thery C, Ostrowski M, Segura E. Membrane vesicles as conveyors of immune responses. Nat Rev Immunol 2009; 9(8): 581 – 93. https://doi.org/10.1038/nri2567. 19498381.

[22] Valenti R, Huber V, Iero M, Filipazzi P, Parmiani G, Rivoltini L. Tumor-released microvesicles as vehicles of immunosuppression. Cancer Res 2007; 67(7): 2912 – 5. https://doi.org/10.1158/0008-5472.CAN-07-0520. 17409393.

[23] Viaud S, Thery C, Ploix S, Tursz T, Lapierre V, Lantz O, Zitvogel L, Chaput N. Dendritic cellderived exosomes for cancer immunotherapy: what's next? Cancer Res 2010; 70(4): 1281 – 5. https://doi.org/10.1158/0008-5472.can-09-3276. PubMed PMID; WOS: 000278485700002.

[24] Rak J. Extracellular vesicles — biomarkers and effectors of the cellular interactome in cancer. Front Pharmacol 2013; 4:

[25] Logozzi M, De Milito A, Lugini L, Borghi M, Calabro L, Spada M, Perdicchio M, Marino ML, Federici C, Iessi E, Brambilla D, Venturi G, Lozupone F, Santinami M, Huber V, Maio M, Rivoltini L, Fais S. High levels of exosomes expressing CD63 and caveolin-1 in plasma of melanoma patients. PLoS One 2009; 4(4): e5219 https://doi.org/10.1371/journal.pone.0005219. 19381331. PMCID: 2667632.

[26] Peinado H, Aleckovic M, Lavotshkin S, Matei I, Costa-Silva B, Moreno-Bueno G, Hergueta-Redondo M, Williams C, Garcia-Santos G, Ghajar C, Nitadori-Hoshino A, Hoffman C, Badal K, Garcia BA, Callahan MK, Yuan J, Martins VR, Skog J, Kaplan RN, Brady MS, Wolchok JD, Chapman PB, Kang Y, Bromberg J, Lyden D. Melanoma exosomes educate bone marrow progenitor cells toward a pro-metastatic phenotype through MET. Nat Med 2012; 18(6): 883 - 91. https://doi.org/10.1038/nm.2753. 22635005. PMCID: 3645291.

[27] Kharaziha P, Ceder S, Li Q, Panaretakis T. Tumor cell-derived exosomes: a message in a bottle. Biochim Biophys Acta 2012; 1826(1): 103 - 11. Epub 2012/04/17 https://doi.org/10.1016/j.bbcan.2012.03.006 22503823.

[28] Hoshino A, Costa-Silva B, Shen TL, Rodrigues G, Hashimoto A, Tesic Mark M, Molina H, Kohsaka S, Di Giannatale A, Ceder S, Singh S, Williams C, Soplop N, Uryu K, Pharmer L, King T, Bojmar L, Davies AE, Ararso Y, Zhang T, Zhang H, Hernandez J, Weiss JM, Dumont-Cole VD, Kramer K, Wexler LH, Narendran A, Schwartz GK, Healey JH, Sandstrom P, Labori KJ, Kure EH, Grandgenett PM, Hollingsworth MA, de Sousa M, Kaur S, Jain M, Mallya K, Batra SK, Jarnagin WR, Brady MS, Fodstad O, Muller V, Pantel K, Minn AJ, Bissell MJ, Garcia BA, Kang Y, Rajasekhar VK, Ghajar CM, Matei I, Peinado H, Bromberg J, Lyden D. Tumour exosome integrins determine organotropic metastasis. Nature 2015; 527(7578): 329 - 35. https://doi.org/10.1038/nature15756. 26524530.

[29] Aline F, Bout D, Amigorena S, Roingeard P, Dimier-Poisson I. Toxoplasma gondii antigenpulsed-dendritic cell-derived exosomes induce a protective immune response against T. gondii infection. Infect Immun 2004; 72(7): 4127 - 37. https://doi.org/10.1128/IAI.72.7.4127-4137.2004. 15213158. PMCID: PMC427397.

[30] Karlsson M, Lundin S, Dahlgren U, Kahu H, Pettersson I, Telemo E. "Tolerosomes" are produced by intestinal epithelial cells. Eur J Immunol 2001; 31(10): 2892 - 900. https://doi.org/10.1002/1521-4141(200110)31: 10<2892:: AID-IMMU2892>3.0.CO; 2-I. 11592064.

[31] Frangsmyr L, Baranov V, Nagaeva O, Stendahl U, Kjellberg L, Mincheva-Nilsson L. Cytoplasmic microvesicular form of Fas ligand in human early placenta: switching the tissue immune privilege hypothesis from cellular to vesicular level. Mol Hum Reprod 2005; 11(1): 35 - 41. https://doi.org/10.1093/molehr/gah129. 15579659.

[32] Kim SH, Bianco N, Menon R, Lechman ER, Shufesky WJ, Morelli AE, Robbins PD. Exosomes derived from genetically modified DC expressing FasL are anti-inflammatory and immunosuppressive. Mol Ther 2006; 13(2): 289 - 300. https://doi.org/10.1016/j.ymthe.2005.09.015. 16275099.

[33] Kim SH, Lechman ER, Bianco N, Menon R, Keravala A, Nash J, Mi Z, Watkins SC, Gambotto A, Robbins PD. Exosomes derived from IL-10-treated dendritic cells can suppress inflammation and collagen-induced arthritis. J Immunol 2005; 174(10): 6440 - 8. 15879146.

[34] Colino J, Snapper CM. Exosomes from bone marrow dendritic cells pulsed with diphtheria toxoid preferentially induce type 1 antigen-specific IgG responses absence of free antigen. J Immunol 2006; 177(6): 3757 - 62. PubMed PMID; WOS: 000240475300029.

[35] Colino J, Snapper CM. Dendritic cell-derived exosomes express a *Streptococcus pneumoniae* capsular polysaccharide type 14 cross-reactive antigen that induces protective immunoglobulin responses against pneumococcal infection in mice. Infect Immun 2007; 75(1): 220 - 30. https://doi.org/10.1128/iai.01217-06. PubMed PMID; WOS: 000243230500023.

[36] Viaud S, Terme M, Flament C, Taieb J, Andre F, Novault S, Escudier B, Robert C, Caillat-Zucman S, Tursz T, Zitvogel L, Chaput N. Dendritic cell-derived exosomes promote natural killer cell activation and proliferation: a role for NKG2D ligands and IL-15R alpha. PLoS One 2009; 4(3). https://doi.org/10.1371/journal.pone.0004942. PubMed PMID; WOS: 000265499200006.

[37] Hao S, Bai O, Li F, Yuan J, Laferte S, Xiang J. Mature dendritic cells pulsed with exosomes stimulate efficient cytotoxic T-lymphocyte responses and antitumour immunity. Immunology 2007; 120(1): 90 - 102. https://doi.org/10.1111/j.1365-2567.2006.02483.x. PubMed PMID; WOS: 000242662500011.

[38] Yang X, Meng S, Jiang H, Zhu C, Wu W. Exosomes Derived from Immature Bone Marrow Dendritic Cells Induce Tolerogenicity of Intestinal Transplantation in Rats. J Surg Res 2011; 171(2): 826 - 32. https://doi.org/10.1016/j.jss.2010.05.021. PubMed PMID; WOS: 000296957900080.

[39] Peche H, Renaudin K, Beriou G, Merieau E, Amigorena S, Cuturi MC. Induction of tolerance by exosomes and short-term immunosuppression in a fully MHC-mismatched rat cardiac allograft model. Am J Transplant 2006; 6(7): 1541 - 50. https://doi.org/10.1111/j.1600-6143.2006.01344.x. PubMed PMID; WOS: 000238465400010.

[40] Peche H, Heslan M, Usal C, Amigorena S, Cuturi MC. Presentation of donor major histocompatibility complex antigens by bone marrow dendritic cell-derived exosomes modulates allograft rejection. Transplantation 2003; 76(10): 1503 - 10. https://doi.org/10.1097/01.tp.0000092494.75313.38. PubMed PMID; WOS: 000186833400022.

[41] Bianco NR, Kim SH, Ruffner MA, Robbins PD. Therapeutic effect of exosomes from indoleamine 2,3-dioxygenase-positive dendritic cells in collagen-induced arthritis and delayed-type hypersensitivity disease models. Arthritis Rheum 2009; 60(2): 380 - 9. https://doi.org/10.1002/art.24229. PubMed PMID; WOS: 000263276400011.

[42] Monleon I, Martinez-Lorenzo MJ, Monteagudo L, Lasierra P, Taules M, Iturralde M, Pineiro A, Larrad L, Alava MA, Naval J, Anel A. Differential secretion of Fas ligand- or APO2 ligand/TNF-related apoptosis-inducing ligand-carrying microvesicles during activation-induced death of human T cells. J Immunol 2001; 167(12): 6736 - 44. https://doi.org/10.4049/jimmunol.167.12.6736. PubMed PMID; WOS: 000172613400007.

[43] Munich S, Sobo-Vujanovic A, Buchser WJ, Beer-Stolz D, Vujanovic NL. Dendritic cell exosomes directly kill tumor cells and activate natural killer cells via TNF superfamily ligands. Oncoimmunology 2012; 1(7): 1074 - 83. https://doi.org/10.4161/onci.20897. PubMed PMID; WOS: 000316279900008.

[44] Zuccato E, Blott EJ, Holt O, Sigismund S, Shaw M, Bossi G, Griffiths GM. Sorting of Fas ligand to secretory lysosomes

is regulated by mono-ubiquitylation and phosphorylation. J Cell Sci 2007; 120(1); 191-9. https://doi.org/10.1242/jcs. 03315. PubMed PMID; WOS; 000243723800019.

[45] Beauvillain C, Ruiz S, Guiton R, Bout D, Dimier-Poisson I. A vaccine based on exosomes secreted by a dendritic cell line confers protection against T. gondii infection in syngeneic and allogeneic mice. Microbes Infect 2007; 9(14-15); 1614-22. https://doi.org/10.1016/j. micinf.2007.07.002. PubMed PMID; WOS; 000252333100014.

[46] Giri PK, Schorey JS. Exosomes derived from M-bovis BCG infected macrophages activate antigen-specific CD4(+) and CD8(+) T cells in vitro and in vivo. PLoS One 2008; 3(6). https://doi.org/10.1371/journal.pone.0002461. PubMed PMID; WOS; 000263280700042.

[47] Keryer-Bibens C, Pioche-Durieu C, Villemant C, Souquere S, Nishi N, Hirashima M, Middeldorp J, Busson P. Exosomes released by EBV-infected nasopharyngeal carcinoma cells convey the viral Latent Membrane Protein 1 and the immunomodulatory protein galectin 9. BMC Cancer 2006; 6. https://doi.org/10.1186/1471-2407-6-283. PubMed PMID; WOS; 000243656700001.

[48] Testa JS, Apcher GS, Comber JD, Eisenlohr LC. Exosome-driven antigen transfer for MHC class Ⅱ presentation facilitated by the receptor binding activity of influenza hemagglutinin. J Immunol 2010; 185(11); 6608-16. https://doi.org/10.4049/jimmunol.1001768. PubMed PMID; WOS; 000284311500026.

[49] Barr F, Lambright DG. Rab GEFs and GAPs. Curr Opin Cell Biol 2010; 22(4); 461-70. https://doi.org/10.1016/j.ceb.2010.04.007. 20466531. PMCID; PMC2929657.

[50] Somsel Rodman J, Wandinger-Ness A. Rab GTPases coordinate endocytosis. J Cell Sci 2000; 113 (Pt 2); 183-92, 10633070.

[51] Frasa MA, Koessmeier KT, Ahmadian MR, Braga VM. Illuminating the functional and structural repertoire of human TBC/RABGAPs. Nat Rev Mol Cell Biol 2012; 13(2); 67-73. https://doi.org/10.1038/nrm3267. 22251903.

[52] Hsu C, Morohashi Y, Yoshimura S, Manrique-Hoyos N, Jung S, Lauterbach MA, Bakhti M, Gronborg M, Mobius W, Rhee J, Barr FA, Simons M. Regulation of exosome secretion by Rab35 and its GTPase-activating proteins TBC1D10A-C. J Cell Biol 2010; 189(2); 223-32. https://doi.org/10.1083/jcb.200911018. 20404108. PMCID; 2856897.

[53] Pan X, Eathiraj S, Munson M, Lambright DG. TBC-domain GAPs for Rab GTPases accelerate GTP hydrolysis by a dual-finger mechanism. Nature 2006; 442(7100); 303-6. https://doi.org/10.1038/nature04847. 16855591.

[54] Shurtleff MJ, Temoche-Diaz MM, Karfilis KV, Ri S, Schekman R. Y-box protein 1 is required to sort microRNAs into exosomes in cells and in a cell-free reaction. elife 2016; 5; e19276https://doi.org/10.7554/eLife.19276. 27559612. PMCID; PMC5047747.

[55] Lo Cicero A, Stahl PD, Raposo G. Extracellular vesicles shuffling intercellular messages; for good or for bad. Curr Opin Cell Biol 2015; 35; 69-77. https://doi.org/10.1016/j.ceb.2015.04.013. 26001269.

[56] Pardoll DM. The blockade of immune checkpoints in cancer immunotherapy. Nat Rev Cancer 2012; 12(4); 252-64. https://doi.org/10.1038/nrc3239. 22437870. PMCID; PMC4856023.

[57] Soung YH, Ford S, Zhang V, Chung J. Exosomes in cancer diagnostics. Cancers (Basel) 2017; 9(1); 8. https://doi.org/10.3390/cancers9010008. 28085080. PMCID; PMC5295779.

[58] Koliha N, Heider U, Ozimkowski T, Wiemann M, Bosio A, Wild S. Melanoma affects the composition of blood cell-derived extracellular vesicles. Front Immunol 2016; 7; 282. https://doi.org/10.3389/fimmu.2016.00282. 27507971. PMCID; PMC4960424.

[59] Koliha N, Wiencek Y, Heider U, Jungst C, Kladt N, Krauthauser S, Johnston IC, Bosio A, Schauss A, Wild S. A novel multiplex bead-based platform highlights the diversity of extracellular vesicles. J Extracell Vesicles 2016; 5; 29975. https://doi.org/10.3402/jev.v5.29975. 26901056. PMCID; PMC4762227.

[60] Groot Kormelink T, Arkesteijn GJ, Nauwelaers FA, van den Engh G, Nolte-'t Hoen EN, Wauben MH. Prerequisites for the analysis and sorting of extracellular vesicle subpopulations by high-resolution flow cytometry. Cytometry A 2016; 89(2); 135-47. https://doi.org/10.1002/cyto.a.22644. 25688721.

[61] van der Vlist EJ, Nolte-'t Hoen EN, Stoorvogel W, Arkesteijn GJ, Wauben MH. Fluorescent labeling of nano-sized vesicles released by cells and subsequent quantitative and qualitative analysis by high-resolution flow cytometry. Nat Protoc 2012; 7(7); 1311-26. https://doi.org/10.1038/nprot.2012.065. 22722367.

[62] Nolte-'t Hoen EN, Buschow SI, Anderton SM, Stoorvogel W, Wauben MH. Activated T cells recruit exosomes secreted by dendritic cells via LFA-1. Blood 2009; 113(9); 1977-81. https://doi.org/10.1182/blood-2008-08-174094. 19064723.

[63] Nolte-'t Hoen EN, van der Vlist EJ, de Boer-Brouwer M, Arkesteijn GJ, Stoorvogel W, Wauben MH. Dynamics of dendritic cell-derived vesicles; high-resolution flow cytometric analysis of extracellular vesicle quantity and quality. J Leukoc Biol 2013; 93(3); 395-402. Epub 2012/12/19, https://doi.org/10.1189/jlb.0911480. 23248328.

[64] Arraud N, Linares R, Tan S, Gounou C, Pasquet JM, Mornet S, Brisson AR. Extracellular vesicles from blood plasma; determination of their morphology, size, phenotype and concentration. J Thromb Haemost 2014; 12(5); 614-27. https://doi.org/10.1111/jth.12554. 24618123.

[65] Chandler WL. Measurement of microvesicle levels in human blood using flow cytometry. Cytometry B Clin Cytom 2016; 90(4); 326-36. https://doi.org/10.1002/cyto.b.21343. 26606416.

[66] Inal JM, Kosgodage U, Azam S, Stratton D, Antwi-Baffour S, Lange S. Blood/plasma secretome and microvesicles. Biochim Biophys Acta 2013; 1834(11); 2317-25. https://doi.org/10.1016/j.bbapap.2013.04.005. 23590876.

[67] Kambayashi T, Laufer TM. Atypical MHC class Ⅱ-expressing antigen-presenting cells; can anything replace a dendritic cell? Nat Rev Immunol 2014; 14(11); 719-30. https://doi.org/10.1038/nri3754. 25324123.

[68] Turpin D, Truchetet ME, Faustin B, Augusto JF, Contin-Bordes C, Brisson A, Blanco P, Duffau P. Role of extracellular vesicles in autoimmune diseases. Autoimmun Rev 2016; 15(2); 174-83. https://doi.org/10.1016/j.autrev.2015.11.004. 26554931.

[69] Willms E, Johansson HJ, Mager I, Lee Y, Blomberg KE, Sadik M, Alaarg A, Smith CI, Lehtio J, El Andaloussi S, Wood MJ, Vader P. Cells release subpopulations of exosomes with distinct molecular and biological properties. Sci Rep

2016; 6: 22519. https://doi.org/10.1038/srep22519. 26931825. PMCID: PMC4773763.

[70] Akagi T, Kato K, Kobayashi M, Kosaka N, Ochiya T, Ichiki T. On-chip immunoelectrophoresis of extracellular vesicles released from human breast cancer cells. PLoS One 2015; 10(4). https://doi.org/10.1371/journal.pone.0123603. 25928805. PMCID: PMC4415775.

[71] Caivano A, Laurenzana I, De Luca L, La Rocca F, Simeon V, Trino S, D'Auria F, Traficante A, Maietti M, Izzo T, D'Arena G, Mansueto G, Pietrantuono G, Laurenti L, Musto P, Del Vecchio L. High serum levels of extracellular vesicles expressing malignancy-related markers are released in patients with various types of hematological neoplastic disorders. Tumour Biol 2015; 36(12): 9739–52. https://doi.org/10.1007/s13277-015-3741-3. 26156801.

[72] van Eijndhoven MA, Zijlstra JM, Groenewegen NJ, Drees EE, van Niele S, Baglio SR, Koppers-Lalic D, van der Voorn H, Libregts SF, Wauben MH, de Menezes RX, van Weering JR, Nieuwland R, Visser L, van den Berg A, de Jong D, Pegtel DM. Plasma vesicle miRNAs for therapy response monitoring in Hodgkin lymphoma patients. JCI Insight 2016; 1(19): e89631. https://doi.org/10.1172/jci.insight.89631. 27882350. PMCID: PMC5111516.

[73] Ostenfeld MS, Jensen SG, Jeppesen DK, Christensen LL, Thorsen SB, Stenvang J, Hvam ML, Thomsen A, Mouritzen P, Rasmussen MH, Nielsen HJ, Orntoft TF, Andersen CL. miRNA profiling of circulating EpCAM(+) extracellular vesicles: promising biomarkers of colorectal cancer. J Extracell Vesicles 2016; 5: 31488. https://doi.org/10.3402/jev.v5.31488. 27576678. PMCID: PMC5005366.

[74] Xiao W, Mindrinos MN, Seok J, Cuschieri J, Cuenca AG, Gao H, Hayden DL, Hennessy L, Moore EE, Minei JP, Bankey PE, Johnson JL, Sperry J, Nathens AB, Billiar TR, West MA, Brownstein BH, Mason PH, Baker HV, Finnerty CC, Jeschke MG, Lopez MC, Klein MB, Gamelli RL, Gibran NS, Arnoldo B, Xu W, Zhang Y, Calvano SE, McDonald-Smith GP, Schoenfeld DA, Storey JD, Cobb JP, Warren HS, Moldawer LL, Herndon DN, Lowry SF, Maier RV, Davis RW, Tompkins RG. A genomic storm in critically injured humans. J Exp Med 2011; 208(13): 2581–90. https://doi.org/10.1084/jem.20111354. 22110166. PMCID: PMC3244029.

[75] Moore EE. Claude H. Organ, Jr. memorial lecture: splanchnic hypoperfusion provokes acute lung injury via a 5-lipoxygenase-dependent mechanism. Am J Surg 2010; 200(6): 681–9. https://doi.org/10.1016/j.amjsurg.2010.05.010. 21146002. PMCID: PMC3031087.

[76] Kojima M, Gimenes-Junior JA, Chan TW, Eliceiri BP, Baird A, Costantini TW, Coimbra R. Exosomes in postshock mesenteric lymph are key mediators of acute lung injury triggering the macrophage activation via Toll-kike receptor 4. FASEB J 2018; 32(1): 97–110. https://doi.org/10.1096/fj.201700488R. 28855278.

[77] Ying W, Riopel M, Bandyopadhyay G, Dong Y, Birmingham A, Seo JB, Ofrecio JM, Wollam J, Hernandez-Carretero A, Fu W, Li P, Olefsky JM. Adipose tissue macrophagederived exosomal miRNAs can modulate in vivo and in vitro insulin sensitivity. Cell 2017; 171(2): 372–84.e12. https://doi.org/10.1016/j.cell.2017.08.03528942920.

[78] Kamerkar S, LeBleu VS, Sugimoto H, Yang S, Ruivo CF, Melo SA, Lee JJ, Kalluri R. Exosomes facilitate therapeutic targeting of oncogenic KRAS in pancreatic cancer. Nature 2017; 546(7659): 498–503. https://doi.org/10.1038/nature22341. 28607485. PMCID: PMC5538883.

[79] Deitch EA. Gut lymph and lymphatics: a source of factors leading to organ injury and dysfunction. Ann N Y Acad Sci 2010; 1207(Suppl 1): E103–11. https://doi.org/10.1111/j.1749-6632.2010.05713.x. 20961300.

[80] Deitch EA, Adams C, Lu Q, Lu DZ. A time course study of the protective effect of mesenteric lymph duct ligation on hemorrhagic shock-induced pulmonary injury and the toxic effects of lymph from shocked rats on endothelial cell monolayer permeability. Surgery 2001; 129(1): 39–47. Epub 2001/01/10. 11150032.

[81] Senthil M, Watkins A, Barlos D, Xu DZ, Lu Q, Abungu B, Caputo F, Feinman R, Deitch EA. Intravenous injection of trauma-hemorrhagic shock mesenteric lymph causes lung injury that is dependent upon activation of the inducible nitric oxide synthase pathway. Ann Surg 2007; 246(5): 822–30. Epub 2007/10/31 https://doi.org/10.1097/SLA.0b013e3180caa3af. 17968175.

[82] Betteridge JD, Armbruster SP, Maydonovitch C, Veerappan GR. Inflammatory bowel disease prevalence by age, gender, race, and geographic location in the U.S. military health care population. Inflamm Bowel Dis 2013; 19(7): 1421–7. https://doi.org/10.1097/MIB.0b013e318281334d. 23518811.

[83] Wagnerova A, Babickova J, Liptak R, Vlkova B, Celec P, Gardlik R. Sex differences in the effect of resveratrol on DSS-induced colitis in mice. Gastroenterol Res Pract 2017; 2017. https://doi.org/10.1155/2017/8051870. 28465680. PMCID: PMC5390549.

[84] Kim KW, Song JH. Emerging roles of lymphatic vasculature in immunity. Immune Netw 2017; 17(1): 68–76. https://doi.org/10.4110/in.2017.17.1.68. 28261022. PMCID: PMC5334124.

[85] Wang Y, Oliver G. Current views on the function of the lymphatic vasculature in health and disease. Genes Dev 2010; 24(19): 2115–26. https://doi.org/10.1101/gad.1955910. 20889712. PMCID: PMC2947764.

[86] AlSharari SD, Bagdas D, Akbarali HI, Lichtman PA, Raborn ES, Cabral GA, Carroll FI, Mc-Gee EA, Damaj MI. Sex differences and drug dose influence the role of the alpha7 nicotinic acetylcholine receptor in the mouse dextran sodium sulfate-induced colitis model. Nicotine Tob Res 2017; 19(4): 460–6. https://doi.org/10.1093/ntr/ntw245. 27639096.

[87] Kojima M, Costantini TW, Eliceiri BP, Chan TW, Baird A, Coimbra R. Gut epithelial cellderived exosomes trigger post-trauma immune dysfunction. J Trauma Acute Care Surg 2017; 84(2): 257–264. Epub 2017/12/02, https://doi.org/10.1097/ta.0000000000001748. 29194317.

[88] Morishita K, Coimbra R, Langness S, Eliceiri BP, Costantini TW. Neuroenteric axis modulates the balance of regulatory T cells and T-helper 17 cells in the mesenteric lymph node following trauma/hemorrhagic shock. Am J Physiol Gastrointest Liver Physiol 2015; 309(3): G202–8. Epub 2015/06/06, https://doi.org/10.1152/ajpgi.00097.2015. 26045612.

[89] Morishita K, Costantini TW, Eliceiri B, Bansal V, Coimbra R. Vagal nerve stimulation modulates the dendritic cell profile in posthemorrhagic shock mesenteric lymph. J Trauma Acute Care Surg 2014; 76(3): 610–7. discussion 7-8, https://doi.org/10.1097/ta.0000000000000137. 24553526.

[90] Morishita K, Costantini TW, Ueno A, Bansal V, Eliceiri B, Coimbra R. A pharmacologic approach to vagal nerve

stimulation prevents mesenteric lymph toxicity after hemorrhagic shock. J Trauma Acute Care Surg 2015; 78(1): 52-8. discussion 8-9, https://doi.org/10.1097/ta.0000000000000489. 25539203.

[91] Ionac M. One technique, two approaches, and results: thoracic duct cannulation in small laboratory animals. Microsurgery 2003; 23(3): 239-45. https://doi.org/10.1002/micr.10136. 12833325.

[92] Chavan SS, Pavlov VA, Tracey KJ. Mechanisms and therapeutic relevance of neuroimmune communication. Immunity 2017; 46(6): 927-42. https://doi.org/10.1016/j.immuni.2017.06.008. 28636960. PMCID: PMC5578398.

[93] Costantini TW, Bansal V, Krzyzaniak M, Putnam JG, Peterson CY, Loomis WH, Wolf P, Baird A, Eliceiri BP, Coimbra R. Vagal nerve stimulation protects against burn-induced intestinal injury through activation of enteric glia cells. Am J Physiol Gastrointest Liver Physiol 2010; 299(6): G1308-18. https://doi.org/10.1152/ajpgi.00156.2010. 20705905. PMCID: PMC3774266.

[94] Lowry DM, Morishita K, Eliceiri BP, Bansal V, Coimbra R, Costantini TW. The vagus nerve alters the pulmonary dendritic cell response to injury. J Surg Res 2014; 192(1): 12-8. https://doi.org/10.1016/j.jss.2014.06.012. 25005822.

[95] Costantini TW, Putnam JG, Sawada R, Baird A, Loomis WH, Eliceiri BP, Bansal V, Coimbra R. Targeting the gut barrier: identification of a homing peptide sequence for delivery into the injured intestinal epithelial cell. Surgery 2009; 146(2): 206-12. https://doi.org/10.1016/j.surg.2009.05.007. 19628075. PMCID: PMC4251594.

[96] Koh TJ, DiPietro LA. Inflammation and wound healing: the role of the macrophage. Expert Rev Mol Med 2011; 13. https://doi.org/10.1017/S1462399411001943. 21740602. PMCID: PMC3596046.

[97] Silva AM, Teixeira JH, Almeida MI, Goncalves RM, Barbosa MA, Santos SG. Extracellular vesicles: immunomodulatory messengers in the context of tissue repair/regeneration. Eur J Pharm Sci 2017; 98: 86-95. https://doi.org/10.1016/j.ejps.2016.09.017. 27644894.

[98] Larouche J, Sheoran S, Maruyama K, Martino MM. Immune regulation of skin wound healing: mechanisms and novel therapeutic targets. Adv Wound Care 2018; 7(7): 209-31. https://doi.org/10.1089/wound.2017.0761. 29984112. PMCID: PMC6032665.

[99] Novak ML, Koh TJ. Phenotypic transitions of macrophages orchestrate tissue repair. Am J Pathol 2013; 183(5): 1352-63. https://doi.org/10.1016/j.ajpath.2013.06.034. 24091222. PMCID: PMC3969506.

[100] Patel DB, Santoro M, Born LJ, Fisher JP, Jay SM. Towards rationally designed biomanufacturing of therapeutic extracellular vesicles: impact of the bioproduction microenvironment. Biotechnol Adv 2018; 36: 2051-9. https://doi.org/10.1016/j.biotechadv.2018.09.001. 30218694.

[101] Thomou T, Mori MA, Dreyfuss JM, Konishi M, Sakaguchi M, Wolfrum C, Rao TN, Winnay JN, Garcia-Martin R, Grinspoon SK, Gorden P, Kahn CR. Adipose-derived circulating miRNAs regulate gene expression in other tissues. Nature 2017; 542(7642): 450-5. https://doi.org/10.1038/nature21365. 28199304. PMCID: PMC5330251.

[102] Stoner SA, Duggan E, Condello D, Guerrero A, Turk JR, Narayanan PK, Nolan JP. High sensitivity flow cytometry of membrane vesicles. Cytometry A 2016; 89(2): 196-206. Epub 2015/10/21, https://doi.org/10.1002/cyto.a.2278726484737.

第 15 章

代谢综合征中的外泌体
Exosomes in metabolic syndrome

Soazig Le Lay[a,b], Ramaroson Andriantsitohaina[a,b], M. Carmen Martinez[a,b]

[a]SOPAM, U1063, INSERM, UNIV ANGERS, SFR ICAT, Bat IRIS-IBS, Angers, France; [b]Angers University Hospital, Angers, France

一、概述

正如 WHO 最近报道所指出的,生活方式的改变,如越来越多的久坐不动导致缺乏身体活动、富含脂肪和葡萄糖的高能量食物的摄入增加,导致包括肿瘤、慢性呼吸系统疾病、心血管疾病和糖尿病在内的非传染性疾病增加[1]。遗传和许多环境因素,如睡眠不足、吸烟和(或)饮酒或干扰内分泌的物质,似乎也与这些慢性疾病的发生有关。更详细地说,与超重、高血压和生化改变(主要是血脂异常和高血糖)相关的一些问题的存在,导致心肌梗死、脑卒中和外周动脉疾病等动脉粥样硬化性心血管疾病的风险增加了大约 2 倍。这些改变的结合定义了代谢综合征(metabolic syndrome,MetS),包括腹部肥胖、胰岛素抵抗(insulin resistance,IR)、血压(blood pressure,BP)升高和由低水平 HDL-胆固醇和高水平三酰甘油组成的肥胖相关血脂异常。

尽管各种健康组织都在努力定义 MetS,但在血压值、显示中心肥胖的腰围或血浆 HDL 水平方面仍存在一些差异。然而,中心性肥胖和 IR 似乎是描述 MetS 患者的主要和初步筛查工具(图 15-1)。事实上,在所有国家中,无论经济水平,MetS 的流行率都在增加,这表明了 MetS 管理在临床和公共卫生中的重要性。在西方国家,MetS 患病率的增加与肥胖的增加直接相关。例如,据估计,MetS 的患病率在所有成年人中约占 25%,在高龄人群中发病率更高。然而,最近的数据凸显了年轻人的患病率在增加[2]。

二、MetS 的不同组分

定义 MetS 的五个标准相互交叉,因此很难采用独立的标准来评估。如上所述,由于 MetS 患者经常伴有肥胖和 IR,因此这两种标准对 MetS 的影响似乎比高血压和血脂异常更大[3]。

(一) 肥胖

在 MetS 患者中,中心性或内脏性肥胖是其增加 IR 发展风险的重要因素之一,而 IR 将促进心脏脂肪堆积、动脉粥样硬化和高血压[4,5]。更详细地说,脂肪细胞及脂肪组织间质细胞,包括促炎巨噬细胞[6],产生促动脉粥样硬化的脂肪因子,如 IL-6、TNFα 和 MCP-1,涉及氧化应激和慢性炎症的发生[7]。这些影响是可逆的,如减肥手术后与巨噬细胞浸润减少

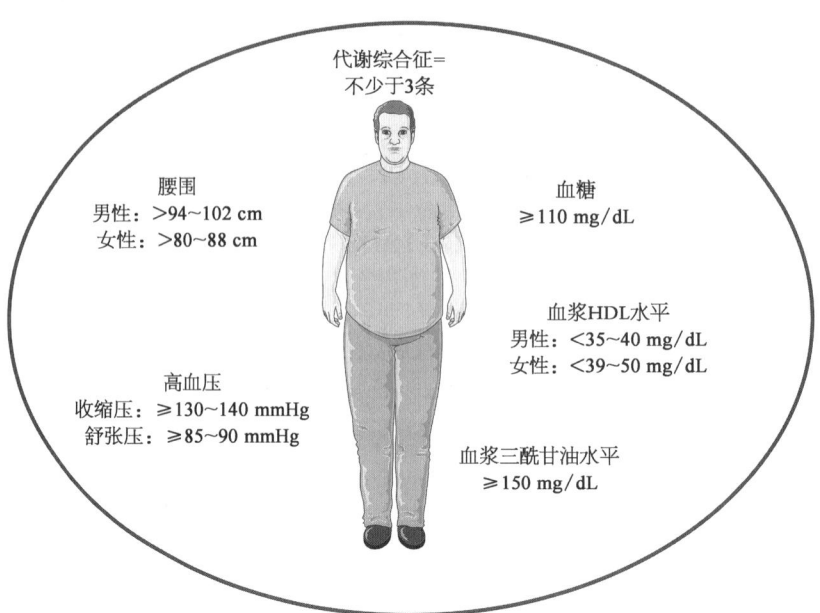

图 15-1 代谢综合征依据以下协会的诊断标准：WHO,世界卫生组织；NCEP‑ATPⅢ,国家胆固醇教育计划——成人治疗。IDF,国际糖尿病联盟；HDL,高密度脂蛋白

相关的促炎分子产生的减少[8]。

（二）血脂异常

两项 MetS 标准涉及脂质紊乱：一方面,三酰甘油血浆浓度的增加；另一方面,HDL 胆固醇浓度的下降[5,9]。这些脂质紊乱直接反映了饱和脂肪酸、部分氢化不饱和脂肪酸和糖类的过度消耗[10]。体外实验表明,脂肪酸或低密度脂蛋白超载诱导肝细胞凋亡[11]。在体外,已经表明脂肪酸或低密度脂蛋白(low density lipoprotein，LDL)超载会诱导肝细胞凋亡[11]。此外,喂食高脂肪饮食(high-fat diet，HFD)的动物在肝脏中会积聚脂质,在某些情况下会导致肝硬化[12]。最后,渗透到血管壁的单核细胞-巨噬细胞中 LDL 的积累促使它们转化为泡沫细胞,从而导致动脉粥样硬化斑块的形成[13]。

（三）动脉高压

在 MetS 期间,收缩压和舒张压的升高反映了不同系统之间复杂的相互作用。事实上,脂肪组织分泌血管紧张素Ⅱ可以刺激醛固酮的产生,而醛固酮对血压的控制起着至关重要的作用[14]。此外,在高胰岛素血症患者中,交感神经系统的活动增加[15],主要加剧了颈动脉体的激活[16],这可能导致高血压的发展。

（四）IR 和糖尿病

胰岛素受体被其配体激活导致信号级联反应,负责增加糖原合成、葡萄糖摄取和蛋白质合成以增加能量储存。然而，在某些病理生理情况下，该信号通路失效导致胰岛素在靶组织（脂肪组织、肝脏、血管内皮和骨骼肌）中的代谢作用降低，也称为 IR。IR 的特征是脂肪细胞中脂肪酸的动员，这些脂肪酸将在骨骼肌中积累。在肝脏中，IR 会增加糖原分解和糖异生，从而导致高血糖。对于内皮，IR 会减少 NO 的产生并增加血管收缩，从而导致高血压[17]。最后，IR 是 2 型糖尿病（type 2 diabetes mellitus，T2DM）的主要原因，其特征是空腹高血糖。从长远来看，血液中高浓度的葡萄糖会影响导致其衰竭的某些组织和器官（眼睛、神经系统、心脏、血管、肾脏等）。所有这些数据表明，一个恶性循环已经形成，所有这些因素都有助于 MetS 的发生和维持。

三、胞外囊泡：MetS 成分的生物标志物

定义 MetS 的风险因素通常是内在相关的，因此有助于 MetS 的发生和维持。虽然通常很难区分每个单独的 MetS 成分的贡献，但临床研究表明它们参与外泌体的产生，这表明这些小 EV 可用作代谢并发症的预后和（或）诊断生物标志物（表 15-1）。

表 15-1 外泌体作为代谢并发症诊断/预后的潜在生物标志物

	特　征	参考文献
肥胖	肥胖患者循环外泌体增加	[18,19]
	循环外泌体和 HOMA IR 之间的正相关	[20,21]
血脂异常	饱和脂肪酸暴露增强了脂肪细胞、肝细胞和肌肉细胞的外泌体分泌	[22-24]
	循环外泌体和血清甘油三酯升高之间的正相关	[25]
高血压	大鼠注射血管紧张素Ⅱ增加血清外泌体	[26]
	RAAS 激活后增加尿液外泌体	[27]
	钠转运体表达水平与高血压发生的相关性	[27,28]
T2DM	糖尿病患者循环外泌体增加	[21,29]
	红细胞源性的外泌体特异性增加	[21]
	IR 增强外泌体的分泌	[21]

注：HOMA，稳态模型评估；RAAS，肾素-血管紧张素-醛固酮系统；T2DM，2 型糖尿病；IR，胰岛素抵抗。

（一）肥胖

内脏肥胖被认为是最有害的 MetS 成分之一，因为它与 IR 高度相关，后者有利于异位脂质积累、动脉粥样硬化和高血压。此外，肥胖的特征是慢性低度炎症状态，其特征是促炎巨噬细胞浸润[8]。

其他研究人员和我们已经发现，循环微囊泡和外泌体浓度都随着肥胖而升高，并与身体质量指数（body mass index，BMI）相关，这表明脂肪组织源性的 EV 可能有助于这种循环 EV 浓度的增加[18,19]。临床前研究已经证实脂肪细胞能够大量分泌外泌体，而且在脂肪超

载条件下会增强分泌[22,30]。尽管有证据表明人体循环中存在脂肪细胞源性的外泌体[31],但脂肪源性的外泌体在整个循环外泌体池中的贡献尚不清楚,主要是由于缺乏可靠和特异性的标志物来识别特定脂肪源性的外泌体。尽管如此,网膜脂肪组织释放的外泌体数量与稳态模型评估(homeostasis model assessment,HOMA)IR指数之间建立了正相关,提示脂肪源性的外泌体在T2DM的产生中发挥了作用[20,21]。

(二) 血脂异常

高胆固醇血症和高甘油三酯血症通常联想到富含脂质和葡萄糖的饮食。肝细胞、肌肉细胞或脂肪细胞在体外于高葡萄糖或脂质浓度作用下会增强外泌体的分泌[22-24]。特别是,棕榈酸为一种已知介导炎症和IR过程的饱和脂肪酸,其处理细胞后产生的外泌体能诱导肝细胞纤维化激活和肌肉细胞IR[24]。与其他代谢参数相比,在MetS患者中,循环外泌体数量与血清三酰甘油升高的相关性最强,表明脂肪酸超载也将有利于人体EV的分泌[25]。

(三) 高血压

高血压是最重要的心血管危险因素之一,有利于巨噬细胞浸润血管。事实上,MetS中发生的动脉压升高反映了不同调节系统之间复杂的相互作用。脂肪组织分泌的血管紧张素Ⅱ参与了醛固酮的产生,从而调节动脉压力。由高胰岛素血症引起的交感神经系统激活也会导致高血压。

尽管不同的出版物报道了高血压动物模型中大EV(即微囊泡)的循环浓度增加[32],并证明了它们作为人类动脉粥样硬化血栓形成病理的预测/诊断标志物的潜力[33],但数量有限的研究侧重于循环外泌体在高血压动物模型中高血压的背景。一项研究报道称,高血压大鼠在输注血管紧张素Ⅱ后,血清外泌体增加,当体外培养内皮细胞时,外泌体能够上调炎症标志物的表达水平[26]。这些结果表明,高血压中发生的内皮损伤可能部分是由循环外泌体携带的物质诱导的。此外,研究报道了肾素-血管紧张素-醛固酮系统激活后尿液外泌体含量的改变[27]。特别是,外泌体钠转运蛋白的表达水平与高血压的发展密切相关[27,28],这揭示了应用尿液外泌体评估高血压方面的前景。

(四) IR和T2DM

T2DM与循环中较高水平的大(微囊泡)和小(外泌体)囊泡相关[21,29],尤其是糖尿病患者红细胞源性外泌体的比例显著增加[21]。此外,这些作者还证明了IR状态增强了EV的分泌,从而确定了一个恶性循环,T2DM的主要风险因素肥胖可以启动EV分泌,这可以进一步受到IR和相关慢性炎症的影响。

(五) 聚集所有MetS元素

MetS的五个确定性标准的紧密联系使得难以单独确定每个标准的参与程度。到目前为止,只有循环微囊泡亚类通过流式细胞术对MetS进行了表型分析。与健康受试者相比,MetS患者的血小板、内皮、红细胞源性微囊泡循环量似乎更高[34,35]。此外,组织因子阳性的微囊泡与 MetS 的成分有关[36]，而胱抑素 C 阳性的 EV 与肥胖发展的代谢并发症有关[37]。

四、胞外囊泡：MetS 的生物学效应

（一）外泌体与肥胖代谢并发症：脂肪源性外泌体的作用是什么？

近来，Li 等[38]和 Nie 等[39]的研究表明，肥胖患者循环外泌体 miR-29a 和 miR-194 水平升高与人体心功能受损密切相关，包括射血分数和心力衰竭生物标志物 N 端前体 b 型利钠肽水平。此外，用来自肥胖患者的循环外泌体体外治疗小鼠心肌细胞可诱发心肌细胞线粒体失活，在饲喂 HFD 的小鼠中也得到类似结果。这些数据突显出，外泌体 miRNA(miR-29a 和 miR-194)都可以成为对抗肥胖引起的心功能障碍的令人关注的靶点。

大量研究表明，脂肪组织释放的外泌体可以作为脂肪与其他细胞和组织之间的交流方式(图 15-2)。这种外泌体介导的交换网络最近在脂肪组织中得到了说明，尽管基因被破坏，caveolin-1 蛋白仍被证明可以利用这些外泌体在内皮细胞和脂肪细胞之间进行运输，从而取代脂肪细胞中的 caveolin-1 蛋白水平[40]。

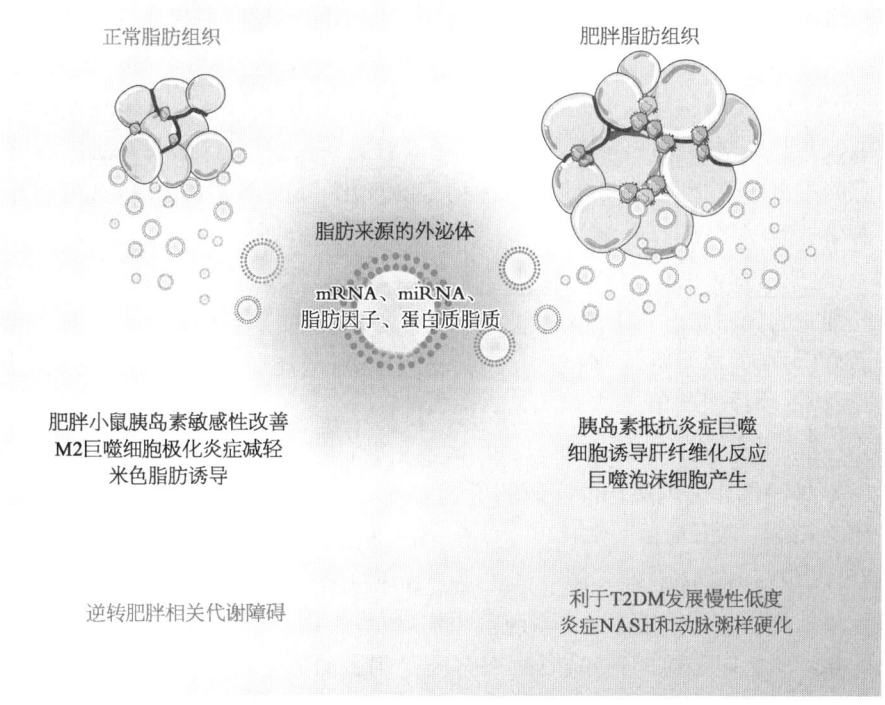

图 15-2 脂肪组织源性的外泌体的代谢作用。来自瘦脂肪组织的外泌体具有保护作用，包括逆转与肥胖相关的代谢功能障碍；而来自肥胖脂肪组织的外泌体有利于 T2DM、慢性低度炎症、NASH 和动脉粥样硬化的发展

这种基于外泌体的细胞物质交换并不限于蛋白质，因为脂肪组织来源的外泌体 miRNA 已被证明可调节肝脏和肌肉中的基因表达，从而通过传递循环 miRNA 来调节体内胰岛素

的敏感性[41,42]。先前的报道实际上已经确定了肥胖脂肪源性外泌体诱导 IR 状态和巨噬细胞活化的能力[43,44]。这种促炎反应可能与 TLR4 信号通路的激活有关,因为对该受体无效的小鼠不受肥胖脂肪源性外泌体的有害影响[43]。不同的脂肪源性外泌体已被证明参与了这种免疫反应,包括炎性脂肪细胞因子[19,45]或特定的 miRNA,如 miR-155,它们可能通过靶向细胞因子信号通路的关键调节因子,即细胞因子信号转导抑制因子 1(suppressor of cytokine signaling 1,SOCS1)[42,44]或 miR-99b,反向抑制肝脏中的成纤维细胞生长因子 21(fibroblast growth factor 21,FGF21)[41]。

有趣的是,来自内脏脂肪组织的外泌体,而不是来自皮下脂肪组织的外泌体,通过下调 ATP 结合盒转运体(ABCA1 和 ABCG1)介导的胆固醇外排诱导巨噬泡沫细胞的产生[46]。同样,只有来自 HFD 喂养小鼠的内脏脂肪组织源性外泌体增加了促炎巨噬细胞表型和细胞因子的分泌。这些作用伴随着 NF-κB-p65 通路的激活。值得注意的是,静脉注射 HFD 内脏脂肪组织源性外泌体明显促进了高脂血症载脂蛋白 E 缺陷小鼠的动脉粥样硬化,而不影响其血脂和体重。这项研究表明,HFD 内脏脂肪组织源性外泌体通过调节巨噬细胞泡沫细胞形成和促炎极化,具有促动脉粥样硬化的作用。

与肥胖条件下产生的外泌体相比,瘦脂肪源性外泌体显示出有益的作用。因此,从瘦小鼠的脂肪组织巨噬细胞中获得的外泌体在给予肥胖小鼠后改善了其葡萄糖耐量和胰岛素敏感性[42]。这些作者认为,这些作用是由外泌体过表达的 miR-155 介导。因为与对照相比,miR-155 KO 动物对胰岛素敏感且对葡萄糖耐受。用脂肪干细胞来源的外泌体治疗肥胖小鼠也可改善胰岛素敏感性,减少肥胖和减轻肝脏脂肪变性[47]。这些外泌体能够激活饮食诱导的肥胖小鼠白色脂肪组织中 M2 巨噬细胞的极化,减少炎症和褐变,这可能是通过外泌体携带的活性 STAT3 对精氨酸酶-1 的反式激活作用。

总之,这些结果说明了脂肪源性外泌体的复杂性,它聚集了蛋白质、遗传物质和脂质,反映了生产细胞的代谢状态。因此,这些脂肪源性外泌体所携带的多种因子很可能参与了基质血管成分(包括内皮细胞、巨噬细胞、前脂肪细胞等)与脂肪细胞之间的交互作用,诱导对组织/细胞靶点的代谢作用。

(二) 外泌体作为内皮功能障碍的促进者

正如 Zamani 等所评价的那样[48],心脏、内皮和血管细胞能够产生含有多种分子的外泌体,包括可以转移到受体细胞并调节其功能的 miRNA。其他类型的细胞如脂肪细胞和肝细胞可以释放外泌体并作用于心血管细胞。即使在基线状态下(未受刺激),也已证明可以通过外泌体在细胞之间传递信息。例如,来自未受刺激的人主动脉平滑肌细胞的外泌体携带参与自噬过程调节的 miRNA-221/222,诱导人内皮细胞中 LC3Ⅱ、ATG5 和 Beclin-1 表达下调,反映了对内皮自噬的抑制作用[49]。相比之下,其他作者已经表明,富含 miR-143 和 miR-145 的内皮外泌体调节平滑肌细胞中的基因表达,并通过减少动脉粥样硬化小鼠模型中的动脉粥样硬化病变进程来起到保护作用[50]。总之,这些数据说明了血管平滑肌细胞和内皮细胞之间对话的复杂性。

最近,有研究描述了糖尿病 *db/db* 小鼠血清的外泌体对内皮功能的直接影响。事实上,内化外泌体进入完整主动脉的内皮细胞会严重损害非糖尿病 db/+小鼠主动脉的内皮依赖性松弛。有趣的是,这些外泌体携带一种降低 L-精氨酸可用性的酶——精氨酸酶 1,它是内皮中 eNOS 介导 NO 产生的底物,导致 NO 的生物利用度降低。当精氨酸酶 1 被沉默时,db/db 源性外泌体的血管有害作用显著减少,表明糖尿病小鼠外泌体诱导内皮功能障碍的细胞机制[47]。此外,在糖尿病期间,心肌细胞源性外泌体抑制内皮细胞增殖、迁移和管状形成,从而在 T2DM 大鼠模型中产生抗血管生成作用。这些作用是由富含 miR-320 的外泌体介导的[51]。

(三)外泌体在血压调节中的作用

自发性高血压大鼠(spontaneously hypertensive rat,SHR)的循环外泌体可以调节血压正常大鼠的血压。事实上,SHR 产生的外泌体显著增加了 Wistar-Kyoto(WKY)大鼠的收缩压和胸主动脉的结构变化,而 WKY 产生的外泌体降低了 SHR 的这些指标。此外,SHR 产生的外泌体显著增加了 WKY 左心室的重量和血管周围纤维化,而 SHR 中 WKY 产生的外泌体显著降低了纤维化而不是心室重量。这项工作强调了循环外泌体在调节血压中的关键作用[52]。

此外,将来自 SHR 主动脉的外膜成纤维细胞的外泌体与 WKY 大鼠产生的外泌体进行比较。有趣的是,来自 SHR 而非 WKY 大鼠的外泌体促进了血管平滑肌细胞的迁移。此外,来自 SHR 的外泌体增加了两种大鼠品系(WKY 和 SHR)血管平滑肌细胞中血管紧张素Ⅱ和血管紧张素转换酶(angiotensin converting enzyme,ACE)的含量和活性。这些作用被能够阻断外泌体产生的中性鞘磷脂酶抑制剂 GW4869、血管紧张素Ⅱ1 型受体拮抗剂或血管紧张素转化酶抑制剂所阻止。总之,这些结果表明 ACE 通过外泌体从 SHR 的外膜成纤维细胞转移到血管平滑肌细胞,导致其迁移增加[53]。

据报道,SHR 或 WKY 大鼠外泌体效应之间的差异可能至少部分与其 miRNA 含量有关。对 SHR 和 WKY 大鼠血浆外泌体 miRNA 表达谱的分析表明,从 SHR 和 WKY 分离的总体小 RNA 中 miRNA 的百分比没有显著差异。然而,与 WKY 外泌体相比,SHR 和 WKY 外泌体之间有 27 种 miRNA 差异表达显著,其中 SHR 外泌体中 23 种上调和 4 种下调[54]。

来自血管紧张素Ⅱ诱发的高血压大鼠的循环外泌体与血管紧张素Ⅱ体外处理的巨噬细胞产生的外泌体产生相似的结果,即 ICAM1 在人冠状动脉内皮细胞中过度表达。这些影响与来自高血压大鼠的外泌体中 miR-17 水平降低有关,miR-17 是 ICAM1 表达的负调节因子。这些数据表明,来自巨噬细胞的外泌体将促炎信息传递给内皮细胞[26]。

(四)外泌体作为促进脂质紊乱的载体

饱和脂肪酸可以增强脂肪细胞、肝细胞和肌肉细胞的外泌体分泌[22,24,55]。已知这类脂肪酸特别有害,因为它们通过增强神经酰胺和二酰基甘油的合成而诱导 IR。接触棕榈酸后分泌的外泌体确实富含神经酰胺,并能够将这些脂毒性脂质转移到肌肉细胞或巨噬细胞中[24,55]。富含脂质的外泌体也显示出纤维化和炎症特性,如肥胖脂肪细胞源性外泌体能够诱导肝细胞的促纤维化反应的[56]。总而言之，这些数据强调了外泌体在非酒精性脂肪性肝炎的发展中可能发挥的潜在作用及其用于诊断及预后目的以评估该疾病的进展[55]。

由于外泌体富含胆固醇和其他脂质，一些作者评估了它们是否可能参与动脉粥样硬化过程。在外泌体通过磷脂酰丝氨酸受体内化后，由活化的人 $CD4^+$ T 淋巴细胞产生的外泌体诱导胆固醇聚积到 THP-1 单核细胞中[57]。有趣的是，由于在外泌体处理的单核细胞中发现的脂滴含有游离胆固醇和胆固醇酯，并且这可能发生在动脉粥样硬化斑块内，这些数据表明，外泌体可能被认为是胆固醇过量条件下的动脉粥样硬化因素[57]。

五、外泌体作为宿主与微生物群之间新的交流方式

过去十年强调了肠道微生物群在代谢并发症发展中的重要性。微生物群失调与肥胖和肝脏疾病的严重程度有关。EV 可能代表一种新的通信模式，因为它们将作为代谢中转在宿主与其微生物群之间传递信息。因此，肠上皮细胞产生富含一些小 RNA 的外泌体，这些小 RNA 将被细菌内化，从而调节生长和微生物基因的表达模式[57]。相比之下，从肥胖小鼠肠道微生物群中分离的外泌体在体外和体内模型中诱导 IR[58]。因此，EV 在将宿主与其微生物群联系起来的复杂通信中扮演新的角色。

六、总结

总之，这些数据表明，外泌体可以代表心脏代谢疾病的预测生物标志物，并通过其介导细胞间通信的能力参与代谢功能障碍的发展。更好地了解外泌体的组成及其作用可能会导致设计创新策略来调节其生物合成和作用。这些可以带来医疗实践的变化，从传统方法转变为基于对外泌体成分和生物活性更好了解的个性化医疗。

致谢

本章得到了 INSERM，Université d'Angers（France），the Société Francophone du Diabète 和 Région Pays de Loire（Mibiogate）的支持。

（余奇 译，覃丽 审校）

参考文献

[1] collaborators NCDC. NCD Countdown 2030: worldwide trends in non-communicable disease mortality and progress towards sustainable development goal target 3.4. Lancet 2018; 392(10152): 1072-88.
[2] Nolan PB, et al. Prevalence of metabolic syndrome and metabolic syndrome components in young adults: a pooled analysis. Prev Med Rep 2017; 7: 211-5.
[3] Alberti KG, et al. Harmonizing the metabolic syndrome: a joint interim statement of the International Diabetes Federation Task Force on Epidemiology and Prevention; National Heart, Lung, and Blood Institute; American Heart Association; World Heart Federation; International Atherosclerosis Society; and International Association for the Study of Obesity. Circulation 2009; 120(16): 1640-5.
[4] Brede S, et al. Clinical scenario of the metabolic syndrome. Visc Med 2016; 32(5): 336-41.
[5] Han TS, Wu FC, Lean ME. Obesity and weight management in the elderly: a focus on men. Best Pract Res Clin Endocrinol Metab 2013; 27(4): 509-25.
[6] Weisberg SP, et al. Obesity is associated with macrophage accumulation in adipose tissue. J Clin Invest 2003; 112(12): 1796-808.
[7] Le Lay S, et al. Oxidative stress and metabolic pathologies: from an adipocentric point of view. Oxid Med Cell Longev 2014; 2014: 908539.
[8] Cancello R, et al. Increased infiltration of macrophages in omental adipose tissue is associated with marked hepatic

lesions in morbid human obesity. Diabetes 2006; 55(6): 1554 - 61.
[9] Grundy SM. Adipose tissue and metabolic syndrome: too much, too little or neither. Eur J Clin Invest 2015; 45(11): 1209 - 17.
[10] Kastorini CM, Panagiotakos DB. Dietary patterns and prevention of type 2 diabetes: from research to clinical practice; a systematic review. Curr Diabetes Rev 2009; 5(4): 221 - 7.
[11] Gan LT, et al. Hepatocyte free cholesterol lipotoxicity results from JNK1-mediated mitochondrial injury and is HMGB1 and TLR4-dependent. J Hepatol 2014; 61(6): 1376 - 84.
[12] Marengo A, Rosso C, Bugianesi E. Liver cancer: connections with obesity, fatty liver, and cirrhosis. Annu Rev Med 2016; 67: 103 - 17.
[13] Expert Dyslipidemia Panel of the International Atherosclerosis Society Panel Memebers. An International Atherosclerosis Society Position Paper: global recommendations for the management of dyslipidemia — full report. J Clin Lipidol 2014; 8(1): 29 - 60.
[14] Bomback AS, Klemmer PJ. Interaction of aldosterone and extracellular volume in the pathogenesis of obesity-associated kidney disease: a narrative review. Am J Nephrol 2009; 30(2): 140 - 6.
[15] Lambert EA, et al. Should the sympathetic nervous system be a target to improve cardiometabolic risk in obesity? Am J Physiol Heart Circ Physiol 2015; 309(2): H244 - 58.
[16] Ribeiro MJ, et al. Carotid body denervation prevents the development of insulin resistance and hypertension induced by hypercaloric diets. Diabetes 2013; 62(8): 2905 - 16.
[17] Lopes HF, et al. Visceral adiposity syndrome. Diabetol Metab Syndr 2016; 8: 40.
[18] Stepanian A, et al. Microparticle increase in severe obesity: Not related to metabolic syndrome and unchanged after massive weight loss. Obesity (Silver Spring) 2013; 21(11): 2236 - 43.
[19] Amosse J, et al. Phenotyping of circulating extracellular vesicles (EVs) in obesity identifies large EVs as functional conveyors of macrophage migration inhibitory factor. Mol Metab 2018; 18: 134 - 42.
[20] Kranendonk ME, et al. Human adipocyte extracellular vesicles in reciprocal signaling between adipocytes and macrophages. Obesity (Silver Spring) 2014; 22(5): 1296 - 308.
[21] Freeman DW, et al. Altered extracellular vesicle concentration, cargo and function in diabetes mellitus. Diabetes 2018; 67(11): 2377 - 88.
[22] Durcin M, et al. Characterisation of adipocyte-derived extracellular vesicle subtypes identifies distinct protein and lipid signatures for large and small extracellular vesicles. J Extracell Vesicles 2017; 6(1): 1305677.
[23] Lee YS, et al. Exosomes derived from palmitic acid-treated hepatocytes induce fibrotic activation of hepatic stellate cells. Sci Rep 2017; 7(1): 3710.
[24] Aswad H, et al. Exosomes participate in the alteration of muscle homeostasis during lipidinduced insulin resistance in mice. Diabetologia 2014; 57(10): 2155 - 64.
[25] Kobayashi Y, et al. Circulating extracellular vesicles are associated with lipid and insulin metabolism. Am J Physiol Endocrinol Metab 2018; 315(4): E574 - 82.
[26] Osada-Oka M, et al. Macrophage-derived exosomes induce inflammatory factors in endothelial cells under hypertensive conditions. Hypertens Res 2017; 40(4): 353 - 60.
[27] Qi Y, et al. Activation of the endogenous renin-angiotensin-aldosterone system or aldosterone administration increases urinary exosomal sodium channel excretion. J Am Soc Nephrol 2016; 27(2): 646 - 56.
[28] van der Lubbe N, et al. The phosphorylated sodium chloride cotransporter in urinary exosomes is superior to prostasin as a marker for aldosteronism. Hypertension 2012; 60(3): 741 - 8.
[29] Li S, et al. Cell-derived microparticles in Patients with type 2 diabetes mellitus: a systematic review and meta-analysis. Cell Physiol Biochem 2016; 39(6): 2439 - 50.
[30] Lazar I, et al. Adipocyte exosomes promote melanoma aggressiveness through fatty acid oxidation: a novel mechanism linking obesity and cancer. Cancer Res 2016; 76(14): 4051 - 7.
[31] Connolly KD, et al. Evidence for adipocyte-derived extracellular vesicles in the human circulation. Endocrinology 2018; 159(9): 3259 - 67.
[32] Lopez Andres N, et al. Increased microparticle production and impaired microvascular endothelial function in aldosterone-salt-treated rats: protective effects of polyphenols. PLoS One 2012; 7(7): e39235.
[33] Boulanger CM, et al. Extracellular vesicles in coronary artery disease. Nat Rev Cardiol 2017; 14(5): 259 - 72.
[34] Agouni A, et al. Endothelial dysfunction caused by circulating microparticles from patients with metabolic syndrome. Am J Pathol 2008; 173(4): 1210 - 9.
[35] Helal O, et al. Increased levels of microparticles originating from endothelial cells, platelets and erythrocytes in subjects with metabolic syndrome: relationship with oxidative stress. Nutr Metab Cardiovasc Dis 2011; 21(9): 665 - 71.
[36] Diamant M, et al. Elevated numbers of tissue-factor exposing microparticles correlate with components of the metabolic syndrome in uncomplicated type 2 diabetes mellitus. Circulation 2002; 106(19): 2442 - 7.
[37] Kranendonk ME, et al. Extracellular vesicle markers in relation to obesity and metabolic complications in patients with manifest cardiovascular disease. Cardiovasc Diabetol 2014; 13: 37.
[38] Li F, et al. Exosomal microRNA-29a mediates cardiac dysfunction and mitochondrial inactivity in obesity-related cardiomyopathy. Endocrine 2019; 63(3): 480 - 8.
[39] Nie H, Pan Y, Zhou Y. Exosomal microRNA-194 causes cardiac injury and mitochondrial dysfunction in obese mice. Biochem Biophys Res Commun 2018; 503(4): 3174 - 9.
[40] Crewe C, et al. An endothelial-to-adipocyte extracellular vesicle axis governed by metabolic state. Cell 2018; 175(3): 695 - 708, e13.
[41] Thomou T, et al. Adipose-derived circulating miRNAs regulate gene expression in other tissues. Nature 2017; 542 (7642): 450 - 5.
[42] Ying W, et al. Adipose tissue macrophage-derived exosomal miRNAs can modulate in vivo and in vitro insulin

sensitivity. Cell 2017; 171(2): 372-84, e12.
[43] Deng ZB, et al. Adipose tissue exosome-kike vesicles mediate activation of macrophage-induced insulin resistance. Diabetes 2009; 58(11): 2498-505.
[44] Zhang Y, et al. Adipocyte-derived microvesicles from obese mice induce M1 macrophage phenotype through secreted miR-155. J Mol Cell Biol 2016; 8(6): 505-17.
[45] Kranendonk ME, et al. Effect of extracellular vesicles of human adipose tissue on insulin signaling in liver and muscle cells. Obesity (Silver Spring) 2014; 22(10): 2216-23.
[46] Xie Z, et al. Adipose-derived exosomes exert proatherogenic effects by regulating macrophage foam cell formation and polarization. J Am Heart Assoc 2018; 7(5).
[47] Zhang H, et al. Serum exosomes mediate delivery of arginase 1 as a novel mechanism for endothelial dysfunction in diabetes. Proc Natl Acad Sci U S A 2018; 115(29): E6927-36.
[48] Zamani P, et al. The therapeutic and diagnostic role of exosomes in cardiovascular diseases. Trends Cardiovasc Med 2018; 29(6): 313-23.
[49] Li L, et al. Human aortic smooth muscle cell-derived exosomal miR-221/222 inhibits autophagy via a PTEN/Akt signaling pathway in human umbilical vein endothelial cells. Biochem Biophys Res Commun 2016; 479(2): 343-50.
[50] Hergenreider E, et al. Atheroprotective communication between endothelial cells and smooth muscle cells through miRNAs. Nat Cell Biol 2012; 14(3): 249-56.
[51] Wang X, et al. Cardiomyocytes mediate anti-angiogenesis in type 2 diabetic rats through the exosomal transfer of miR-320 into endothelial cells. J Mol Cell Cardiol 2014; 74: 139-50.
[52] Otani K, et al. Plasma exosomes regulate systemic blood pressure in rats. Biochem Biophys Res Commun 2018; 503(2): 776-83.
[53] Tong Y, et al. Exosome-mediated transfer of ACE (angiotensin-converting enzyme) from adventitial fibroblasts of spontaneously hypertensive rats promotes vascular smooth muscle cell migration. Hypertension 2018; 72(4): 881-8.
[54] Liu X, et al. miRNA profiling of exosomes from spontaneous hypertensive rats using nextgeneration sequencing. J Cardiovasc Transl Res 2019; 12(1): 75-83.
[55] Hirsova P, et al. Lipid-induced signaling causes release of inflammatory extracellular vesicles from hepatocytes. Gastroenterology 2016; 150(4): 956-67.
[56] Koeck ES, et al. Adipocyte exosomes induce transforming growth factor beta pathway dysregulation in hepatocytes: a novel paradigm for obesity-related liver disease. J Surg Res 2014; 192(2): 268-75.
[57] Zakharova L, Svetlova M, Fomina AF. T cell exosomes induce cholesterol accumulation in human monocytes via phosphatidylserine receptor. J Cell Physiol 2007; 212(1): 174-81.
[57a] Liu S, et al. The host shapes the gut microbiota via fecal microRNA. Cell Host Microbe 2016; 19(1): 32-43.
[58] Choi Y, et al. Gut microbe-derived extracellular vesicles induce insulin resistance, thereby impairing glucose metabolism in skeletal muscle. Sci Rep 2015; 5, 15878.

第 16 章

外泌体在妊娠与生殖医学中的作用潜力
Potential role of exosomes in reproductive medicine and pregnancy

Soumyalekshmi Nair[a], Carlos Salomon[a,b,c]

[a]Exosome Biology Laboratory, Centre for Clinical Diagnostics, UQ centre for Clinical Research, Royal Brisbane and Women's Hospital, The University of Queensland, St Lucia, QLD, Australia, [b]Department of Clinical Biochemistry and Immunology, University of Concepción, Concepción, Chile, [c]Department of Obstetrics and Gynecology, Ochsner Baptist Hospital, New Orleans, LA, United States

一、概述

妊娠是一种独特的生理状态，其特征是母体为了满足和维持胚胎或胎儿生长发育而做出的多种生理性改变，包括内分泌、代谢、心血管、血液和免疫系统的变化，从而维持胎儿的正常生长和发育。上述生理性改变在时间和空间上的协调发生对获得良好的妊娠结局至关重要。同时，不同组织器官释放的因子在这一生理过程中也起着关键的调节作用。胎盘作为妊娠期间的主要器官，可以释放多种激素、生长因子、细胞因子、miRNA和蛋白质，而这些物质对母胎的健康尤为重要。近年来，随着EV领域的研究不断推进，尤其是被称为"外泌体"的纳米级囊泡改变了人们对细胞间交流的认知。更有趣的是，在正常和有子痫前期、妊娠糖尿病、胎儿生长受限和早产等并发症的妊娠期间，胎盘均会分泌大量外泌体进入母体循环，并在妊娠生理多个方面发挥重要作用，包括胎儿-母体间的信号传递。

二、胞外囊泡的多样性、生成和分泌

在过去的几十年，EV因其新颖、有效的细胞交流方式引起科研人员极大的兴趣[1]。起初，EV被认为是细胞的"碎片"，但后来的研究证实其可以与特定的靶细胞相互作用，并调节后者的生物功能[2]。典型的EV为脂质双分子层，是由细胞释放到胞外环境的100～1 000 nm大小不等的囊泡[3]。值得注意的是，其囊内装配了多种信使分子，包括蛋白质、脂质、RNA和DNA。几乎每一种细胞都可分泌EV，这些囊泡可通过生理屏障，并在多种体液包括血液、尿液、唾液、母乳和CSF中富集[4]。EV由不同来源和不同形态的异质囊泡群体组成而种类繁多。具体而言，根据其大小和来源可分为三个亚类，包括：① 外泌体（50～150 nm）；② 微囊泡（0.2～1 μm）；③ 凋亡小体（巨囊泡，超过1 μm）[5]。外泌体是细胞通过内吞途径形成的纳米微泡。外泌体的生成始于细胞膜内陷而形成的MVB，之后，多泡体进一步内陷形成ILV。有趣的是，据报道，ILV可通过选择性包装机制，将蛋白质、miRNA等分子内容物载入其囊内[6,7]。而后，腔内小泡通过胞外分泌途径释放至胞外环境，继而形成

"外泌体"。因此,外泌体富含内吞通路的蛋白,如 CD63、CD9、CD81、TSG101 和凋亡相关基因 2 互作蛋白 X(apoptosis-linked gene 2 - interacting protein X,ALIX)。除了这些蛋白标志物,典型的杯状外形、在梯度浓度的蔗糖溶液中浮力密度范围为 1.13~1.19 g/mL 也可将外泌体与其他 EV 区别开来[1,8,9]。其他种类的 EV 如微囊泡通过质膜的出芽或脱落机制产生,凋亡小体来自凋亡的细胞[10,11]。表 16-1 概括总结了不同类型 EV 的生成、特征和功能。

表 16-1 不同类型 EV 的生成、特点及功能

类型	生成机制	大小	代表蛋白[a]	内容物	提取方法[b]	已知功能
外泌体	与晚期内体内的腔内囊泡一致;通过多泡体与细胞膜融合分泌至胞外;依赖或非依赖 ESCRT 蛋白(脂蛋白、跨膜蛋白、Rab GTP 酶、SNARE)参与外泌体的生成	典型的外泌体直径为 50~150 nm,与电镜下腔内囊泡相近	跨膜蛋白(CD81、CD63、CD9),ESCRT 组成成分,ALIX,TSG101,同线蛋白,鞭毛蛋白,整合素,解聚素,金属基质蛋白酶结构域蛋白 10,ADAM10,HSC70,HSPA8,HSPC7[13-15]	蛋白质,miRNA,lncRNA,小片段非核 DNA,线粒体,内质网和高尔基体成分蛋白[13,14]	差速离心和 100 000 g 超速离心 90 分钟;差异梯度离心(蔗糖或碘二醇溶液),超滤,尺寸排阻色谱法,使用抗体或者商业试剂盒(沉淀法)[16,17]	通过将内容物传递给受体细胞完成细胞间的信息交流[18,19]、免疫调节[20,21]、肿瘤进展与转移[22,23]
微囊泡	多种机制以胞膜出芽的形式生成,如早期胞内体囊泡的分泌,细胞内 Ca^{2+} 水平升高,细胞骨架的重构,磷脂酶 D2 的活化[1]	典型的微囊泡直径较大,可至几微米,小的如外泌体大小即<150 nm	CD63,CD9,HSC70/HSPA8/HSPC7,flotillin - 1,KIF23,RACGAP,CSE1L,ARF6,EMMPRIN[13-15]	蛋白质,miRNA,mRNA,小片段 DNA[114]	差速离心。以 10 000 g 的离速离心 40 分钟可获得微囊泡	参与细胞间信息传递、炎症和免疫、肿瘤进展和侵袭[24,25]
凋亡小体	由将死细胞凋亡形成。凋亡细胞经历形态变化,如胞膜起泡、胞膜薄弱处向外突出形成微管棘或凋亡棘突,这些结构从胞膜脱落,形成凋亡小体	>1 μm	CD63,CD9,HSC70/HSPA8/HSPC7,α-actinin - 4/ACTN4/ACTN4,GP96,HSP90B1/ENPL,磷脂酰丝氨酸,组蛋白,钙连蛋白,细胞色素 c,CX3CL1,ICAM - 3,唾液酰化和糖基化配体 MHC Ⅱ[13-15,26]	细胞核,蛋白质,细胞器[14]	差速离心。以 2 000 g 的离速离心 20 分钟可获得凋亡小体[15]。以 400 g 的离速离心去除细胞,再用 1.2 μm 的过滤器过滤也可获得凋亡小体[27]	传递炎症因子和损伤相关的分子片段,促进炎症,参与调节免疫细胞对细菌和病毒感染的免疫反应[26]

注:[a] 蛋白质的表达可因 EV 的来源、蛋白质分析方法的不同而有所差异。
[b] EV 的提取方法可因提取原料如体液或细胞培养液以及实验目的而不同。

外泌体的功能和作用机制

外泌体载有多种生物分子,包括蛋白质(胞浆蛋白和膜结合蛋白)、mRNA、非编码 RNA(如 miRNA 和长非编码 RNA 或 lncRNA)、DNA 片段和脂质,而这些分子则可能代表其源细胞的组成成分。通过携带的遗传信息或有效的信号分子,外泌体介导了其源细胞与相邻细胞或者远端受体细胞间的信号传递。此外,得益于具有通过生理屏障如内皮细胞[30]和血脑屏障[31]的功能,外泌体可在多种体液中富集[28,29],而该功能则赋予了外泌体成为理想治疗手段的潜力。值得注意的是,外泌体膜上存在特定的细胞表面分子,如差异表达的整合素,这将有助于其靶向作用于不同的受体细胞[33,34]。

靶细胞可以以不同的方式摄取外泌体。某些情况下,外泌体和靶细胞膜蛋白之间经典的受体-配体相互作用可以激活下游信号通路,从而改变靶细胞的功能[37,36]。其他情况下,外泌体的内化可以由不同的机制来介导,如吞噬作用、网格蛋白介导的内吞作用、小泡蛋白依赖的内吞作用、微胞饮作用以及脂筏介导的摄取[37]。此外,外泌体通过膜与膜间的直接融合,实现内容物向靶细胞内的转移也在既往研究中被报道[38,39]。然而,外泌体内容物(如蛋白质和 miRNA)影响或改变靶细胞生物行为的机制尚需进一步的研究。有趣的是,有研究报道外泌体中的蛋白质可通过改变磷酸化过程激活或抑制信号通路,从而完成细胞[18]之间遗传信息的传递。至于外泌体中的 miRNA,它们可以改变某些特定靶蛋白的表达,并改变受体细胞的表型[40,41]。图 16-1 为 EV 生成、外泌体结构及其与靶细胞相互作用的示意图。

三、妊娠期外泌体的来源和功能

外泌体通过调节包括母体免疫反应和代谢适应在内的多个生理过程,在妊娠中起到关键的作用[42,43]。已有研究表明,妊娠期外周循环中外泌体总量随着妊娠周而逐渐增加[44],并在妊娠期并发症如妊娠糖尿病(gestational diabetes mellitus,GDM)和子痫前期(preeclampsia,PE)中显著增加[45,46]。到目前为止,母体循环中外泌体的确切来源、内容物和功能尚未完全了解,仍需进一步探索。然而,胎盘作为妊娠期的主要器官,其分泌的外泌体最早便可在妊娠 6 周时于母体外周循环中被发现[44]。值得注意的是,在正常和异常的妊娠中,来自胎盘的外泌体是胎盘与其他母体组织进行信息交流的重要纽带。

(一)胎盘来源的外泌体

胎盘是一种独特的胎儿-母体器官,分泌维持妊娠所必需的激素和分子,并通过交换营养物质、氧气和代谢废物,在母胎之间起着关键的连接作用。胎盘绒毛是胎盘的基本功能单位,由三种主要的滋养层细胞所组成:① 绒毛滋养层细胞;② 绒毛外滋养层细胞(extravillous cytotrophoblast,EVT);③ 合体滋养层细胞(syncytiotrophoblast,STB)(由绒毛滋养层细胞融合而成)[47],而每组细胞的功能差异较大。胎盘可释放多种激素,如胎盘生长激素、胎盘泌乳激素、雌激素和孕酮,以及炎症因子如 TNF-α 和皮质醇等,这些激素的分泌与母体妊娠生理变化协调一致,以满足胎儿生长发育的需求[48,49]。除了激素和细胞因子,胎盘在整个妊娠期还会向母体外周循环释放大量的 EV。这些 EV 主要来自胎盘的合体

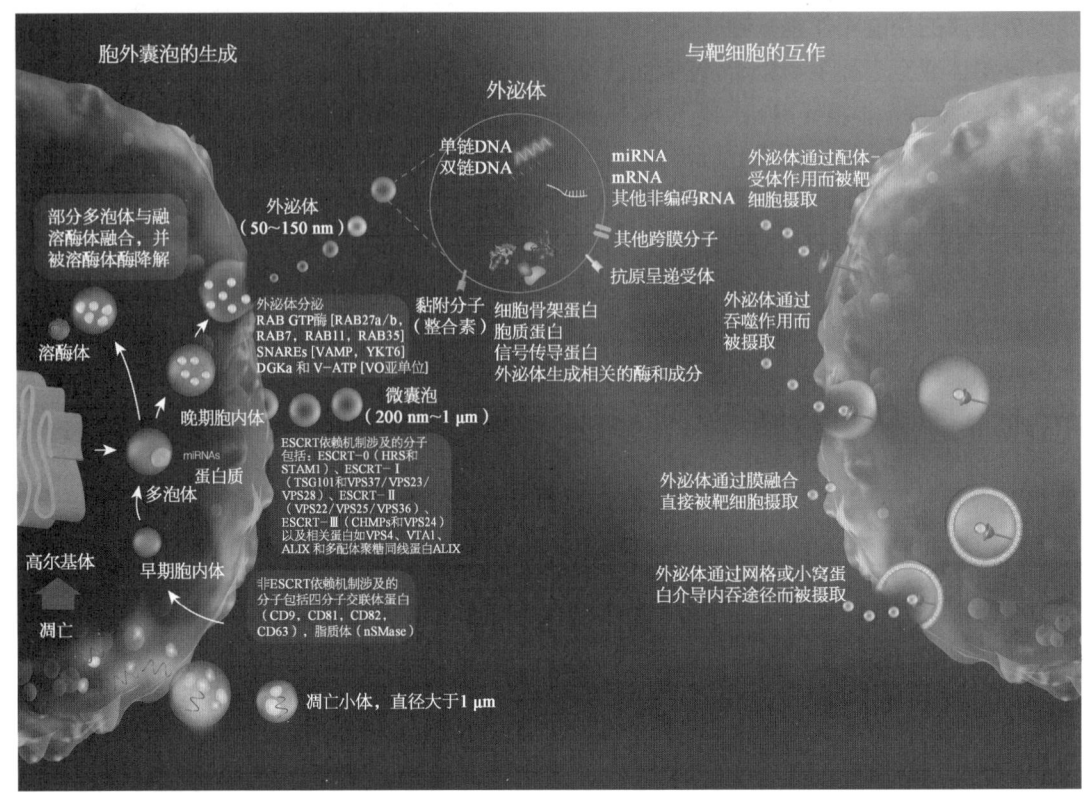

图 16-1 EV 生成、结构组成及功能示意图。EV 有不同的亚群：① 由胞内体形成的外泌体(50～150 nm)；② 由质膜直接出芽形成的微囊泡(200 nm～1 μm)；③ 死亡细胞凋亡形成的凋亡小体(大于 1 μm)。外泌体的形成始于质膜的内陷形成早期胞内体。早期胞内体通过膜内陷，在其囊内形成特异性包被有蛋白质、脂质、核酸等内容物的 ILV，从而成熟为晚期胞内体。包含 ILV 的晚期胞内体称为 MVB，它既可以与溶酶体融合而被降解，也可以与质膜融合而被释放到胞外环境。外泌体形成所需要的依赖和不依赖 ESCRT 机制的重要蛋白质和参与外泌体分泌的蛋白质已罗列在示意图中。外泌体膜表面存在跨膜受体和黏附分子，囊内载有多种蛋白质，包括胞质蛋白、细胞骨架蛋白、信号转导蛋白、外泌体形成基质蛋白以及包括单链和双链 DNA、mRNA 和非编码 RNA 在内的多种核酸。至于作用机制，外泌体可通过受体-配体相互作用机制介导下游信号的传递，或经过吞噬作用、网格蛋白或小窝蛋白介导的内吞作用被靶细胞摄取，或直接与靶细胞膜融合释放其内容物进入靶细胞，从而影响靶细胞功能

扫描二维码查看彩图

滋养细胞层，目前已鉴定出四个主要的亚群。它们是：① 外泌体(30～100 nm)；② MV(100 nm～1 μm，也称 STB 微颗粒)；③ 合胞核聚集物(20～500 μm，囊泡内为细胞排出的老化核)；④ 凋亡小体(1～4 μm)[51]。其他来源的外泌体，如卵泡液、子宫内膜、胚胎和滋养细胞，可能会影响女性的生育能力、受精卵的着床和妊娠早期，而胎盘合体滋养细胞来源的外泌体则是影响妊娠中晚期的关键因素[51,52]。此外，通过识别 HLA-G 抗原，也已在母体循环、早期妊娠胎盘外植体和 EVT 样细胞系 Swan71 细胞鉴定出绒毛外滋养细胞来源的外泌体[20,52,54]（HLA-G 在 EVT 上表达，而在 STB 上不表达）。

需要指出的是，不同类型胎盘来源的 EV，其生成机制、生物学功能和对母体的影响是不尽相同的。有趣的是，外泌体具有独特的生成机制，因为其生成源于胞内体途径，且存在多

种选择性机制可将分子内容物如蛋白质和 miRNA 等装配至其囊泡中[6]。此外,大量文献表明外泌体在细胞间信息交流中可能发挥重要的作用[1,55]。与非妊娠相比,妊娠期循环中外泌体的浓度更高,且浓度会随妊娠周而逐步增加,在妊娠晚期达到最高浓度[44,56]。

胎盘内的微环境,如氧分压和葡萄糖浓度可以调节胎盘来源外泌体的生成和分泌。低氧分力或缺氧可增加胎盘来源外泌体的分泌,并改变其内容物以及对靶细胞功能的影响[57]。同样,高浓度的葡萄糖可以增加胎盘细胞来源外泌体的分泌[58]。导致这一现象的确切机制目前尚不清楚。然而,有研究证实,在缺氧条件下,HIF 可以调节外泌体生成的过程[59,60];而在葡萄糖存在的情况下,细胞内 Ca^{2+} 通道的激活可能在调节内体途径中发挥作用[61,62]。

(二) 胎盘外泌体的鉴定和提取

研究表明,胎盘来源的外泌体占妊娠期循环外泌体总量的 10%~25%[63]。如何将胎盘来源的外泌体与其他细胞类型的外泌区别开来,尤其是如何从总外泌体种群中将其提取出来显得至关重要。胎盘来源的外泌体可以通过识别胎盘碱性磷酸酶(placental alkaline phosphatase,PLAP)蛋白进行特异性的鉴定,而该蛋白为膜整合蛋白且主要表达于 STB 细胞膜表面[64,65]。此外,PLAP 在胎盘的大多数滋养层细胞中均有表达[66],包括原代细胞滋养层细胞[67]和从早期绒毛膜绒毛中分离出来的 ED27 滋养层样细胞[68]。已有多种技术被用于检测和定量分析循环总外泌中的 PLAP$^+$ 外泌体。Dragovic 等利用荧光 NTA 对胎盘灌洗液中的 PLAP$^+$ 外泌体进行了鉴定分析,其方法是使用抗 PLAP 抗体包被免疫磁珠富集 PLAP$^+$ 外泌体,然后用偶联抗 PLAP 抗体的量子点(Qdot)标记它们[69]。同样,也有使用免疫荧光 NTA 与耦合 CD63$^+$ 和 PLAP$^+$ 抗体的量子点标记法对母体循环中的胎盘外泌体进行定量分析[63,70]。此外,也有使用商用 PLAP ELISA 试剂盒对母体循环中胎盘来源的外泌体表达谱进行鉴定分析[44,71]。有趣的是,Lai 等描述了可使用抗 PLAP 抗体包膜磁珠的免疫亲和捕获从母体循环中分泌的 PLAP$^+$ 外泌体[72]。最近,研究报道了使用金包被的氧化铁纳米多孔立方体可直接分离 PLAP$^+$ 外泌体(无须预分离外泌体)[73],该方法为外泌体检测的临床开发开辟了新的途径。然而,从母体循环中分离出特定的胎盘来源的外泌体极具挑战性,因为母体循环中胎盘来源外泌体的水平较低(约 15%,且与妊娠周相关),其膜表面的 PLAP 表达相对较低,且高度依赖所使用的 PLAP 抗体的特异性。已有多个实验研究了胎盘来源外泌体在妊娠中的作用,包括从母体血浆/血清、细胞培养液(原代和细胞系)、胎盘灌注液以及胎盘外植体中分离胎盘来源的外泌体(表 16-2 展示了研究胎盘来源外泌体的实验和分离方法)。母体血浆是纯化和分析包括外泌体在内胎盘来源 EV 最广泛采用的体液。从母体血浆中获得外泌体最常用的分离方法是使用蔗糖缓冲液或碘二沙醇密度梯度离心法[44,45,63]。提取完成后,再使用上述描述的任何一种方法,从总外泌体中定量分析胎盘来源的外泌体[44,67,70,71]。胎盘外泌体可以从原代滋养细胞、滋养细胞系(如 BeWo、JEG-3 和 HTR8 细胞)和胎盘外植体的培养基中分离出来。从细胞培养基中分离外泌体最常用的方法是先序惯离心,然后接着进行超速离心或密度梯度离心[74,88,94]。另一个引人注意的胎盘来源外泌体分离和分析模型则是基于胎盘子叶双灌注的胎盘灌注系统。通过各种 EV 的分离方法，包括超速离心法和滤过法，可以富集灌洗液中 EV 和去除混杂的红细胞[69,81,95,96]。从生物体液中分离出的胎盘来源外泌体，可通过体内和体外模型对其内容物进行量化和分析，并确定其对靶细胞生物活性的影响。

表 16-2 研究胎盘来源外泌体具有代表性的实验模型和外泌体提取方法

实验模型	外泌体提取方法	主 要 发 现	参考文献
人原代滋养细胞和 JEG-3 细胞	超速离心和密度梯度离心法	外泌体可传递 C19MC miRNA 并调节病毒感染的免疫反应	[74]
Bewo 和 Jurkat 细胞	超速离心法	外泌体中的 miR-517a-3p 靶向作用于 NK 细胞并调控其活性	[75]
滋养细胞培养液和外植体培养液	密度梯度离心法	胎盘可通过外泌体分泌免疫调节分子	[20]
Sw71 人滋养细胞	超速离心和超滤	滋养细胞来源外泌体具有促炎作用	[53]
孕早期原代滋养细胞	差速离心和密度梯度离心法	高糖(25 mM)和低氧条件下，外泌体的分泌量显著增加。与对照组相比，外泌体可诱导 HUVEC 细胞分泌细胞因子	[76]
Sw71 人滋养细胞	超速离心法，差速离心和密度梯度离心法	描绘培养滋养细胞分泌的外泌体形态和蛋白质组学特征	[77]
原代滋养细胞培养液	超速离心和密度梯度离心法	原代滋养细胞分泌的外泌体囊内 miRNA 的主要部分为 C19MC miRNA	[78]
胎盘来源绒毛滋养细胞	差速离心，Exoquick 试剂盒，超滤和超速离心法	外泌体富含合胞素-1 和合胞素-2，而 PE 来源的外泌体中合胞素-2 含量减少	[79]
细胞滋养层细胞	密度梯度离心法	缺氧条件下外泌体的分泌增加，细胞滋养层细胞来源外泌体可提高 EVT 细胞迁移能力	[57]
血浆	密度梯度离心法	在孕 6 周时外周循环可鉴定出胎盘来源的外泌体，且其含量会随着孕周的增加而增加	[44]
外植体培养液	超速离心和密度梯度离心法	胎盘来源外泌体中含活性 FasL 和 TRAIL 蛋白，在孕期免疫调节方面可能起到一定的作用	[80]
体外胎盘双向灌注液	超速离心法	通过 NTA 和荧光 NTA 对外泌体的特点进行了描绘	[81]
Bewo 细胞株	超滤和免疫分离法	胎盘特有的 miRNA 可通过外泌体分泌到细胞外	[82]
外植体培养液，原代滋养细胞和 Bewo 细胞株	密度梯度离心法和超滤法	胎盘来源外泌体含 syncytin-1，并在免疫抑制方面起到一定的作用	[83]
血浆和体外胎盘双向灌注液	超滤法	分析了体外通过流式细胞分析技术研究血浆 EV 的难点和局限性	[84]
外植体培养液	超滤法和密度梯度离心法	人胎盘可分泌载有 NKG2D 配体的外泌体	[85]
人妊娠早期 EVT 细胞株和 HTR8 细胞株	ExoQuick 试剂盒	aPL 可通过 TLR4 受体诱导 miR-146a-3p 的表达上调，而后者则促进细胞分泌 IL-8	[86]

续 表

实验模型	外泌体提取方法	主 要 发 现	参考文献
血浆	密度梯度离心法	妊娠期糖尿病和正常孕妇外周循环外泌体含量随孕周的增加而增加。妊娠期糖尿病孕妇的外泌体会显著促进内皮细胞释放促炎因子	[71]
血浆	超速离心法	子痫前期孕妇外周循环总外泌体中胎盘来源外泌体的分布以及其在子痫前期发病所起到的作用	[87]
JEG-3 和 HTR-8/SVneo 细胞株	密度梯度离心法	描绘了外泌体蛋白质内容物的特点,并报道外泌体可促进血管平滑肌细胞的迁移能力	[88]
血浆和 EVT 细胞	密度梯度离心法	与 1% 氧浓度相比,在 8% 氧浓度条件下,EVT 细胞来源的外泌体可显著提高细胞的迁移能力	[89]
血浆	尺寸排阻色谱法和超速离心法,尺寸排阻色谱超速离心法	胎盘来源外泌体可抑制 T 细胞信号成分的表达,并识别 FasL 和 PD-L1 在免疫调节中的作用	[90]
体外胎盘双向灌注液和血浆	超速离心法	血浆合体滋养细胞来源和胎盘来源外泌体含活性 eNOS 合成酶,而在 PE 中该酶的水平下降	[91]
血浆	密度梯度离心法	从 PE 患者血浆外泌体中鉴定出差异表达的 miRNA(hsa-miR-486-1-5P 和 hsa-miR-486-2-5P)	[45]
血浆	密度梯度离心法	孕期 12%~15% 的外周循环外泌体来自胎盘。而孕妇的 BMI 越高,该比例越低	[63]
外植体培养液	超速离心法	人胎盘来源纳米囊泡注入孕鼠 24 小时,可出现在孕鼠肺、肝脏和肾脏中。胎盘来源的纳米囊泡可与内皮细胞快速发生作用并介导血管的舒张	[92]
血浆	密度梯度离心法	对比分析胎儿生长受限和小于胎龄儿胎盘来源外泌体的表达谱	[70]
血浆和胎盘合胞体脂质筏	ExoQuick 试剂盒,密度梯度离心法	研究了片段内皮素经外泌体对血管的作用在子痫前期病理生理中所扮演的角色	[93]

(三)胎盘来源外泌体在体内的分布及对靶细胞的影响

胎盘分泌的外泌体一旦进入循环,便可被运送到各种靶细胞,并在介导胎盘和其他器官之间的交叉对话中发挥重要的作用。Tong 等证明,将来自妊娠早期人胎盘的外泌体注射到小鼠体内后,可靶向作用于包括肺、肝和肾在内的特定器官,并可通过 NO 信号通路与肠系膜内皮细胞的相互作用,导致血管舒张[92]。Miranda 等发现胎儿循环中存在人胎盘来源的外泌体,并证实其与胎儿生长有关[70]。此外,来自家畜的研究证实了绵羊脐带血中胎盘来源外泌体的存在,并评估了通过外泌体转运 miRNA 的可能[97]。这表明外泌体可能参与母胎之间的双向物质交换,即母体细胞或分子向胎儿循环的转运,反之亦然。母胎物质交换对正常妊娠和不良妊娠中母胎之间信号的传递非常重要,而外泌体可通过代偿机制为保护胎儿提供额外机制[98,99]。然而,胎盘来源外泌体通过胎盘屏障的机制尚不清楚。同时,在胎儿系统中发现的母体外泌体对胎儿生长和发育的影响有待进一步研究。

越来越多的证据表明胎盘来源的外泌体对其靶细胞功能的影响,并证实其在介导胎盘形成和母胎血管系统发育中细胞间的信息传递方面发挥重要作用。母胎之间循环的建立是胎盘形成过程中的关键事件,它始于 EVT 细胞的侵袭,并在妊娠 10 周内完成。EVT 的侵袭重塑了子宫螺旋动脉(spiral artery,SpA),并使母体的血液流入绒毛间隙。早孕期的终末阶段,胎盘以细胞滋养层融合为特征,形成具有多核的合体滋养层,该合体滋养层沐浴在母体血液、可溶性蛋白和营养物质中,并覆盖大部分的胎盘表面[100]。因此,与 EVT 和合体滋养细胞直接接触的母体血液,接收了由这些细胞分泌的绝大部分 EV,包括外泌体。研究表明,外泌体信号通路与 EVT 侵袭、滋养细胞融合、内皮细胞迁移和螺旋动脉重铸相关[79,88,89,101,102]。

特别是低氧分压下胎盘细胞滋养层外泌体促进了 EVT(HTR-8)的迁移,这可能是胎盘对缺氧的反应[57]。此外,从胎盘 MSC 提取的外泌体在体内和体外实验中都可增加内皮细胞的迁移和促进血管管腔的形成,提示胎盘血管的自我改造[57,103]。来自胎盘细胞系、JEG-3(绒毛膜肿瘤细胞系)和 HTR-8/SVneo(EVT 细胞系)的外泌体的蛋白质组学特性表明,与 JEG-3 细胞相比,HRT8/SVneo 外泌体中参与调节细胞迁移的蛋白质比例更高[88]。有趣的是,研究表明,外泌体参与类二十烷糖的跨细胞代谢[104,105],并可携带磷脂酶和游离脂肪酸[104]。这些外泌体在被靶细胞内化时可影响后者的代谢通路,并导致各种病理生理情况的发生[105]。图 16-2 展示合体滋养层外泌体的生成、细胞外环境对外泌体生成机制的影响及外泌体对靶细胞功能产生的影响。

胎盘来源外泌体的免疫调节作用及其对胎儿发育可能提供的免疫耐受作用已被广泛研究。有趣的是,大量参与妊娠免疫调节的分子与胎盘细胞外泌体的生成密切相关,并以活性状态与外泌体一起分泌到胞外。这包括免疫调节分子,如 Fas 配体(Fas ligand,FasL)、肿瘤坏死因子相关凋亡诱导配体(TNF-related apoptosis-inducing ligand,TRAIL)、NKG2D 配体和一些 B7 免疫调节配体家族成员,这些分子与淋巴细胞中的受体结合,介导免疫反应,并为胎儿提供免疫豁免[20,80,85,90,106]。此外,免疫抑制分子如 HLA-G[20,89]和 syncitin-1[83]也与外泌体一起分泌至胞外,介导免疫耐受和妊娠期细胞因子由 Th1 相向 Th2 相转移。也有报道表明,外泌体可诱导促炎症反应并介导妊娠期全身炎症[53,54]。例如,胎盘来源外泌体可增加单核细胞从母体系统到母胎界面的募集,并可增加促炎细胞因子如 IL-1β、IL-6、serpin-e1、粒细胞/单核细胞集落刺激因子和 TNF-α 的释放[54]。外泌体膜上的纤连蛋白与巨噬细胞表面的 α5β1 整合素结合,介导了这种效应[53]。

外泌体影响靶细胞行为的另一种重要途径是以自身为媒介将 miRNA 传递至靶细胞。19 号染色体 miRNA 簇(C19MC)是一个由 46 个 miRNA 组成的 miRNA 簇,仅在人类胎盘中表达[78]。然而,C19MC 对胎盘健康和妊娠的重要性尚不清楚。Delorme Axford 等报道了 C19MC miRNA,即 miR-512-3p 和 miR-517-3p,可通过外泌体介导的旁分泌传递滋养细胞之间的病毒抵抗力,并通过诱导自噬来抑制胎盘细胞中的病毒复制[74]。另一种 C19MC miRNA,miR-517a-3p 由胎盘来源外泌体携带,被母体免疫细胞内化后,通过

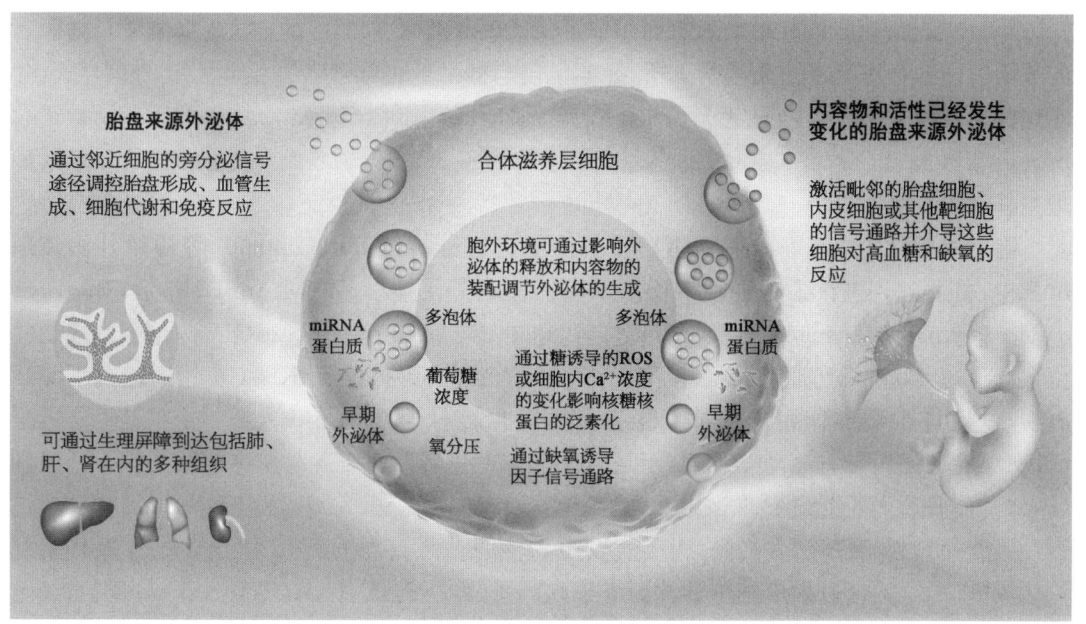

图 16-2 合胞滋养细胞来源外泌体生成、影响其生成的胞外因素及对靶细胞的作用示意图。合胞滋养细胞释放的外泌体可以与邻近的胎盘细胞、内皮细胞和免疫细胞相互作用,介导胎盘形成、胎盘血管生成、细胞代谢和免疫应答。此外,胎盘来源外泌体可以通过生理屏障,到达包括肺、肝和肾在内的各种器官。胞外环境,如高糖和低氧可以影响外泌体的生成,释放和囊内成分。高糖通过诱导 ROS 的释放、增加细胞内 Ca^{2+} 浓度和改变异质核糖核蛋白(heterogeneous nuclear ribonucleoprotein,hnRNP)的泛素化来影响外泌体的释放和生物活性。缺氧可诱导 ROS 和 HIF 信号传导从而影响外泌体的生成

NO/cGMP 信号通路,调节后者的活化和增殖[94]。

四、外泌体与妊娠并发症

(一) GDM

GDM 是首次在妊娠期间发现的任何程度的葡萄糖耐受不良,与母亲和后代近期和远期不良结局相关,并对公共卫生产生显著影响[107]。GDM 的代谢功能障碍包括胰腺胰岛素分泌不足、肝脏葡萄糖生成受到抑制以及骨骼肌葡萄糖摄取减少[108]。GDM 的特点是血糖控制不良或高血糖、组织缺氧和机体炎症或细胞因子的表达发生改变,这将导致胎儿-母体血管形成和胎盘形成发生缺陷[109]。如前所述,与非糖尿病内环境相比,体外缺氧和较高浓度葡萄糖的条件下,可诱导胎盘细胞分泌更高浓度的外泌体[76,89]。此外,低氧可以改变外泌体的生物活性。更有趣的是,研究报道,缺氧诱导的外泌体可以增加炎性细胞因子即 TNF-α 和 IL-6 的释放,并减弱靶细胞的迁移能力[89]。高糖诱导的外泌体可促进内皮细胞释放促炎细胞因子,包括 IL-6 和 TNF-α[76]。Salomon 等在一项纵向队列研究中发现,GDM 患者的胎盘来源外泌体在整个妊娠期其浓度均高于正常孕妇,同时还发现 GDM 女性的血浆外泌体可促进内皮细胞促炎细胞因子(GM-CSF、IL-4、IL-6、IL-8、IFN-γ 和 TNF-α)的表达[71]。此外,有研究采用定量、信息独立获取[全理论质谱序列窗口获取(sequential windowed acquisition of all theoretical mass spectra，SWATH）]的方法对源自 GDM 患者的外泌体内容物进行蛋白质组学分析，并鉴定出与糖耐量正常患者外泌体主要的差异蛋白。在这些蛋白中，最重要的是钙/钙调素依赖蛋白激酶Ⅱβ（calcium/calmodulin-dependent protein kinase Ⅱ beta，CAMK2β）和 Pappalysin-1（PAPP-A），而这些蛋白与 GDM 的病理生理有关[110]。

除了对 GDM 患者外泌体内蛋白质的特征进行分析，Almohammadi 等还对外泌体中 miRNA 的表达谱进行了研究，结果发现 GDM 患者外泌体中 C19MC miRNA 簇，如 miR-518a-5p、miR-518b、miR-518c、miR-518e、miR-520c-3p 和 miR-525-5p 的表达发生上调[111]。Nair 等还通过二代测序技术对绒毛来源外泌体的 miRNA 表达谱进行了测序分析，并鉴定出靶向作用于葡萄糖稳态和胰岛素信号通路的 miRNA。该研究还分析了 GDM 绒毛来源外泌体对骨骼肌葡萄糖摄取的影响，发现胎盘来源外泌体可改变正常妊娠和 GDM 骨骼肌对葡萄糖的摄取[112]。

肥胖是包括 GDM 在内的代谢疾病发生的核心[113]，较高的 BMI 可导致母体循环中外泌体浓度升高，并促进内皮细胞释放促炎细胞因子、IL-6、IL-8 和 TNF-α[63]。脂肪细胞来源外泌体在妊娠代谢中发挥着重要作用，并参与肥胖向 GDM 的发展[114]。近来的研究表明，脂肪细胞来源外泌体的蛋白质表达谱不尽相同，且已证实其可影响胎盘细胞的代谢通路。有趣的是，脂肪细胞外泌体可影响胎盘细胞糖酵解和糖异生相关基因的表达，提示其在 GDM 胎盘营养物质的运输和胎儿过度生长方面可能发挥重要作用[115]。GDM 另一个重要的病理生理改变是高糖诱导的、以内皮功能障碍为特征的胎盘血管形成不良[109]。Saez 等报道，高糖条件下内皮细胞来源外泌体可改变内皮细胞的活性和迁移能力[116]。此外，GDM 内皮细胞来源外泌体可调控 L-精氨酸/NO 信号通路，并以旁分泌的方式在胎儿胎盘血管系统中扩展 GDM 的病理表型[117]。总之，这些研究证实了外泌体种类和活性与 GDM 病理生理之间的潜在联系。虽然外泌体内容物和活性在不同 GDM 孕妇中有所差异，但其作为诊断或治疗该并发症靶点所具备的潜能仍值得更进一步的研究。

（二）PE

PE 是一种潜在的、危险性的胎盘相关性疾病，也是导致孕产妇和胎儿死亡的主要原因[118]。胎盘形成不良，包括螺旋动脉重铸障碍导致胎盘缺氧、母体高血压和蛋白尿以及母体血栓-炎症系统调节异常是 PE 病理生理的特征[118,119]。包括胎盘源性小泡在内的循环微粒分泌增加，增强机体炎症反应，是 PE 发病的关键病理生理过程[120,121]。此外，胎盘源性囊泡内容物中蛋白质和 miRNA 的表达发生改变，其内的组织因子、内啡肽和 fms 样酪氨酸激酶（fms-like tyrosine kinase，Flt-1）表达也升高，这些特征是子痫前期发病的关键[95]。子痫前期患者的胎盘来源外泌体浓度明显高于正常对照组，且其内 hsa-miR-486-1-5p 和 hsa-miR-486-2-5p 的表达也增加[45]。此外，有报道称，合体滋养细胞来源外泌体携带的 miR-141 可抑制 T 细胞增殖，并介导母体对胎儿的免疫耐受，且 miR-141 在子痫前期胎盘中表达上调，参与子痫前期的病理生理过程[122]。有趣的是，Chaparro 等[123]报道，与正常孕妇相比，PE 患者唾液和牙龈沟液内 sFlt-1 水平明显升高，且牙龈沟液内胎盘来源外泌体也明显升高。

通过分析胎盘来源外泌体在各种靶细胞中的作用,外泌体在 PE 发病中的具体作用已被广泛证实。如前所述,缺氧会增加胎盘外泌体的分泌,而缺氧诱导的外泌体进而会促进促炎因子的释放,并降低靶细胞的迁移能力[76,89]。此外,体外实验证实胎盘来源的外泌体可影响内皮细胞的迁移,而这些改变可导致螺旋动脉重铸障碍和胎盘形成不良[67,102]。外泌体分泌量和内容物的改变也会影响其介导的母体免疫调节,进而导致母体并发症,如 PE 和宫内生长受限(intrauterine growth restriction,IUGR)的发生[20,79,106]。关于 IUGR,已有研究报道母体和胎儿循环中胎盘的外泌体不同于正常组,并认为在胎儿生长受限总外泌体中胎盘来源外泌体的含量较低[70]。整体上,外泌体参与了 PE 的多种病理生理过程,如母体全身炎症反应、血栓凝血功能、胎盘形成、胎盘氧化应激和血管重塑等,并有望成为诊断和判断 PE 预后的生物标志物[124]。

(三)早产

早产是一种与妊娠相关的并发症,可对胎儿的出生和新生儿的生长产生近期和远期不良影响[125]。较少有研究分析早产中外泌体的种类、含量或生物活性。有趣的是,有研究认为早产外泌体的浓度比足月妊娠(>36 周时)低 1.8 倍[126]。最近有研究分析了外泌体在诱导胎膜早衰和无菌性炎症,并将信号传递至母体组织中的作用[127]。在动物模型中,晚孕期的外泌体携带炎症介质,可以以旁分泌的形式介导临产和分娩[128]。早产孕妇血浆外泌体蛋白质内容物与足月分娩孕妇相比存在差异,而这些差异蛋白主要富集在与炎症和代谢相关的通路上[129]。此外,早产与足月产孕妇循环外泌体 miRNA 成分也存在差异,这些差异与 miRNA 的靶标与 TGF-β 信号通路、p53 和糖皮质激素受体信号通路相关[130]。需要指出的是,早产羊水来源外泌体的浓度和蛋白质成分的差异也在既往研究中被报道[131]。此外,外泌体在预测和治疗支气管肺发育不良(bronchopulmonary dys plasia,BPD)方面的研究也在进行中,而 BPD 是早产儿常见的病理状态[132,133]。总而言之,这些研究表明外泌体可能影响启动分娩的分子机制,并可作为预测早产的生物标志物[134]。然而,外泌体在影响与分娩启动相关信号通路中的作用还有待进一步研究。

五、总结

外泌体通过内吞途径产生的纳米级 EV,在细胞间信息传递中发挥重要作用。外泌体信号通路涉及妊娠的各个方面,如母体代谢、炎症适应、母胎血管的重构和胎盘形成。而在与妊娠相关的各种病理状态方面,外泌体的浓度、内容物及活性的差异均已见既往报道。外泌体能在细胞间传递关键信息,从而具备临床转化应用的潜力,并使其成为极有吸引力的可预测和治疗相关疾病的生物标志物和靶点。改进纯化胎盘来源外泌体的方法,了解其参与调控妊娠相关的重要分子机制,将有助于外泌体在生殖医学中的临床应用。

致谢

C.S. 受 Lions Medical Research Foundation,National Health and Medical Research

Council(NHMRC；1114013），Diabetes Australia，Fondo Nacional de Desarrollo Científico y Tecnológico(FONDECYT 1170809)资助. S. N. 获得 University of Queensland，funded by the Commonwealth Government of Australia 研究培训计划奖学金.

（白宇翔 译，郭尚春 审校）

参考文献

[1] Colombo M, Raposo G, Théry C. Biogenesis, secretion, and intercellular interactions of exosomes and other extracellular vesicles. Annu Rev Cell Dev Biol 2014；30：255-89.
[2] Lee TH, et al. Microvesicles as mediators of intercellular communication in cancer — the emerging science of cellular 'debris'. Semin Immunopathol 2011；33(5)：455-67.
[3] Tkach M, Théry C. Communication by extracellular vesicles：where we are and where we need to go. Cell 2016；164(6)：1226-32.
[4] S ELA, et al. Extracellular vesicles：biology and emerging therapeutic opportunities. Nat Rev Drug Discov 2013；12(5)：347-57.
[5] Tkach M, Kowal J, Théry C. Why the need and how to approach the functional diversity of extracellular vesicles. PhilosophicalPhilos Trans R Soc B 2017；373(1737)：20160479.
[6] Villarroya-Beltri C, et al. sorting it out：regulation of exosome loading. Semin Cancer Biol 2014；28：3-13.
[7] Villarroya-Beltri C, et al. Sumoylated hnRNPA2B1 controls the sorting of miRNAs into exosomes through binding to specific motifs. Nat Commun 2013；4：2980.
[8] Hessvik NP, Llorente A. Current knowledge on exosome biogenesis and release. Cell Mol Life Sci 2018；75(2)：193-208.
[9] Colombo M, et al. Analysis of ESCRT functions in exosome biogenesis, composition and secretion highlights the heterogeneity of extracellular vesicles. J Cell Sci 2013；126(24)：5553-65.
[10] Muralidharan-Chari V, et al. ARF6-regulated shedding of tumor cell-derived plasma membrane microvesicles. Curr Biol 2009；19(22)：1875-85.
[11] Hauser P, Wang S, Didenko VV. Apoptotic bodies：selective detection in extracellular vesicles. Methods Mol Biol 2017；1554：193-200.
[12] Kowal J, Tkach M, Thery C. Biogenesis and secretion of exosomes. Curr Opin Cell Biol 2014；29：116-25.
[13] Tkach M, Kowal J, Thery C. Why the need and how to approach the functional diversity of extracellular vesicles. Philos Trans R Soc Lond B Biol Sci 2018；373(1737)：20160479.
[14] Greening DW, et al. Proteomic insights into extracellular vesicle biology-defining exosomes and shed microvesicles. Expert Rev Proteomics 2017；14(1)：69-95.
[15] Kowal J, et al. Proteomic comparison defines novel markers to characterize heterogeneous populations of extracellular vesicle subtypes. Proc Natl Acad Sci U S A 2016；113(8)：E968-77. https：//doi.org/10.1080/14789450.2017.1260450.
[16] Lobb RJ, et al. Optimized exosome isolation protocol for cell culture supernatant and human plasma. J Extracell Vesicles 2015；4：27031.
[17] Li P, et al. Progress in exosome isolation techniques. Theranostics 2017；7(3)：789-804.
[18] Al-Nedawi K, et al. Intercellular transfer of the oncogenic receptor EGFRvIII by microvesicles derived from tumour cells. Nat Cell Biol 2008；10(5)：619-24.
[19] Valadi H, et al. Exosome-mediated transfer of mRNAs and microRNAs is a novel mechanism of genetic exchange between cells. Nat Cell Biol 2007；9(6)：654-9.
[20] Kshirsagar SK, et al. Immunomodulatory molecules are released from the first trimester and term placenta via exosomes. Placenta 2012；33(12)：982-90.
[21] Williams JL, et al. Serum exosomes in pregnancy-associated immune modulation and neuroprotection during CNS autoimmunity. Clin Immunol 2013；149(2)：236-43.
[22] Zhong H, et al. Induction of a tumour-specific CTL response by exosomes isolated from heattreated malignant ascites of gastric cancer patients. Int J Hyperthermia 2011；27(6)：604-11.
[23] Taylor DD, Gerçel-Taylor C. Tumour-derived exosomes and their role in cancer-associated T-cell signalling defects. Br J Cancer 2005；92(2)：305-11.
[24] Warmoes M, Lam SW, van der Groep P, Jaspers JE, et al. Secretome proteomics reveals candidate non-invasive biomarkers of BRCA1 deficiency in breast cancer. Oncotarget 2016；7：63537-48.
[25] Tricarico C, Clancy J, D'Souza-Schorey C. Biology and biogenesis of shed microvesicles. Small GTPases 2016；8(4)：220-32.
[26] Caruso S, Poon IKH. Apoptotic cell-derived extracellular vesicles：more than just debris. Front Immunol 2018；9：1486.
[27] Reich III CF, Pisetsky DS. The content of DNA and RNA in microparticles released by Jurkat and HL-60 cells undergoing in vitro apoptosis. Exp Cell Res 2009；315(5)：760-8. https：//doi.org/10.1016/j.yexcr.2008.12.014.
[28] Andre F, et al. Malignant effusions and immunogenic tumour-derived exosomes. Lancet 2002；360(9329)：295-305.
[29] Lässer C, et al. Human saliva, plasma and breast milk exosomes contain RNA：uptake by macrophages. J Transl Med 2011；9：9.
[30] An T, et al. Exosomes serve as tumour markers for personalized diagnostics owing to their important role in cancer

[31] Alvarez-Erviti L, et al. Delivery of siRNA to the mouse brain by systemic injection of targeted exosomes. Nat Biotechnol 2011; 29(4): 341-5.
[32] Kojima R, et al. Designer exosomes produced by implanted cells intracerebrally deliver therapeutic cargo for Parkinson's disease treatment. Nat Commun 2018; 9(1): 1305.
[33] Paolillo M, Schinelli S. Integrins and exosomes, a dangerous liaison in cancer progression. Cancer 2017; 9(8): 95.
[34] Hoshino A, et al. Tumour exosome integrins determine organotropic metastasis. Nature 2015; 527(7578): 329-35.
[35] Ashiru O, et al. Natural killer cell cytotoxicity is suppressed by exposure to the human NKG2D ligand MICA*008 that is shed by tumor cells in exosomes. Cancer Res 2010; 70(2): 481-9.
[36] Segura E, et al. CD8+ dendritic cells use LFA-1 to capture MHC-peptide complexes from exosomes in vivo. J Immunol 2007; 179(3): 1489-96.
[37] Mulcahy LA, Pink RC, Carter DR. Routes and mechanisms of extracellular vesicle uptake. J Extracell Vesicles 2014; 3: https://doi.org/10.3402/jev.v3.24641.
[38] Parolini I, et al. Microenvironmental pH Is a key factor for exosome traffic in tumor cells. J Biol Chem 2009; 284(49): 34211-22.
[39] Montecalvo A, et al. Mechanism of transfer of functional microRNAs between mouse dendritic cells via exosomes. Blood 2012; 119(3): 756-66.
[40] Ying W, et al. Adipose tissue macrophage-derived exosomal miRNAs can modulate in vivo and in vitro insulin sensitivity. Cell 2017; 171(2): 372-84. e12.
[41] Yu Y, et al. Adipocyte-derived exosomal MiR-27a induces insulin resistance in skeletal muscle through repression of PPARgamma. Theranostics 2018; 8(8): 2171-88.
[42] Nair S, Salomon C. Extracellular vesicles and their immunomodulatory functions in pregnancy. Semin Immunopathol 2018; 40(5): 425-37.
[43] Mitchell MD, et al. Placental exosomes in normal and complicated pregnancy. Am J Obstet Gynecol 2015; 213(4, Supplement): S173-81.
[44] Sarker S, et al. Placenta-derived exosomes continuously increase in maternal circulation over the first trimester of pregnancy. J Transl Med 2014; 12: 204.
[45] Salomon C, Guanzon D, Romero KS, Longo S, Correa P, Illanes SE, Rice GE. Placental exosomes as early biomarker of preeclampsia — potential role of exosomal microRNAs across gestation. J Clin Endocrinol Metab 2017; 102(9): 3182-94. https://doi.org/10.1210/jc.2017-00672.
[46] Salomon C, et al. The role of placental exosomes in gestational diabetes mellitus. In: Sobrevia L, editor. Gestational diabetes-causes, diagnosis and treatment. IntechOpen; 2013. https://doi.org/10.5772/55298.
[47] Castellucci M, et al. The development of the human placental villous tree. Anat Embryol 1990; 181(2): 117-28.
[48] Freemark M. Placental hormones and the control of fetal growth. J Clin Endocrinol Metabol 2010; 95(5): 2054-7.
[49] Freemark M. Regulation of maternal metabolism by pituitary and placental hormones: roles in fetal development and metabolic programming. Horm Res Paediatr 2006; 65: 41-9. (Suppl. 3).
[50] Adam S, et al. Review: fetal-maternal communication via extracellular vesicles - Implications for complications of pregnancies. Placenta 2017; 54: 83-8.
[51] Tannetta D, et al. Extracellular vesicles and reproduction-promotion of successful pregnancy. Cell Mol Immunol 2014; 11(6): 548-63.
[52] Tong M, Chamley LW. Placental extracellular vesicles and feto-maternal communication. Cold Spring Harb Perspect Med 2015; 5(3): a023028.
[53] Atay S, Gercel-Taylor C, Taylor DD. Human trophoblast-derived exosomal fibronectin induces pro-inflammatory IL-1beta production by macrophages. Am J Reprod Immunol 2011; 66(4): 259-69.
[54] Atay S, et al. Trophoblast-derived exosomes mediate monocyte recruitment and differentiation. Am J Reprod Immunol 2011; 65(1): 65-77.
[55] Thery C, Zitvogel L, Amigorena S. Exosomes: composition, biogenesis and function. Nat Rev Immunol 2002; 2(8): 569-79.
[56] Nardi Fda S, et al. High levels of circulating extracellular vesicles with altered expression and function during pregnancy. Immunobiology 2016; 221(7): 753-60.
[57] Salomon C, et al. Hypoxia-induced changes in the bioactivity of cytotrophoblast-derived exosomes. PLoS One 2013; 8(11): e79636.
[58] Salomon C, et al. Oxygen tension regulates glucose-induced biogenesis and release of different subpopulations of exosome vesicles from trophoblast cells: a gestational age profile of placental exosomes in maternal plasma with gestational diabetes mellitus. Placenta 2015; 36(4): 488.
[59] Zhang W, et al. HIF-1-mediated production of exosomes during hypoxia is protective in renal tubular cells. Am J Physiol Renal Physiol 2017; 313(4): F906-13.
[60] King HW, Michael MZ, Gleadle JM. Hypoxic enhancement of exosome release by breast cancer cells. BMC Cancer 2012; 12: 421.
[61] Savina A, et al. Exosome release is regulated by a calcium-dependent mechanism in K562 cells. J Biol Chem 2003; 278(22): 20083-90.
[62] MacDonald PE, Eliasson L, Rorsman P. Calcium increases endocytotic vesicle size and accelerates membrane fission in insulin-secreting INS-1 cells. J Cell Sci 2005; 118(Pt 24): 5911-20.
[63] Elfeky O, et al. Influence of maternal BMI on the exosomal profile during gestation and their role on maternal systemic inflammation. Placenta 2017; 50: 60-9. https://doi.org/10.1016/j.placenta.2016.
[64] Vongthavaravat V, et al. Isolated elevation of serum alkaline phosphatase level in an uncomplicated pregnancy: a case report. Am J Obstet Gynecol 2000; 183(2): 505-6.

[65] Leitner K, et al. Placental alkaline phosphatase expression at the apical and basal plasma membrane in term villous trophoblasts. J Histochem Cytochem 2001; 49(9): 1155-64.

[66] Bashiri A, et al. Positive placental staining for alkaline phosphatase corresponding with extreme elevation of serum alkaline phosphatase during pregnancy. Arch Gynecol Obstet 2007; 275(3): 211-4.

[67] Salomon C, et al. A gestational profile of placental exosomes in maternal plasma and their effects on endothelial cell migration. PLoS One 2014; 9(6): e98667.

[68] Kniss DA, et al. ED(27) trophoblast-kike cells isolated from first-trimester chorionic villi are genetically identical to HeLa cells yet exhibit a distinct phenotype. Placenta 2002; 23(1): 32-43.

[69] Dragovic RA, et al. Isolation of syncytiotrophoblast microvesicles and exosomes and their characterisation by multicolour flow cytometry and fluorescence nanoparticle tracking analysis. Methods 2015; 87: 64-74.

[70] Miranda J, et al. Placental exosomes profile in maternal and fetal circulation in intrauterine growth restriction — Liquid biopsies to monitoring fetal growth. Placenta 2018; 64: 34-43.

[71] Salomon C, et al. Gestational diabetes mellitus is associated with changes in the concentration and bioactivity of placenta-derived exosomes in maternal circulation across gestation. Diabetes 2016; 65(3): 598-609.

[72] Lai A, et al. Optimized specific isolation of placenta-derived exosomes from maternal circulation. Methods Mol Biol 2018; 1710: 131-8.

[73] Boriachek K, et al. Avoiding pre-isolation step in exosome analysis: direct isolation and sensitive detection of exosomes using gold-koaded nanoporous ferric oxide nanozymes. Anal Chem 2019; 91: 3827-34.

[74] Delorme-Axford E, et al. Human placental trophoblasts confer viral resistance to recipient cells. Proc Natl Acad Sci U S A 2013; 110(29): 12048-53.

[75] Kambe S, et al. Human exosomal placenta-associated miR-517a-3p modulates the expression of PRKG1 mRNA in Jurkat cells1. Biol Reprod 2014; 91(5): 129. 1-11.

[76] Rice GE, et al. The effect of glucose on the release and bioactivity of exosomes from first trimester trophoblast cells. J Clin Endocrinol Metab 2015; 100(10): E1280-8.

[77] Atay S, et al. Morphologic and proteomic characterization of exosomes released by cultured extravillous trophoblast cells. Exp Cell Res 2011; 317(8): 1192-202.

[78] Donker RB, et al. The expression profile of C19MC microRNAs in primary human trophoblast cells and exosomes. Mol Hum Reprod 2012; 18(8): 417-24.

[79] Vargas A, et al. Syncytin proteins incorporated in placenta exosomes are important for cell uptake and show variation in abundance in serum exosomes from patients with preeclampsia. FASEB J 2014; 28(8): 3703-19.

[80] Stenqvist AC, et al. Exosomes secreted by human placenta carry functional Fas ligand and TRAIL molecules and convey apoptosis in activated immune cells, suggesting exosomemediated immune privilege of the fetus. J Immunol 2013; 191(11): 5515-23.

[81] Dragovic RA, et al. Sizing and phenotyping of cellular vesicles using nanoparticle tracking analysis. Nanomedicine 2011; 7(6): 780-8. https://doi.org/10.1016/j.nano.2011.04.003.

[82] Luo SS, et al. Human villous trophoblasts express and secrete placenta-specific microRNAs into maternal circulation via exosomes. Biol Reprod 2009; 81(4): 717-29.

[83] Tolosa JM, et al. The endogenous retroviral envelope protein syncytin-1 inhibits LPS/PHAstimulated cytokine responses in human blood and is sorted into placental exosomes. Placenta 2012; 33(11): 933-41.

[84] Dragovic RA, et al. Multicolor flow cytometry and nanoparticle tracking analysis of extracellular vesicles in the plasma of normal pregnant and pre-eclamptic women. Biol Reprod 2013; 89(6): 151.

[85] Hedlund M, et al. Human placenta expresses and secretes NKG2D ligands via exosomes that down-modulate the cognate receptor expression: evidence for immunosuppressive function. J Immunol 2009; 183(1): 340-51.

[86] Gysler SM, et al. Antiphospholipid antibody-induced miR-146a-3p drives trophoblast interleukin-8 secretion through activation of Toll-kike receptor 8. Mol Hum Reprod 2016; 22(7): 465-74.

[87] Pillay P, et al. Placental exosomes and pre-eclampsia: maternal circulating levels in normal pregnancies and, early and late onset pre-eclamptic pregnancies. Placenta 2016; 46: 18-25.

[88] Salomon C, et al. Extravillous trophoblast cells-derived exosomes promote vascular smooth muscle cell migration. Front Pharmacol 2014; 5: 175.

[89] Truong G, et al. Oxygen tension regulates the miRNA profile and bioactivity of exosomes released from extravillous trophoblast cells — liquid biopsies for monitoring complications of pregnancy. PLoS One 2017; 12(3): e0174514.

[90] Sabapatha A, Gercel-Taylor C, Taylor DD. Specific isolation of placenta-derived exosomes from the circulation of pregnant women and their immunoregulatory consequences. Am J Reprod Immunol 2006; 56(5-6): 345-55.

[91] Motta-Mejia C, et al. placental vesicles carry active endothelial nitric oxide synthase and their activity is reduced in preeclampsia. Hypertension 2017; 70(2): 372-81.

[92] Tong M, et al. Placental nano-vesicles target to specific organs and modulate vascular tone in vivo. Hum Reprod 2017; 32(11): 2188-98.

[93] Ermini L, et al. A single sphingomyelin species promotes exosomal release of endoglin into the maternal circulation in preeclampsia. Sci Rep 2017; 7(1): 12172.

[94] Kambe S, et al. Human exosomal placenta-associated miR-517a-3p modulates the expression of PRKG1 mRNA in Jurkat cells. Biol Reprod 2014; 91(5): 129.

[95] Tannetta DS, et al. Characterisation of syncytiotrophoblast vesicles in normal pregnancy and pre-eclampsia: expression of Flt-1 and endoglin. PLoS One 2013; 8(2): e56754.

[96] Gardiner C, et al. Extracellular vesicle sizing and enumeration by nanoparticle tracking analysis. J Extracell Vesicles 2013; 2; https://doi.org/10.3402/jev.v2i0.19671.

[97] Cleys ER, et al. Identification of microRNAs in exosomes isolated from serum and umbilical cord blood, as well as placentomes of gestational day 90 pregnant sheep. Mol Reprod Dev 2014; 81(11): 983-93.

[98] Jeanty C, Derderian SC, MacKenzie TC. Maternal-fetal cellular trafficking: clinical implications and consequences. Curr Opin Pediatr 2014; 26(3): 377-82.
[99] Kallenbach LR, et al. Maternal background strain influences fetal-maternal trafficking more than maternal immune competence in mice. J Reprod Immunol 2011; 90(2): 188-94.
[100] Burton GJ, Jauniaux E, Charnock-Jones DS. Human early placental development: potential roles of the endometrial glands. Placenta 2007; 28: S64-9. Suppl A.
[101] Salomon C, et al. Hypoxia regulates the response of trophoblast-derived exosomes to hyperglycemia and displays a difference placental exosome profile in plasma from patients with gestational diabetes mellitus. Reprod Sci 2015; 22: 257a-8a.
[102] Salomon C, et al. Exosomal signaling during hypoxia mediates microvascular endothelial cell migration and vasculogenesis. PLoS One 2013; 8(7): e68451.
[103] Zhang HC, et al. Microvesicles derived from human umbilical cord mesenchymal stem cells stimulated by hypoxia promote angiogenesis both in vitro and in vivo. Stem Cells Dev 2012; 21: 3289-97.
[104] Subra C, et al. Exosomes account for vesicle-mediated transcellular transport of activatable phospholipases and prostaglandins. J Lipid Res 2010; 51(8): 2105-20.
[105] Record M, et al. Exosomes as new vesicular lipid transporters involved in cell-cell communication and various pathophysiologies. Biochim Biophys Acta 2014; 1841(1): 108-20.
[106] Frangsmyr L, et al. Cytoplasmic microvesicular form of Fas ligand in human early placenta: switching the tissue immune privilege hypothesis from cellular to vesicular level. Mol Hum Reprod 2005; 11(1): 35-41.
[107] Metzger BE, Coustan DR. Summary and recommendations of the Fourth International Workshop-Conference on Gestational Diabetes Mellitus. The Organizing Committee. Diabetes Care 1998; 21(Suppl 2): B161-7.
[108] Catalano PM. Trying to understand gestational diabetes. Diabet Med 2014; 31(3): 273-81.
[109] Desoye G, Hauguel-de Mouzon S. The human placenta in gestational diabetes mellitus. The insulin and cytokine network. Diabetes Care 2007; 30(Suppl 2): S120-6.
[110] Jayabalan N, et al. Quantitative proteomics by SWATH-MS suggest an association between circulating exosomes and maternal metabolic changes in gestational diabetes mellitus. Proteomics 2018; 19: e1800164.
[111] Almohammadi D, et al. C19MC miRNA signatures of placenta-derived exosomes in women diagnosed with gestational diabetes mellitus. In: Diabetes programing-genes and gestation. Endocrine Society; 2016. p. OR27-4.
[112] Nair S, et al. Human placental exosomes in gestational diabetes mellitus carry a specific set of miRNAs associated with skeletal muscle insulin sensitivity. Clin Sci 2018; 132: 2451-67.
[113] Catalano PM, et al. Longitudinal changes in glucose metabolism during pregnancy in obese women with normal glucose tolerance and gestational diabetes mellitus. Am J Obstet Gynecol 1999; 180(4): 903-16.
[114] Jayabalan N, et al. Cross talk between adipose tissue and placenta in obese and gestational diabetes mellitus pregnancies via exosomes. Front Endocrinol (Lausanne) 2017; 8: 239.
[115] Jayabalan N, et al. Adipose tissue exosomal proteomic profile reveals a role on placenta glucose metabolism in gestational diabetes mellitus. J Clin Endocrinol Metab 2018; 104: 1735-52. p. jc.2018-01599-jc.2018-01599.
[116] Saez T, et al. Fetoplacental endothelial exosomes modulate high d-glucose-induced endothelial dysfunction. Placenta 2018; 66: 26-35.
[117] Saez T, et al. Human umbilical vein endothelium-derived exosomes play a role in foetoplacental endothelial dysfunction in gestational diabetes mellitus. Biochim Biophys Acta 2018; 1864(2): 499-508.
[118] Redman CW, Sargent IL. Latest advances in understanding preeclampsia. Science 2005; 308(5728): 1592-4.
[119] Laresgoiti-Servitje E. A leading role for the immune system in the pathophysiology of preeclampsia. J Leukoc Biol 2013; 94(2): 247-57.
[120] Germain SJ, et al. Systemic inflammatory priming in normal pregnancy and preeclampsia: the role of circulating syncytiotrophoblast microparticles. J Immunol 2007; 178.
[121] Gohner C, Plosch T, Faas MM. Immune-modulatory effects of syncytiotrophoblast extracellular vesicles in pregnancy and preeclampsia. Placenta 2017; 60: S41-51.
[122] Ospina-Prieto S, et al. MicroRNA-141 is upregulated in preeclamptic placentae and regulates trophoblast invasion and intercellular communication. Transl Res 2016; 172: 61-72.
[123] Chaparro A, et al. Placental biomarkers and angiogenic factors in oral fluids of patients with preeclampsia. Prenat Diagn 2016; 36(5): 476-82.
[124] Pillay P, et al. Placenta-derived exosomes: potential biomarkers of preeclampsia. Int J Nanomedicine 2017; 12: 8009-23.
[125] Menon R. Preterm birth: a global burden on maternal and child health. Pathog Glob Health 2012; 106(3): 139-40.
[126] Taylor DD, Akyol S, Gercel-Taylor C. Pregnancy-associated exosomes and their modulation of T cell signaling. J Immunol 2006; 176(3): 1534-42.
[127] Menon R, et al. Histological evidence of oxidative stress and premature senescence in preterm premature rupture of the human fetal membranes recapitulated in vitro. Am J Pathol 2014; 184(6): 1740-51.
[128] Sheller-Miller S, et al. Exosomes cause preterm birth in mice: evidence for paracrine signaling in pregnancy. Sci Rep 2019; 9(1): 608.
[129] Menon R, et al. Quantitative proteomics by SWATH-MS of maternal plasma exosomes determine pathways associated with term and preterm birth. Endocrinology 2019; 160: 639-50.
[130] Menon R, et al. Circulating exosomal miRNA profile during term and preterm birth pregnancies: a longitudinal study. Endocrinology 2019; 160(2): 249-75.
[131] Dixon CL, et al. Amniotic fluid exosome proteomic profile exhibits unique pathways of term and preterm labor. Endocrinology 2018; 159(5): 2229-40.
[132] Lesage F, Thebaud B. Nanotherapies for micropreemies: stem cells and the secretome in bronchopulmonary dysplasia.

Semin Perinatol 2018;42(7):453-8.
[133] Lal CV, et al. Exosomal microRNA predicts and protects against severe bronchopulmonary dysplasia in extremely premature infants. JCI insight 2018;3(5):e93994.
[134] Salomon C, et al. Placental exosomes during gestation: liquid biopsies carrying signals for the regulation of human parturition. Curr Pharm Des 2018;24(9):974-82.

第 17 章

外泌体在呼吸系统疾病中的作用
Exosomes in respiratory disease

Shamila D. Alipoor[a], Esmaeil Mortaz[b,c]

[a]Molecular Medicine Department, Institute of Medical Biotechnology, National Institute of Genetic Engineering and Biotechnology (NIGEB), Tehran, Iran, [b]Clinical Tuberculosis and Epidemiology Research Center, National Research Institute of Tuberculosis and Lung Diseases (NRITLD), Shahid Beheshti University of Medical Sciences, Tehran, Iran, [c]Department of Immunology, Faculty of Medicine, Shahid Beheshti University of Medical Sciences, Tehran, Iran

    细胞-细胞间的信息交流是多细胞生物的主要特征。肺为一对复杂器官,肺实质和气道结构中存在大量细胞。因此,细胞内通信对发挥和维持肺部的最佳功能至关重要[1]。

    细胞内通信由多种机制介导,如直接接触细胞或基于分泌分子的作用。近期研究报道了与此相关的第三种机制,即引入外泌体在活细胞间发挥信息传递作用[2]。外泌体的发现刷新了大众对机体重要功能(如生理和信号协调)的认知。

    外泌体是一种几乎由所有细胞分泌的直径在 30~100 nm 的小囊泡,包含 RNA(mRNA 和非编码 RNA)、DNA(mtDNA、ssDNA 和 dsDNA)、蛋白质、脂质、脂质介质等物质(图 17-1)。外泌体分泌可促进细胞释放选择性分子源进行信息传递,在胞内发挥特定调节作用并去除多余分子。例如,外泌体诱捕可触发各种细胞信号传导过程,促进靶细胞生长,或在肿瘤微环境中促进细胞侵袭和肿瘤生长[3]。

    外泌体最早发现于 20 世纪 80 年代中期,是一种产生于成熟绵羊网织红细胞的囊性小泡,主要作用在于消除部分膜结合蛋白和多余细胞成分[4-6]。所述结构最初被认为是细胞排除代谢废物的"垃圾桶",但后期的深入研究表明,B 细胞衍

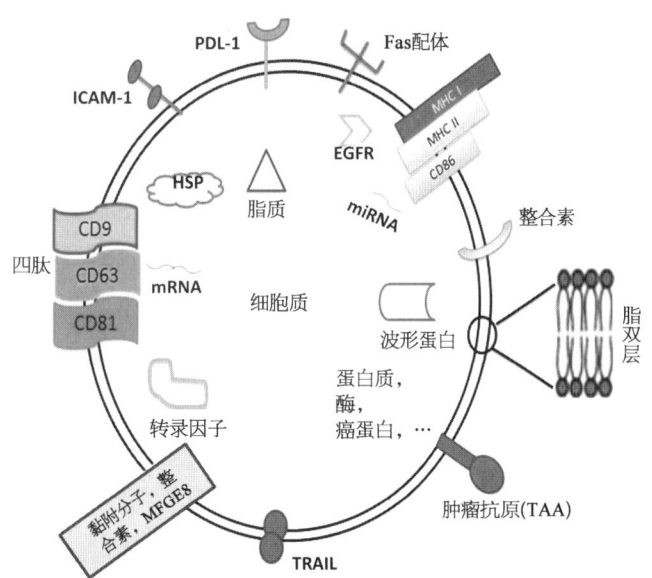

图 17-1　外泌体常见组成示意图。外泌体是一种由细胞分泌至胞外并存在于宿主细胞内的膜性小囊泡,包括蛋白质、脂类、核酸等。HSP,热休克蛋白;miRNA,微 RNA;TAA,肿瘤相关抗原;TRAIL,肿瘤坏死因子相关凋亡诱导配体;ICAM-1,细胞间黏附分子 1;PD-L1,程序性死亡配体 1;MHC,主要组织相容性复合体;EGFR,表皮生长因子受体

生外泌体具有免疫调节作用,并能刺激 T 细胞[7,8]。后续研究提示外泌体可参与众多生理和病理过程,如运载传染源、致瘤性、免疫调节以及介导神经退行性疾病进程[9,10]。

外泌体研究的转折点在于:这些微泡可通过其功能性核酸(如线粒体 DNA、信使 RNA 以及在受体细胞中起作用的非编码小 miRNA)参与细胞间遗传信息交换[11]。2007 年,一项研究首次报道肥大细胞(mast cell,MC)衍生外泌体中含有>1 200 个 mRNA,后者 mRNA 在传递至受体细胞后可转化为蛋白质[12]。同时,既往研究已证实不同源性外泌体中存在不同的 miRNA 和 mRNA[11]。

外泌体生物学分子载物的类型可因其来源细胞及释放外泌体时细胞的生理状况不同而有所区别。一般而言,外泌体含有四磷酸钠、整合素、MHC、黏附分子、膜转运蛋白、脂筏、膜转运蛋白和融合蛋白,前述类型通常用于表示所检测外泌体的含量。

同时,外泌体亦可携带代谢酶、细胞骨架蛋白、信号转导蛋白、脂质介质(如胆固醇、甘油二酯、磷脂)、伴随分子、前列腺素和白三烯(leukotriene,LT)。四跨膜蛋白分子如 CD63、CD81、CD9 和 HSP70 均为普遍存在的外泌体蛋白,并被视为外泌体标记物[13]。

ExoCarta 为外泌体蛋白质、RNA 和脂质数据库[14]。基于该数据库,在不同物种外泌体中已鉴定出 4 563 个蛋白质、194 个脂质体、1 639 个 mRNA 和 764 个 miRNA[14]。

应用脂质双层分子包裹可保护外泌体内容物(如蛋白质和 miRNA),使其免于降解,因而可存在于体液中。该特性可维持外泌体保持相对较长和稳定的存在时间,进而为研究者提供大量有关原始细胞生理状态的信息[15]。另一方面,外泌体可包裹功能性分子,有利于将多种成分同时传递至受体细胞[16]。

外泌体存在于几乎所有体液,如尿液、血浆、母乳、支气管肺泡灌洗(bronchoalveolar lavage,BAL)、唾液、精液、羊水、腹水、滑液、母乳和 CSF 中。因此,外泌体在医学应用领域受到越来越多的关注。

外泌体具有循环稳定性、低免疫原性和生物相容性等特性,提示其作为小 RNA、信号分子或药物传递系统的可行性[17,18]。此外,鉴于外泌体组成可因细胞生理或病理状况而有所区别,其有望作为诊疗监测的生物标志物,这使外泌体在近年来颇受关注[19]。

外泌体可对其他细胞发挥自分泌、旁分泌和内分泌作用,进而发挥治疗性功能[20]。例如,在细胞治疗中,MSC 和其他祖细胞源性外泌体可在细胞保护、血管生成和再生效应方面发挥类似于其亲本细胞的特性和活性,提示外泌体在"无细胞治疗"技术中的潜在价值[21]。

在本章中,我们将重点探讨外泌体在肺部微环境中的作用,包括其在肺功能和呼吸系统疾病病理条件中的作用。

一、外泌体在肺部微环境和肺部疾病发病中的作用

肺病为全世界范围内常见疾病的死亡原因。空气污染、吸烟、有毒物质及传染因素在所述疾病的发病率持续攀升中扮演着重要角色。

肺部上下气道的支气管和肺泡上皮细胞(alveolar epithelial cell,AEC)是暴露于外部环境的最大表面积的结构,为抵御环境污染物的第一道防线。

人体暴露于有毒烟剂、微生物或有毒气体可导致气道损伤,诱导各种肺部疾病,如肺癌、哮喘或慢性阻塞性肺疾病(chronic obstructive pulmonary disease,COPD)。一方面,气道发挥肺保护功能可通过一系列机制实现,包括机械屏障、黏液纤毛系统(基于酶)和天然免疫系统中的分泌型 IgA;另一方面,呼吸道黏膜中的 DC 网络可捕获入侵微生物,并将其转移至引流淋巴结。经过细支气管,肺泡巨噬细胞(alveolar macrophage,AM)可在肺部微环境(富含 IgG、纤维连接蛋白、补体成分、表面活性成分和其他防御成分)中诱捕入侵颗粒。基于病原体负荷状况,其他炎症细胞,尤其是中性粒细胞,可被招募至感染部位。气道微环境中的过度炎症反应可诱导上皮细胞损伤,从而导致上皮细胞炎症免疫反应和表型改变。所述改变可导致"上皮-间质转化(epithelial-mesenchymal transition,EMT)",诱导气道重塑,进而促进 COPD、肺癌或支气管哮喘等病理性改变。

基于前述理解,肺部细胞网络(如上皮细胞、内皮细胞、免疫细胞和间充质细胞)中的旁分泌细胞间通信在呼吸系统微环境的生理稳态和病理状态的协调中发挥着重要作用。

外泌体在细胞内和旁分泌通信中发挥重要作用,因此在近年来颇受关注。

例如,Admyer 等于 2003 年首次报道了健康人群 BAL 中存在含有主要组织相容性抗原和共刺激分子的外泌体[22]。

所述外泌体包含 miRNA、功能性 RNA 和蛋白质,可将其功能性载物递送至影响细胞内稳态或生理条件的其他细胞中。例如,AM 衍生外泌体可通过传递 miR-223 促进原始单核细胞的分化[23]。上皮细胞来源外泌体中膜黏蛋白的存在可改变外泌体表面电荷和结构特性,从而影响肺固有免疫系统的局部黏液纤毛防御机制[24]。此外,亦有研究证实外泌体可通过传递信号分子在气道炎症途径的调节中发挥关键作用。例如,巨噬细胞衍生外泌体可传递细胞因子信号传送阻抑物(suppressor of cytokine signaling,SOCS)1,导致 AEC 中信号转导和转录活化因子(signal transducer and activator of transcription,STAT)的活性降低[25]。与此同时,据报道,外泌体在哮喘细胞间串扰和疾病最终表型的机制中亦发挥着重要作用[26]。在过敏性气道炎症中,上皮细胞可释放具有促炎作用的外泌体[27]。气道上皮细胞衍生外泌体对人流感病毒具有中和作用,其原因在于前者可运载黏蛋白和 α2,6-唾液酸转移酶[28](图 17-2)。

外泌体亦可参与气道应激反应。在肺结节病中,外泌体可促进如 INF-γ、IL-13 和 CXCL-8 等促炎因子在呼吸环境中的产生,进而诱发炎症反应[29]。此外,机体感染状况亦可对外泌体分泌和载物类型产生一定影响。例如,感染分枝杆菌的巨噬细胞可分泌富含 HSP-70 的外泌体[30]。前述外泌体可招募免疫细胞并活化免疫系统。与此同时,病理状况亦可改变外泌体的 miRNA 含量[31-33]。前述途径均可最终诱导细胞应激反应。

而在缺氧性肺动脉高压中,间充质基质细胞通过外泌体介导的旁分泌机制抵御肺部炎症,发挥保护作用[34]。几乎所有呼吸细胞,如肺上皮细胞、成纤维细胞、内皮细胞(endothelial cell,EC)和各种免疫细胞,均可向胞外释放外泌体,参与多种生理过程并维持肺部平衡。本章节后续部分将继续讨论所述外泌体的具体作用。

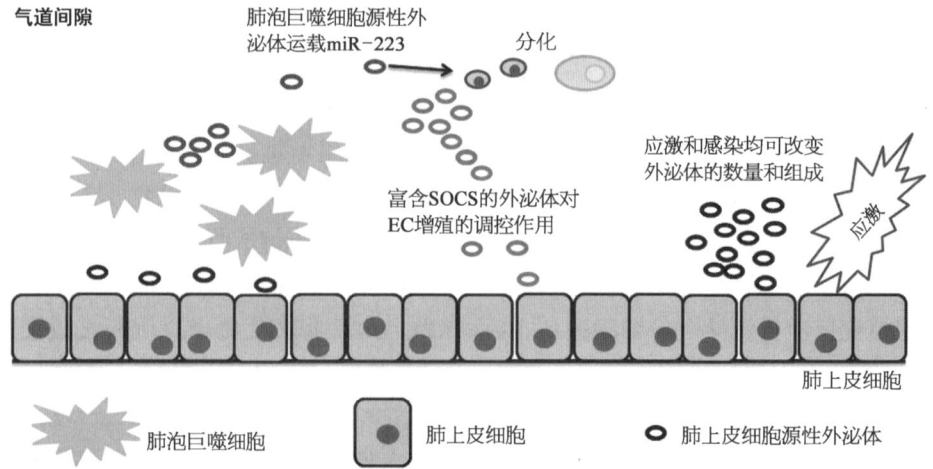

图 17-2 应激性气道生理条件下的外泌体。呼吸道中多种呼吸细胞类型均可释放外泌体。暴露于各种类型的应激(如感染或氧化应激)均可改变外泌体的组成并增强其分泌。损伤巨噬细胞源性外泌体含有多种促炎细胞因子,可影响免疫效果。肺泡巨噬细胞源性外泌体可通过运载 miR-223 调控胞内稳态和分化,并通过向肺上皮细胞传递 SOCS 蛋白调节炎症信号。肺 EC 衍生外泌体释放到血液中,并在应激条件下运载改性生物分子

二、肺部微环境中效应免疫细胞和结构细胞衍生外泌体的作用

肺结构细胞可释放外泌体,进而在肺部健康或疾病发展过程中发挥重要作用[35]。所述外泌体在微调肺部微环境的细胞内通信中发挥着至关重要的作用[1,32]。

既往一项研究发现,在肺部病理状态下,肺组织结构细胞释放外泌体增多且含量发生一定改变[32]。在肺结构细胞中,气道平滑肌细胞(airway smooth muscle cell,ASMC)、杯状细胞和上皮细胞为参与病理变化的关键细胞。然而,目前尚无有关 ASMC 或杯状细胞衍生外泌体的研究[36],而肺泡或支气管上皮细胞(bronchial epithelial cell,BEC)释放外泌体在形态(大小和形状)上存在一定差异[37]。

AEC 衍生外泌体可包裹包括黏蛋白和唾液酸在内的重要分子,参与天然免疫机制,进而介导气道炎症的调节[37]。

机械应力和细胞因子如 IL-13 均可促进 BEC 释放外泌体,并诱导 BEC 衍生外泌体组成的改变。受机械应力刺激的 BEC 可进一步释放出含有组织因子(tissue factor,TF)来源的外泌体,从而触发 TF 信号。所述外泌体亦可促进单核细胞的增殖[38]。同时,哮喘患者支气管收缩时的机械应力可诱导 BEC 分泌外泌体[38]。此外,支气管成纤维细胞衍生外泌体含有 TGF-2,在外泌体摄取后可诱导 BEC 增殖[39]。

淋巴细胞是机体免疫功能的关键因子,在肺部微环境的应激反应和炎症反应中作用显著。B 细胞作为 APC,在无 IgE 和 T 淋巴细胞介导的情况下,可诱发哮喘反应[40]。

IFN-γ 或产生 IL-4 的 B 淋巴细胞亦可参与原始 T0 淋巴细胞向 T1 淋巴细胞或 T2

淋巴细胞的分化。此外,B 型调节(Breg)细胞可下调高反应性气道的炎症反应[41],并通过招募天然 Treg($CD4^+$、$CD25^+$、$FoxP3^+$ 细胞)到肺部,在缓解哮喘病理状态下的过敏性炎症中发挥重要作用[42]。

既往已有大量研究表明,B 细胞可产生外泌体。B 细胞衍生外泌体与其亲本表型存在相似性,可表达 MHC、整合素(β1 和 β2)以及 CD40、CD80 和 CD86 等共刺激分子[26]。所述外泌体可通过提呈抗原肽诱导 T 细胞应答[43],亦可通过诱导 HSP70 表达促进 DC 细胞成熟[44]。B 细胞源性外泌体含有桦木肽(betv1 衍生肽)可诱导 T 细胞增殖及 IL-5 和 IL-13 的合成。所述外泌体的相关反应类似于 B 细胞和 T 细胞直接相互作用时的反应。另有研究发现无须细胞间接触,B 细胞源性外泌体可在肺部免疫调节中的重要作用[43]。

T 淋巴细胞亦可释放外泌体[45-47],但其生物活性目前尚未被完全了解[48]。T 细胞分泌的外泌体为碟形外泌体,含有 Src 样酪氨酸激酶、MHC、CD3、黏附分子 CD2、溶酶体相关膜蛋白 1(lysosomal-associated membrane protein 1,LAMP-1)、趋化因子受体 CXCR4、淋巴细胞功能相关抗原-1(lymphocyte function-associated antigen-1,LFA-1)和 T 细胞受体亚单位[45,48]。

TCR 激活可诱导 T 细胞产生外泌体。然而,有丝分裂信号如佛波醇酯和离子酶素的刺激并无法诱导外泌体的释放,因此 T 细胞产生外泌体为高度调控的过程[45]。

活化 T 细胞亦可通过 Fas 配体途径促进外泌体分泌,上调基质金属蛋白酶 9 的表达,促进小鼠肺肿瘤细胞侵袭[49]。T 调节(Treg;$CD8^+$、$CD45^+$ 细胞)以及 $CD4^+$ T 细胞可促进具有抗肿瘤活性的外泌体释放,抑制肺部微环境中 $CD8^+$ 细胞毒性 T 淋巴细胞的分泌[46]。

活化 $CD3^+$ T 细胞可通过外泌体与非活性自体 T 细胞相互作用。事实上,由活化 $CD3^+$ T 细胞和 IL-2 共同产生的外泌体可在非活性自体 $CD3^+$ T 细胞中诱导细胞增殖并促进独特细胞因子谱的产生[50]。

嗜酸性粒细胞为在肺部微环境中产生、储存和释放一系列免疫介质的主要粒细胞,如趋化因子、脂质介质、经典嗜酸性粒细胞蛋白,包括嗜酸性粒细胞过氧化物酶(eosinophil peroxidase,EPX)、嗜酸性粒细胞阳离子蛋白(eosinophil cationic protein,ECP)、嗜酸性粒细胞衍生神经毒素(eosinophil-derived neurotoxin,EDN)和主要碱性蛋白(major basic protein,MBP)。因此,前述细胞在哮喘、过敏等炎症病理状态中发挥着重要作用[51]。

嗜酸性粒细胞可通过整个囊泡的内化机制摄取外泌体。此外,在释放嗜酸性粒细胞特征蛋白载物,如 MBP 和嗜酸性粒细胞过氧化物酶(eosinophil peroxidase,EPO)的同时,嗜酸性粒细胞亦可释放碟形外泌体[52]。同时,嗜酸性粒细胞衍生外泌体亦可携带参与不同细胞功能的蛋白质,包括具有抗真菌和抗菌活性的 S100 蛋白(S100A8 和 S100A9)[53]、参与蛋白质折叠的 HSP70、细胞黏附分子(如整合素)、丝聚蛋白和骨膜蛋白以及代谢酶[52]。前述外泌体具有与亲本细胞相似的活性,可诱发组织损伤,在肺部微环境的应激反应和肺部平衡调节中作用显著。

此外,基于对呼吸道病原体和组织损伤的免疫反应,MC 在维持肺部健康中发挥重要作用。然而,在哮喘、肺纤维化、肺动脉高压、COPD、急性呼吸窘迫综合征(acute respiratory distress syndrome,ARDS)和肺癌等不适当、持续性活化的背景下,MC 可触发炎症和重塑组织结构,驱动疾病进程[54]。

活化的 MC 可释放过敏和促炎介质,如组胺、前列腺素、LT、TNF-α 和 IL-13,促进肺部微环境中的先天性和适应性免疫应答[55,56]。同时,通过不同机制(包括外泌体产生),MC 可与肺部微环境(包括气道结构细胞和其他炎症细胞)相互作用。外泌体来源于肺部微环境中其他免疫细胞对 MC 的摄取,可影响其表型和生物活性。例如,DC 摄取 MC 衍生外泌体可诱导共刺激 MHC Ⅱ 类分子、CD80、CD86 和 CD40 的表达,促使 DC 向 T 细胞呈现抗原[57]。所述外泌体还可刺激 B 淋巴细胞和 T 淋巴细胞产生细胞因子[58]。

同时,MC 衍生外泌体可通过细胞表面受体触发细胞信号传导。例如,在无 T 细胞参与的过程中,外泌体可通过 B 细胞的 CD40 表面配体促进 IgE 的产生[59]。此外,骨髓源性肥大细胞(bone marrow-derived mast cell,BMMC)可释放携带表面 CD63 和 OX40L 的外泌体,并通过与相应配体连接,诱导原始 T 细胞向 T2 细胞增殖和分化。既往研究已证实外泌体亦可通过传递特定载物影响 T 细胞功能[60]。

众所周知,DC 是一种可实现抗原加工并提呈至 T 细胞的特异性 APC。同时,鉴于其吞噬能力,DC 可促进先天免疫[61]。

DC 可释放具有亲本性质的外泌体,并在其表面表达 MHC 以及共刺激分子 CD86 和 CD54。此类外泌体可通过其表面 MHC 分子刺激 T 细胞[36]。此外,DC 亦可通过表面 CD86 诱导 T 细胞的增殖和分化,并通过表面 CD54 与 T 淋巴细胞的 LFA-1 相互作用[62]。

DC 衍生外泌体可通过将过敏原提呈至相关细胞而诱导 T2 反应[63]。同时,外泌体的酶性载物可将 LTA4 转化为其他 LT,如 LTB4 和 LTC4[64]。此外,DC 衍生外泌体的酶性载物可产生花生四烯酸(5-酮基二十碳四烯酸、KETE 和 LTB4)的脂质代谢物,后者可作为促炎症代谢物并触发粒细胞和白细胞向炎症部位的迁移[62]。

三、外泌体在肺疾病中的作用

在后续章节中,我们将进一步回顾外泌体在哮喘、COPD、肺结节病和肺结核等肺部疾病发生、发展和治疗中的作用和功能。

(一)哮喘

哮喘是一种异质性慢性气道疾病,以非特异性刺激诱导的可逆性气道阻塞为特征[65]。目前针对哮喘的病理生理学认知有限,大大局限了哮喘的临床治疗,挑战巨大。哮喘表型众多,且具有不同病理生理学机制。临床已定义两种类型的哮喘(T2 和非 T2),然而多数研究者认为哮喘是一种综合征而非单一性疾病[66]。针对哮喘的几大研究项目旨在将基于表型的哮喘分类与其病理生理学机制相关联,从而确定预测药物疗效的哮喘类型[67]。

哮喘主要表现为活化 $CD4^+$ T 细胞促炎细胞因子对环境过敏原(如感染或空气污染物)的病理生理学效应。IL-4、IL-5、IL-13 等介体的释放可促进 MC、Th2 细胞和嗜酸性粒细胞的活化,进而诱发气道可逆性阻塞、重塑和高反应性[26]。

在哮喘中,来源于先天性和适应性免疫系统的多种细胞可参与诱发肺上皮细胞的炎症反应。支气管组织和哮喘气道黏液中存在大量淋巴细胞、浆细胞、嗜酸性粒细胞和中性粒细胞。过敏原诱导哮喘发作时,IgE 介导的支气管气流迅速减少,并可能伴有晚期 IgE 介导反应和持续 4～8 小时的支气管气流减少[56]。

同时,在哮喘的发病过程中,确定便捷的生物标志物至关重要,以便定义患者亚群,从而确保在恰当的时间为合适的患者提供妥当的药物治疗。

从患者角度考虑,其必要性不言而喻。此外,当目前的钝性措施如血液嗜酸性粒细胞无法区分潜在病理生理过程的差异时,其对医疗保健提供者至关重要[26]。

外泌体的相关研究为哮喘患者的诊断和治疗监测中生物标志物的发现提供了新的思维方式。另外,针对外泌体在细胞内通信中的作用,其对哮喘的病理学发挥着不可忽视的作用。因此,考虑外泌体在哮喘病理条件中的作用对于理解其内在机制具有重要意义。

外泌体在哮喘中的作用

就外泌体的生物学和结构特性而言,这些微泡在哮喘病理生物学中的作用是无可争辩的事实。在哮喘的病理生理学中,炎症是主要的致病因素,外泌体可通过调节免疫细胞功能,进而在募集、激活或分化水平上促进慢性炎症过程。在哮喘的发病过程中,大量免疫细胞和结构细胞可释放出外泌体,如 DC 嗜酸性粒细胞、T 细胞、上皮细胞或 BEC 等。DC 可产生并释放携带共刺激分子和 MHC Ⅰ类和 Ⅱ类分子的外泌体,并可触发变应原特异性 T2 细胞作为其亲本细胞[68]。

一项既往研究在哮喘患者的 BAL 中检测到含有黏蛋白-1 标记物的外泌体,提示其 BEC 起源[69]。所述外泌体可诱导靶细胞表达 CXCL-8 和 LT-C4[27]。另外,IL-13 可以一种相互作用的方式促进气道上皮细胞释放外泌体,后者可反过来促进未分化肺巨噬细胞的增殖[70]。有趣的是,在哮喘小鼠模型中,应用 GW4869 抑制外泌体的产生,缓解了该模型中哮喘特征的诱发[26]。

含有嗜酸性蛋白(如 EPO、MBP 和 ECP)的嗜酸性粒细胞源性外泌体可通过自分泌或旁分泌功能模拟其亲本细胞在哮喘炎症过程中的作用[52]。

在哮喘患者中,嗜酸性粒细胞产生和释放的外泌体数量大于健康受试者细胞释放的相应数量。所述外泌体可增加炎症介质的产生,如受体嗜酸性粒细胞中的趋化因子、ROS 和 NO。同时,其还可上调嗜酸性粒细胞中黏附分子的表达,如细胞间黏附分子 1(intercellular adhesion molecule 1,ICAM-1)和整合素 2[71],从而增强所述细胞的迁移能力,后者在哮喘的发展过程中至关重要[72]。有趣的是,健康受试者的嗜酸细胞源性外泌体对哮喘嗜酸细胞的功能并无明显影响[73]。

与此同时,外泌体亦可防止过敏反应的发生和发展[74]。通过鼻内给药,耐受小鼠 BAL 液中外泌体可抑制其致敏反应,该发现揭示了外泌体疫苗在治疗哮喘和其他过敏性疾病方面的潜力[74]。同时,CD8$^+$T 细胞产生的外泌体被抗原特异性抗体包被并含有 miR-150。T 细胞摄取此类外泌体可诱导小鼠抗原性耐受[75]。

此外,MC 衍生外泌体可通过其表面 FcεRI 结合并降低血清游离 IgE 水平,进而限制 MC 活化[76]。基于其 TGF-β2 含量,哮喘患者成纤维细胞来源外泌体对上皮细胞增殖具有促进作用。同时,哮喘成纤维细胞外泌体 TGF-β2 水平低于正常人群的相应水平[39]。

脂多糖刺激中性粒细胞释放外泌体,对 ASMC 的增殖和重塑具有一定影响[77]。

人体气道中 MC 与 ASMC 的相互作用可调节炎症,引发哮喘症状。MC-ASMC 的相互作用可增强 ASMC 细胞因子分泌,从而导致 MC 招募的增多,最终促进哮喘的发生[78]。无须直接接触,MC 与 ASMC 的相互作用可通过 MC 衍生外泌体诱发哮喘的发生并促进其发展。因此,MC 衍生外泌体或其他可溶性因子的缺失有助于缓解刺激性哮喘反应[1]。

哮喘外泌体中的 miRNA 含量亦发生了一定变化。哮喘患者外泌体失调的 miRNA 与患者部分临床特征,如嗜酸性粒细胞计数或 FEV1 相关[79],且大多与气道完整性相关的信号通路有关。此外,SA 患者不同的外泌体 miRNA 谱与 TGF-β 信号通路、ErbB 信号通路、局灶黏附[80]及 IL-13 介导的事件有关[33]。

(二)肺癌

肺癌为全球最常见的肿瘤之一。现阶段在肺癌诊疗方面已取得重大进展,然而其仍然是全球肿瘤相关死亡的主要原因。肺癌全球控制的主要挑战为早期诊断方法缺乏以及对其潜在病理生理机制的了解有限。

就细胞内通信中的外泌体生理学特征及功能而言,其可影响受体细胞的生理学过程,从而导致肿瘤等病理状况的发生[81]。

肿瘤细胞可产生和释放外泌体。从肿瘤细胞分泌的外泌体被称为肿瘤源性外泌体(tumor-derived exosome,TEX)[82]。

TEX 为肿瘤微环境中的主要串扰机制,可促进肿瘤细胞的自身生长和生存。事实上,肿瘤恶性程度的决定因素为肿瘤微环境中的分子和细胞成分[83],外泌体根据其含量参与肿瘤微环境的调控。

肿瘤细胞来源外泌体可通过传递多种免疫刺激因子和免疫抑制因子以及诱导靶细胞重编癌蛋白,从其亲本细胞传递大量致瘤信息。例如,TEX 含有 K-RAS 和 MET 或致癌 miRNA,进而促进其他健康细胞的肿瘤发生和发展[84]。

通过诱导播散肿瘤细胞转移至靶部位,TEX 在制造转移前生态位并促进转移方面发挥着关键作用[85,86],这主要归因于 TEX 表面整合素的表达[87]。然而,TEX 可通过调节 NK 细胞活性并促进其表面受体,如杀伤细胞凝集素样受体 K1(KLRK1 或 NKG2D)的表达,进而诱导抗肿瘤免疫应答[88,89]。此外,TEX 可调节 EMT、肿瘤相关成纤维细胞功能和血管生成。

肺癌相关 TEX 可诱导转移前炎症反应。例如,肺癌相关 TEX 通过其 miR-21 和 miR-29a 载物与免疫细胞的细胞内 Toll 样受体(Toll-like receptor,TLR)结合,进而激活 NF-κB,最终导致肿瘤细胞转移和肿瘤生长[90](图 17-3)。

1. 外泌体在肺癌免疫细胞功能中的作用

在小鼠肺癌模型中,TEX 可导致肺组织中 NK 细胞的百分率降低[91]。同时,肺癌患者肺组织中 NK 细胞活性亦呈降低趋势[92];而 NK 细胞可通过其 C 型凝集素样受体 NKG2D 触发针对肿瘤细胞的细胞毒性途径[93]。通过将 TGF-β1 转移至 NK 细胞,TEX 可有助于降低该受体表达,从而降低 NK 细胞的毒性激活[94]。通过促进肿瘤细胞表面 NKG2D 配体

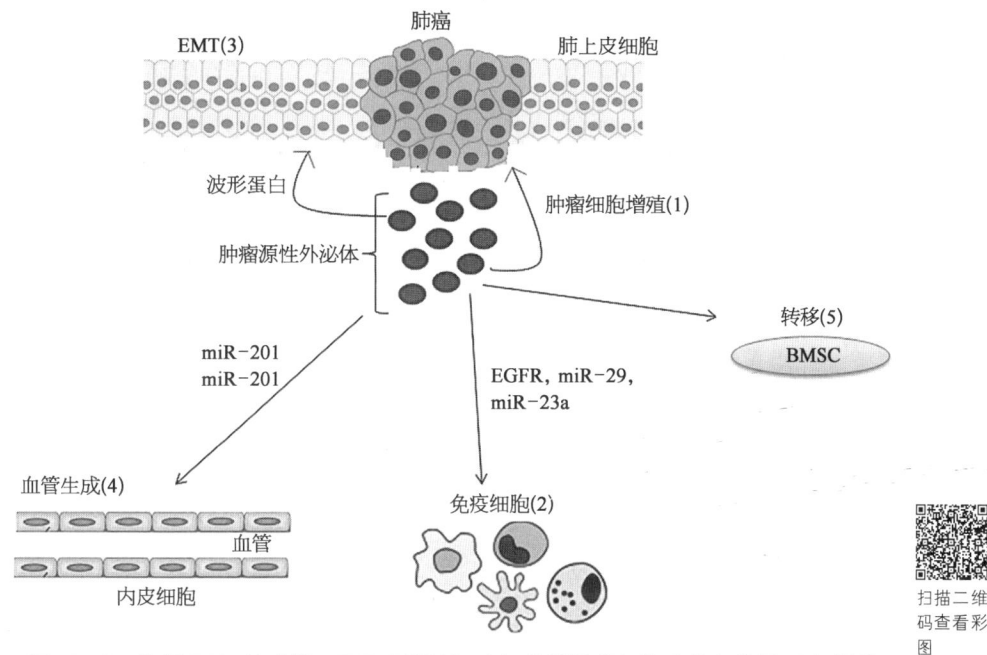

图 17-3 肺部 TEX 的功能。TEX 可通过:(1) 促进肿瘤细胞生长和发展;(2) 调节免疫反应;(3) 调节 EMT;(4) 血管生成;(5) 诱导骨髓祖细胞转移影响肿瘤微环境

脱落,TEX 还可下调 NKG2D 表达,进而导致受体脱敏和内化[95]。

此外,肺癌组织中的 miR-23a 载物可直接与 CD107a 分子结合,保护 NK 免受细胞毒性颗粒相关损伤[96]。TEX 亦可通过影响 IL-2 相关途径[97]、穿孔素或细胞周期蛋白 D3 的产生[91]以及 Janus 激酶 3(Jak3)的激活[91],依赖其他机制干扰 NK 细胞的抗肿瘤活性。

肿瘤相关外泌体在肿瘤微环境中可诱导免疫细胞极化和分化。DC 可在肿瘤部位表现出不同的表型和活性,进而发挥潜在促癌或抑癌作用。DC 的功能基于肿瘤微环境的性质,后者机制复杂而意义重大。实际上,DC 通常通过诱导和维持抗肿瘤免疫而发挥作用。然而,肿瘤微环境可能会促使 DC 发挥促癌作用,因此 DC 的抗原提呈功能在肿瘤的发展过程中可能会降低或丧失。在肿瘤微环境中,DC 亦可分化为免疫抑制性/耐受性调节性 DC,进而降低效应 T 细胞的功能,促进肿瘤发生。肿瘤中 DC 功能紊乱可能与多种机制有关,但值得肯定的是,肿瘤来源外泌体可传递大量分子,在其中发挥着重要作用。

一项既往研究报道,约 80% 肺癌活检组织分离的外泌体具有诱导耐受性 DC 和调节性 T 细胞的潜能,主要归因于其可传递 EGFR,并可导致肿瘤抗原特异性 $CD8^+$ 细胞活性的抑制[98]。TEX 中 miR-203a 可降低 DC 表面 TLR4 表达,进而导致下游细胞因子 TNF-α 和 IL-12 水平的降低[98]以及细胞免疫功能缺陷和 DC 功能障碍[99]。TEX 亦可通过其 TGF-β1 载物干扰 DC 成熟的进程,并诱导 MDSC 的产生[100]。MDSC 是一种来源于骨髓的、具有异质性和未成熟性的细胞群体,在肿瘤中表现出巨大的增殖潜能,且具有显著的抑制 T 细胞增殖的潜力,并可频繁分泌 TGF-β 和前列腺素 E2 等免疫抑制性细胞因子[100]。同时,TEX 可诱导 $CD14^+$ 单核细胞向 MDSC 而非 DC 分化[100]。TEX 表面 HSP72 可通过 STAT3 途径增强 MDSC 的抑制活性,并促进 MDSC 自分泌 IL-6 的产生[101]。TEX 与单核细胞的相互作用可导致单核细胞未成熟状态的维持,共刺激分子[102]和人类白细胞抗原 DR 下调或丢失,而对单核细胞表面 CD14 表达无明显影响[103]。小鼠肺癌模型 TEX 的注射可显著增加肺内 MDSC 募集,促进肺转移。此外,TEX 具有促进肿瘤转移的潜能,主要归因于其 MyD88 载物因子参与 TLR 信号通路的整合和转导[104]。

既往研究证实,通过传递功能性受体酪氨酸激酶、触发 MAPK 通路并抑制相关半胱天冬酶凋亡,TEX 可促进单核细胞前体产生 TAM[105]。在肺癌中,TAM 可诱导 STAT3 活化并促进肿瘤进展[105]。同时,TAM 与肿瘤细胞的相互作用主要由 TEX 介导。此外,TAM 衍生外泌体亦可运载相关因子,维持炎症生态位内 TAM 的存活,发挥互补支撑性作用[106]。与此同时,TAM 衍生外泌体具备特异性蛋白质组学特征,后者表现出较高的蛋白水解活性[107]。总体而言,肿瘤微环境中存在不同类型的、具有不同功能的癌性外泌体,后者在促进肿瘤发生发展方面意义重大。

2. 外泌体在肺癌 EMT 中的作用

EMT 是导致肿瘤发生和转移的重要过程。在此过程中,上皮细胞丢失细胞极性和细胞黏附特性,而获得间充质细胞迁移特性[108],使其发生远处迁移,从而促进肿瘤细胞转移和肿瘤进展[108]。

既往一项研究从高转移性肺癌患者血清中分离获得 TEX,发现其可诱导人 BEC 的 EMT[109]。TEX 中波形蛋白表达水平升高,波形蛋白为Ⅲ型中间丝蛋白家族成员,广泛表达于间充质细胞中,是 EMT 的相关标志物[110]。既往研究已报道波形蛋白水平与肺癌肿瘤细胞转移和侵袭潜能的关联性[111]。此外,在前列腺癌[112]和胃癌[113]中已检测到该标志物的异常表达。

在肺癌中,通过改变 VAV2-Rac1 通路和黏着斑激酶活性,波形蛋白可进一步诱导肿瘤细胞黏附特性的变化[113]。

TGF-β 诱导上皮腺癌 A549 细胞 EMT 的进程可进一步改变前述细胞中外泌体载物的类型[114]。与上皮样 A549 细胞相比,间充质样 A549 细胞释放外泌体含有更高水平的 β-catenin、波形蛋白、E-钙黏蛋白和 miR-23a。同时,外泌体 miR-23a 载物可直接靶向 E-cadherin,并以 smad 依赖途径调节 TGF-β 诱导的 A549 细胞 EMT[115]。

3. 外泌体在肺癌血管生成中的作用

血管生成和血管网络形成是肿瘤进展和转移的关键过程,该过程与众多调节机制相关。然而,值得肯定的是,外泌体通过转移血管生成因子(包括 VEGF、TGF 和成纤维细胞生长因子)在血管形成中发挥重要作用。

肿瘤微环境中缺氧等致病因素的存在可诱导具有特异性载物的外泌体的产生与释放,获得诱导血管生成的能力,进而促使细胞缓解肿瘤微环境中的应激状态[115]。

例如,在 CL1-5 肺腺肿瘤细胞中,缺氧条件通过增加伴有载物 miR-23a 表达增强的外泌体的产生而诱导血管生成。外泌体 miR-23a 载物可直接靶向脯氨酰羟化酶(prolyl hydroxylase,PHD)1 和 2,导致 HIF-1 在 EC 中积累。此外,外泌体 miR-23a 亦可通过靶向紧密连接蛋白 ZO-1 增加血管通透性和肿瘤细胞跨内皮迁移[116]。

与此同时,组织金属蛋白酶抑制物(tissue inhibitor of metalloproteinase,TIMP)-1 在肺癌的进展和转移中作用显著[117]。通过调节 PI3K/Akt/HIF-1 途径,TIMP-1 在肺腺肿瘤细胞中的过表达可增强前述细胞及其衍生外泌体中致瘤性 miR-210 的表达。此外,所述外泌体可通过下调 EC 摄取 Ephrin A3,促进血管生成[117]。

有研究检测肺癌患者血清中 miR-210 的表达水平,发现其明显高于健康人群[118]。肺癌外泌体中 EGFR 载物可触发 EC 中 EGFR 依赖性反应,导致 VEGFR-2 的自分泌激活并促进血管生成[119]。有趣的是,在大鼠严重肢体缺血的模型中,将肺癌患者分离外泌体注射至模型大鼠可显著增强 VEGFR-2 的表达,增加血管生成,并改善血流[120]。

4. 外泌体在肺癌转移中的作用

近年来,TEX 在转移前生态位(pre-metastatic niche,PMN)形成和转移发展中的作用受到越来越多的关注[121]。Janowska Wieczorek 等在 2005 年首次报道了外泌体在肺癌转移中的重要性[122]。

在肺癌转移前阶段,血管生成素 2(Angpt2)、MMP3 和 MMP10 的上调可增加肺部血管通透性和血管渗漏,该过程可由外泌体调控。此外,黑色素瘤衍生 TEX 可通过转移和过度表达 BM 祖细胞中的癌基因 MET,并通过增加肺 PMN 中促血管生成 c-Kit$^+$Tie2$^+$细胞群,将骨髓祖细胞重编为促血管表型,从而增加肺部血管的通透性[123]。血管渗漏可进一步促进外渗,促进 CTC 逃逸至转移前部位[124],导致肿瘤细胞转移和肿瘤进展。

事实上,黑色素瘤 TEX 在肺癌转移过程中发挥着重要作用,后者与黑色素瘤的转移能力有关。有趣的是,与低转移性黑色素瘤相比,高转移性黑色素瘤来源 TEX 可对肺部造成更大负担[123]。例如,未试验小鼠给予黑色素瘤 TEX 注射 24 小时内表现出肺部驻留,且 TEX 诱导转移前部位的肺上皮细胞通透性增加。该效应与 TEX 注射部位转移前生态位效应分子,如 S100A8、s100A9 和 TNF-α 的表达上调有关[125]。同时,TEX 给药亦可诱发炎症反应和 ECM 相关黑色素瘤基因的上调[123]。

与此同时,基于外泌体的作用,血小板在肺癌的发生发展、血管生成和转移中亦发挥着重要作用。血小板衍生外泌体(platelet-derived exosome,PMV)穿梭整合素 α2β(CD41)可促进小鼠肿瘤细胞增殖和肿瘤进展[122]。

此外,肺癌外泌体小 RNA 可诱导上皮细胞 TLR3 活化,进而激发趋化因子的产生和后续炎症免疫细胞在肺部的募集,最终促进转移前生态位的形成[126]。

外泌体表面整合素为靶细胞选择的决定性因素。表面整合素特定谱可直接将 TEX 引致特定器官,诱导转移性器官的亲和性[87]。例如,携带上调 s100 基因摄取外泌体与表面 α6α4 整合素异二聚体的肺成纤维细胞可逆向促进肺 PMN 的形成[87]。

携带表面整合素 α6β4 和 α6β1 的外泌体(如 4175-LuT 乳腺肿瘤细胞源性)可促进肺转移,并优先富集于肺部层粘连蛋白丰富区[87]。

NSCLC 常见转移部位为引起溶骨性病变的骨骼[127]。在 NSCLC 中,EGFR 上调的肿瘤细胞[128],释放的外泌体含有双调蛋白(amphiregulin,AREG)(一种 EGFR 配体)[129],可在破骨细胞前触发 EGFR 途径,并增强 RANKL 和蛋白水解酶的表达,进而引发恶性循环,最终导致溶骨性骨转移[128]。相反,高转移性骨肿瘤源性外泌体通常转移至肺部,并加速肿瘤细胞的转移[130]。

肺为最常见的转移靶器官之一,转移性肺肿瘤发病率高于原发性肺癌[130]。目前对所述组织特异性转移的分子机制尚未完全可知,但 TEX 可能在这一过程中发挥关键作用。为探究肿瘤微环境中外泌体特异性功能驱动肺转移的确切机制,尚需进一步研究。

(三)肺结核

结核分枝杆菌(mycobacterium tuberculosis,MTB)可使个体维持带菌生存状态数年,而不表现任何"潜伏性结核病"的临床症状,这已成为阻碍该病根治的一大顽固性特性[131]。

直至 2010 年,一些研究通过蛋白质印迹法证实,MTB 感染的巨噬细胞源性外泌体中存在分枝杆菌蛋白。

既往研究已应用综合蛋白质组学分析鉴定结核分枝杆菌活菌或死菌感染巨噬细胞中外泌体的蛋白质含量。结果显示所述外泌体中发现 41 种分枝杆菌蛋白簇的结合[132]。对前述蛋白簇的进一步分析提示存在高度免疫原性分枝杆菌蛋白,包括抗原 SAT‐6(Rv3875)、Ag85 复合物(Rv3804c、Rv1886c 和 Rv0129c)、MPT64(1980c)和 MPT63(1926c)[133]。

后续研究进一步分析了结核(tuberculosis,TB)患者的血清外泌体,并鉴定出 20 种分枝杆菌蛋白,主要包括 85b、BfrB、GlcB 和 Mpt64 抗原[134]。有趣的是,血清外泌体标记物如 MPT64 有助于鉴别肺结核和肺外结核[134]。

针对活动性和潜伏性结核病鉴别的研究同样证实了一些特异性外泌体标志物的存在[134]。在地方种群中发现潜伏性结核病的可能性意义重大,有助于高危人群的监测和感染传播的控制。

结核分枝杆菌培养 CFP 处理后巨噬细胞的外泌体成分可有助于激活先天性和获得性免疫应答。所述外泌体的大部分蛋白质载物与结核分枝杆菌感染巨噬细胞分离外泌体中的蛋白质出现重叠。以上结果提示携带结核分枝杆菌抗原载体的外泌体可为 CFP 结核病疫苗的研制提供合适方法[135]。

与此同时,外泌体可参与 PAMP 并以此方式调节免疫应答[136]。结核分枝杆菌可诱导感染巨噬细胞对 INF‐γ 产生部分耐药性。该作用基于结核分枝杆菌相关的 PAMP(如 19 kDa 脂蛋白和聚阿拉伯糖半乳糖−分枝菌酸复合物),后者与巨噬细胞受体(如 TLR 2)结合并导致 INF‐γ 反应性抑制[137]。该过程可通过结核分枝杆菌感染巨噬细胞源性外泌体所模拟[138]。

事实上,以含有分枝杆菌成分的外泌体处理巨噬细胞对 IFN‐γ 刺激的反应有限,提示外泌体可作为 PAMP 的载体并导致靶细胞中宿主免疫反应的抑制[139]。

有趣的是,结核分枝杆菌感染可调节宿主 miRNA 的表达[133]。应用毒性结核分枝杆菌 H37Rv 和无毒结核分枝杆菌 BCG 感染人巨噬细胞后,相应诱导 miRNA 表达模式在两种结核分枝杆菌活菌之间无明显差异;而应用结核分枝杆菌死菌感染产生的 miRNA 表达模式却表现出显著差异[140]。这一结果揭示了细胞内活菌对宿主细胞 miRNA 网络的积极影响。

另外,结核分枝杆菌感染巨噬细胞后,外泌体 miRNA 的数量和含量发生显著变化。巨噬细胞源性单核细胞(macrophage-derived monocyte，MDM)感染BCG后，可诱导BCG感染MDM源性特异性外泌体miRNA的表达，后者miRNA主要参与宿主代谢和能量产生[32]。此外，大于100 mRNA为结核分枝杆菌感染细胞源性外泌体所特有，后者主要参与宿主免疫应答的调节[141]。总之，上述研究发现强调了外泌体mRNA与miRNA在结核病中的功能和诊断潜力。

（四）COPD

COPD以慢性进行性气流阻塞为特征，伴有炎性细胞浸润、肺泡壁增厚，最终导致肺实质和上皮损伤。COPD的主要特征是炎症反应[142,143]，外泌体该病理状态下可发挥显著作用[143]。

肺气肿以肺实质EC损伤为主[144]。在稳定期COPD患者中，内皮源性外泌体的产生在疾病活动期呈增加趋势，且其水平与肺部损伤和气流受限显著相关。外泌体微粒可携带血管内皮钙黏蛋白、血小板EC黏附分子和E-选择素[145]。上述发现提示了外泌体在COPD肺损伤和病理生理中的作用。气道暴露于香烟烟雾(cigarette smoke，CS)等刺激物后可诱发上皮细胞损伤和COPD的发生，其机制主要包括肺毛细血管的破坏、上皮细胞的衰老、恶化以及气道重塑的相互作用，最终导致肺功能的丧失[146]。受损上皮细胞可产生一系列炎症介质，如TNF-α、IL-1α、GMCSF、TGF-β和CXCL-8，进而通过自分泌和旁分泌发挥生物学效应。

因而，TGF-β可进一步促进肌成纤维细胞的分化和纤维化发展，并诱导气道重塑[147]。值得注意的是，外泌体至少在一定限度上可调节前述炎症介质的旁分泌作用[148]。肺上皮细胞持续暴露于CS可诱导AAT1富集外泌体的分泌。其中，CCN1作为一种细胞外基质相关蛋白，在重塑和修复过程中具有重要作用[149]，并可通过WNT信号通路增强CXCL-8的表达[150]。因此，AAT1富集外泌体可通过旁分泌诱导CXCL-8分泌，进而促进炎症细胞(如中性粒细胞)向肺间质或肺实质的募集，最终导致肺组织纤维化[150]。此外，CS亦可增加肺上皮细胞分泌外泌体的水平[151]。有研究发现，约1.5%的COPD患者患有α1抗胰蛋白酶(alpha 1 anti-trypsin，AAT1)缺乏症[145]。AAT1是一种糖蛋白丝氨酸蛋白酶抑制剂，可保护肺部免受炎症损伤[152]。上皮细胞快速摄取的外泌体可介导AAT1从肺EC向肺泡上皮细胞和肺腔中的转运。基于肺内皮屏障的有效转运，AAT1富集外泌体可抵御CS暴露风险，发挥一定的保护作用[153]。COPD的关键症状为EMT，后者可导致小气道重塑和纤维化[154]。EMT可伴随着大气道的血管生成，进而导致癌前基质生态位的形成[155]。针对外泌体在生物活性分子调节和细胞内通信中的生物学作用，既往研究已证实外泌体在EMT过程中的关键作用[155]。COPD进展通常伴随着小气道壁增厚，以及上皮-间充质营养单位(epithelial mesenchymal trophic unit，EMTU)成纤维细胞介导的修复和重塑。其中，EMTU由一层上皮细胞、基底膜区(basement membrane zone，BMZ)和包括成纤维细胞在内的间充质细胞组成[1]。重塑过程是损伤/应激上皮与下层成纤维细胞间相互作用的结果，可导致间充质细胞的增殖和重塑，该过程受到外泌体的高度调控。除作为COPD病理生理学的重要驱动因素外，外泌体亦可作为COPD病情进展或改善的生物标志物[145]。同时，

COPD 的肺 EC 损伤程度可能与循环外泌体水平存在相关性。有研究报道外泌体的 miRNA 水平与骨骼肌损伤程度相关,前者可作为骨骼肌功能障碍的潜在生物标志物[156],且 COPD 患者 BAL 液中 5 种外泌体 miRNA 的表达差异与疾病程度相关。前述 miRNA 可靶向核糖体 s6 蛋白激酶(s6 kinase,S6K),其中 S6K 为 TORC1 信号通路的一部分,是骨骼肌萎缩的重要调节因子。这一重要发现提示外泌体 miRNA 作为一种无创性诊断生物标志物的潜力,有助于预测 COPD 的进展状况和治疗结局[156]。

(五)肺结节病

肺结节病是一种系统性和炎症性疾病,主要靶向器官为肺部。结节病主要特征为非干酪样肉芽肿(non-caseating granuloma,NCG)和干扰素诱导 T 细胞在受累靶器官中的聚集,导致炎症和组织损伤,尤其在肺部[157]。结节病的病因目前尚未完全可知。然而,根据结节病病理生理学的分子特征,外泌体在结节病炎症的发生和发展中可发挥关键作用。与健康人群相比,结节病患者 BAL 液中外泌体的数量呈增长趋势。结节病患者 BAL 液分离外泌体可增加 PBMC 中 IFN-γ 和 IL-13 的表达水平[158],以及上皮细胞 CXCL-8 生成[29]。此外,结节病患者血清和 BAL 液外泌体中的外泌体 miRNA 表达谱存在明显差异[159]。综上,外泌体在结节病炎症发生和发展中的潜在作用不容忽视。然而,未来仍有必要进一步开展深入的应用研究,以证实外泌体在结节病治疗中的应用前景。

(六)其他呼吸系统疾病

除上述肺部疾病外,本综述同时对其他肺疾病中外泌体的功能进行阐述。

例如,缺氧条件下,促炎介质和活化巨噬细胞表达增加,可导致缺氧性肺动脉高压的发展[34]。

缺氧可诱发内质网(endoplasmic reticulum,ER)应激,导致肺上皮细胞分泌大量的外泌体。此类外泌体含有大量 caspase-3,可激活 AM 并促进炎症反应,导致肺损伤。前述发现提示外泌体可参与肺上皮细胞和巨噬细胞间的相互作用,进而介导组织损伤进程[160]。

特发性肺纤维化(idiopathic pulmonary fibrosis,IPF)是一种以进行性肺纤维化为特征性病理改变,最终导致肺功能不可逆性下降的慢性肺疾病[161]。例如,与健康受试者相比,IPF 患者外泌体中抗纤维化 miRNA(如 miR-141)水平降低,纤维化 miRNA(如 miR-7)水平升高。有趣的是,miR-7 上调程度与疾病负荷间,以及 miR-125b 上调与轻型病症间存在显著相关性。前述发现提示了外泌体 miRNA 作为生物标志物在 IPF 发病机制中的潜在作用[162]。

囊性纤维化(cystic fibrosis,CF)是一种进行性肺疾病,以囊性纤维化跨膜传导调节蛋白(cystic fibrosis transmembrane conductance regulator,CFTR)基因缺陷为主要特征,后者可影响氯通道活性,导致气道中性粒细胞显著增多和黏液淤滞[163]。鉴于 CF 患者 BEC 分泌的外泌体增多,因此生物流体中外泌体可作为 CF 无创诊断的疾病生物标志物,具有潜在价值[164]。

此外,以伴持续性细菌感染的 CF 患者为研究对象,其外泌体检测发现脯氨酰内肽酶

(prolyl endopeptidase，PE)呈高水平。

PE 酶可参与中性粒细胞从胶原合成趋化性三肽 ProGly - Pro(PGP)的过程[165]。PE 酶由外泌体携带气道上皮细胞分泌。同时，LPS 可通过 TLR4 促进 PE 的产生和释放。

CF 患者的高炎症状态可能部分归因于 PE 酶水平的升高[165]。

此外，在肠道生物学中，胃肠上皮和基侧膜外泌体的分泌与抗原表达存在一定关联，而 TLR4 信号可显著促进胆管上皮和肠上皮外泌体的管腔释放，并在感染后呈增加趋势[166]。未来研究有必要进一步探究 CF 患者外泌体释放的不同途径。根据其来源细胞的类型和生理状况，气道上皮细胞源性外泌体在尺寸和物理性质上存在差异，这一特征有助于发挥对异常病理变化的诊断作用[37]。例如，在 CF 患者中，外泌体表面黏蛋白的数量和类型会发生一定改变，表现为黏液分泌过多。黏蛋白表面蛋白可决定外泌体的个体大小和表面电荷。

此外，CF 患者外泌体 miRNA 和蛋白含量的变化在一定程度上反映了炎症刺激后的细胞变化。上述发现提示外泌体在促进 CF 气道微环境中高炎症状态中的作用[167]。

当前 CF 研究的主要目的之一为恢复 CFTR 基因功能，随着外泌体作为药物传递载体的出现，前述基因的功能得到了广泛应用[163]。以外泌体为载体成功地将 CFTR 基因转移至人 CFTR 缺陷的鼻上皮细胞，并促进该细胞 CFTR 功能以剂量依赖的方式恢复[163]。来自 CFTR 阳性的 Calu - 3 细胞或应用过表达 GFP 质粒标记的 CFTR(GFP - CFTR)腺病毒载体转导的 A549 细胞源性外泌体可将 GFP - CFTR 糖蛋白和 mRNA(GFP - CFTR)包裹并转移至靶细胞中，并可纠正人 CF 细胞的遗传性缺陷[163]。

四、外泌体在呼吸系统疾病中的临床应用：临床试验和未来展望

外泌体在维持呼吸微环境稳态和维持肺部正常功能方面发挥着重要作用。在肺组织中，外泌体包含从结构细胞到免疫细胞的多种细胞类型。前述外泌体的数量和含量因疾病状态不同而有所区别，并可携带不同疾病的特异性成分。基于此，我们认为外泌体可为各种呼吸系统疾病的诊疗监测提供新型生物学标志物，亦可发挥治疗性干预作用。

目前，MSC 源性外泌体已被报道具有创伤愈合和组织修复潜能，尤其在肺组织生成过程中[164]。MSC 衍生外泌体颇受关注，其原因在于此类外泌体的抗凋亡和抗炎特性[168]在治疗肺部慢性炎症方面颇具成效[168]。此类外泌体可促进肺组织再生和伤口愈合，在减轻和改善哮喘气道重塑方面具有一定效果[168]。

在 ARDS 动物模型中，MSC 衍生外泌体可诱导损伤肺泡中角质细胞生长因子 (keratinocyte growth factor，KGF)的表达，提高蛋白通透性，进而减轻肺部炎症[169]。应用外泌体治疗 ARDS 的临床试验目前正在进行中[170]。

既往一项Ⅰ期临床试验利用负载肿瘤抗原的 DC 源性外泌体(dexosomes)进行 NSCLC 免疫治疗[171]。该项试验结果表明：所述外泌体可诱导患者先天性和适应性免疫应答，并证实"dexosome 疗法"的安全性和可行性，可作为当前肿瘤或其他肺部炎症疾病治疗的良好替代方案。

当然，该疗法对疾病稳定性和长期生存率的影响尚需进一步研究。

同时，外泌体还有其他功能，可用其设置"陷阱"，抑制免疫反应。例如，MC 衍生外泌体

可通过其表面 FCεR1 受体捕获无血清 IgE，进而抑制 MC 的持续激活。此外，$CD8^+$ 细胞源性外泌体可诱导小鼠产生抗原特异性耐受，减轻变应性接触性皮炎（allergic contact dermatitis，ACD）[75]。鉴于外泌体含量可反映其亲本细胞畸变，且其在体液中的稳定性，可作为肺癌"液体活检"的生物标志物，极具潜力[172]。以外泌体为基础的生物标志物可绕过需手术的组织活检，是一种无创诊断途径[172]。既往研究已在肺癌患者血清和血浆中检测出 miRNA 和蛋白质等外泌体生物标志物。此外，基于微阵列的肺癌患者血清外泌体 miRNA 分析表明，miR-21 和 miR-4257 上调与肺癌复发显著相关[173]。另一项研究纳入了 276 例 NSCLC 患者，其血清外泌体蛋白分析表明 NY-ESO-1 等与患者生存存在关联性[174]。

既往一项研究提示 NSCLC TEX 中 EGFR 表达增强[175]。同时，该研究显示在肺癌患者中，两种抑癌基因 miRNA（miR-51 和 miR-373）水平均降低，且该趋势与患者的预后不良有关[175]。

此外，肺癌患者外泌体 miRNA 分析显示，与健康受试者相比，miR-378a、miR-379、miR-139-5p、miR-200b-5p[70]、miR-21[173]、miR-155[173]、miR-23b、miR-10b-5p[173] 和 miR-4257[173] 的表达水平均存在差异。

与此同时，研究者认为外泌体 miRNA 可作为肺癌治疗评价的标志物。例如，有研究发现分别靶向 p21 和 DR5 mRNA 的致瘤性 miR-208a 和 miR-1246 为放疗抵抗的标志物[176]。

基于 TEX 的生物标志物在肺癌诊疗监测中具有更高的灵敏度、特异性及无创的优势，然而其仍面临众多挑战。具体而言，其关键局限性在于缺乏统一标准化的外泌体分离方法，以及肿瘤源性外泌体异质性的存在[177]。然而，结合肺癌 TEX 中 miRNA 和蛋白质载物信息与下一代测序和蛋白质组学分析，推动基于 TEX 的肺癌诊断或治疗进展，仍不失为一项极具意义的研究课题。

近期，有学者提出利用表面增强拉曼光谱（surface-enhanced Raman spectroscopy，SERS）和主成分分析（principle component analysis，PCA）相结合的方法进行外泌体表面蛋白质和脂质分子的表征。脂类和蛋白质均有其特定拉曼光谱。因而，不同表面脂类和蛋白质形态的肿瘤细胞或正常细胞外泌体的拉曼光谱亦可能存在一定差异。应用该方法，其在肺癌 TEX 与正常细胞外泌体鉴别中的灵敏度和特异性分别为 95.3% 和 97.3%[178]。诚然，目前外泌体的传统检测方法尚存在一定挑战，如肿瘤源性外泌体的异质性以及对大量高浓度样本的要求，前述方法不失为一良策，值得临床实践的推广与应用[178]。

既往一项研究通过纳入 46 例晚期非小细胞肺癌患者，对 1 369 个血清外泌体蛋白质进行质谱定量，结果显示 CD91 为肺腺癌的外泌体抗原分子[179]。

同样地，另一项研究引入多变量 EV 阵列（EV 阵列）作为 NSCLC 诊断的一种潜在补充策略。该研究应用此法，引入一组外泌体表面蛋白标记物（$n=30$；包括 CD91、CD317 和 EGFR）进行鉴别诊断，其特异性达 75%[180]。

既往一项研究通过对 NSCLC 患者尿液外泌体进行蛋白质组学质谱分析，发现外泌体中富含亮氨酸的 α-2-糖蛋白 1（lucien rich alpha-2-glycoprotein 1，LRG1）的表达明显高于正常人群，LRG1 在 NSCLC 组织中亦呈高表达[181]。同时，其他标记物（如 CD171、

CD151 和 tetra-spanin 8)亦被证实为 NSCLC 诊断的潜在外泌体生物标志物[182]。

除诊断应用外,外泌体可作为合适载体,将药物或核酸运载至靶器官,该用途同样备受关注。例如,有实验构建小鼠肺癌模型,应用牛乳外泌体负载 Aferin-A 进行药物递送。结果发现载 Aferin-A 外泌体在小鼠肺癌模型中可发挥一定抑瘤作用[183]。

另外,脑内皮细胞系(bEND.3)源性外泌体可透过血脑屏障,在体内给药和降低脑肿瘤 VEGF 水平方面效果颇为显著[184]。

基于上述理解,我们不难发现外泌体具有其独特的生物学特性,有望成为肿瘤治疗新策略开发的重要靶点。考虑到肿瘤源性外泌体可运载肿瘤特异性抗原,前者在抗肿瘤疫苗研制中潜力巨大[185]。

外泌体的靶向性选择具有亲器官性,且其依赖于整合素介导的信号传导[87]。因此,通过诱饵肽阻断整合素可有助于抑制外泌体融合和摄取,进而抑制肿瘤进展[186]。

肺癌免疫治疗的最新进展之一为肿瘤微环境中炎症信号和 T 细胞活化负性调节因子(如 PD-1 和 PD-L1)的阻断。外泌体已被证实在这其中发挥了重要的调节作用[174]。

同时,阻断外泌体分泌或抑制外泌体介导的细胞串扰策略可能在抑制适宜肿瘤生长的肿瘤微环境发展中发挥一定作用[185]。

值得注意的是,外泌体可通过调节肿瘤微环境中的抗炎信号而显著提高肺癌免疫治疗的疗效[187]。

综上所述,外泌体具有特异性靶向性、体积小、传导信号和运载生物分子等特性,以及穿透生物屏障的能力。因而,外泌体可在肿瘤诊断生物标志物、肿瘤治疗、药物递送和肿瘤免疫治疗等更广泛的医学应用中发挥重要作用。

总体而言,当前研究进展已证实外泌体在肺部微环境中细胞串扰及致病性中的作用。外泌体可作为疾病无创诊断策略,亦可作为一种新型潜在途径用于肺部疾病的治疗。

目前,外泌体在分离和纯化上仍存在一定局限性。然而,在不久的将来,外泌体有望在肿瘤诊治中发挥重要作用。当然,在将基于外泌体的技术向临床应用转化之前,外泌体应用的局限性尚待进一步的临床研究。

(张文梅 译,周晓辉 审校)

参考文献

[1] Alipoor SD, et al. Exosomes and exosomal miRNA in respiratory diseases. Mediators Inflamm 2016;2016,5628404.
[2] Raposo G, Stoorvogel W. Extracellular vesicles: exosomes, microvesicles, and friends. J Cell Biol 2013;200(4):373-83.
[3] Clark DJ, et al. Triple SILAC quantitative proteomic analysis reveals differential abundance of cell signaling proteins between normal and lung cancer-derived exosomes. J Proteomics 2016;133:161-9.
[4] Johnstone RM, et al. Vesicle formation during reticulocyte maturation. Association of plasma membrane activities with released vesicles (exosomes). J Biol Chem 1987;262(19):9412-20.
[5] Pan BT, Johnstone RM. Fate of the transferrin receptor during maturation of sheep reticulocytes in vitro: selective externalization of the receptor. Cell 1983;33(3):967-78.
[6] Trams EG, et al. Exfoliation of membrane ecto-enzymes in the form of micro-vesicles. Biochim Biophys Acta 1981;645(1):63-70.
[7] Bhatnagar S, Schorey JS. Exosomes released from infected macrophages contain *Mycobacterium avium* glycopeptidolipids and are proinflammatory. J Biol Chem 2007;282(35):25779-89.
[8] Kourembanas S. Exosomes: vehicles of intercellular signaling, biomarkers, and vectors of cell therapy. Annu Rev Physiol 2015;77:13-27.
[9] Jan AT, et al. Perspective insights of exosomes in neurodegenerative diseases: a critical appraisal. Front Aging Neurosci

2017; 9: 317.
[10] Quek C, Hill AF. The role of extracellular vesicles in neurodegenerative diseases. Biochem Biophys Res Commun 2017; 483(4): 1178-86.
[11] Eissa NT. The exosome in lung diseases: message in a bottle. J Allergy Clin Immunol 2013; 131(3): 904-5.
[12] Valadi H, et al. Exosome-mediated transfer of mRNAs and microRNAs is a novel mechanism of genetic exchange between cells. Nat Cell Biol 2007; 9(6): 654.
[13] Tickner JA, et al. Functions and therapeutic roles of exosomes in cancer. Front Oncol 2014; 4: 127.
[14] Mathivanan S, Simpson RJ. ExoCarta: a compendium of exosomal proteins and RNA. Proteomics 2009; 9(21): 4997-5000.
[15] Cheng L, et al. Exosomes provide a protective and enriched source of miRNA for biomarker profiling compared to intracellular and cell-free blood. J Extracell Vesicles 2014; 3(1): 23743.
[16] Hough KP, et al. Exosomes in immunoregulation of chronic lung diseases. Allergy 2017; 72(4): 534-44.
[17] Samanta S, et al. Exosomes: new molecular targets of diseases. Acta Pharmacol Sin 2018; 39(4): 501-13.
[18] Barile L, Vassalli G. Exosomes: therapy delivery tools and biomarkers of diseases. Pharmacol Ther 2017; 174: 63-78.
[19] Masyuk AI, Masyuk TV, Larusso NF. Exosomes in the pathogenesis, diagnostics and therapeutics of liver diseases. J Hepatol 2013; 59(3): 621-5.
[20] Andaloussi ELS, et al. Extracellular vesicles: biology and emerging therapeutic opportunities. Nat Rev Drug Discov 2013; 12(5): 347-57.
[21] Barile L, et al. Extracellular vesicles from human cardiac progenitor cells inhibit cardiomyocyte apoptosis and improve cardiac function after myocardial infarction. Cardiovasc Res 2014; 103(4): 530-41.
[22] Admyre C, et al. Exosomes with major histocompatibility complex class II and co-stimulatory molecules are present in human BAL fluid. Eur Respir J 2003; 22(4): 578-83.
[23] Ismail N, et al. Macrophage microvesicles induce macrophage differentiation and miR-223 transfer. Blood 2012; 121: 984-95. https://doi.org/10.1182/blood-2011-08-374793.
[24] Rose MC, Voynow JA. Respiratory tract mucin genes and mucin glycoproteins in health and disease. Physiol Rev 2006; 86(1): 245-78.
[25] Fujita Y, et al. Extracellular vesicles in lung microenvironment and pathogenesis. Trends Mol Med 2015; 21(9): 533-42.
[26] Mortaz E, et al. Exosomes in severe asthma: update in their roles and potential in therapy. Biomed Res Int 2018; 2018: 2862187.
[27] Kulshreshtha A, et al. Proinflammatory role of epithelial cell-derived exosomes in allergic airway inflammation. J Allergy Clin Immunol 2013; 131(4): 1194-203, 1203.e1-14.
[28] Kesimer M, et al. Characterization of exosome-kike vesicles released from human tracheobronchial ciliated epithelium: a possible role in innate defense. FASEB J 2009; 23(6): 1858-68.
[29] Qazi KR, et al. Proinflammatory exosomes in bronchoalveolar lavage fluid of patients with sarcoidosis. Thorax 2010; 65(11): 1016-24.
[30] Cordazzo C, et al. Rapid shedding of proinflammatory microparticles by human mononuclear cells exposed to cigarette smoke is dependent on Ca^{2+} mobilization. Inflamm Res 2014; 63(7): 539-47.
[31] Alipoor SD, et al. miR-1224 expression is increased in human macrophages after infection with Bacillus Calmette-Guerin (BCG). Iran J Allergy Asthma Immunol 2018; 17(3): 250-7.
[32] Alipoor SD, et al. Bovis Bacillus Calmette-Guerin (BCG) infection induces exosomal miRNA release by human macrophages. J Transl Med 2017; 15(1): 105.
[33] Levänen B, et al. Altered microRNA profiles in bronchoalveolar lavage fluid exosomes in asthmatic patients. J Allergy Clin Immunol 2013; 131(3): 894-903, e8.
[34] Lee C, et al. Exosomes mediate the cytoprotective action of mesenchymal stromal cells on hypoxia-induced pulmonary hypertension. Circulation 2012; 126(22): 2601-11.
[35] Merluzzi S, et al. Mast cells, basophils and B cell connection network. Mol Immunol 2015; 63(1): 94-103.
[36] Théry C, et al. Indirect activation of naïve CD4+ T cells by dendritic cell-derived exosomes. Nat Immunol 2002; 3(12): 1156.
[37] Kesimer M, Gupta R. Physical characterization and profiling of airway epithelial derived exosomes using light scattering. Methods 2015; 87: 59-63.
[38] Park JA, et al. Tissue factor-bearing exosome secretion from human mechanically stimulated bronchial epithelial cells in vitro and in vivo. J Allergy Clin Immunol 2012; 130(6): 1375-83.
[39] Haj-Salem I, et al. Fibroblast-derived exosomes promote epithelial cell proliferation through TGF-β2 signalling pathway in severe asthma. Allergy 2018; 73(1): 178-86.
[40] De Vooght V, et al. B-kymphocytes as key players in chemical-induced asthma. PLoS ONE 2013; 8(12): e83228.
[41] Natarajan P, Guernsey LA, Schramm CM. Regulatory B cells in allergic airways disease and asthma. In: Regulatory B cells. Springer; 2014. p.207-25.
[42] Harris DP, et al. Reciprocal regulation of polarized cytokine production by effector B and T cells. Nat Immunol 2000; 1(6): 475.
[43] Admyre C, et al. B cell-derived exosomes can present allergen peptides and activate allergen-specific T cells to proliferate and produce TH2-kike cytokines. J Allergy Clin Immunol 2007; 120(6): 1418-24.
[44] Clayton A, et al. Induction of heat shock proteins in B-cell exosomes. J Cell Sci 2005; 118(Pt 16): 3631-8.
[45] Blanchard N, et al. TCR activation of human T cells induces the production of exosomes bearing the TCR/CD3/zeta complex. J Immunol 2002; 168(7): 3235-41.
[46] Zhang H, et al. CD4(+) T cell-released exosomes inhibit CD8(+) cytotoxic T-kymphocyte responses and antitumor immunity. Cell Mol Immunol 2011; 8(1): 23-30.

[47] Peters PJ, et al. Molecules relevant for T cell-target cell interaction are present in cytolytic granules of human T lymphocytes. Eur J Immunol 1989; 19(8): 1469-75.
[48] Ventimiglia LN, Alonso MA. Biogenesis and function of T cell-derived exosomes. Front Cell Dev Biol 2016; 4: 84.
[49] Cai Z, et al. Activated T cell exosomes promote tumor invasion via Fas signaling pathway. J Immunol 2012; 188(12): 5954-61.
[50] Wahlgren J, et al. Activated human T cells secrete exosomes that participate in IL-2 mediated immune response signaling. PLoS ONE 2012; 7(11): e49723.
[51] Stone KD, Prussin C, Metcalfe DD. IgE, mast cells, basophils, and eosinophils. J Allergy Clin Immunol 2010; 125(2): S73-80.
[52] Mazzeo C, et al. Exosome secretion by eosinophils: a possible role in asthma pathogenesis. J Allergy Clin Immunol 2015; 135(6): 1603-13.
[53] Lässer C, et al. Exosomes in the nose induce immune cell trafficking and harbour an altered protein cargo in chronic airway inflammation. J Transl Med 2016; 14(1): 181.
[54] Virk H, Arthur G, Bradding P. Mast cells and their activation in lung disease. Transl Res 2016; 174: 60-76.
[55] Brightling CE, et al. Mast-cell infiltration of airway smooth muscle in asthma. N Engl J Med 2002; 346(22): 1699-705.
[56] Rossios C, et al. Impaired innate immune gene profiling in airway smooth muscle cells from chronic cough patients. Biosci Rep 2017; 37(6), BSR20171090.
[57] Skokos D, et al. Mast cell-dependent exosomes induce phenotypic and functional maturation of dendritic cells and elicit specific immune responses in vivo. J Immunol 2003; 170(6): 3037-45.
[58] Tkaczyk C, et al. In vitro and in vivo immunostimulatory potential of bone marrow-derived mast cells on B-and T-kymphocyte activation. J Allergy Clin Immunol 2000; 105(1): 134-42.
[59] Gauchat J-F, et al. Induction of human IgE synthesis in B cells by mast cells and basophils. Nature 1993; 365(6444): 340.
[60] Li F, et al. Mast cell-derived exosomes promote Th2 cell differentiation via OX40L-OX40 ligation. J Immunol Res 2016; 2016: 3623898.
[61] Iwasaki A, Medzhitov R. Control of adaptive immunity by the innate immune system. Nat Immunol 2015; 16(4): 343.
[62] Esser J, et al. Exosomes from human macrophages and dendritic cells contain enzymes for leukotriene biosynthesis and promote granulocyte migration. J Allergy Clin Immunol 2010; 126(5): 1032-40, e4.
[63] Vallhov H, et al. Dendritic cell-derived exosomes carry the major cat allergen Fel d 1 and induce an allergic immune response. Allergy 2015; 70(12): 1651-5.
[64] Liu Y, Cao X. Characteristics and significance of the pre-metastatic niche. Cancer Cell 2016; 30(5): 668-81.
[65] Gelb AF, Christenson SA, Nadel JA. Understanding the pathophysiology of the asthma-chronic obstructive pulmonary disease overlap syndrome. Curr Opin Pulm Med 2016; 22(2): 100-5.
[66] Lambrecht BN, Hammad H. The immunology of asthma. Nat Immunol 2015; 16(1): 45.
[67] Lötvall J, et al. Asthma endotypes: a new approach to classification of disease entities within the asthma syndrome. J Allergy Clin Immunol 2011; 127(2): 355-60.
[68] Admyre C, et al. Exosomes-nanovesicles with possible roles in allergic inflammation. Allergy 2008; 63(4): 404-8.
[69] Torregrosa Paredes P, et al. Bronchoalveolar lavage fluid exosomes contribute to cytokine and leukotriene production in allergic asthma. Allergy 2012; 67(7): 911-9.
[70] Cazzoli R, et al. microRNAs derived from circulating exosomes as noninvasive biomarkers for screening and diagnosing lung cancer. J Thorac Oncol 2013; 8(9): 1156-62.
[71] Canas JA, et al. Exosomes from eosinophils autoregulate and promote eosinophil functions. J Leukoc Biol 2017; 101(5): 1191-9.
[72] Sastre B, et al. Novel modulators of asthma and allergy: exosomes and microRNAs. Front Immunol 2017; 8: 826.
[73] Lässer C. Exosomal RNA as biomarkers and the therapeutic potential of exosome vectors. Expert Opin Biol Ther 2012; 12(Suppl. 1): S189-97.
[74] Prado N, et al. Exosomes from bronchoalveolar fluid of tolerized mice prevent allergic reaction. J Immunol 2008; 181(2): 1519-25.
[75] Rebane A, Akdis CA. MicroRNAs in allergy and asthma. Curr Allergy Asthma Rep 2014; 14(4): 424.
[76] Xie G, et al. Mast cell exosomes can suppress allergic reactions by binding to IgE. J Allergy Clin Immunol 2018; 141(2): 788-91.
[77] Dvorak AM. Degranulation and recovery from degranulation of basophils and mast cells. In: Ultrastructure of mast cells and basophils. Karger Publishers; 2005. p.205-51.
[78] Liu L, Yang J, Huang Y. Human airway smooth muscle cells express eotaxin in response to signaling following mast cell contact. Respiration 2006; 73(2): 227-35.
[79] Francisco-Garcia A, et al. LSC abstract-altered small RNA cargo in severe asthma exosomes. Eur Respiratory Soc 2016; 48: PP101.
[80] Suzuki M, et al. Altered circulating exosomal RNA profiles detected by next-generation sequencing in patients with severe asthma. Eur Respiratory Soc 2016; 48: PA3410.
[81] Andre F, et al. Exosomes for cancer immunotherapy. Ann Oncol 2004; 15(Suppl 4): iv141-4.
[82] Muller L, et al. Tumor-derived exosomes regulate expression of immune function-related genes in human T cell subsets. Sci Rep 2016; 6: 20254.
[83] Haratani K, et al. Tumor immune microenvironment and nivolumab efficacy in EGFR mutation-positive non-small cell lung cancer based on T790M status after disease progression during EGFR-TKI treatment. Ann Oncol 2017; 28(7): 1532-9.
[84] Sun T, et al. Role of exosomal noncoding RNAs in lung carcinogenesis. Biomed Res Int 2015; 2015: 125807.
[85] Zhang Y, Wang XF. A niche role for cancer exosomes in metastasis. Nat Cell Biol 2015; 17(6): 709-11.

[86] Sceneay J, Smyth MJ, Möler A. The pre-metastatic niche: finding common ground. Cancer Metastasis Rev 2013; 32(3-4): 449-64.
[87] Hoshino A, et al. Tumour exosome integrins determine organotropic metastasis. Nature 2015; 527(7578): 329.
[88] Théry C, Ostrowski M, Segura E. Membrane vesicles as conveyors of immune responses. Nat Rev Immunol 2009; 9(8): 581.
[89] Viaud S, et al. Dendritic cell-derived exosomes promote natural killer cell activation and proliferation: a role for NKG2D ligands and IL-15Rα. PLoS ONE 2009; 4(3), e4942.
[90] Fabbri M, et al. MicroRNAs bind to Toll-kike receptors to induce prometastatic inflammatory response. Proc Natl Acad Sci 2012; 109(31): E2110-6.
[91] Whiteside TL. Immune modulation of T-cell and NK (natural killer) cell activities by TEXs (tumour-derived exosomes). Portland Press Limited; 2013.
[92] Szczepanski MJ, et al. Blast-derived microvesicles in sera from patients with acute myeloid leukemia suppress natural killer cell function via membrane-associated transforming growth factor-β1. Haematologica 2011; 96(9): 1302-9.
[93] Malmberg K-J, et al. Natural killer cell-mediated immunosurveillance of human cancer. Semin Immunol 2017; 31: 20-9.
[94] Berchem G, et al. Hypoxic tumor-derived microvesicles negatively regulate NK cell function by a mechanism involving TGF-β and miR23a transfer. Oncoimmunology 2016; 5(4): e1062968.
[95] Clayton A, et al. Human tumor-derived exosomes down-modulate NKG2D expression. J Immunol 2008; 180(11): 7249-58.
[96] Cohnen A, et al. Surface CD107a/LAMP-1 protects natural killer cells from degranulationassociated damage. Blood 2013; 122(8): 1411-8.
[97] Filipazzi P, et al. Recent advances on the role of tumor exosomes in immunosuppression and disease progression. Semin Cancer Biol 2012; 22(4): 342-9.
[98] Huang S-H, et al. Epidermal growth factor receptor-containing exosomes induce tumor-specific regulatory T cells. Cancer Invest 2013; 31(5): 330-5.
[99] Zhou M, et al. Pancreatic cancer derived exosomes regulate the expression of TLR4 in dendritic cells via miR-203. Cell Immunol 2014; 292(1-2): 65-9.
[100] Chen W, et al. Tumor-related exosomes contribute to tumor-promoting microenvironment: an immunological perspective. J Immunol Res 2017; 2017: 1073947.
[101] Chalmin F, et al. Membrane-associated Hsp72 from tumor-derived exosomes mediates STAT3-dependent immunosuppressive function of mouse and human myeloid-derived suppressor cells. J Clin Invest 2010; 120(2): 457-71.
[102] Yang C, et al. Tumor-derived exosomes confer antigen-specific immunosuppression in a murine delayed-type hypersensitivity model. PLoS ONE 2011; 6(8), e22517.
[103] Valenti R, et al. Tumor-released microvesicles as vehicles of immunosuppression. Cancer Res 2007; 67(7): 2912-5.
[104] Liu Y, et al. Contribution of MyD88 to the tumor exosome-mediated induction of myeloid derived suppressor cells. Am J Pathol 2010; 176(5): 2490-9.
[105] Song X, et al. Cancer cell-derived exosomes induce mitogen-activated protein kinase-dependent monocyte survival by transport of functional receptor tyrosine kinases. J Biol Chem 2016; 291: 8453-64. https://doi.org/10.1074/jbc.M116.716316.
[106] Ades PA. A controversial step forward: a commentary on the 2013 ACC/AHA guideline on the treatment of blood cholesterol to reduce atherosclerotic cardiovascular risk in adults. Coron Artery Dis 2014; 25(4): 360.
[107] Zhu Y, et al. A comprehensive proteomics analysis reveals a secretory path- and status-dependent signature of exosomes released from tumor-associated macrophages. J Proteome Res 2015; 14(10): 4319-31.
[108] Lamouille S, Xu J, Derynck R. Molecular mechanisms of epithelial-mesenchymal transition. Nat Rev Mol Cell Biol 2014; 15(3): 178.
[109] Rahman MA, et al. Lung cancer exosomes as drivers of epithelial mesenchymal transition. Oncotarget 2016; 7(34): 54852.
[110] Satelli A, Li S. Vimentin in cancer and its potential as a molecular target for cancer therapy. Cell Mol Life Sci 2011; 68(18): 3033-46.
[111] Havel LS, et al. Vimentin regulates lung cancer cell adhesion through a VAV2-Rac1 pathway to control focal adhesion kinase activity. Oncogene 2015; 34(15): 1979.
[112] Wei J, et al. Overexpression of vimentin contributes to prostate cancer invasion and metastasis via src regulation. Anticancer Res 2008; 28(1A): 327-34.
[113] Otsuki S, et al. Vimentin expression is associated with decreased survival in gastric cancer. Oncol Rep 2011; 25(5): 1235-42.
[114] Kim J, et al. Exosome cargo reflects TGF-β1-mediated epithelial-to-mesenchymal transition (EMT) status in A549 human lung adenocarcinoma cells. Biochem Biophys Res Commun 2016; 478(2): 643-8.
[115] Cao M, et al. MiR-23a regulates TGF-β-induced epithelial-mesenchymal transition by targeting E-cadherin in lung cancer cells. Int J Oncol 2012; 41(3): 869-75.
[116] Hsu YL, et al. Hypoxic lung cancer-secreted exosomal miR-23a increased angiogenesis and vascular permeability by targeting prolyl hydroxylase and tight junction protein ZO-1. Oncogene 2017; 36(34): 4929-42.
[117] Chang Y-H, et al. Down-regulation of TIMP-1 inhibits cell migration, invasion, and metastatic colonization in lung adenocarcinoma. Tumour Biol 2015; 36(5): 3957-67.
[118] Rabinowits G, et al. Exosomal microRNA: a diagnostic marker for lung cancer. Clin Lung Cancer 2009; 10(1): 42-6.
[119] Al-Nedawi K, et al. Endothelial expression of autocrine VEGF upon the uptake of tumor-derived microvesicles containing oncogenic EGFR. Proc Natl Acad Sci 2009; 106(10): 3794-9.

[120] Sheu J-J, et al. Administered circulating microparticles derived from lung cancer patients markedly improved angiogenesis, blood flow and ischemic recovery in rat critical limb ischemia. J Transl Med 2015; 13(1): 59.
[121] Lobb RJ, Lima LG, Möller A. Exosomes: key mediators of metastasis and pre-metastatic niche formation. Semin Cell Dev Biol 2017; 67: 3-10.
[122] Janowska-Wieczorek A, et al. Microvesicles derived from activated platelets induce metastasis and angiogenesis in lung cancer. Int J Cancer 2005; 113(5): 752-60.
[123] Peinado H, et al. Melanoma exosomes educate bone marrow progenitor cells toward a prometastatic phenotype through MET. Nat Med 2012; 18(6): 883.
[124] Peinado H, et al. Pre-metastatic niches: organ-specific homes for metastases. Nat Rev Cancer 2017; 17(5): 302-17.
[125] Hiratsuka S, et al. The S100A8 - serum amyloid A3 - TLR4 paracrine cascade establishes a pre-metastatic phase. Nat Cell Biol 2008; 10(11): 1349.
[126] Liu Y, et al. Tumor exosomal RNAs promote lung pre-metastatic niche formation by activating alveolar epithelial TLR3 to recruit neutrophils. Cancer Cell 2016; 30(2): 243-56.
[127] Taverna S, et al. Amphiregulin contained in NSCLC-exosomes induces osteoclast differentiation through the activation of EGFR pathway. Sci Rep 2017; 7(1): 3170.
[128] Dempke WC, Suto T, Reck M. Targeted therapies for non-small cell lung cancer. Lung Cancer 2010; 67(3): 257-74.
[129] Higginbotham JN, et al. Amphiregulin exosomes increase cancer cell invasion. Curr Biol 2011; 21(9): 779-86.
[130] Macklin R, et al. Extracellular vesicles secreted by highly metastatic clonal variants of osteosarcoma preferentially localize to the lungs and induce metastatic behaviour in poorly metastatic clones. Oncotarget 2016; 7(28): 43570.
[131] Velayati AA, et al. Populations of latent *Mycobacterium tuberculosis* lack a cell wall: isolation, visualization, and whole-genome characterization. Int J Mycobacteriol 2016; 5(1): 66-73.
[132] Giri PK, et al. Proteomic analysis identifies highly antigenic proteins in exosomes from *M. tuberculosis*-infected and culture filtrate protein-treated macrophages. Proteomics 2010; 10(17): 3190-202.
[133] Kruh-Garcia NA, Wolfe LM, Dobos KM. Deciphering the role of exosomes in tuberculosis. Tuberculosis (Edinb) 2015; 95(1): 26-30.
[134] Kruh-Garcia NA, et al. Detection of *Mycobacterium tuberculosis* peptides in the exosomes of patients with active and latent *M. tuberculosis* infection using MRM-MS. PLoS ONE 2014; 9(7): e103811.
[135] Booton R, Lindsay MA. Emerging role of MicroRNAs and long noncoding RNAs in respiratory disease. Chest J 2014; 146(1): 193-204.
[136] Schorey JS, et al. Exosomes and other extracellular vesicles in host-pathogen interactions. EMBO Rep 2015; 16(1): 24-43.
[137] Fortune SM, et al. Mycobacterium tuberculosis inhibits macrophage responses to IFN-gamma through myeloid differentiation factor 88-dependent and -independent mechanisms. J Immunol 2004; 172(10): 6272-80.
[138] Singh PP, et al. Exosomes released from *M. tuberculosis* infected cells can suppress IFN-γ mediated activation of naïve macrophages. PLoS ONE 2011; 6(4): e18564.
[139] Singh PP, et al. Exosomes released from *M. tuberculosis* infected cells can suppress IFNgamma mediated activation of naive macrophages. PLoS ONE 2011; 6(4): e18564.
[140] Furci L, et al. Alteration of human macrophages microRNA expression profile upon infection with *Mycobacterium tuberculosis*. Int J Mycobacteriol 2013; 2(3): 128-34.
[141] Singh PP, Li L, Schorey JS. Exosomal RNA from *Mycobacterium tuberculosis*-infected cells is functional in recipient macrophages. Traffic 2015; 16(6): 555-71.
[142] Pearson M. Is the primary mechanism underlying COPD: inflammation or ischaemia? COPD: J Chron Obstruct Pulmon Dis 2013; 10(4): 536-41.
[143] Barnes PJ, Shapiro S, Pauwels R. Chronic obstructive pulmonary disease: molecular and cellularmechanisms. Eur Respir J 2003; 22(4): 672-88.
[144] Kratzer A, et al. Endothelial cell adhesion molecule CD146: implications for its role in the pathogenesis of COPD. J Pathol 2013; 230(4): 388-98.
[145] Takahashi T, Kubo H. The role of microparticles in chronic obstructive pulmonary disease. Int J Chron Obstruct Pulmon Dis 2014; 9: 303.
[146] Di Stefano A, et al. Cellular and molecular mechanisms in chronic obstructive pulmonary disease: an overview. Clin Exp Allergy 2004; 34(8): 1156-67.
[147] Ardekani AM, Naeini MM. The role of microRNAs in human diseases. Avicenna J Med Biotechnol 2010; 2(4): 161.
[148] Li CJ, et al. Novel proteolytic microvesicles released from human macrophages after exposure to tobacco smoke. Am J Pathol 2013; 182(5): 1552-62.
[149] Moon H-G, et al. CCN1 secretion and cleavage regulate the lung epithelial cell functions after cigarette smoke. Am J Physiol Lung Cell Mol Physiol 2014; 307(4): L326-37.
[150] Chew LP, et al. Fast detection of common geometric substructure in proteins. J Comput Biol 1999; 6(3-4): 313-25.
[151] Letsiou E, et al. Pathologic mechanical stress and endotoxin exposure increases lung endothelial microparticle shedding. Am J Respir Cell Mol Biol 2015; 52(2): 193-204.
[152] Sorroche PB, et al. Alpha-1 antitrypsin deficiency in COPD patients: a cross-sectional study. Archivos de Bronconeumología (English Edition) 2015; 51(11): 539-43.
[153] Lockett AD, et al. Active trafficking of alpha 1 antitrypsin across the lung endothelium. PLoS ONE 2014; 9(4): e93979.
[154] Sohal SS, Walters EH. Role of epithelial mesenchymal transition (EMT) in chronic obstructive pulmonary disease (COPD). Respir Res 2013; 14(1): 120.
[155] Vella LJ. The emerging role of exosomes in epithelial-mesenchymal-transition in cancer. Front Oncol 2014; 4: 361.
[156] Donaldson A, et al. Increased skeletal muscle-specific microRNA in the blood of patients with COPD. Thorax 2013;

68: 1140-9. https://doi.org/10.1136/thoraxjnl-2012-203129.
[157] Maertzdorf J, et al. Common patterns and disease-related signatures in tuberculosis and sarcoidosis. Proc Natl Acad Sci 2012; 109(20): 7853-8.
[158] Lin J, et al. Exosomes: novel biomarkers for clinical diagnosis. Scientific World J 2015; 2015: 657086.
[159] Kishore A, et al. Detection of exosomal miRNA in pulmonary sarcoidosis. Eur Respir J 2014; 44(Suppl 58): 199.
[160] Moon H, et al. Lung epithelial cell-derived extracellular vesicles activate macrophage-mediated inflammatory responses via ROCK1 pathway. Cell Death Dis 2015; 6(12), e2016.
[161] Ley B, Collard HR, King Jr. TE. Clinical course and prediction of survival in idiopathic pulmonary fibrosis. Am J Respir Crit Care Med 2011; 183(4): 431-40.
[162] Minnis P, et al. Serum exosomes from IPF patients display a fibrotic miRNA profile that correlates to clinical measures of disease severity. Eur Respiratory Soc 2015; 46: PA3845.
[163] Vituret C, et al. Transfer of the cystic fibrosis transmembrane conductance regulator to human cystic fibrosis cells mediated by extracellular vesicles. Hum Gene Ther 2016; 27(2): 166-83.
[164] Porro C, et al. Isolation and characterization of microparticles in sputum from cystic fibrosis patients. Respir Res 2010; 11(1): 94.
[165] Szul T, et al. Toll-kike receptor 4 engagement mediates prolyl endopeptidase release from airway epithelia via exosomes. Am J Respir Cell Mol Biol 2016; 54(3): 359-69.
[166] Hu G, et al. Release of luminal exosomes contributes to TLR4-mediated epithelial antimicrobial defense. PLoS Pathog 2013; 9(4): e1003261.
[167] Batson B, et al. Qualitative and quantitative changes of gel forming mucins and exosomes in response to infection and inflammation in the airways. In: C60. All about cystic fibrosis. American Thoracic Society; 2016. p. A5565.
[168] Huang L, et al. Exosomes in mesenchymal stem cells, a new therapeutic strategy for cardiovascular diseases? Int J Biol Sci 2015; 11(2): 238.
[169] Zhu YG, et al. Human mesenchymal stem cell microvesicles for treatment of *Escherichia coli* endotoxin-induced acute lung injury in mice. Stem Cells 2014; 32(1): 116-25.
[170] Wilson JG, et al. Mesenchymal stem (stromal) cells for treatment of ARDS: a phase 1 clinical trial. Lancet Respir Med 2015; 3(1): 24-32.
[171] Morse MA, et al. A phase I study of dexosome immunotherapy in patients with advanced non-small cell lung cancer. J Transl Med 2005; 3(1): 9.
[172] Soung YH, et al. Exosomes in cancer diagnostics. Cancer 2017; 9(1): 8.
[173] Dejima H, et al. Exosomal microRNA in plasma as a non-invasive biomarker for the recurrence of non-small cell lung cancer. Oncol Lett 2017; 13(3): 1256-63.
[174] Sandfeld-Paulsen B, et al. Exosomal proteins as prognostic biomarkers in non-small cell lung cancer. Mol Oncol 2016; 10(10): 1595-602.
[175] Alipoor SD, et al. The roles of miRNAs as potential biomarkers in lung diseases. Eur J Pharmacol 2016; 791: 395-404.
[176] Reclusa P, et al. Exosomes genetic cargo in lung cancer: a truly Pandora's box. Transl Lung Cancer Res 2016; 5(5): 483.
[177] Zöller M. Exosomes in cancer disease. In: Cancer gene profiling. Springer; 2016. p.111-49.
[178] Park J, et al. Exosome classification by pattern analysis of surface-enhanced Raman spectroscopy data for lung cancer diagnosis. Anal Chem 2017; 89(12): 6695-701.
[179] Ueda K, et al. Antibody-coupled monolithic silica microtips for highthroughput molecular profiling of circulating exosomes. Sci Rep 2014; 4: 6232.
[180] Jakobsen KR, et al. Exosomal proteins as potential diagnostic markers in advanced nonsmall cell lung carcinoma. J Extracell Vesicles 2015; 4(1): 26659.
[181] Li Y, et al. Proteomic identification of exosomal LRG1: a potential urinary biomarker for detecting NSCLC. Electrophoresis 2011; 32(15): 1976-83.
[182] Sandfeld-Paulsen B, et al. Exosomal proteins as diagnostic biomarkers in lung cancer. J Thorac Oncol 2016; 11(10): 1701-10.
[183] Munagala R, et al. Bovine milk-derived exosomes for drug delivery. Cancer Lett 2016; 371(1): 48-61.
[184] Yang T, et al. Exosome delivered anticancer drugs across the blood-brain barrier for brain cancer therapy in Danio rerio. Pharm Res 2015; 32(6): 2003-14.
[185] Inamdar S, Nitiyanandan R, Rege K. Emerging applications of exosomes in cancer therapeutics and diagnostics. Bioeng Transl Med 2017; 2(1): 70-80.
[186] Wu YJ, et al. Targeting α V-integrins decreased metastasis and increased survival in a nude rat breast cancer brain metastasis model. J Neurooncol 2012; 110(1): 27-36.
[187] Whiteside TL. Tumor-derived exosomes and their role in cancer progression. In: Advances in clinical chemistry. Elsevier; 2016. p.103-41.

第 18 章

外泌体在视网膜疾病中的作用
Exosomes in retinal diseases

Sarah R. Weber, Mi Zhou, Yuanjun Zhao, Jeffrey M. Sundstrom

Department of Ophthalmology, Penn State College of Medicine, Hershey, PA, United States

一、概述

视网膜是位于眼后部的一种专项分化的感觉组织(图 18-1),其功能是感知光线,并以电信号的形式将图像传递给大脑。视网膜由多层细胞组成,主要类型包括光感受器、水平细胞、双极细胞、无长突细胞和神经节细胞。光感受器层的外层是单层的有丝分裂后细胞,称为视网膜色素上皮(retinal pigment epithelium,RPE)细胞(图 18-1)。此类细胞执行着许多特定功能,对维持视神经视网膜的健康至关重要。

视网膜的血液供应有两个来源:视网膜中央动脉,供应视网膜内层;脉络膜,位于视网膜和巩膜之间的血管层,供应视网膜外层。Bruch 膜由多层细胞外基质组成,与多种视网膜疾病的发病密切相关。Bruch 膜的外层由脉络膜毛细血管的基底膜构成(图 18-1)。Bruch 膜的最内层由 RPE 基底膜构成,中间三层则由胶原纤维和弹性纤维构成。

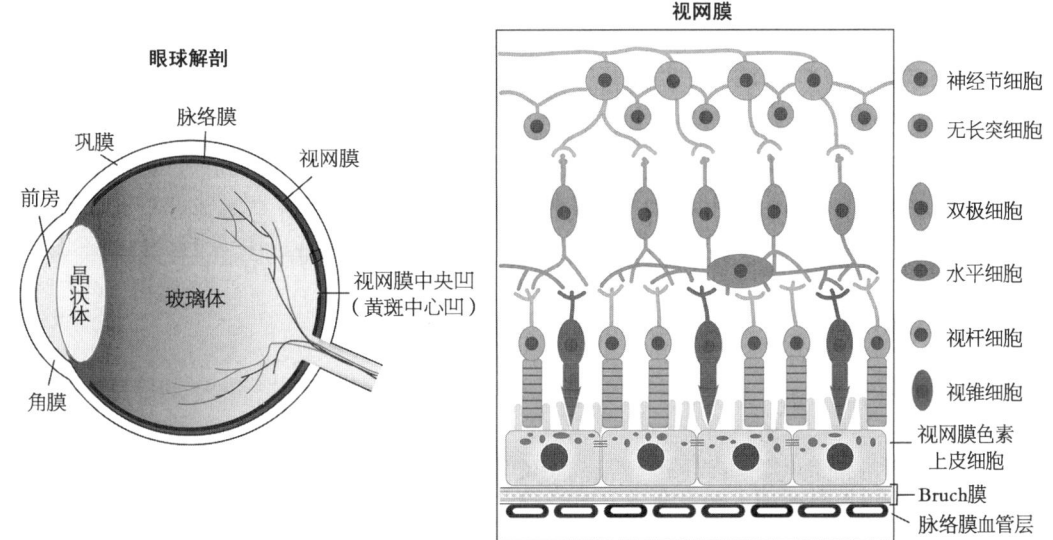

扫描二维码查看彩图

图 18-1 左:全眼横断面解剖图。右:视网膜细胞层示意图,方框区左侧为排列顺序

由于视网膜的本质属性,从伦理角度出发,对患者的视网膜进行活检取材十分困难。因此,对视网膜组织或细胞的直接研究通常来自尸体供眼、动物模型或细胞培养研究,而这些

均不能反映活体状态。另一种可以直接分析患者组织的方法是测试眼内液,通常获取眼内液后对其进行蛋白组学检测,以完成对患者病变组织的分子生物学分析。玻璃体液是最毗邻视网膜组织的生物液体(因此常常被用于视网膜疾病患者的检测)。当然,患者的房水也常被用于研究。这两种体液均可在手术期间或临床检查中安全地从患者身上获得。虽然房水和玻璃体都被认为含有与视网膜疾病相关的蛋白质,而且它们在蛋白质组中确实也表现出一些重叠,但总的来说,它们的蛋白质成分似乎是截然不同的。基于解剖学因素和大量研究表明,玻璃体中存在与视网膜疾病相关的蛋白,故相比房水,我们更推荐玻璃体液活检,因为它毗邻视网膜。

最近在无视网膜血管疾病患者的玻璃体中发现了大量的外泌体(EV的一种亚类),证实了玻璃体液可以反映视网膜疾病的这一假说。这一发现在没有眼部疾病的尸体供眼和小鼠中也得到了验证。房水中也发现了外泌体的存在。

不论是对于健康还是疾病的细胞,EV均在细胞间的通信中发挥作用。大多数类型的细胞都能分泌EV,所以其功能在很多系统中被广泛应用。由于EV在许多病理过程中大量存在并且发挥着不可或缺的作用,因此它们经常被当作生物标志物的来源。基于EV的疗法也是一个新兴的研究领域。尽管这些研究领域不断扩大,但眼部EV的研究却没有跟上步伐。我们对EV在视网膜疾病中的作用缺乏了解,尽管已有相关研究证实玻璃体中含有大量外泌体对其邻近的视网膜有潜在作用。幸运的是,关于EV在疾病中一般机制的研究为我们提供了有价值的发现,这有助于视网膜病理的初步研究。这些研究包括氧化应激、ER应激、炎症和免疫反应、血管生成和肿瘤,这些研究将会在下面的章节中分别进行概述。更多的推论可以从EV参与其他器官系统的发病过程中得到,而这些过程能反映在眼和视网膜疾病中。在接下来的章节中,我们将酌情纳入符合这些标准的EV研究。

EV是一组异质性的囊泡,通常根据其大小、表面标志或生物发生机制分成不同的亚类。因为研究人员在扩大目前关于这些囊泡的知识库,因此这些分类标准在过去几年中一直在变动。EV有两个主要的类型:外泌体和微囊泡。外泌体起源于内涵体,直径50～150 nm;而微囊泡是从质膜上脱落的,通常直径在50～500 nm。在本章中,我们将根据原始研究中对EV的分类来定义外囊泡亚型,并使用通用术语"EV"来指代未指定的囊泡和统称外泌体和微囊泡。

二、一般发病机制

(一) 氧化应激

氧化应激是指细胞内存在的具有生物分子破坏性的ROS数量增加。正常的新陈代谢产生ROS,它们被抗氧化物质或酶所拮抗。ROS的产生超过细胞抗氧化能力时,细胞内氧化还原平衡便会紊乱,导致疾病的发生。

遗传性和老年性黄斑变性的病理变化与氧化应激的水平升高有关。在这些疾病中,视网膜细胞的逐渐退化导致了失明。黄斑变性的特征是在视网膜或RPE下形成沉积物。在年龄相关性黄斑变性(age-related macular degeneration,AMD)中,这些沉积物被称为玻璃膜疣。当沉积物数量和体积增加时,它们就会融合在一起,从而阻碍其上细胞获取营养。最终,大片视网膜组织萎缩并死亡,这种病变被称为地图状萎缩(geographic atrophy,GA),并称为晚期干性 AMD;而湿性 AMD 的定义则是:来自脉络膜的异常形成的新生血管(neovascularization,NV)通过 Bruch 膜断裂的缝隙生长到视网膜内(图 18-2)。

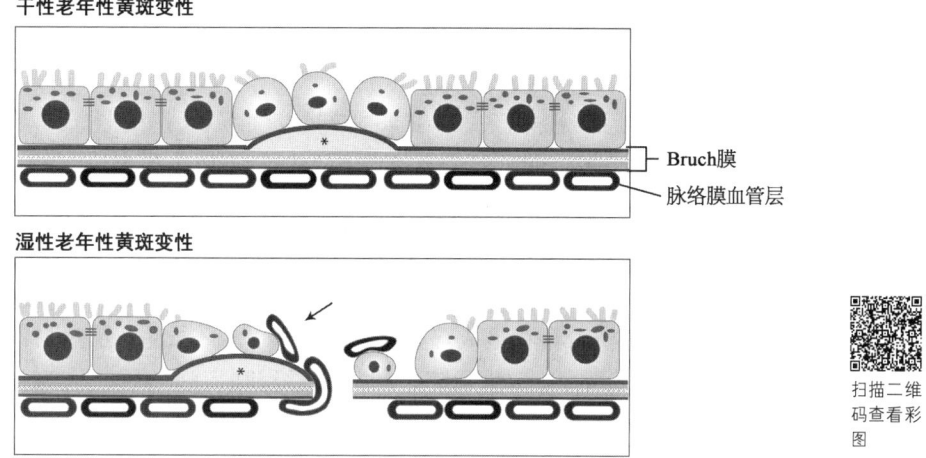

星号(*)表示玻璃膜疣;箭头表示新生血管。

图 18-2　干性和湿性老年性黄斑变性的病理示意图

AMD 的发生与产生氧化应激的环境因素有关。与氧化应激损伤相关的黄斑变性病损,多数情况下与 RPE 细胞的损伤相关。氧化应激引起细胞坏死后细胞的残骸碎片等堆积,最终导致 AMD 的玻璃膜疣和 GA。此外,氧化分子的积累可能破坏 RPE 调节血管生成的能力,导致 NV。多项研究已经证明了外泌体在这些氧化应激诱导的 RPE 变化中具有潜在的作用。例如,在一项使用 ARPE-19 细胞的研究中,Wang 等检测了暴露于 CS 中的有毒成分(已知的 AMD 危险因素)对 RPE 的影响,发现了外泌体标志物 CD63、CD81 和 LAMP2 均有所增加。在 AMD 患者的玻璃膜疣中也发现了这三种蛋白。

外泌体对确诊为 GA 的 AMD 患者中同样具有一定作用。最近,Shah 等提出 EV 可能是造成 RPE 长距离损伤的介质,最终造成了 GA。从那些受氧化应激损伤的原代培养的 RPE 细胞中获取的 EV,如果直接作用于受体的 RPE 单层,将会引起其屏障功能的损伤。这种效应是由组蛋白去乙酰化酶 6 介导的,该酶调节了氧化应激介导的自噬反应。

其他研究人员已经证明了在氧化应激条件下的外泌体有促血管生成的潜在作用。众所周知,ROS 能刺激 VEGF 的表达,而 VEGF 是促进视网膜疾病如黄斑变性和糖尿病视网膜病变(diabetic retinopathy,DR)血管生成的主要因素。研究表明,ARPE-19 细胞在氧化应激条件下分泌的外泌体数量增加,这些囊泡内容物更有利于血管生成,使更多的 VEGF 受体,如 VEGFR-1、VEGFR-2 膜蛋白和微囊化信使(m)RNA 的表达增加,造成更强的诱导体外血管生成的能力。ARPE-19 细胞受到氧化应激损伤后,其分泌的外泌体内蛋白质的磷酸化状态发生改变,研究发现这些蛋白质与细胞凋亡、细胞存活和代谢途径有关。

我们需要进一步研究 EV 在视网膜病理下的氧化应激中作用,但从 RPE 源性外泌体研究来看,外囊泡和氧化应激是有内在联系的。

(二)内质网应激

蛋白质生物合成和降解之间的平衡以及正确折叠蛋白质的能力都是维持细胞内稳态的关键因素。ER 是这些过程的主调节器,当它们失去平衡时,内质网应激发生。细胞对内质网应激的反应是激活下游信号通路,统称为未折叠蛋白反应(unfolded protein response,UPR),其目的是通过适当的蛋白质折叠、翻译(终止)、加速降解(如果损伤无法修复)或凋亡来恢复平衡。

ER 应激与多种视网膜疾病有关。在多种遗传性视网膜变性(inherited retinal degenerations,IRD)中,突变的、错误折叠的蛋白质可能在 ER 中积累,从而引起应激反应。造成 IRD 的基因突变包括:编码视紫红质、光感受器维生素 A 结合蛋白、碳酸酐酶Ⅳ和纤维蛋白-3 的基因。其他引起 IRD 的突变,如 ELOVL 脂肪酸延伸酶 4、磷酸二酯酶 6B 和 Usherin 蛋白,这些反应与 ER 应激和 UPR 介质的上调有关。IRD 和 AMD 都具有沉积物的特征,而沉积物是由蛋白质聚集物组成,这显示了蛋白质代谢紊乱。虽然目前缺乏直接证据证明外泌体参与了这些情况,但其他系统中的类似过程和疾病的研究已为我们积累了大量证据。

最近研究发现,ER 应激增加外泌体的释放。其他研究表明,在中枢神经系统的神经退行性疾病中,外泌体在朊病毒的传播和聚集中起着重要作用。这些疾病的特点是不溶性蛋白质聚集物的异常积累,如阿尔茨海默病中的 β 淀粉样蛋白斑块、帕金森病中的 α-突触核蛋白聚集,以及多种朊病毒病中的朊蛋白斑块。已有研究证明,外泌体分泌的多种 Aβ 肽,有助于阿尔茨海默病 β-淀粉样斑块的形成以及促进在培养的胶质细胞中的蛋白聚集。在阿尔茨海默病和帕金森病中形成聚集的 Tau 蛋白也可以通过外泌体分泌,来自阿尔茨海默病患者的 CSF 来源的外泌体已被证明在体外增加 Tau 蛋白聚集。同样,α-突触核蛋白可以通过外泌体分泌,并且外泌体相关形式的 a-突触核蛋白比其自由形式对受体细胞的毒性更大。朊病毒蛋白也被证明与外泌体有关,最近发现刺激外泌体分泌可增加细胞间朊病毒传播。除了分泌和毒性,外泌体还可能在这些疾病中发挥沉积形成的作用。这些病与黄斑变性的沉积形成具有一致性,即可能视网膜变性与神经退行性疾病的沉积物的形成机制相似。在 AMD 尸体供眼中,已在视网膜下沉积物中鉴定出 129 种蛋白质,其中 20% 的成分与阿尔茨海默斑块和 AMD 沉积物相同。IRD 中的沉积物在表型和成分上与 AMD 相似,并且在至少一个 IRD 中的沉积物中发现了淀粉样肽。因此,外泌体可能在黄斑变性的沉积形成中起着类似的作用。

除了在传播病理变化中的潜在作用,外泌体还可能在维持蛋白质平衡方面发挥作用。分子伴侣如 HSP,是维持蛋白质平衡的主要参与者,因为它们有助于蛋白质折叠的过程,并帮助折叠不当的蛋白质降解。因此,HSP 在应激反应中被上调。Takeuchi 等研究表明分子伴侣 HSP40、HSP70 和 HSP90 是通过外泌体分泌的。重要的是,含有这些蛋白质的外泌体减少了神经退行性疾病模型中的蛋白聚集形成,有助于维持蛋白质平衡。有研究观察到,在 AMD 中视网膜的 HSP 表达增加,RPE 中的 HSP 表达降低。

另一种较小的伴侣蛋白,αB-晶状体蛋白,是由 RPE 通过外泌体分泌的,对邻近的光感受器具有神经保护作用。在 RPE 培养中,抑制 αB-结晶蛋白的表达致使外泌体分泌受阻,突显了αB-晶状体蛋白与外泌体的整体相互作用。αB-晶状体蛋白具有广泛的降低蛋白质聚集的能力，并与许多神经退行性疾病有关，包括阿尔茨海默病、帕金森病和朊病毒病。也有人提出，αB-晶状体蛋白可能是AMD的生物标志物，因为有研究显示它在AMD患者的RPE中表达升高，且在一定程度上与疾病的严重程度相关。在对玻璃膜疣的蛋白质组学分析中发现，αB-晶状体蛋白是最具有差异性的蛋白质之一。由于αB-晶状体蛋白与外泌体关系密切，并与异常蛋白聚集的疾病相关，αB-晶状体蛋白可能是通过外泌体介导ER应激机制在黄斑变性中发挥作用。

这些来自视网膜细胞和其他系统的研究结果表明，ER应激对视网膜病理的影响可能在一定程度上是由外泌体介导的。除了在疾病状态下发挥作用，外泌体还可能在视网膜细胞中维持蛋白质稳态和预防因ER应激而加重的疾病方面发挥作用。

（三）炎症和免疫反应

虽然眼球内部基本呈现免疫豁免的状态，但是异常的炎症反应或免疫反应也能引起或加重多种视网膜疾病。炎症反应可以引起多种疾病，如葡萄膜炎、AMD和DR（炎症是多种致病因素之一）。

葡萄膜炎是葡萄膜的一种炎症，可以根据受影响的特定结构以及炎症的原因分成不同亚类。在这里，我们关注的是影响视网膜的自身免疫性葡萄膜炎。

葡萄膜炎是葡萄膜受到T淋巴细胞活化损伤所引起，其特征是眼内液及血清内细胞因子的含量发生变化。众所周知，RPE在眼睛中具有免疫抑制和抑制T细胞活性的功能，而且研究表明，EV在其他系统中可介导免疫活性。最新研究显示，RPE源性EV可能在介导葡萄膜炎炎症中发挥作用。Knickelbein等研究证明RPE源性EV与来自非感染性葡萄膜炎患者的外周血单个核细胞一起培养可以抑制T细胞的增殖。当与单核细胞一起培养时，RPE源性EV增加了单核细胞的数量，这些单核细胞属于已知的调节非感染性葡萄膜炎患者免疫反应的亚群。来自其他细胞类型的EV也可能发挥类似的免疫抑制作用。Bai等最近证明了MSC源性外泌体在自身免疫性葡萄膜视网膜炎大鼠模型中有治疗作用。具体来说，他们发现在眼周注射MSC源性外泌体，可以通过减少免疫细胞（包括T细胞）进入眼睛的迁移来抑制疾病程度。

与葡萄膜炎相比，免疫激活和炎症也在AMD中起到作用，虽然表现没有那么明显。多项研究表明，补体成分的遗传多态性与AMD有一定的联系。在对AMD供体黄斑的Bruch膜和脉络膜组织的蛋白质组学分析中发现，大多数鉴定的蛋白质都参与到免疫或防御中。在眼内负责众多免疫调节的细胞，即RPE，同样是AMD中主要受影响的细胞类型。RPE能分泌调节分子（如肿瘤生长因子β），并在细胞膜上表达补体调节蛋白。炎症在AMD进展中的作用可能部分是由外泌体介导的。RPE表达的补体调节蛋白有CD59和CD46。在一项关于AMD眼黄斑的研究中发现，这些蛋白水平在有病理改变的区域下降。在使用补体触发化合物处理的ARPE-19细胞中，CD59和CD46水平也降低了。由于上清液中CD59和CD46染色的增加与外泌体标志物显著重叠，本研究的作者提出，这些蛋白应该是由RPE通过外泌体释放的。这进一步证实了外泌体在RPE免疫调节中可能会发生作用，已有证据显示，再用促炎细胞因子刺激后，RPE 源性 EV 数量普遍增加。

在 AMD 和 DR 中，因失去分裂能力而衰老的衰老细胞，似乎具有影响炎症的作用。衰老的一个主要表现为衰老相关分泌表型（senescence associated secretory phenotype，SASP）表达上调，而这部分的特征是促炎因子和其他分子的表达上调。有实验证实，在暴露于氧化应激的 ARPE-19 细胞中，SASP 标记的表达增加。此外，衰老的 ARPE-19 细胞显示 VEGF 表达增加，补体因子 H（complement factor H，CFH）表达减少。由于 RPE 分泌的 VEGF 在湿性 AMD 中促进新生血管生成，故 CFH 的多态性与 AMD 的易感性相关，因此本研究的结果提示 RPE 衰老与 AMD 的病理密切相关。SASP 还被证明在缺血视网膜病变的小鼠模型中发挥病理作用，在该模型中，玻璃体内注入 SASP 抑制剂可降低视网膜 NV。在同一项研究中，从增生型糖尿病视网膜病变（proliferative diabetic retinopathy，PDR）患者的玻璃体中鉴定出 SASP 标志物，包括纤溶酶原激活物抑制物 1、IL-6、IL-8 和 VEGF。玻璃体中 SASP 标志物的水平，包括 IL-6、IL-8 和 CC 类趋化因子 2，也被证明与该疾病中 NV 的驱动因子 VEGF 密切相关。越来越多的证据表明，EV 在衰老中起着重要的作用，因此它们可能在导致 AMD 和 DR 的衰老变化中发挥作用。目前已证明 EV 的分泌随着衰老而增加，这可能是衰老细胞清除无用 DNA 的一种机制。如上所述，SASP 与多种促炎细胞因子的上调有关。最新研究表明，许多细胞因子，包括许多与 SASP 相关的细胞因子与 EV 的协同分泌有关，且这种协同作用是动态的和系统依赖性的。

基于外泌体在其他系统炎症中的既定作用，以及视网膜色素上皮细胞分泌的外泌体、衰老和 EV 相关细胞因子的新证据表明，外泌体可能在多种视网膜疾病中促进免疫激活和炎症反应。

（四）视网膜和脉络膜血管生成

异常血管形成，称为 NV，发生在许多视网膜疾病中，往往导致严重的视力损伤。根据新形成的病理血管，与视网膜疾病相关的 NV 命名为视网膜型或脉络膜型。视网膜 NV 发生于 DR、早产儿视网膜病变、视网膜静脉阻塞和其他视网膜病变；而脉络膜 NV 是渗出性 AMD、其他黄斑变性、近视和创伤等疾病的特征性表现。虽然在解剖学上是不同的，但这两种类型的 NV 都是由共同的血管生成因子驱动，并且受到共同的抗血管生成因子抑制。视网膜中的主要血管生成因子包括 VEGF、成纤维细胞生长因子（fibroblast growth factor，FGF）-2、血管生成素和 Tie2、Wnt 和基质金属蛋白酶（matrix metalloproteinase，MMP）；而抗血管生成因子包括色素上皮源性因子（pigment epithelium derived factor，PEDF）、血管抑素和内皮抑素。虽然目前有关外泌体调控视网膜或脉络膜 NV 的研究较少，但是来自其他领域的大量证据表明，EV 在其他系统的血管生成中起着不可或缺的作用。

RPE 源性外泌体是大多数研究 EV 在视网膜或脉络膜 NV 中作用的焦点。最新研究表明，ARPE-19 细胞源性外泌体中的 VEGFR 蛋白和 mRNA 在应激下增加，并能在体外刺激血管生成。RPE 源性外泌体也可能有介导抗血管生成的特性。Naga 等研究发现，玻璃体内注射的抗 VEGF 抗体贝伐单抗能够穿透视网膜被视网膜色素上皮细胞吸收，它们似乎是从 RPE 中通过外泌体释放出来的。抗血管生成因子 PEDF 由 RPE 细胞顶端分泌，以防止视网膜发生异常的血管生成，该因子在 RPE 源性外泌体中被鉴定出来，并在顶端分泌的囊泡中存在的比例更大。已有研究证实，另一种具有抗血管生成特性的蛋白质，即过氧化物酶体增殖物激活受体 γ，被证明在 PDR 患者的玻璃体和房水中升高。由于过氧化物酶增殖物激活受体 γ 存在于体循环血浆外泌体中，因此推测其也可能在眼内液中与外泌体相关。

其他研究也评估了来自其他细胞类型的外泌体对视网膜的影响。在低氧条件下培养的 MSC 源性外泌体可减少玻璃体内注射氧化诱导视网膜病变小鼠模型的视网膜缺血。在激光诱导的脉络膜 NV 小鼠模型中，视网膜星形胶质细胞来源的外泌体含有抗血管生成分子，能够抑制视网膜血管的渗漏和脉络膜 NV。在该模型中，RPE 源性外泌体没有这些作用。

关于 EV 参与 NV 的进一步证据来自其他系统。驱动视网膜和脉络膜 NV 的多种血管生成因子已在外泌体或其他 EV 中被发现。肿瘤来源的外泌体已被证明能够向其他细胞输送 VEGF 和类似的生长因子以及促血管生成 mRNA 和 miRNA。此外，来自健康细胞的外泌体已被证明能刺激 VEGF mRNA 在体外的表达。微囊相关的 VEGF 已被证明比游离 VEGF 更能持续激活 VEGF 受体，并对贝伐单抗不敏感，导致 EV 相关 VEGF 诱导无法阻断 VEGF 信号。在胶质母细胞瘤模型中，用血管生成因子 FGF-2 也观察到类似的效果。在这项研究中，与单独使用 FGF-2 相比，胶质母细胞瘤衍生的外泌体富含 FGF-2 共受体，并刺激血管形成增加。在外囊泡中也发现了 Tie2 信号组分。具体来说，血管生成素（angiopoietin，Ang）1 和 Ang2 蛋白已被证明是在外泌体中分泌的，而较大的 EV 已被证明含有 Ang1 mRNA。许多研究已经报道了外泌体分泌 Wnt 信号通路组分，并且已经证明很大一部分活性 Wnt 通路组分是由这些囊泡分泌的。MMP 也是血管生成的关键因素，因为它们降解 ECM，使新的血管生长。活性 MMP 以前已经在外泌体上被鉴定出来。研究表明，用肿瘤细胞分泌的外泌体处理可以刺激受体细胞分泌多种 MMP 和 VEGFA。研究还发现，肿瘤细胞衍生的过表达 MMP-13 的外泌体可以刺激血管生成。

虽然对视网膜和脉络膜 NV 的研究有限，但初步研究表明，EV 在视网膜疾病的 NV 中起着重要作用。上述的理论可以通过 EV 在其他系统中促血管生成的能力证实，且值得进一步研究 EV 对视网膜与脉络膜血管新生的作用。

（五）肿瘤

外泌体被公认在肿瘤中发挥着作用，而且在不同的器官系统中，外泌体对肿瘤生态影响的证据不断增加。它们已被证明在肿瘤中介导免疫反应，影响肿瘤的微环境，并促进肿瘤转移。例如，来自 APC 的外泌体已被证明可促进小鼠对抗肿瘤的免疫应答。在肿瘤微环境中，有研究观察到双向囊泡效应。在一项研究中，前列腺肿瘤细胞分泌的外泌体可激活肿瘤微环境中的成纤维细胞；而在另一项研究中，来自肿瘤相关成纤维细胞的外泌体可诱导乳腺肿瘤细胞源性外泌体发生肿瘤前侵袭性改变。肿瘤细胞来源的外泌体能够通过促进 ECM 降解、定向器官和建立转移前龛帮助转移。

除了这些功能研究，外泌体也越来越多地被作为肿瘤的生物标志物进行研究，外泌体的 miRNA 通常是研究的重点。外泌体的作用是保护这些在肿瘤中经常失调的核酸。越来多的证据表明，miRNA 的功能作用与上述外泌体的功能类似。虽然与肿瘤领域的一般情况相比有局限性，但一些证据表明外泌体 miRNA 在葡萄膜黑色素瘤中存在调节障碍。葡萄膜黑色素瘤是最常见的原发性眼内肿瘤，起源于黑色素细胞。它的预后很差，大约一半的患者死于肿瘤转移，患者的 5 年生存率低。最常见的转移器官是肝脏（90%）。Eldh 等的一项研究在葡萄膜黑色素瘤患者的肝脏灌注液中发现了黑色素瘤特异性标志物黑色素-A 阳性的外泌体，表明肿瘤来源的外泌体到达了这些患者的转移部位。与黑色素瘤细胞系相比，这些小泡的 miRNA 含量分析显示了不同的 miRNA 装载。另一项研究检查了葡萄膜黑色素瘤患者的玻璃体、玻璃体外泌体和血清中的 miRNA，并将它们与非病理性对照患者进行了比较。他们发现，在至少 2/3 的样本中，有 32 个差异表达的 miRNA，其中大多数变化都在玻璃体和玻璃体外泌体中发生。

外泌体在肿瘤方面被广泛研究，这项研究的结果可以指导对眼部肿瘤的进一步研究。最近对葡萄膜黑色素瘤中 miRNA 失调的研究为外泌体在眼部的研究应用奠定了基础。

三、基于外泌体的治疗方法

除了上述发现表明外泌体导致了视网膜病理改变，其他一些数据也证明了外泌体对视网膜有治疗作用。这些研究大多关注的是 MSC 源性外泌体。这些囊泡往往比干细胞本身更受青睐，因为 MSC 的治疗效果似乎主要来自它们分泌的可溶性因子，而且使用非细胞的方法避免了细胞移植固有的安全性问题。一些研究已经检查了 MSC 源性外泌体在视网膜中的作用。Mead 等观察到在大鼠视神经挤压模型中，玻璃体内注射骨髓来源的 MSC 外泌体后，视网膜神经节细胞的存活率和轴突再生增加。在原代视网膜细胞培养中，这些囊泡显示出神经保护作用。同样，Yu 等观察到在激光诱导的视网膜病变小鼠模型中，玻璃体内注射 MSC 源性外泌体后，激光损伤、凋亡和炎症减少。如上所述，MSC 源性外泌体也通过抑制炎症细胞向眼睛迁移的方法来减轻实验性自身免疫性葡萄膜炎大鼠模型的严重程度。在自身免疫性葡萄膜炎小鼠模型中，MSC 源性 EV 可预防疾病的发生和抑制免疫细胞的激活。

除了作为治疗本身，外泌体可能能够加强其他已经在使用的治疗技术。Wassmer 等证明，在小鼠玻璃体内注射外泌体相关腺病毒（adeno-associated virus，AAV）2 后，相对于传统的 AAV2 介导的转染，外泌体相关 AAV2 可以更好地使基因传递到视网膜。作为最近被美国 IRD 批准的首个基因疗法，这些发现为未来人类视网膜疾病的应用提供了一个基础框架。

由于 EV 在视网膜疾病中的作用才刚刚被发现，它们在这些条件下的治疗应用也才刚刚开始。根据我们提到的研究，基于 EV 的疗法是未来治疗视网膜疾病的一个有希望的选项。

四、总结

从其他领域可以明显看出，EV 在健康和疾病中都发挥着不可或缺的作用。虽然数据表明外泌体在视网膜健康和疾病中的直接作用才刚刚开始积累，但来自其他领域的推论已为我们提供了初步证据，并为进一步的研究提供了前提。大量研究已经揭示了 EV 在视网膜疾病和其他组织疾病普遍病理机制中的作用，这些机制包括氧化应激、ER 应激、炎症和免疫反应、血管生成和肿瘤发生。最新的研究表明，EV 对视网膜也有治疗作用。为了扩大和加深对这些主题的理解，我们需要更多进一步的研究。

（李文哲　徐泽全　黄扬　译，吴文灿　审校）

参考文献

[1] Van der Lelij A, Rothova A. Diagnostic anterior chamber paracentesis in uveitis: a safe procedure? Br J Ophthalmol 1997; 81(11): 976-9.
[2] Ghodasra DH, et al. Safety and feasibility of quantitative multiplexed cytokine analysis from office-based vitreous aspiration. Invest Ophthalmol Vis Sci 2016; 57(7): 3017-23.
[3] Ecker SM, Hines JC, Pfahler SM, Glaser BM. Aqueous cytokine and growth factor levels do not reliably reflect those levels found in the vitreous. Mol Vis 2011; 17: 2856-63.
[4] Aiello LP, et al. Vascular endothelial growth factor in ocular fluid of patients with diabetic retinopathy and other retinal disorders. N Engl J Med 1994; 331(22): 1480-7.
[5] Zhao Y, et al. Liquid biopsy of vitreous reveals an abundant vesicle population consistent with the size and morphology of exosomes. Transl Vis Sci Technol 2018; 7(3): 6.
[6] Schori C, et al. The proteomic landscape in the vitreous of patients with age-related and diabetic retinal disease. Invest Ophthalmol Vis Sci 2018; 59(4): AMD31-40.
[7] Klaassen I, et al. Identification of proteins associated with clinical and pathological features of proliferative diabetic retinopathy in vitreous and fibrovascular membranes. PLoS One 2017; 12(11): e0187304.
[8] Nobl M, et al. Proteomics of vitreous in neovascular age-related macular degeneration. Exp Eye Res 2016; 146: 107-17.
[9] Bromberg-White JL, et al. Identification of VEGF-independent cytokines in proliferative diabetic retinopathy vitreous. Invest Ophthalmol Vis Sci 2013; 54: 6472-80.
[10] Dismuke WM, et al. Human aqueous humor exosomes. Exp Eye Res 2015; 132: 73-7.
[11] Tetta C, et al. Extracellular vesicles as an emerging mechanism of cell-to-cell communication. Endocrine 2013; 44(1): 11-9.
[12] Mallocci M, et al. Extracellular vesicles: mechanisms in human health and disease. Antioxid Redox Signal 2018; 30(6): 813-56.
[13] van Niel G, D'Angelo G, Raposo G. Shedding light on the cell biology of extracellular vesicles. Nat Rev Mol Cell Biol 2018; 19: 213-28.
[14] Schieber M, Chandel NS. ROS function in redox signaling and oxidative stress. Curr Biol 2014; 24(10): R453-62.
[15] Wang W, et al. Genetic and environmental factors strongly influence risk, severity and progression of age-related macular degeneration. Signal Transduct Target Ther 2016; 1: 16016.
[16] Brantley MA, Umfress AC, Sternberg P. Mechanisms of oxidative stress in retinal injury. In: Schachat AP, editor. Ryan's retina. Elsevier Inc; 2018.
[17] Beatty S, et al. The role of oxidative stress in the pathogenesis of age-related macular degeneration. Surv Ophthalmol 2000; 45(2): 115-34.
[18] Wang AL, et al. Changes in retinal pigment epithelium related to cigarette smoke: possible relevance to smoking as a risk factor for age-related macular degeneration. PLoS One 2009; 4(4): e5304.
[19] Wang AL, et al. Autophagy and exosomes in the aged retinal pigment epithelium: possible relevance to drusen formation and age-related macular degeneration. PLoS One 2009; 4(1): e4160.
[20] Shah N, et al. Extracellular vesicle-mediated long-range communication in stressed retinal pigment epithelial cell monolayers. Biochim Biophys Acta Mol basis Dis 2018; 1864(8): 2610-22.
[21] Lee JY, et al. HDAC6 controls autophagosome maturation essential for ubiquitin-selective quality-control autophagy. EMBO J 2010; 29(5): 969-80.
[22] Fay J, et al. Reactive oxygen species induce expression of vascular endothelial growth factor in chondrocytes and human articular cartilage explants. Arthritis Res Ther 2006; 8(6): R189.
[23] Amadio M, Govoni S, Pascale A. Targeting VEGF in eye neovascularization: what's new?: a comprehensive review on current therapies and oligonucleotide-based interventions under development. Pharmacol Res 2016; 103: 253-69.
[24] Atienzar-Aroca S, et al. Oxidative stress in retinal pigment epithelium cells increases exosome secretion and promotes angiogenesis in endothelial cells. J Cell Mol Med 2016; 20(8): 1457-66.
[25] Biasutto L, et al. Retinal pigment epithelium (RPE) exosomes contain signaling phosphoproteins affected by oxidative stress. Exp Cell Res 2013; 319(13): 2113-23.
[26] Hetz C. The unfolded protein response: controlling cell fate decisions under ER stress and beyond. Nat Rev Mol Cell Biol 2012; 13(2): 89-102.
[27] Li S, et al. Secretory defect and cytotoxicity: the potential disease mechanisms for the retinitis pigmentosa (RP)-associated interphotoreceptor retinoid-binding protein (IRBP). J Biol Chem 2013; 288(16): 11395-406.
[28] Gorbatyuk MS, et al. Restoration of visual function in P23H rhodopsin transgenic rats by gene delivery of BiP/Grp78. Proc Natl Acad Sci U S A 2010; 107(13): 5961-6.

[29] Rebello G, et al. Apoptosis-inducing signal sequence mutation in carbonic anhydrase IV identified in patients with the RP17 form of retinitis pigmentosa. Proc Natl Acad Sci U S A 2004; 101(17): 6617-22.

[30] Marmorstein LY, et al. Aberrant accumulation of EFEMP1 underlies drusen formation in Malattia Leventinese and age-related macular degeneration. Proc Natl Acad Sci U S A 2002; 99(20): 13067-72.

[31] Karan G, et al. Loss of ER retention and sequestration of the wild-type ELOVL4 by Stargardt disease dominant negative mutants. Mol Vis 2005; 11: 657-64.

[32] Yang LP, et al. Activation of endoplasmic reticulum stress in degenerating photoreceptors of the rd1 mouse. Invest Ophthalmol Vis Sci 2007; 48(11): 5191-8.

[33] Tucker BA, et al. Patient-specific iPSC-derived photoreceptor precursor cells as a means to investigate retinitis pigmentosa. elife 2013; 2: e00824.

[34] Kanemoto S, et al. Multivesicular body formation enhancement and exosome release during endoplasmic reticulum stress. Biochem Biophys Res Commun 2016; 480(2): 166-72.

[35] Lim YJ, Lee SJ. Are exosomes the vehicle for protein aggregate propagation in neurodegenerative diseases? Acta Neuropathol Commun 2017; 5(1): 64.

[36] Rajendran L, et al. Alzheimer's disease beta-amyloid peptides are released in association with exosomes. Proc Natl Acad Sci U S A 2006; 103(30): 11172-7.

[37] Dinkins MB, et al. Exosome reduction in vivo is associated with lower amyloid plaque load in the 5XFAD mouse model of Alzheimer's disease. Neurobiol Aging 2014; 35(8): 1792-800.

[38] Saman S, et al. Exosome-associated tau is secreted in tauopathy models and is selectively phosphorylated in cerebrospinal fluid in early Alzheimer disease. J Biol Chem 2012; 287(6): 3842-9.

[39] Wang Y, et al. The release and trans-synaptic transmission of Tau via exosomes. Mol Neurodegener 2017; 12(1): 5.

[40] Emmanouilidou E, et al. Cell-produced alpha-synuclein is secreted in a calcium-dependent manner by exosomes and impacts neuronal survival. J Neurosci 2010; 30(20): 6838-51.

[41] Danzer KM, et al. Exosomal cell-to-cell transmission of alpha synuclein oligomers. Mol Neurodegener 2012; 7: 42.

[42] Cheng L, Zhao W, Hill AF. Exosomes and their role in the intercellular trafficking of normal and disease associated prion proteins. Mol Asp Med 2018; 60: 62-8.

[43] Guo BB, Bellingham SA, Hill AF. Stimulating the release of exosomes increases the intercellular transfer of prions. J Biol Chem 2016; 291(10): 5128-37.

[44] Yuyama K, Yamamoto N, Yanagisawa K. Accelerated release of exosome-associated GM1 ganglioside (GM1) by endocytic pathway abnormality: another putative pathway for GM1-induced amyloid fibril formation. J Neurochem 2008; 105(1): 217-24.

[45] Grey M, et al. Acceleration of alpha-synuclein aggregation by exosomes. J Biol Chem 2015; 290(5): 2969-82.

[46] Booij JC, et al. The dynamic nature of Bruch's membrane. Prog Retin Eye Res 2010; 29(1): 1-18.

[47] Sohn EH, et al. Comparison of drusen and modifying genes in autosomal dominant radial drusen and age-related macular degeneration_Fibulin 3 IHC. Retina 2015; 35(1): 48-57.

[48] Hartl FU, Bracher A, Hayer-Hartl M. Molecular chaperones in protein folding and proteostasis. Nature 2011; 475 (7356): 324-32.

[49] Takeuchi T. Non-cell autonomous maintenance of proteostasis by molecular chaperones and its molecular mechanism. Biol Pharm Bull 2018; 41(6): 843-9.

[50] Takeuchi T, et al. Intercellular chaperone transmission via exosomes contributes to maintenance of protein homeostasis at the organismal level. Proc Natl Acad Sci U S A 2015; 112(19): E2497-506.

[51] Kaarniranta K, et al. Heat shock proteins as gatekeepers of proteolytic pathways-implications for age-related macular degeneration (AMD). Ageing Res Rev 2009; 8(2): 128-39.

[52] Nordgaard CL, et al. Proteomics of the retinal pigment epithelium reveals altered protein expression at progressive stages of age-related macular degeneration. Invest Ophthalmol Vis Sci 2006; 47(3): 815-22.

[53] Sreekumar PG, et al. alphaB crystallin is apically secreted within exosomes by polarized human retinal pigment epithelium and provides neuroprotection to adjacent cells. PLoS One 2010; 5(10): e12578.

[54] Gangalum RK, et al. Inhibition of the expression of the small heat shock protein alphaBcrystallin inhibits exosome secretion in human retinal pigment epithelial cells in culture. J Biol Chem 2016; 291(25): 12930-42.

[55] Horwitz J. The function of alpha-crystallin in vision. Semin Cell Dev Biol 2000; 11(1): 53-60.

[56] De S, et al. Human retinal pigment epithelium cell changes and expression of alphaB-crystallin: a biomarker for retinal pigment epithelium cell change in age-related macular degeneration. Arch Ophthalmol 2007; 125(5): 641-5.

[57] Crabb JW, et al. Drusen proteome analysis: an approach to the etiology of age-related macular degeneration. Proc Natl Acad Sci U S A 2002; 99(23): 14682-7.

[58] Horai R, Caspi RR. Cytokines in autoimmune uveitis. J Interf Cytokine Res 2011; 31(10): 733-44.

[59] Kaestel CG, et al. The immune privilege of the eye: human retinal pigment epithelial cells selectively modulate T-cell activation in vitro. Curr Eye Res 2005; 30(5): 375-83.

[60] Jorgensen A, et al. Human retinal pigment epithelial cell-induced apoptosis in activated T cells. Invest Ophthalmol Vis Sci 1998; 39(9): 1590-9.

[61] Kim SH, et al. Exosomes derived from IL-10-treated dendritic cells can suppress inflammation and collagen-induced arthritis. J Immunol 2005; 174(10): 6440-8.

[62] Bianco NR, et al. Therapeutic effect of exosomes from indoleamine 2,3-dioxygenase-positive dendritic cells in collagen-induced arthritis and delayed-type hypersensitivity disease models. Arthritis Rheum 2009; 60(2): 380-9.

[63] Robbins PD, Morelli AE. Regulation of immune responses by extracellular vesicles. Nat Rev Immunol 2014; 14(3): 195-208.

[64] Knickelbein JE, et al. Modulation of immune responses by extracellular vesicles from retinal pigment epithelium. Invest Ophthalmol Vis Sci 2016; 57(10): 4101-7.

[65] Bai L, et al. Effects of mesenchymal stem cell-derived exosomes on experimental autoimmune uveitis. Sci Rep 2017; 7(1): 4323.
[66] Hageman GS, et al. Extended haplotypes in the complement factor H (CFH) and CFH-related (CFHR) family of genes protect against age-related macular degeneration: characterization, ethnic distribution and evolutionary implications. Ann Med 2006; 38(8): 592-604.
[67] Edwards AO, et al. Complement factor H polymorphism and age-related macular degeneration. Science 2005; 308(5720): 421-4.
[68] Klein RJ, et al. Complement factor H polymorphism in age-related macular degeneration. Science 2005; 308(5720): 385-9.
[69] Yuan X, et al. Quantitative proteomics: comparison of the macular Bruch membrane/choroid complex from age-related macular degeneration and normal eyes. Mol Cell Proteomics 2010; 9(6): 1031-46.
[70] Hirsch L, et al. TGF-beta2 secretion from RPE decreases with polarization and becomes apically oriented. Cytokine 2015; 71(2): 394-6.
[71] Chen M, Forrester JV, Xu H. Synthesis of complement factor H by retinal pigment epithelial cells is down-regulated by oxidized photoreceptor outer segments. Exp Eye Res 2007; 84(4): 635-45.
[72] Luo C, et al. Complement expression in retinal pigment epithelial cells is modulated by activated macrophages. Exp Eye Res 2013; 112: 93-101.
[73] Ebrahimi KB, et al. Oxidized low-density-kipoprotein-induced injury in retinal pigment epithelium alters expression of the membrane complement regulatory factors CD46 and CD59 through exosomal and apoptotic bleb release. Adv Exp Med Biol 2014; 801: 259-65.
[74] Coppe JP, et al. The senescence-associated secretory phenotype: the dark side of tumor suppression. Annu Rev Pathol 2010; 5: 99-118.
[75] Marazita MC, et al. Oxidative stress-induced premature senescence dysregulates VEGF and CFH expression in retinal pigment epithelial cells: implications for age-related macular degeneration. Redox Biol 2016; 7: 78-87.
[76] Ford KM, D'Amore PA. Molecular regulation of vascular endothelial growth factor expression in the retinal pigment epithelium. Mol Vis 2012; 18: 519-27.
[77] Oubaha M, et al. Senescence-associated secretory phenotype contributes to pathological angiogenesis in retinopathy. Sci Transl Med 2016; 8(362): 362ra144.
[78] Zhou J, Wang S, Xia X. Role of intravitreal inflammatory cytokines and angiogenic factors in proliferative diabetic retinopathy. Curr Eye Res 2012; 37(5): 416-20.
[79] Takasugi M. Emerging roles of extracellular vesicles in cellular senescence and aging. Aging Cell 2018; 17(2).
[80] Lehmann BD, et al. Senescence-associated exosome release from human prostate cancer cells. Cancer Res 2008; 68(19): 7864-71.
[81] Takahashi A, et al. Exosomes maintain cellular homeostasis by excreting harmful DNA from cells. Nat Commun 2017; 8: 15287.
[82] Fitzgerald W, et al. A system of cytokines encapsulated in extracellular vesicles. Sci Rep 2018; 8(1): 8973.
[83] Vavvas D, et al. In: Schachat AP, editor. Basic mechanisms of pathologic retinal and choroidal angiogenesis, in Ryan's retina. Elsevier Inc. p. 639-55.
[84] Campochiaro PA. Molecular pathogenesis of retinal and choroidal vascular diseases. Prog Retin Eye Res 2015; 49: 67-81.
[85] Rousseau B, et al. Involvement of fibroblast growth factors in choroidal angiogenesis and retinal vascularization. Exp Eye Res 2003; 77(2): 147-56.
[86] Hu Y, et al. Pathogenic role of the Wnt signaling pathway activation in laser-induced choroidal neovascularization. Invest Ophthalmol Vis Sci 2013; 54(1): 141-54.
[87] Drenser KA. Wnt signaling pathway in retinal vascularization. Eye Brain 2016; 8: 141-6.
[88] Das A, et al. Retinal neovascularization is suppressed with a matrix metalloproteinase inhibitor. Arch Ophthalmol 1999; 117(4): 498-503.
[89] Mori K, et al. Pigment epithelium-derived factor inhibits retinal and choroidal neovascularization. J Cell Physiol 2001; 188(2): 253-63.
[90] Drixler TA, et al. Angiostatin inhibits pathological but not physiological retinal angiogenesis. Invest Ophthalmol Vis Sci 2001; 42(13): 3325-30.
[91] Bai YJ, et al. Antiangiogenesis effects of endostatin in retinal neovascularization. J Ocul Pharmacol Ther 2013; 29(7): 619-26.
[92] Aboul Naga SH, et al. Intracellular pathways following uptake of bevacizumab in RPE cells. Exp Eye Res 2015; 131: 29-41.
[93] Klingeborn M, et al. Directional exosome proteomes reflect polarity-specific functions in retinal pigmented epithelium monolayers. Sci Rep 2017; 7(1): 4901.
[94] Katome T, et al. Expression of intraocular peroxisome proliferator-activated receptor gamma in patients with proliferative diabetic retinopathy. J Diabetes Complicat 2015; 29(2): 275-81.
[95] Looze C, et al. Proteomic profiling of human plasma exosomes identifies PPARgamma as an exosome-associated protein. Biochem Biophys Res Commun 2009; 378(3): 433-8.
[96] Moisseiev E, et al. Protective effect of intravitreal administration of exosomes derived from mesenchymal stem cells on retinal ischemia. Curr Eye Res 2017; 42: 1-10.
[97] Hajrasouliha AR, et al. Exosomes from retinal astrocytes contain antiangiogenic components that inhibit laser-induced choroidal neovascularization. J Biol Chem 2013; 288(39): 28058-67.
[98] Konstantinell A, et al. Secretomic analysis of extracellular vesicles originating from polyomavirus-negative and polyomavirus-positive Merkel cell carcinoma cell lines. Proteomics 2016; 16(19): 2587-91.

[99] Janowska-Wieczorek A, et al. Microvesicles derived from activated platelets induce metastasis and angiogenesis in lung cancer. Int J Cancer 2005; 113(5): 752-60.

[100] Feng Q, et al. A class of extracellular vesicles from breast cancer cells activates VEGF receptors and tumour angiogenesis. Nat Commun 2017; 8: 14450.

[101] Monteforte A, et al. (*) Glioblastoma exosomes for therapeutic angiogenesis in peripheral ischemia. Tissue Eng Part A 2017; 23(21-22): 1251-61.

[102] Ju R, et al. Angiopoietin-2 secretion by endothelial cell exosomes: regulation by the phosphatidylinositol 3-kinase (PI3K)/Akt/endothelial nitric oxide synthase (eNOS) and syndecan-4/syntenin pathways. J Biol Chem 2014; 289(1): 510-9.

[103] Goetzl EJ, et al. Altered cargo proteins of human plasma endothelial cell-derived exosomes in atherosclerotic cerebrovascular disease. FASEB J 2017; 31(8): 3689-94.

[104] Tang XD, et al. Mesenchymal stem cell microvesicles attenuate acute lung injury in mice partly mediated by Ang-1 mRNA. Stem Cells 2017; 35(7): 1849-59.

[105] Beckett K, et al. Drosophila S2 cells secrete wingless on exosome-kike vesicles but the wingless gradient forms independently of exosomes. Traffic 2013; 14(1): 82-96.

[106] Gross JC, et al. Active Wnt proteins are secreted on exosomes. Nat Cell Biol 2012; 14(10): 1036-45.

[107] Korkut C, et al. Trans-synaptic transmission of vesicular Wnt signals through Evi/Wntless. Cell 2009; 139(2): 393-404.

[108] Luga V, et al. Exosomes mediate stromal mobilization of autocrine Wnt-PCP signaling in breast cancer cell migration. Cell 2012; 151(7): 1542-56.

[109] Zhang L, Wrana JL. The emerging role of exosomes in Wnt secretion and transport. Curr Opin Genet Dev 2014; 27: 14-9.

[110] Shimoda M, Khokha R. Proteolytic factors in exosomes. Proteomics 2013; 13(10-11): 1624-36.

[111] Chowdhury R, et al. Cancer exosomes trigger mesenchymal stem cell differentiation into pro-angiogenic and pro-invasive myofibroblasts. Oncotarget 2015; 6(2): 715-31.

[112] You Y, et al. Matrix metalloproteinase 13-containing exosomes promote nasopharyngeal carcinoma metastasis. Cancer Sci 2015; 106(12): 1669-77.

[113] Ruivo CF, et al. The biology of cancer exosomes: insights and new perspectives. Cancer Res 2017; 77(23): 6480-8.

[114] Zitvogel L, et al. Eradication of established murine tumors using a novel cell-free vaccine: dendritic cell-derived exosomes. Nat Med 1998; 4(5): 594-600.

[115] Webber J, et al. Cancer exosomes trigger fibroblast to myofibroblast differentiation. Cancer Res 2010; 70(23): 9621-30.

[116] Hoshino D, et al. Exosome secretion is enhanced by invadopodia and drives invasive behavior. Cell Rep 2013; 5(5): 1159-68.

[117] Mu W, Rana S, Zoller M. Host matrix modulation by tumor exosomes promotes motility and invasiveness. Neoplasia 2013; 15(8): 875-87.

[118] Peinado H, et al. Melanoma exosomes educate bone marrow progenitor cells toward a prometastatic phenotype through MET. Nat Med 2012; 18(6): 883-91.

[119] Salehi M, Sharifi M. Exosomal miRNAs as novel cancer biomarkers: challenges and opportunities. J Cell Physiol 2018; 233(9): 6370-80.

[120] Kujala E, Makitie T, Kivela T. Very long-term prognosis of patients with malignant uveal melanoma. Invest Ophthalmol Vis Sci 2003; 44(11): 4651-9.

[121] Diener-West M, et al. Development of metastatic disease after enrollment in the COMS trials for treatment of choroidal melanoma: collaborative ocular melanoma study group report No. 26. Arch Ophthalmol 2005; 123(12): 1639-43.

[122] Eldh M, et al. MicroRNA in exosomes isolated directly from the liver circulation in patients with metastatic uveal melanoma. BMC Cancer 2014; 14: 962.

[123] Ragusa M, et al. miRNA profiling in vitreous humor, vitreal exosomes and serum from uveal melanoma patients: pathological and diagnostic implications. Cancer Biol Ther 2015; 16(9): 1387-96.

[124] Volarevic V, et al. Mesenchymal stem cell-derived factors: immuno-modulatory effects and therapeutic potential. Biofactors 2017; 43(5): 633-44.

[125] Mead B, Tomarev S. Bone marrow-derived mesenchymal stem cells-derived exosomes promote survival of retinal ganglion cells through miRNA-dependent mechanisms. Stem Cells Transl Med 2017; 6(4): 1273-85.

[126] Yu B, et al. Exosomes derived from MSCs ameliorate retinal laser injury partially by inhibition of MCP-1. Sci Rep 2016; 6: 34562.

[127] Shigemoto-Kuroda T, et al. MSC-derived extracellular vesicles attenuate immune responses in two autoimmune murine models: type 1 diabetes and uveoretinitis. Stem Cell Rep 2017; 8(5): 1214-25.

[128] Wassmer SJ, et al. Exosome-associated AAV2 vector mediates robust gene delivery into the murine retina upon intravitreal injection. Sci Rep 2017; 7: 45329.

第 19 章

MSC 外泌体在再生医学中的应用
MSC-exosomes in regenerative medicine

Yueyuan Zhou[a,b], Nobuyoshi Kosaka[a,d], Zhongdang Xiao[b], and Takahiro Ochiya[a,c]

[a]Division of Molecular and Cellular Medicine, National Cancer Center Research Institute, Tokyo, Japan, [b]State Key Laboratory of Bioelectronics, School of Biological Science and Medical Engineering, Southeast University, Nanjing, China, [c]Department of Molecular and Cellular Medicine, Institute of Medical Science, Tokyo Medical University, Tokyo, Japan, [d]Department of Translational Research for Extracellular Vesicles, Institute of Medical Science, Tokyo Medical University, Tokyo, Japan

一、概述

再生医学旨在通过应用工程学和生命科学原理促进再生,从而恢复患病和受损组织及整个器官的功能。再生医学的策略包括使用材料、种子细胞以及它们的多种组合以促进组织愈合,并重建缺失或受损的组织和器官[1]。当前再生医学领域的趋势是使用干细胞,包括间充质干细胞(mesenchymal stem cell,MSC)。MSC 是多功能的非造血成体干细胞,最早由 Friedenstein 等于 20 世纪 60 年代在骨髓中鉴定出来[2]。MSC 具有多种特性,包括归巢到受损组织、多系分化潜能、集落形成和自我更新[3,4]。由于具有这些特性,MSC 作为一种有前景的、基于细胞的疗法在再生医学领域中得到了研究者的广泛关注,被用于治疗受伤的、功能异常的组织和器官(图 19-1)。研究者最初认为 MSC 迁移至损伤部位,植入并随后

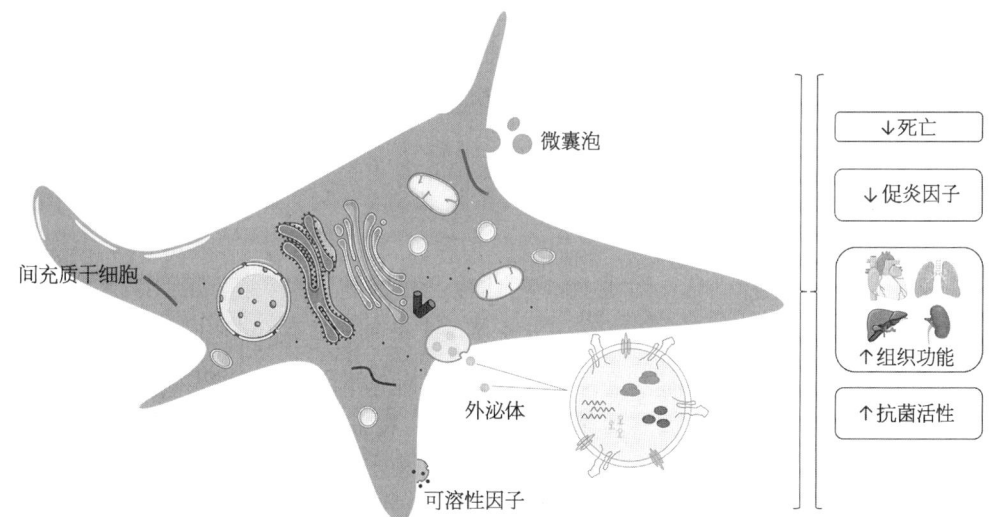

扫描二维码查看彩图

图 19-1 MSC 在再生医学中应用的概述

分化为靶细胞进行组织再生而发挥其治疗作用[3]。然而，最近的一些研究表明，MSC 的有益作用不仅归因于它们的分化潜能，更主要归因于其旁分泌活性，因为只有小部分被移植的 MSC 能够存活并与周围现有的细胞在宿主组织损伤部位处进行融合[5-7]。MSC 的旁分泌功能是通过分泌可溶性因子和释放 EV（如外泌体）来发挥的。事实上，这些可溶性因子（包括生长因子、趋化因子和细胞因子）可以减少细胞、增强神经元存活和分化、限制局部炎症并调节免疫应答[8-10]。最近的研究表明，MSC 释放的 EV 在这些细胞的生理功能中可能也发挥了关键作用，至少部分地对 MSC 的治疗效果作出了贡献[11-13]。

二、来源于间充质基质细胞的外泌体

EV 包括一组异质的纳米脂质双层膜囊泡，可由多种类型细胞分泌，包括 T 细胞、B 细胞、DC、肥大细胞、内皮细胞、神经元细胞、肿瘤细胞、胚胎细胞和 MSC[14,15]。根据 EV 的来源、大小、形态和内容物分为几个亚群：外泌体、微泡等。外泌体生物发生的经典观点认为，外泌体最初是通过内体膜内陷形成的 MVB 产生的。事实上，就其生化组成和表型而言，外泌体本身包括相当异质的种群，这由其细胞来源决定。随着研究的不断进展，外泌体和 EV 领域的术语不断地被定义和完善。最近，研究者发现外泌体至少包含三个亚群，它们具有独特的 N-糖基化、蛋白质、脂质、DNA 和 RNA 谱以及生物物理特性[16]。在研究绵羊网织红细胞成熟过程的期间，研究者首次发现了直径 40～150 nm 的外泌体，其密度为 1.09～1.19 g/mL。最初，外泌体被认为是细胞碎片或一种排泄细胞代谢废物的手段，但也有研究证明它们是一种细胞间通信机制，并参与多种生理和病理过程。

外泌体被包裹在脂质双层膜中，该膜保护它们的内容物免于降解，且使外泌体能够在组织中长距离移动并被受体细胞内化。外泌体膜富含膜联蛋白、四跨膜蛋白（如 CD9、CD63 和 CD81）和 HSP（包括 HSP60、HSP70 和 HSP90）。外泌体内生物活性成分包括多种 RNA（如 mRNA、miRNA、premiRNA 和长-非编码 RNA）、DNA、脂质和可转移到靶细胞的可溶性蛋白质[18-20]。

外泌体的成分是特定于细胞类型的，通常受亲代细胞的生理或病理状态、调节其分泌的外部刺激以及涉及其生物发生的分子机制影响[21,22]。此外，已有研究表明，源自 MSC 的外泌体可以继承其亲代细胞的多能性，从而促进组织修复和再生[23-25]。研究发现，一些表面受体（CD29、CD44、CD73 和 CD105）、信号分子（参与 BMP、MAPK 和 PPAR 受体细胞信号通路的调节）、黏附分子和 MSC 相关标志物有助于增强 MSC 来源外泌体的治疗作用[26,27]。同样，在急性肾损伤模型中，MSC 衍生的外泌体减少了细胞凋亡，并增加了细胞增殖，其部分原因是通过外泌体介导的 RNA 转移[28]。近期，研究者通过高分辨率蛋白质组学分析区分了 MSC 衍生的外泌体和微泡[29]。简而言之，由 MSC 产生的外泌体可通过转运外源性生物活性物质和化学分子充当靶向递送系统用于无细胞再生医学。另外，从年轻和老年宿主获得的 MSC 来源的外泌体显示出不同的 miRNA 表达模式，这表明外泌体是评估亲代细胞状态的生物标志物的候选物[30,31]。因此，在当前基于干细胞疗法的再生医学中，MSC-外泌体有望作为生物标志物用于移植细胞的鉴定。

三、MSC‑EV 在再生医学中的应用

由于具有明显的生物学功能,如归巢到受损或炎症组织、多系分化和免疫调节作用,MSC 在再生医学中被广泛应用。然而,在外泌体移植、归巢和分化的长期安全性方面仍然存在许多挑战。基于 MSC 的再生医学疗法的临床局限性包括免疫排斥、遗传不稳定、存活率低和功能受限。此外,MSC 移植后形成肿瘤是其主要的风险[32]。MSC 的体外扩增、大规模生产、存储、交付以及质量控制的标准应得到验证和确认[33]。

近年来,因为与细胞、合成纳米颗粒和单分子相比具有许多优越性,MSC‑外泌体在无细胞再生治疗中显示出巨大的潜力。与 MSC 相比,外泌体具有一定的优势,例如,缺乏细胞核以避免肿瘤性转化;增强的稳定性,可以在体内长期保存和长程转移生物活性分子;用靶向分子更容易进行表面修饰;能够负载小分子、蛋白质和 RNA。同时,外泌体也可以用不同的受体或抗体进行工程改造,以将治疗药物转移至特定的细胞和组织中。由于外泌体是细胞分泌的,它们具有良好的生物相容性和全身生物分布性[34,35]。此外,外泌体拥有各种类型的生物活性分子,使其能够同时发挥不同的治疗机制,这是传统的小单分子无法实现的。因此,我们在这里探讨外泌体在再生医学中应用的分子机制。

(一)神经再生

在探讨 MSC‑外泌体与神经系统疾病关系之前,我们首先讨论干细胞治疗神经系统疾病的现状。目前,干细胞疗法被认为是多种神经系统疾病有前景的治疗方案,包括脑卒中、帕金森病、肌萎缩侧索硬化和亨廷顿病[36]。下面,我们介绍使用 MSC‑外泌体作为神经疾病治疗策略的相关研究。AD 的病理特征在于 β 淀粉样肽(Aβ)生成与清除之间的不平衡导致 Aβ 在大脑中积聚。脑啡肽酶(neprilysin,NEP)是大脑中最重要的 Aβ 降解酶。研究表明,人脂肪组织 MSC 来源的外泌体含有大量的酶活性 NEP,并且可以同时降低共培养后神经母细胞瘤细胞内部及其分泌的 Aβ 水平,这可能作为 AD 的治疗方法[37]。同样,从人类脱落乳牙(human exfoliated deciduous teeth,SHED)牙髓干细胞分离的外泌体在 3D 培养环境中抑制了 6‑羟基多巴胺氢溴酸盐(6‑OHDA)诱导的多巴胺能神经元的凋亡,这表明从 SHED 衍生的外泌体是一种有前景的帕金森病新型治疗手段[38]。在大鼠脑卒中模型中全身应用骨髓间充质干细胞来源的外泌体能够通过促进神经突触重塑,增加神经和血管生成,显著改善功能恢复[39]。类似的研究也表明,MSC‑外泌体可恢复神经系统损伤、长期保护神经和增强血管生成。这些作用与外泌体在小鼠脑卒中模型中调节局部缺血后的免疫反应类似[40]。Ophelders 等发现,MSC‑外泌体通过减少缺氧‑缺血性损伤后的神经后遗症来保护脑功能[41]。另一项研究已证明 MSC‑外泌体可显著改善炎症诱导的神经元变性、减少小胶质细胞增生和预防反应性星形胶质细胞增生,从而改善持久的认知功能[42]。

与 MSC‑外泌体相关的 miRNA 在神经再生过程中也发挥着重要作用。Xin 等发现在大鼠脑卒中模型中 MSC‑外泌体将 miR‑133b 转移至神经元和星形胶质细胞,随后促进了神经突重塑和功能恢复[43]。Xin 等报道了富含 miR‑17‑92 簇的 MSC‑外泌体通过靶向 PTEN 激活 PI3K/Akt/mTOR/GSK‑3β 信号通路增强少突胶质细胞生成,促进神经发生,

增强神经可塑性并促进神经系统恢复[44]。由外伤性（视神经病变）或退行性眼病引起的视网膜神经节细胞(retinal ganglion cell，RGC)及其轴突丧失是失明的主要原因之一。骨髓间充质干细胞来源的外泌体显著促进了 RGC 的存活及其轴突的再生，同时部分防止了 RGC 轴突的丧失和功能障碍。这些外泌体将其内容物转移到视网膜内层，其发挥的作用与内含的 miRNA 有关[45]。颅脑损伤(traumatic brain injury，TBI)涉及由瞬时外力导致的一系列颅内继发性病理和(或)功能改变，是全球范围内导致死亡和长期残疾的主要原因[46]。研究发现，骨髓 MSC-外泌体可在 TBI 后诱导大鼠病灶边界区和齿状回的内皮细胞以及未成熟/成熟神经元增殖，并减少神经炎症[47]。在另一个 TBI 小鼠模型中，MSC-外泌体抑制了 TBI 后的神经炎症，并治疗了模式分离和空间学习障碍。因此，这些外泌体打断了组织破坏和炎症的自我延续周期[48]。MSC-外泌体可能通过靶向神经源"龛"抑制星形胶质细胞和小胶质细胞的活化，并促进神经发生而减少神经炎症，这些作用有助于 TBI 后神经组织修复和功能恢复[49]。

尽管最新的研究表明，MSC-外泌体可改善神经功能恢复，促进神经发生和减少神经炎症，但其中确切的细胞和分子机制尚不清楚。因此，未来应该进行机制研究，以充分利用 MSC-外泌体并发掘其在神经再生中的潜力。

（二）心血管再生

心血管疾病不仅在发达国家还是在全世界都是主要的致死和致残因素[50]。心血管疾病发病的主要原因是脉管系统的损害。脉管系统的损害会导致逐渐积聚的动脉粥样硬化斑块部分阻塞血管，继而阻塞远端心肌，并在心肌需血量增加时导致心肌局部缺血。血管快速灌注对预防缺血性心肌梗死至关重要。但是，血管再灌注可能会导致其他损害。2010 年，Lai 等首次报道了 MSC-外泌体在心血管再生中的应用。在小鼠模型中，从人类胚胎干细胞衍生的 MSC 条件培养液(conditioned medium，CM)中分离出的外泌体可通过缩小心肌缺血/再灌注损伤期间的梗死面积发挥心脏保护作用。随后，同一小组的另一项研究表明，在心肌梗死小鼠模型中使用 MSC-外泌体治疗可缩小心肌梗死面积，提升 NADH 和 ATP 水平，并降低氧化应激反应。同时，MSC-外泌体在心肌缺血/再灌注过程中增加了磷酸化 AKT 和磷酸化 GSK-3β 的水平，同时降低了磷酸化 c-JNK 的水平。因此，MSC-外泌体可以通过恢复生物能，降低氧化应激和激活促进生存信号通路改善心脏功能[52]。其他研究人员发现，在心肌内应用 MSC 衍生的外泌体显著促进了血流恢复，减小了心肌梗死面积，并保留了心脏的收缩和舒张功能。因此，MSC-外泌体通过刺激新生血管保护心脏组织[53]。另外，研究报道，MSC-外泌体显著促进了人脐静脉内皮细胞成管，抑制 T 细胞功能，减少心肌梗死面积，并保护心脏的收缩和舒张功能，从而刺激了新生血管形成并抑制了炎症反应[54]。

近年来，各种研究聚焦于 MSC-外泌体递送的 miRNA 在心血管再生中的作用。研究表明，来自 MSC-外泌体递送的 miR-221 下调了 p53 的表达，并上调了凋亡调控因子(p53 and upregulated modulator of apoptosis，PUMA) 的表达，因此显著发挥了心脏保护作用[55]。该小组的另一项研究报道，MSC-外泌体不仅在体外转送 miR-19a，并可在体内转移 miR-19a 至缺血心肌，通过降低磷酸酶和张力蛋白同源物（phosphatase and tensin homolog，PTEN）的表达以及抑制随后激活 AKT 和 ERK 信号通路产生更强大的心脏保护作用[56]。Li 等发现在大鼠心肌梗死模型中，MSC-外泌体抑制了心脏纤维化和炎症，并改善了心脏功能。此外，他们证实了 MSC-外泌体和 MSC 具有相似的 miRNA 表达谱，这表明 MSC-外泌体可以替代 MSC 进行心脏修复。此外，MSC-外泌体中存在的几种特异性和关键性的 miRNA 与 MSC 中的 miRNA 显著不同，这表明 MSC-外泌体在心脏再生中的作用甚至可能比 MSC 更好。例如，MSC-外泌体和 MSC 中 miR-29 的表达均增加，而 miR-34 的表达均降低可能是 MSC-外泌体发挥治疗作用的原因。然而与 MSC 相比，miR-21 和 miR-15 在外泌体中的表达明显降低，这有助于解释相对于 MSC，外泌体具有更好的心肌修复作用[57]。但是，另一项关于外泌体 miR-21 的研究表明，由于富含 miR-21 的分泌性外泌体旁分泌作用增强，人子宫内膜来源的 MSC（endometrium-derived MSC，EnMSC）的心脏保护作用优于人骨髓 MSC 和脂肪组织 MSC。anti-miR 拮抗 miR-21 后消除了 EnMSC 的抗凋亡和血管生成作用，这些结果表明外泌体 miR-21 是 EnMSC 通过 PTEN/AKT 途径发挥了心脏保护作用的潜在介质[58]。脓毒症导致多种组织的血液灌注不良，因此通常可以观察到脓毒症患者出现心脏损伤和功能障碍[59]。据报道，MSC-外泌体中包含的 miR-233 减轻了败血症引发的心肌抑制，下调了 Sema3A 和 Stat3 的表达，从而导致炎症反应和细胞死亡的减少[60]。Zhang 等发现用 MSC-外泌体预处理心肌细胞可减少心脏纤维化并提升干细胞的存活率和毛细血管密度，从而改善大鼠心肌梗死模型的心脏功能[61]。

外泌体在心血管疾病中的治疗作用涉及几种途径：① 心肌内注射干细胞产生的外泌体发挥旁分泌作用；② 常驻心脏干细胞可能引起自身或心脏其他类型细胞的自养性刺激；③ 心肌内注射的外泌体可直接影响不同类型的细胞；④ 全身性应用外泌体与心血管系统细胞，如内皮细胞、血液和心肌细胞发生相互作用[62]。

（三）肝再生

肝脏是人体内具有强大再生能力的重要器官，在体内发挥排毒作用。肝脏疾病，包括病毒性肝炎、酒精性肝病、非酒精性脂肪性肝病以及相关的终末期肝病均是全球健康问题。数项研究已经探究了 MSC-外泌体对于肝损伤的治疗作用。Xu 等建立了四氯化碳（CCl_4）诱导的小鼠肝纤维化模型。随后，给小鼠肝脏直接注射人脐带 MSC-外泌体。研究结果表明，移植人脐带 MSC 外泌体通过抑制上皮-间充质转化减少了肝脏表面纤维囊、软化了它们的质地，减轻了肝脏的炎症并减少了胶原蛋白的沉积[63]。在另一个由 CCl_4 诱导的小鼠肝损伤模型的研究中，MSC-外泌体抑制了对乙酰氨基酚（acetaminophen，APAP）和过氧化氢（H_2O_2）诱导的肝细胞凋亡，通过激活增殖和再生反应来对抗毒物诱导的损伤发挥肝脏保护作用。此外，人脐带 MSC-外泌体转移了谷胱甘肽过氧化物酶 1（glutathione peroxidase 1，GPX1）并促进了肝氧化剂损伤后的恢复[65]。在大鼠肝缺血再灌注（ischemia-reperfusion，I/R）损伤模型中，通过下腔静脉全身注射人源性多能干细胞衍生的 MSC-外泌体（human-induced pluripotent stem cell-derived MSC exosomes，hiPSC-MSC-exosomes），抑制了炎症细胞的浸润，减少了炎症因子的释放，缓解了肝脏氧化应激。这些结果表明 hiPSC-

MSC-外泌体通过抑制炎症反应,减弱氧化应激反应和抑制细胞凋亡在 I/R 损伤中发挥肝脏保护作用[66]。Du 等发现在缺血/再灌注损伤模型中,hiPSC-MSC-外泌体抑制了肝细胞坏死和窦性充血。此外,hiPSC-MSC-外泌体促进了原代肝细胞增殖,增加了鞘氨醇激酶的活性和鞘氨醇-1-磷酸(sphingosine-1-phosphate,S1P)的合成[67]。人经血来源的干细胞(menstrual blood-derived stem cell,MenSC)是 MSC 的新型来源,它具有易于收集和分离的优势。研究者发现 MenSC-外泌体能够表达各种细胞因子,如 IL-6 和血管生成素-1,具有减轻暴发性肝衰竭的作用,并且能够减少暴发性肝功能衰竭中肝单核细胞的数量和活性凋亡蛋白 caspase-1 的量[68]。为了应对肝脏损伤,IL-6 介导了急性期反应并诱导细胞保护同时促进细胞有丝分裂。研究已经证实 IL-6 诱导的信号通路在肝再生过程的早期启动、进展和维持中起着至关重要的作用[69]。总之,MSC-外泌体可以抑制炎症因子风暴,抑制细胞凋亡,促进血管生成,提供能量支持,促进肝细胞增殖并有助于胆道恢复以逆转肝衰竭,因此外泌体疗法可能是 MSC 治疗的替代方法。

(四)肾再生

有证据表明肾脏是多种疾病(如高血压、贫血和血脂异常等)的靶器官,当肾脏生理受到损害时,它可以引发或加剧其他病理生理状况,如心血管疾病[70]。在大鼠慢性肾脏疾病(chronic kidney disease,CKD)模型中,MSC 衍生的条件培养基通过减缓 CKD 进程、降低高血压及减小肾小球损伤促进了肾脏的治疗性抢救。该研究表明,旁分泌因子包括 MSC 分泌的细胞因子和外泌体,有助于保护肾脏[71]。在顺铂诱导的大鼠急性肾损伤(acute kidney injury,AKI)模型中,MSC-外泌体的治疗减少了凋亡细胞的数量,抑制了氧化应激和 p38 促分裂原活化蛋白激酶(p38 MAPK)途径的激活。有研究揭示了 MSC-外泌体通过激活 ERK1/2 通路促进了细胞增殖,这表明 MSC-外泌体可以通过减轻氧化应激、减少细胞凋亡及促进细胞增殖来修复顺铂诱导的大鼠 AKI 和 NRK-52E 细胞损伤[72]。此外,Zou 等报道人类 Wharton-Jelly MSC(hWJMSC)产生的外泌体在缺血性 AKI 后急性和慢性阶段均减轻了肾脏损伤。他们观察到应用 hWJMSC-外泌体后减少了肾细胞凋亡,增强了肾细胞增殖能力,下调了 CX3CL1 的表达,同时减少了肾脏中 CD68$^+$ 巨噬细胞的数量。这些结果表明 hWJMSC-外泌体通过抑制 CX3CL1 发挥抗炎活性,从而发挥治疗作用[73]。在肾脏缺血/再灌注损伤后,趋化因子 CCR2 及其受体 CX3CR1 介导调节单核/巨噬细胞运输的信号通路,从而导致炎症相关的肾脏损伤[74]。然而,富含 CCR2 的 MSC-外泌体能够降低游离 CCL2 的浓度,抑制其募集或激活巨噬细胞的能力,从而促进肾脏缺血/再灌注损伤后的修复[75]。有研究发现,另一种细胞因子 IL-10 与 MSC-外泌体的肾脏保护作用有关。在猪代谢综合征和肾动脉狭窄模型中,脂肪组织 MSC 衍生的外泌体缓解了肾脏的炎症、改善了髓质氧合同时抑制了纤维化,而 IL-10 缺失的外泌体肾脏保护性治疗作用被减弱了[76]。此外,由 MSC 外泌体递送的 miRNA 参与了 AKI 的恢复。Collino 等通过敲除 MSC 中的 Drosha 基因降低了外泌体中整体 miRNA 的表达,然后用这种外泌体处理甘油诱导的小鼠 AKI 模型。他们发现整体下调 MSC 外泌体富含的 miRNA 后抑制了外泌体的肾脏再生作用,这表明外泌体介导的 miRNA 传递在肾脏保护功能中起着至关重要的作用[77]。最近

MSC-外泌体已经被应用于临床去评估来源于人脐带血的外泌体在改善Ⅲ级和Ⅳ级CKD进展中的安全性和治疗效果。研究结果显示，应用脐血MSC-外泌体是安全的，可以改善Ⅲ级和Ⅳ级CKD患者的炎症免疫反应并改善整体肾脏功能[78]。综上所述，越来越多的证据表明MSC-外泌体凭借其内含的生物活性物质（包括miRNA和蛋白质）发挥保护肾脏的潜力。

（五）骨骼、软骨和肌肉的再生

骨质疏松症、骨关节炎和类风湿关节炎等病理破坏性骨病是一个重大的全球性健康问题，与患者生活质量的持续下降息息相关[79-81]。据报道，由TNF-α预处理的脂肪组织MSC来源的外泌体可通过抑制Wnt信号通路促进原代成骨细胞的增殖和分化[82]。这些结果表明MSC-外泌体有望用于骨组织再生，并代替直接的干细胞移植进行骨修复和再生。Zhang等报道了人诱导的多能干细胞来源的MSC-外泌体可以通过激活人骨髓MSC中的PI3K/AKT信号通路来增强β-TCP的骨诱导性[83]。另一项研究表明，MSC-外泌体能够在免疫功能完全的大鼠骨软骨缺损模型中促进软骨有序再生。每周关节腔内注射MSC-外泌体可促进早期细胞浸润和增殖，减少修复组织中凋亡细胞的数量，并诱导滑膜巨噬细胞极化为促再生的M2表型从而促进有序的软骨和软骨下骨再生[84]。另外，在$CD9^{-/-}$小鼠股骨骨折模型中，注射MSC-外泌体加速了骨折愈合。外泌体中骨修复相关细胞因子[包括单核细胞趋化蛋白-1(monocyte chemotactic protein-1，MCP-1)、MCP-3和基质细胞衍生因子-1]的含量低于条件培养基，这表明外泌体的部分骨骼修复作用可能由其他成分介导的，如miRNA。MiR-21是一种抗凋亡的miRNA，在MSC-外泌体中含量最高[85]。先前的研究还表明，miR-21通过靶向Smad7(small mothers against decapentaplegic 7)和PI3K/β-catenin途径[87]促进MSC的成骨分化，同时局部注射过表达miR-21的MSC能够促进大鼠骨折愈合[88]。在已建立的大鼠骨软骨缺损模型中，每周一次关节内注射人胚胎MSC衍生的外泌体可改善骨软骨修复的总体外观并提升组织学评分。此外，到12周时，经外泌体处理的缺损处显示出软骨和软骨下骨的完全恢复。修复的组织与未手术的同龄鼠软骨十分相似，具有软骨的特征性表现包括具有良好表面规则性的透明软骨，与相邻软骨的完全结合以及丰富的细胞外基质沉积。相比之下，经PBS处理的骨软骨缺损仅表现出纤维增殖[89]。除了增强成骨作用，hiPSC-MSC-外泌体还能够促进骨质疏松大鼠的血管生成。体外研究结果表明，hiPSC-MSC-外泌体可促进去卵巢大鼠骨髓MSC增殖，提升碱性磷酸酶(alkaline phosphatase，ALP)活性，并上调成骨相关基因的表达[90]。MSC-外泌体促进了骨骼肌再生，软骨和软骨下骨的修复。Nakamura等研究发现人骨髓间充质干细胞分泌的外泌体在体外肌肉损伤模型中增强了成肌作用、血管生成以及骨骼肌的再生。他们还证实了MSC-外泌体中miR-494可能部分促进了肌肉的再生[91]。据报道，MSC-外泌体和心脏特异性过表达的miR-494可保护缺血/再灌注引起的心脏损伤[51,53,92]。通过软骨内骨化途径修复骨缺损的主要挑战包括通过新生血管系统募集间充质祖细胞，祖细胞的软骨分化和肥大成熟以及肥大软骨的重塑[93]。然而，基于外泌体的疗法可以克服其中一个或多个瓶颈。总之，MSC-外泌体在骨缺损微环境中显示出潜在的优势。他们通过其丰富的内容物发挥治疗作用并发挥多重功能。

（六）皮肤再生

皮肤受损后，损坏的组织通过构建皮肤愈合反应的协同生物作用得到修复。伤口愈合是一个复杂的过程，涉及一系列分子和细胞事件，包括细胞迁移、炎症、血管生成、肉芽形成、再上皮化和细胞外基质（extracellular matrix，ECM）重塑[94]。目前的研究集中于 MSC-外泌体对皮肤伤口愈合的促进作用。据报道，骨髓 MSC 来源的外泌体被人脐静脉内皮细胞内化后，通过剂量依赖的方式诱导脐静脉内皮细胞成管增加。此外，这些 MSC-外泌体激活了涉及伤口愈合的多个信号通路，如 AKT、ERK 和 STAT3 通路，并提升了许多生长因子的表达，包括肝细胞生长因子（hepatocyte growth factor，HGF）、IGF-1、神经生长因子（nerve growth factor，NGF）和基质衍生生长因子-1（stromal-derived growth factor-1，SDF-1）。因此，MSC-外泌体显示出以剂量依赖的方式增强了来自正常供体和慢性伤口患者的成纤维细胞的增殖和迁移[95]。研究者还揭示了注射了人诱导的多能干细胞衍生的 MSC-外泌体加速了再上皮化，减少了瘢痕宽度并促进了胶原蛋白的成熟。注射外泌体不仅增加了新生血管的生成，而且促进了它们在伤口部位的成熟。体外结果表明，这些外泌体刺激了人类皮肤成纤维细胞和 HUVEC 的增殖和迁移，并以剂量依赖的方式增加了成纤维细胞 I 型胶原蛋白、III 型胶原蛋白和弹性蛋白的分泌[96]，同时增加了 HUVEC 的成管能力。研究表明，MSC-外泌体中富含的 miRNA 特异性表达模式至少部分负责 MSC-外泌体促进伤口愈合的作用。在伤口愈合过程中，从脐带来源的 MSC 分离出的外泌体包含一组不同的 miRNA（miR-21、miR-23a、miR-125b 和 miR-145），它们通过抑制 TGF-β2/SMAD2 信号通路与负调控成肌纤维细胞的形成相关[97]。另一项研究报道，脂肪组织 MSC-外泌体转移的 miR-125a 抑制了血管新生抑制剂 delta-like 4（DDL4）的表达，并通过促进内皮尖端细胞的形成来调节内皮细胞的血管新生[98]。在大鼠严重烧伤模型中，人脐带 MSC-外泌体中的 miR-181c 通过抑制 TLR4 信号通路有效地减轻了炎症[63]。另外，人脐带 MSC-外泌体促进了 β-catenin 核易位，增加了增殖细胞核抗原、cyclin D3、N-cadherin 和 β-catenin 的表达，同时降低了 E-cadherin 的表达。此外，Wnt4/β-catenin 信号通路的激活增强了血管生成[99]。这些结果表明人脐带 MSC-外泌体在伤口愈合的应用中具有广阔的前景。皮瓣坏死是重建手术中最常见的术后并发症，其主要原因可能是新血管形成不足和促血管生成因子水平降低。研究者已经发现，来自脂肪组织 MSC 的外泌体可以显著提高遭受缺血再灌注损伤皮瓣的存活率和毛细血管密度，而 MSC-外泌体的这种功能可能是通过介导 IL-6/STAT3 途径发挥的[100]。尽管研究者已经确定了 MSC 来源的外泌体对伤口愈合过程的重要性，并且此概念已在该领域的大多数研究中被普遍接受，但外泌体所传递的生物活性分子如何发挥功能的详细机制仍然不清楚。将来我们需要更多的研究来阐明外泌体如何调节伤口愈合过程。

四、再生医学中的外泌体修饰

外泌体已显示出巨大的治疗潜力，可以作为干细胞疗法的替代品，用于再生医学，促进内源性修复。适当修饰外泌体的生物相容性可以增加外泌体治疗的稳定性和功效,同时增加细胞的摄取量。通常外泌体修饰主要涉及用特定的配体修饰其表面并装载治疗剂,如短干扰 RNA(short-interfering RNA,siRNA)、miRNA、DNA、蛋白质和小分子。

(一)外泌体表面工程化

由于脂质双层膜提供的抗降解和抗失活保护,外泌体属于能够长程转移的新型生物活性分子。从理论上讲,外泌体可以被工程化以靶向特定的细胞类型。来自 MSC 的外泌体具有影响组织对损伤、感染和疾病反应的特征。外泌体可以安全有效地输送药物,包括多种化学药品、多肽和遗传分子,并成功治疗了缺血性脑卒中。但是,外泌体在缺血性脑卒中应用的主要障碍是血脑屏障(blood-brain barrier,BBB)[101,102]。田等提出了一种简单、快速、有效的方法,通过生物正交的无铜叠氮炔环加成反应将对整联蛋白具有高亲和力的配体缀合到 MSC-外泌体表面。首先,他们建立了小鼠脑缺血模型。其次,将环缀合的 MSC-外泌体静脉注射,外泌体显示出靶向脑缺血性的病变区域并进入小胶质细胞、神经元和星形胶质细胞。此外,这些预装姜黄素的外泌体还促进了促炎细胞因子的释放和小胶质细胞的激活[103]。

据报道,靶向树突状外泌体与神经元特异性 RVG 肽 Lamp2b 结合能够转移整个血脑屏障的 GAPDH siRNA 和 BACE1。随后,大脑中的 mRNA 和 β-淀粉样蛋白表达被显著抑制[104]。基于 MSC 外泌体在 AD 中的治疗作用[37],这些脂肪组织 MSC 衍生的外泌体可以用 Lamp2b 修饰以靶向受体神经母细胞瘤细胞,从而降低分泌的和细胞内的 Aβ 水平。另一个研究使用 GE11 肽修饰外泌体,该肽在其表面上特异性结合 EGFR,在小鼠模型中将 miRNA 传递给异种移植的乳腺肿瘤细胞[105]。

(二)外泌体成分有效工程化

外泌体脂质双层膜围绕并包含亲水核。基于对外泌体结构的透彻了解,外泌体修饰的另一个重要方面是针对外泌体内容物。目前可以使用两种主要方法将治疗剂(如小分子、蛋白质和核酸)掺入外泌体:主动或被动封装[106,107]。这些不同的方法导致 EV 中不同的搭载效率和不同的药物稳定性。被动装载的策略相对简单,主要分为两种类型:将药物与外泌体或亲代细胞一起孵育。小化学分子的疏水性会导致较高的负载量,因为疏水性药物可以与膜的脂质层相互作用[108]。例如,姜黄素是可形成均一溶液的疏水性多酚化合物。据报道,在蔗糖梯度离心之前,姜黄素可以通过与小鼠淋巴瘤细胞衍生的外泌体在磷酸盐缓冲液(phosphate-buffered saline,PBS)中于 22℃ 孵育 5 分钟而掺入外泌体中,并保护小鼠对抗脂多糖(lipopolysaccharide,LPS)诱导的感染性休克[108]。体内外结果表明,目标特异性是由外泌体决定的,并且通过将姜黄素引导至炎性细胞可以实现姜黄素活性的提升。此外,实验中仅观察到外泌体治疗作用而未观察到毒性作用。同样,过氧化氢酶(一种有效的抗氧化剂)通过在室温下孵育而被搭载到外泌体中。负载过氧化氢酶的外泌体可保护 SNpc 神经元免受小鼠急性脑炎的氧化应激损伤[109]。此外,经共孵育后疏水修饰的 siRNA(hydrophobically modified siRNA,hsiRNA)可有效地加载到 U87 细胞衍生的外泌体中,然后递送至小鼠原代皮质神经元,并有效沉默多达 35% 的目标 mRNA,即 Huntington mRNA[110]。活性药物负载是指电穿孔、超声处理、挤出、冷冻/融化循环、透化和点击化学等方法。

1. 电穿孔

该策略涉及通过对悬浮在导电溶液中的外泌体施加电场,在外泌体膜上形成小孔。电流干扰磷脂双层,导致形成暂时的孔,这些孔允许药物自由扩散到囊泡内部。然后在药物加载之后,外泌体膜的完整性得以恢复。电穿孔已被用于预装载数种类型的内容物,包括 siRNA 和 miRNA。GAPDH 和 BACE1 siRNA 在 400V 和 125 μF 下通过电穿孔进入外泌体,并且保留较多的 siRNA。此外,外泌体转移此 siRNA 成功地敲低了 GAPDH 和 BACE1 的表达[104]。Wahlgren 等的研究显示了相似的结果。他们使用血浆中的外泌体作为向 T 细胞和单核细胞的药物递送系统,并通过电穿孔法向它们预装了针对有丝分裂 MAPK1 的 siRNA[111]。在另一个研究中,通过电穿孔将两个针对 RAD51 和 RAD52 的 siRNA 载入外泌体中,并验证了这些外泌体可将 siRNA 传递至受体细胞并强烈抑制 RAD51 的表达[112]。然而据报道,用 siRNA 对外泌体进行电穿孔会伴随大量的 siRNA 聚集体形成,这可能会导致高估了实际装载到外泌体中的 siRNA 量[113]。

将 miR-155 模拟物通过电穿孔引入外泌体显著增加 miR-155 敲除的小鼠原代肝细胞和肝脏中 miR-155 水平[114]。除了 siRNA 和 miRNA,小分子药物也可以通过电穿孔加载到外泌体中。阿霉素以不超过 20% 的包封效率被电穿孔包封到未成熟 DC 衍生的外泌体中[115]。Johnsen 等报道电穿孔并没有改变脂肪组织 MSC-外泌体诱导多形性胶质母细胞瘤细胞增殖的内源性刺激能力,但会引起外泌体不利的形态变化,包括外泌体的聚集等[116]。

2. 超声处理

在外泌体与药物和蛋白质混合后,可以使用均质器探头对其进行超声处理。超声波探头产生的机械剪切力损害了外泌体膜的完整性,并在膜变形期间使药物扩散到外泌体中。紫杉醇通过超声处理被加载到 RAW264.7 巨噬细胞衍生的外泌体中,其负载能力接近 30%,高于通过孵育(~2%)和电穿孔(~5.5%)达到的负载能力[117]。在另一项研究中,研究者使用几种不同的方法将过氧化氢酶加载到外泌体中,包括超声处理、皂苷处理、冻融循环和挤出。此外,研究已经证实外泌体的表面修饰可能会改变外泌体表面蛋白含量以及脂质双层的组织结构,并导致外泌体与靶细胞膜的相互作用增加。此外,在超声处理和挤压后,外泌体的大量重整和重塑使过氧化氢酶在相对紧密和高度结构化的脂质双层中扩散并导致较高的装载效率[109]。

3. 冻结/解冻周期

将外泌体与药物在室温下孵育后,可以将混合物在 -80°C 或液氮中快速冷冻,然后在室温下解冻。重复此冻结/融化循环至少 3 次,以确保封装的有效性和效率。这种方法可以优化外泌体表面的特性,以降低免疫原性,增加胶体稳定性,并改善外泌体在血液中的半衰期[118]。基于纳米颗粒跟踪分析的研究已表明该策略可诱导外泌体聚集,并导致载药外泌体的粒径分布较宽。此外,与通过和酶在室温下孵育、超声处理、挤压和透化等加载方式相比,冷冻/融化循环预加载过氧化氢酶至外泌体的方法具有中等的加载效率值。然而可能是由于处理后聚集,这些外泌体的尺寸明显更大[109]。

4. 透化

通常,细胞固定后经通透化处理以检测细胞内抗原[119]。由于外泌体的膜在组成和结构上与细胞膜相似,外泌体可以被透化以使其对抗体具有渗透性。通常使用两种通用类型的试剂进行通透处理:有机溶剂,如甲醇;清洁剂如皂素和Triton X - 100[119]。据报道,与无皂苷处理的被动加载方式相比,皂苷辅助渗透使外泌体中的药物负载量增加了11倍[106]。

其他基于外泌体的药物递送方式包括:① 药物负载在从离体亲代细胞分离的幼稚外泌体上;② 用药物装载亲代细胞,然后从细胞分泌的外泌体中释放药物;③ 用编码治疗活性化合物的DNA,或者miRNA和siRNA转染亲本细胞,然后从外泌体中释放它们[120]。之前描述的主动或被动封装策略涉及将药物掺入分离的外泌体中。我们可以在亲本细胞中预装外源性化合物进行被动封装。将小鼠MSC细胞系SR4987与紫杉醇孵育可以释放出大量富含紫杉醇的外泌体[121]。同样,用抗癌药物(紫杉醇、卡铂、依托泊苷和盐酸伊立替康)处理耐药的HepG2细胞,可上调细胞分泌的外泌体表面HSP,从而在细胞内产生良好的免疫原性,诱导HSP特异性NK细胞反应[122]。此外,据报道孔径减小的过滤器连续挤压分解单核细胞或巨噬细胞能够产生载有化学治疗剂的纳米囊泡。这些纳米粒子通过维持质膜蛋白的拓扑结构而具有天然的细胞靶向能力,在体外诱导了TNF-α刺激的内皮细胞死亡,并抑制了体内肿瘤的生长[123]。研究还显示外源化合物可以通过脂质体改造亲代细胞而包装在EV中,并且EV通过多个肿瘤细胞层介导化合物的自主细胞间迁移[124]。最后,从转基因亲代细胞中分离和纯化载有药物的外泌体已普遍用于生产基于外泌体的制剂。通常,将编码miRNA、siRNA、DNA或mRNA序列的DNA通过转染或电穿孔至源细胞中,然后将基因封装到这些亲本细胞分泌的外泌体中(表19-1)。

表19-1 以外泌体为基础的基因递送

亲代细胞	搭载方法	基因生物型	效　果	参考文献
DC	电穿孔	siRNA - GAPDH	体内外敲低GAPDH	[104]
内皮细胞	转染	siRNA	抑制靶细胞荧光素酶表达	[125]
L929成纤维细胞	转染	siRNA - TGF - beta1	抑制小鼠TGF-β1表达,同时抑制生长和转移	[126]
人胚胎肾细胞293T	转染	siRNA - MOR (opioid receptor Mu)	将siRNA递送至脑部同时抑制MOR表达	[127]
MSC	转染	miR - 146b	减少大鼠脑胶质瘤异种移植物的生长	[128]
MSC	转染	Anti - miR - 9	逆转胶质母细胞瘤多形细胞的化学耐药性	[129]
人胚胎肾细胞293	转染	let - 7a	将let-7a传递给表达EGFR的乳腺肿瘤细胞和组织	[105]

续 表

亲代细胞	搭载方法	基因生物型	效果	参考文献
成人肝脏干细胞	转染	miRNA	抑制小鼠肝细胞癌的生长和存活	[130]
人胚胎肾细胞293	转染	miR-124	抑制靶基因	[131]
骨髓间充质干细胞	电穿孔	miR-124	将miR-124递送至梗死部位并保护其免受缺血性损伤	[132]
内皮细胞	转染	miR-195	抑制5-HTT(5-羟色胺)的表达	[133]
脂肪组织MSC	转染	miR-450a-5p	通过抑制WISP2促进脂肪生成	[134]
人Wharton Jelly间充质干细胞	转染	miR-30	通过抑制线粒体功能改善急性肾缺血再灌注损伤	[135]
人胚胎肾细胞293	转染	miR-29a/c	通过阻断血管生成控制胃癌生长	[136]
骨髓间充质干细胞	转染	miR-200b	预防上皮细胞-间充质转化并减轻结肠纤维化	[137]
小鼠心肌细胞	转染	DNA	改变基因表达	[138]
人胚胎肾细胞293，人脐静脉内皮细胞，逆转录病毒端粒化HUVEC,MSC	电穿孔	dsDNA	递送DNA	[139]
人类神经胶质瘤干细胞	转染	DNA	EV穿过完整的血脑屏障	[140]
心球来源干细胞	转染	Y RNA fragment	通过调节IL-10表达和分泌进行心脏保护	[141]
人卵巢肿瘤细胞系ES-2和SKOV3	转染	MMP1 mRNA	诱导间皮细胞凋亡	[142]
人胚胎肾细胞293T	转染	Cytosine deaminase uracil mRNA	抑制神经鞘瘤生长	[143]

通过电穿孔将GAPDH-siRNA和BACE1-siRNA加载到外泌体中能够敲低BACE1 60%的mRNA和62%的蛋白质，这些载有siRNA的外泌体对小鼠阿尔兹海默病具有治疗作用[104]。miRNA可以通过降解mRNA或抑制靶基因的翻译来抑制蛋白表达水平，同时外泌体可以将miRNA传递至靶受体细胞。在体外用表达miR-146b质粒转染的MSC-外泌体降低了神经胶质瘤细胞中EGFR和NF-kB蛋白的表达水平。体内研究结果显示用载有miR-146的外泌体治疗能够减小胶质瘤体积[128]。在另一种神经元疾病中，转染anti-miR-9的MSC产生的外泌体被多形性胶质母细胞瘤(glioblastoma multiforme, GBM)细胞内化后降低了化学转运性基因MDR1在耐化学性GBM细胞中的表达，并增加了GBM细胞的化学敏感性[129]。研究报道从MSC中分离并装载了miR-124的外泌体随后将

miR-124递送至梗死部位，促进皮质神经祖细胞获得神经元身份，并通过强大的皮质神经发生作用防止缺血性损伤[132]。miR-124也参与了亨廷顿病。降低miR-124表达会增加RE1转录因子（RE1-silecing transcription factor，REST）的水平，从而导致关键靶基因（如脑源性神经营养因子）的表达受到抑制[144]。据报道，递送miR-30转染的人Wharton Jelly MSC来源的外泌体至受损的肾小管上皮细胞，可以在受损的大鼠肾脏中恢复miR-30的表达[135]。此外，DNA是另一种可被携带至靶细胞和组织的生物活性分子。将参与慢性粒细胞白血病（chronic myeloid leukemia，CML）发病机制的BCR/ABL杂种基因从供体K562细胞衍生的外泌体转移至中性粒细胞，能够在体外降低中性粒细胞的吞噬活性[145]。Lamichhane等报道外源线性DNA可以通过电穿孔装载到外泌体中，其数量足以使每个囊泡平均产生数百个DNA分子。他们认为外泌体中DNA的装载效率和能力取决于DNA的大小。与长度较大的线性DNA和质粒DNA分子相比，长度小于1 000 bp的线性DNA分子的装载效率更高。研究进一步表明，外泌体将外源DNA递送至受体细胞[139]。除DNA外，微囊泡（包括外泌体）还可以转移mRNA和蛋白质。心球来源细胞的外泌体富含Y RNA的片段，这些外泌体被输送到巨噬细胞并诱导IL-10的产生。而且，这些装载Y RNA的外泌体减小了心肌梗死面积，并在心肌缺血/再灌注损伤后引发了心脏保护反应[141]。总体而言，我们可以将各种编码miRNA、siRNA、DNA和mRNA序列的DNA分子装载到外泌体中，这表明MSC-外泌体代表了再生医学中有前景的DNA"药物"递送系统。

五、MSC-外泌体在再生医学中的临床应用

近来，外泌体已被批准用于一些临床试验，并且基于外泌体的人体治疗方法正在蓬勃发展。由于DC的外泌体对免疫系统的特定调节作用，外泌体有望作为肿瘤疫苗并引发了研究者广泛的关注。研究表明DC-外泌体通过同时提呈MHC-Ⅰ和MHC-Ⅱ来刺激幼稚的$CD4^+$ T细胞和$CD8^+$ T细胞[146,147]。三个Ⅰ期临床试验证实了DC-外泌体在肿瘤治疗中的安全性和可行性。然而，注射的DC-外泌体在刺激MHC限制的T细胞反应中效果有限[148,149]。另一项Ⅱ期临床试验是使用来源于IFN-γ处理的成熟的DC的外泌体进行的。研究已证明通过NKp30激活NK细胞可能是ⅢB/Ⅳ期NSCLC患者的有效免疫调节策略[150]。不幸的是，该试验的目标，即让至少50%的患者在化疗停止后4个月病情无进展，并没有实现。此外，目前已有公司一直致力于DC外泌体的商业用途。Anosys公司已生产用于肿瘤治疗的自体DC-外泌体疫苗。来自MSC、内皮祖细胞、Treg和其他类型细胞的外泌体的其他有效应用包括再生医学和针对非恶性疾病的免疫疗法。源自MSC的外泌体的临床试验正在进行中。另外有两家公司正在开发MSC-外泌体的商业用途[151]。ReNeuron Group PLC在神经和缺血领域中具有实践经验。Capricor公司正在研究外泌体在心脏和肌肉疾病中的治疗作用（http://capricor.com）。

六、局限与挑战

目前，研究已经证明源自MSC的外泌体在各种生理和病理过程中起关键作用。最初研

究中由于 MSC 具有不同的潜力和免疫调节的优势,外泌体在组织修复和再生中作为细胞疗法的备选方案引起了研究者极大的兴趣[152-154]。但是,越来越多的证据表明,MSC 在再生医学中的治疗作用主要源于其旁分泌作用[119,155,156]。外泌体是 MSC 分泌的因子之一,它介导细胞之间的相互作用并模仿亲代细胞的生物学功能。由于具有多种多样且全面的特性,外泌体拥有巨大的潜力可作为基于 MSC 的细胞疗法的替代品。为了将外泌体用于临床试验,我们第一步是准备用于分离外泌体的源细胞。其次,扩展培养系统以获得所需数量的外泌体。然后,必须通过几种方法分离和纯化外泌体。最后,具有治疗潜力的外泌体需要通过静脉内或鼻内给予患者(图 19-2)[104,157,158]。

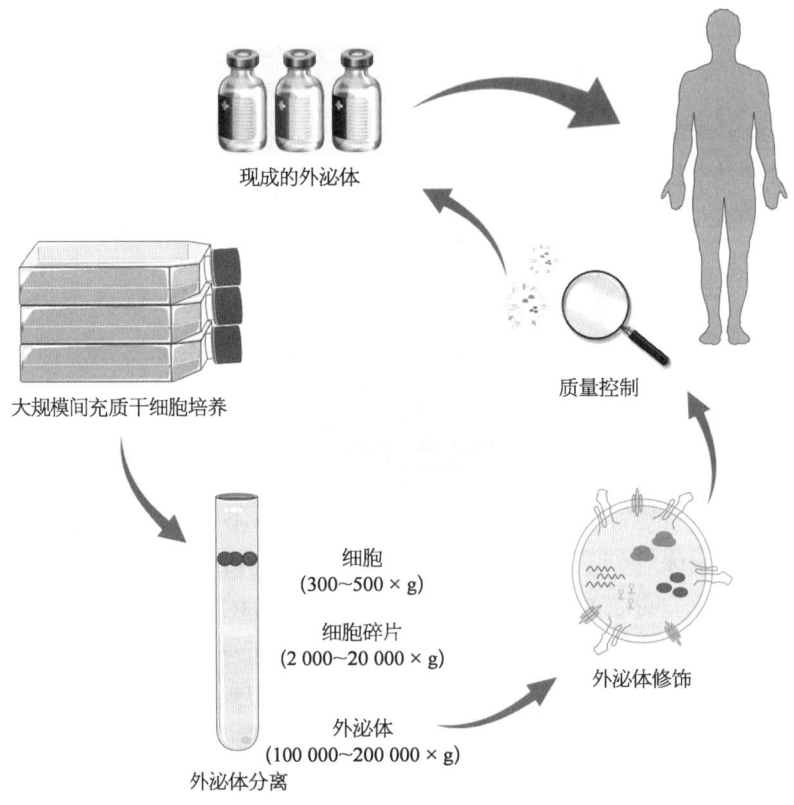

图 19-2 以外泌体为基础疗法的临床应用代表步骤示意图

至于 MSC 外泌体在临床试验中的应用,在生产、修饰、储存、运输和质量控制方面仍然存在一些障碍(表 19-2)。

表 19-2 外泌体临床应用的挑战

问 题	详细的问题
细胞来源	骨髓间充质干细胞类型 培养和刺激状况 自体/外生

续 表

问　　题	详细的问题
修饰	目标分子
	生物活性成分
	标志
质量控制	cGMP（临床良好制造规范）
	同质
	大规模
	活性/效率
	储存和运输

　　对于不同类型和阶段的疾病，在应用外泌体之前，我们需要解决几个问题。例如，外泌体来源应该是哪种干细胞。研究已经证实外泌体的内容物至少部分与亲代细胞类似。因此，可以根据它们的组织起源和治疗目的来选择不同的亲代间充质基质细胞。可以从患者本人或同种异体供体中分离细胞，并应在常见的微环境或特定刺激下培养细胞。MSC在临床上的应用利用了其免疫原性弱的优势，这确定了从同种异体供体获得MSC甚至外泌体的可能性[3]。然后，为了实现精确的靶向递送和（或）增强治疗效果，我们可以用不同的肽或受体修饰外泌体，并且可以将特定类型的治疗物［遗传药物和（或）化学化合物］或其组合加载到外泌体中。我们还需要根据加载的内容物选择加载策略，以确保外泌体的封装效率。此外，我们可能还需要其他标识标记外泌体，以通过体内成像技术追踪外泌体的生物分布及其归巢到的目标组织和器官。另外，为了获得足够数量的外泌体用于临床试验中，第一步我们要离体扩增亲代MSC细胞。据报道，TSAP6对压力具有p53反应，能够增强细胞外泌体的分泌[159]。研究还证明调节某些基因的表达或调节培养环境的pH可能会增加MSC的外泌体分泌量[160-162]。第二步是选择外泌体的分离方法。目前分离和纯化外泌体常用的方法是差速离心、尺寸排阻色谱、聚合物沉淀、免疫磁分离和过滤。

　　差速离心是使用最广泛的分离外泌体的方法[163]，它已被广泛用作从生物体液中分离外泌体[164]。在这种方法中，通过低速离心去除细胞和凋亡碎片，以较高的速度去除较大尺寸的微囊泡，最后通过超速离心沉淀外泌体。但是当来源的生物液体为血浆和血清时，此耗时的过程效率较低[165]。尺寸排阻色谱法（size exclusion chromatography，SEC）是一种基于化合物尺寸的分离方法，其分离效率取决于化合物渗透固定相孔的效率。与差速离心相比，尺寸排阻色谱法完全清除了污染蛋白，因此可实现高产量和稳定的外泌体回收率。尺寸排阻色谱法分离外泌体不利的一面是色谱柱可能会造成污染，并且需要收集大量馏分并进行分析，这包括了一系列耗时的步骤[166]。将与沉淀溶液混合的生物流体在4℃下孵育过夜，然后通过低速离心获得外泌体沉淀。该方法相对容易执行，并且不需要专门的设备或较长的时间。然而，低速离心法的主要费用是购买沉淀试剂盒[167]。免疫磁分离通过将外泌体与特定表面蛋白或抗原结合并附着于珠子来分离外泌体。尽管通过这种免疫亲和方法产率很低，但是与通过其他方法获得的外泌体相比，免疫磁分离获得的外泌体纯度较高。总之，每种方法都有优缺点，外泌体的分离需要不同的样品预处理技术，并且会产生不同纯度和质量的外泌体制剂。用户可以根据预期的下游应用选择外泌体分离方法。未来的研究需要开发新的大规模生产外泌体的方法。外泌体的应用需要临床良好的生产规范（clinical good manufacturing practice，cGMP）标准，包括细胞储存和存储、可扩展性、稳定性、批次和批次跟踪、病原体筛选以及其他进行质量控制的物理、化学和生物学方法[157,168]。除了外泌体的生产和质量控制，未来外泌体研究的其他关键点包括将外泌体治疗与患者病情状况紧密联系起来以及包括毒性和不良反应在内的安全性考虑。因此，研究者应进行大量工作以充分利用 MSC-外泌体并挖掘其在临床和个性化治疗中的潜力。

七、总结和展望

在本章中，我们介绍了来自 MSC 的外泌体的生物学特性和治疗功能，并强调了 MSC-外泌体在再生医学中的临床应用潜力。由于外泌体的生物发生参与细胞间通信的理论已被研究者广为接受，因此与细胞、合成纳米颗粒和单分子相比，外泌体具有多种优越的治疗作用。大多数类型细胞都可以释放外泌体，因此可以将外泌体改造为低免疫原性甚至是非免疫原性状态，并且外泌体具有出色的生物相容性、生物稳定性和安全性。由于缺乏细胞核，相对于整个细胞，外泌体避免了肿瘤转化的风险。外泌体在冷冻/融化循环，长距离运输和长期保存后仍能保持活力，并将生物活性治疗剂包封在膜内，从而保护了治疗剂免于降解和失活。另外，可以用特定的表面受体对外泌体进行遗传修饰，以将外泌体对细胞和器官进行特异性递送。因此，外泌体作为药物递送和基因治疗的载体吸引了很多研究者的关注。对于再生医学，外泌体有望激活受损的细胞和组织，并通过其生物活性成分和功能分子促进损伤恢复。此外，MSC-外泌体可以用作生物标志物鉴定高质量亲代 MSC 并使用当前再生医学方法进行移植。

尽管外泌体在体外和动物模型中的研究数量不断增加并取得了令人鼓舞的结果，但我们仍需要解决和规范将来源于 MSC 的外泌体用于治疗的方法。特别是如何在扩大生产规模以获得足够数量外泌体的同时保持用于临床试验和治疗的外泌体的 cGMP 标准是当前研究的难点。在动物研究和临床前测试中进一步研究 MSC-外泌体的不良反应尤其重要。因此，我们不仅需要探索外泌体新颖的治疗潜力，还必须仔细评估其安全性和有效性。

总而言之，我们应该进行更多的工作来确定源自间充质基质细胞的外泌体促进组织修复和再生的潜在机制。MSC-外泌体的临床前研究取得了令人满意的结果，为再生医学带来了新的希望。

利益冲突

作者声明他们没有利益冲突。

（宋伟　译，何耀华　审校）

参考文献

[1] Bajaj P, Schweller RM, Khademhosseini A, West JL, Bashir R. 3D biofabrication strategies for tissue engineering and

[2] Kassem M, Kristiansen M, Abdallah BM. Mesenchymal stem cells: cell biology and potential use in therapy. Basic Clin Pharmacol Toxicol 2004 Nov; 95(5): 209-14.

regenerative medicine. Annu Rev Biomed Eng 2014; 16: 247-76.

[3] Uccelli A, Moretta L, Pistoia V. Mesenchymal stem cells in health and disease. Nat Rev Immunol 2008; 8(9): 726-36.
[4] Trohatou O, Roubelakis MG. Mesenchymal stem/stromal cells in regenerative medicine: past, present, and future. Cell Reprogram 2017; 19(4): 217-24.
[5] Madrigal M, Rao KS, Riordan NH. A review of therapeutic effects of mesenchymal stem cell secretions and induction of secretory modification by different culture methods. J Transl Med 2014; 12 (1): 260. Available from: http://translational-medicine.biomedcentral.com/articles/10.1186/s12967-014-0260-8. [cited 15 October 2018].
[6] Haynesworth SE, Baber MA, Caplan AI. Cytokine expression by human marrow-derived mesenchymal progenitor cells in vitro: effects of dexamethasone and IL-1α. J Cell Physiol 1996; 166: 585-92. https://doi.org/10.1002/(SICI)1097-4652(199603)166: 3<585:: AIDJCP13> 3.0.CO; 2-6.
[7] Basu J, Ludlow JW. Exosomes for repair, regeneration and rejuvenation. Expert Opin Biol Ther 2016; 16(4): 489-506.
[8] Seki A, Sakai Y, Komura T, Nasti A, Yoshida K, Higashimoto M, et al. Adipose tissue-derived stem cells as a regenerative therapy for a mouse steatohepatitis-induced cirrhosis model. Hepatology 2013; 58(3): 1133-42.
[9] Higashimoto M, Sakai Y, Takamura M, Usui S, Nasti A, Yoshida K, et al. Adipose tissue derived stromal stem cell therapy in murine ConA-derived hepatitis is dependent on myeloidlineage and CD4+ T-cell suppression. Eur J Immunol 2013; 43(11): 2956-68.
[10] Katsuda T, Ochiya T. Potential application of mesenchymal stem cell-derived exosomes as a novel therapeutic drug. Drug Deliv Syst 2014; 29(2): 140-51.
[11] De Jong OG, Van Balkom BWM, Schiffelers RM, Bouten CVC, Verhaar MC. Extracellular vesicles: potential roles in regenerative medicine. Front Immunol 2014; 5: 608. Available from: http://journal.frontiersin.org/article/10.3389/fimmu.2014.00608/abstract. [cited 15 October 2018].
[12] Goradel NH, Jahangiri S, Negahdari B. Effects of mesenchymal stem cell-derived exosomes on angiogenesis in regenerative medicine. Curr Regen Med 2018; 7(1): 46-53.
[13] Cheng L, Zhang K, Wu S, Cui M, Xu T. Focus on mesenchymal stem cell-derived exosomes: opportunities and challenges in cell-free therapy. Stem Cells Int 2017; 2017: 1-10.
[14] Rani S, Ryan AE, Griffin MD, Ritter T. Mesenchymal stem cell-derived extracellular vesicles: toward cell-free therapeutic applications. Mol Ther 2015; 23(5): 812-23.
[15] Keshtkar S, Azarpira N, Ghahremani MH. Mesenchymal stem cell-derived extracellular vesicles: novel frontiers in regenerative medicine. Stem Cell Res Ther 2018; 9(1): 63. Available from: https://stemcellres.biomedcentral.com/articles/10.1186/s13287-018-0791-7. [cited 15 October 2018].
[16] Zhang H, Freitas D, Kim HS, Fabijanic K, Li Z, Chen H, et al. Identification of distinct nanoparticles and subsets of extracellular vesicles by asymmetric flow field-flow fractionation. Nat Cell Biol 2018; 20(3): 332-43.
[17] Pan B-T, Johnstone RM. Fate of the transferrin receptor during maturation of sheep reticulocytes in vitro: selective externalization of the receptor. Cell 1983; 33(3): 967-78.
[18] Stoorvogel W, Kleijmeer MJ, Geuze HJ, Raposo G. The biogenesis and functions of exosomes. Traffic 2002; 3(5): 321-30.
[19] Théry C, Zitvogel L, Amigorena S. Exosomes: composition, biogenesis and function. Nat Rev Immunol 2002; 2: 569.
[20] Valadi H, Ekström K, Bossios A, Sjöstrand M, Lee JJ, Lötvall JO. Exosome-mediated transfer of mRNAs and microRNAs is a novel mechanism of genetic exchange between cells. Nat Cell Biol 2007; 9: 654.
[21] Minciacchi VR, Freeman MR, Di Vizio D. Extracellular vesicles in cancer: exosomes, microvesicles and the emerging role of large oncosomes. Semin Cell Dev Biol 2015; 40: 41-51.
[22] Kalra H, Drummen GPC, Mathivanan S. Focus on extracellular vesicles: introducing the next small big thing. Tikkanen R, editor. Int J Mol Sci 2016; 17(2): 170.
[23] Tan SS, Yin Y, Lee T, Lai RC, Yeo RWY, Zhang B, et al. Therapeutic MSC exosomes are derived from lipid raft microdomains in the plasma membrane. J Extracell Vesicles 2013; 2. https://doi.org/10.3402/jev.v2i0.22614.
[24] Liu S, Liu D, Chen C, Hamamura K, Moshaverinia A, Yang R, et al. MSC transplantation improves osteopenia via epigenetic regulation of notch signaling in lupus. Cell Metab 2015; 22(4): 606-18.
[25] Pashoutan Sarvar D, Shamsasenjan K, Akbarzadehlaleh P. Mesenchymal stem cell-derived exosomes: new opportunity in cell-free therapy. Adv Pharm Bull 2016; 6(3): 293-9.
[26] Kim H-S, Choi D-Y, Yun SJ, Choi S-M, Kang JW, Jung JW, et al. Proteomic analysis of microvesicles derived from human mesenchymal stem cells. J Proteome Res 2012; 11(2): 839-49.
[27] Vallabhaneni KC, Penfornis P, Dhule S, Guillonneau F, Adams KV, Mo YY, et al. Extracellular vesicles from bone marrow mesenchymal stem/stromal cells transport tumor regulatory microRNA, proteins, and metabolites. Oncotarget 2015; 6(7): 4953-67.
[28] Reis LA, Borges FT, Simões MJ, Borges AA, Sinigaglia-Coimbra R, Schor N. Bone marrowderived mesenchymal stem cells repaired but did not prevent gentamicin-induced acute kidney injury through paracrine effects in rats. PLoS One 2012; 7(9): e44092.
[29] Haraszti RA, Didiot M-C, Sapp E, Leszyk J, Shaffer SA, Rockwell HE, et al. High-resolution proteomic and lipidomic analysis of exosomes and microvesicles from different cell sources. J Extracell Vesicles 2016; 5: 32570. https://doi.org/10.3402/jev.v5.32570.
[30] Wang Y, Fu B, Sun X, Li D, Huang Q, Zhao W, et al. Differentially expressed microRNAs in bone marrow mesenchymal stem cell-derived microvesicles in young and older rats and their effect on tumor growth factor-β1-mediated epithelial-mesenchymal transition in HK2 cells. Stem Cell Res Ther 2015; 6: 185.
[31] Lei Q, Liu T, Gao F, Xie H, Sun L, Zhao A, et al. Microvesicles as potential biomarkers for the identification of

senescence in human mesenchymal stem cells. Theranostics 2017; 7(10): 2673-89.
[32] Sakaida I, Terai S, Yamamoto N, Aoyama K, Ishikawa T, Nishina H, et al. Transplantation of bone marrow cells reduces CCl4-induced liver fibrosis in mice. Hepatology 2004; 40(6): 1304-11.
[33] Tögel F, Hu Z, Weiss K, Isaac J, Lange C, Westenfelder C. Administered mesenchymal stem cells protect against ischemic acute renal failure through differentiation-independent mechanisms. Am J Physiol-Ren Physiol 2005; 289(1): F31-42.
[34] Kourembanas S. Exosomes: vehicles of intercellular signaling, biomarkers, and vectors of cell therapy. Annu Rev Physiol 2015; 77(1): 13-27.
[35] Yáñez-Mó M, Siljander PR-M, Andreu Z, Zavec AB, Borràs FE, Buzas EI, et al. Biological properties of extracellular vesicles and their physiological functions. J Extracell Vesicles 2015; 4: 27066. https://doi.org/10.3402/jev.v4.27066.
[36] Yoo J, Kim H-S, Hwang D-Y. Stem cells as promising therapeutic options for neurological disorders. J Cell Biochem 2012; 114(4): 743-53.
[37] Katsuda T, Tsuchiya R, Kosaka N, Yoshioka Y, Takagaki K, Oki K, et al. Human adipose tissue-derived mesenchymal stem cells secrete functional neprilysin-bound exosomes. Sci Rep 2013; 3: 1197.
[38] Jarmalavičiūtė A, Tunaitis V, Pivoraitė U, Venalis A, Pivoriūnas A. Exosomes from dental pulp stem cells rescue human dopaminergic neurons from 6-hydroxy-dopamine-induced apoptosis. Cytotherapy 2015; 17(7): 932-9.
[39] Xin H, Li Y, Cui Y, Yang JJ, Zhang ZG, Chopp M. Systemic administration of exosomes released from mesenchymal stromal cells promote functional recovery and neurovascular plasticity after stroke in rats. J Cereb Blood Flow Metab 2013; 33(11): 1711-5.
[40] Doeppner TR, Herz J, Görgens A, Schlechter J, Ludwig A-K, Radtke S, et al. Extracellular vesicles improve post-stroke neuroregeneration and prevent postischemic immunosuppression. Stem Cells Transl Med 2015; 4(10): 1131-43.
[41] Ophelders DR, Wolfs TG, Jellema RK, Zwanenburg A, Andriessen P, Delhaas T, et al. Mesenchymal stromal cell-derived extracellular vesicles protect the fetal brain after hypoxia-ischemia. Stem Cells Transl Med 2016; 5(6): 754-63.
[42] Drommelschmidt K, Serdar M, Bendix I, Herz J, Bertling F, Prager S, et al. Mesenchymal stem cell-derived extracellular vesicles ameliorate inflammation-induced preterm brain injury. Brain Behav Immun 2017; 60: 220-32.
[43] Xin H, Li Y, Liu Z, Wang X, Shang X, Cui Y, et al. MiR-133b promotes neural plasticity and functional recovery after treatment of stroke with multipotent mesenchymal stromal cells in rats via transfer of exosome-enriched extracellular particles. Stem Cells 2013; 31(12): 2737-46.
[44] Xin H, Katakowski M, Wang F, Qian J-Y, Shuang Liu X, Ali MM, et al. MiR-17-92 cluster in exosomes enhance neuroplasticity and functional recovery after stroke in rats. Stroke 2017; 48(3): 747-53.
[45] Mead B, Amaral J, Tomarev S. Mesenchymal stem cell-derived small extracellular vesicles promote neuroprotection in rodent models of glaucoma. Invest Ophthalmol Vis Sci 2018; 59(2): 702-14.
[46] Menon DK, Schwab K, Wright DW, Maas AI. Position statement: definition of traumatic brain injury. Arch Phys Med Rehabil 2010; 91(11): 1637-40.
[47] Zhang Y, Chopp M, Meng Y, Katakowski M, Xin H, Mahmood A, et al. Effect of exosomes derived from multipluripotent mesenchymal stromal cells on functional recovery and neurovascular plasticity in rats after traumatic brain injury. J Neurosurg 2015; 122(4): 856-67.
[48] Kim D, Nishida H, An SY, Shetty AK, Bartosh TJ, Prockop DJ. Chromatographically isolated CD63(+)CD81(+) extracellular vesicles from mesenchymal stromal cells rescue cognitive impairments after TBI. Proc Natl Acad Sci U S A 2016; 113(1): 170-5.
[49] Yang Y, Ye Y, Su X, He J, Bai W, He X. MSCs-derived exosomes and neuroinflammation, neurogenesis and therapy of traumatic brain injury. Front Cell Neurosci 2017; 11: 55.
[50] Hausenloy DJ, Yellon DM. Myocardial ischemia-reperfusion injury: a neglected therapeutic target. J Clin Invest 2013; 123(1): 92-100.
[51] Lai RC, Arslan F, Lee MM, Sze NSK, Choo A, Chen TS, et al. Exosome secreted by MSC reduces myocardial ischemia/reperfusion injury. Stem Cell Res 2010; 4(3): 214-22.
[52] Arslan F, Lai RC, Smeets MB, Akeroyd L, Choo A, Aguor ENE, et al. Mesenchymal stem cell-derived exosomes increase ATP levels, decrease oxidative stress and activate PI3K/Akt pathway to enhance myocardial viability and prevent adverse remodeling after myocardial ischemia/reperfusion injury. Stem Cell Res 2013; 10(3): 301-12.
[53] Bian S, Zhang L, Duan L, Wang X, Min Y, Hu Y. Extracellular vesicles derived from human bone marrow mesenchymal stem cells promote angiogenesis in a rat myocardial infarction model. J Mol Med 2014; 92(4): 387-97.
[54] Teng X, Chen L, Chen W, Yang J, Yang Z, Shen Z. Mesenchymal stem cell-derived exosomes improve the microenvironment of infarcted myocardium contributing to angiogenesis and anti-inflammation. Cell Physiol Biochem 2015; 37(6): 2415-24.
[55] Yu B, Gong M, Wang Y, Millard RW, Pasha Z, Yang Y, et al. Cardiomyocyte protection by GATA-4 gene engineered mesenchymal stem cells is partially mediated by translocation of miR-221 in microvesicles. PLoS ONE 2013; 8(8): e73304.
[56] Yu B, Kim HW, Gong M, Wang J, Millard RW, Wang Y, et al. Exosomes secreted from GATA-4 overexpressing mesenchymal stem cells serve as a reservoir of anti-apoptotic microRNAs for cardioprotection. Int J Cardiol 2015; 182: 349-60.
[57] Shao L, Zhang Y, Lan B, Wang J, Zhang Z, Zhang L, et al. MiRNA-sequence indicates that mesenchymal stem cells and exosomes have similar mechanism to enhance cardiac repair. Biomed Res Int 2017; 2017: 4150705.
[58] Wang K, Jiang Z, Webster KA, Chen J, Hu H, Zhou Y, et al. Enhanced cardioprotection by human endometrium mesenchymal stem cells driven by exosomal MicroRNA-21. Stem Cells Transl Med 2017; 6(1): 209-22.
[59] Romero-Bermejo FJ, Ruiz-Bailen M, Gil-Cebrian J, Huertos-Ranchal MJ. Sepsis-induced cardiomyopathy. Curr Cardiol Rev 2011; 7(3): 163-83.
[60] Wang X, Gu H, Qin D, Yang L, Huang W, Essandoh K, et al. Exosomal miR-223 contributes to mesenchymal stem

[61] Zhang Z, Yang J, Yan W, Li Y, Shen Z, Asahara T. Pretreatment of cardiac stem cells with exosomes derived from mesenchymal stem cells enhances myocardial repair. J Am Heart Assoc 2016; 5(1): e002856.
[62] Davidson SM, Yellon DM. Exosomes and cardioprotection — a critical analysis. Mol Aspects Med 2018; 60: 104-14.
[63] Li T, Yan Y, Wang B, Qian H, Zhang X, Shen L, et al. Exosomes derived from human umbilical cord mesenchymal stem cells alleviate liver fibrosis. Stem Cells Dev 2013; 22(6): 845-54.
[64] Tan CY, Lai RC, Wong W, Dan YY, Lim S-K, Ho HK. Mesenchymal stem cell-derived exosomes promote hepatic regeneration in drug-induced liver injury models. Stem Cell Res Ther 2014; 5(3): 76.
[65] Yan Y, Jiang W, Tan Y, Zou S, Zhang H, Mao F, et al. hucMSC exosome-derived GPX1 is required for the recovery of hepatic oxidant injury. Mol Ther 2017; 25(2): 465-79.
[66] Nong K, Wang W, Niu X, Hu B, Ma C, Bai Y, et al. Hepatoprotective effect of exosomes from human-induced pluripotent stem cell-derived mesenchymal stromal cells against hepatic ischemia-reperfusion injury in rats. Cytotherapy 2016; 18(12): 1548-59.
[67] Du Y, Li D, Han C, Wu H, Xu L, Zhang M, et al. Exosomes from human-induced pluripotent stem cell-derived mesenchymal stromal cells (hiPSC-MSCs) protect liver against hepatic ischemia/reperfusion injury via activating sphingosine kinase and sphingosine-1-phosphate signaling pathway. Cell Physiol Biochem 2017; 43(2): 611-25.
[68] Chen L, Xiang B, Wang X, Xiang C. Exosomes derived from human menstrual blood-derived stem cells alleviate fulminant hepatic failure. Stem Cell Res Ther 2017; 8: 9.
[69] Fujiyoshi M, Ozaki M. Molecular mechanisms of liver regeneration and protection for treatment of liver dysfunction and diseases. J Hepato-Biliary-Pancreat Sci 2010; 18(1): 13-22.
[70] Torres Crigna A, Daniele C, Gamez C, Medina Balbuena S, Pastene DO, Nardozi D, et al. Stem/stromal cells for treatment of kidney injuries with focus on preclinical models. Front Med 2018; 5: 179.
[71] van Koppen A, Joles JA, van Balkom BWM, Lim SK, de Kleijn D, Giles RH, et al. Human embryonic mesenchymal stem cell-derived conditioned medium rescues kidney function in rats with established chronic kidney disease. Dussaule J-C, editor PLoS ONE 2012; 7(6): e38746.
[72] Zhou Y, Xu H, Xu W, Wang B, Wu H, Tao Y, et al. Exosomes released by human umbilical cord mesenchymal stem cells protect against cisplatin-induced renal oxidative stress and apoptosis in vivo and in vitro. Stem Cell Res Ther 2013; 4(2): 34.
[73] Zou X, Zhang G, Cheng Z, Yin D, Du T, Ju G, et al. Microvesicles derived from human Wharton's jelly mesenchymal stromal cells ameliorate renal ischemia-reperfusion injury in rats by suppressing CX3CL1. Stem Cell Res Ther 2014; 5(2): 40.
[74] Li L, Huang L, Sung S-SJ, Vergis AL, Rosin DL, Rose CE, et al. The chemokine receptors CCR2 and CX3CR1 mediate monocyte/macrophage trafficking in kidney ischemia-reperfusion injury. Kidney Int 2008; 74(12): 1526-37.
[75] Shen B, Liu J, Zhang F, Wang Y, Qin Y, Zhou Z, et al. CCR2 positive exosome released by mesenchymal stem cells suppresses macrophage functions and alleviates ischemia/reperfusion-induced renal injury. Stem Cells Int 2016; 2016: 1-9.
[76] Eirin A, Zhu X-Y, Puranik AS, Tang H, McGurren KA, van Wijnen AJ, et al. Mesenchymal stem cell-derived extracellular vesicles attenuate kidney inflammation. Kidney Int 2017; 92(1): 114-24.
[77] Collino F, Bruno S, Incarnato D, Dettori D, Neri F, Provero P, et al. AKI recovery induced by mesenchymal stromal cell-derived extracellular vesicles carrying microRNAs. J Am Soc Nephrol 2015; 26(10): 2349-60.
[78] Nassar W, El-Ansary M, Sabry D, Mostafa MA, Fayad T, Kotb E, et al. Umbilical cord mesenchymal stem cells derived extracellular vesicles can safely ameliorate the progression of chronic kidney diseases. Biomater Res 2016; 20: 21.
[79] Kowada T, Kikuta J, Kubo A, Ishii M, Maeda H, Mizukami S, et al. In vivo fluorescence imaging of bone-resorbing osteoclasts. J Am Chem Soc 2011; 133(44): 17772-6.
[80] Xie Y, Gao Y, Zhang L, Chen Y, Ge W, Tang P. Involvement of serum-derived exosomes of elderly patients with bone loss in failure of bone remodeling via alteration of exosomal bonerelated proteins. Aging Cell 2018; 17(3): e12758.
[81] Manolagas SC. Steroids and osteoporosis: the quest for mechanisms. J Clin Invest 2013; 123(5): 1919-21.
[82] Lu Z, Chen Y, Dunstan C, Roohani-Esfahani S, Zreiqat H. Priming adipose stem cells with tumor necrosis factor-alpha preconditioning potentiates their exosome efficacy for bone regeneration. Tissue Eng Part A 2017; 23(21-22): 1212-20.
[83] Zhang J, Liu X, Li H, Chen C, Hu B, Niu X, et al. Exosomes/tricalcium phosphate combination scaffolds can enhance bone regeneration by activating the PI3K/Akt signaling pathway. Stem Cell Res Ther 2016; 7(1): 136.
[84] Zhang S, Chu W, Lai R, Hui J, Lee E, Lim S, et al. Human mesenchymal stem cell-derived exosomes promote orderly cartilage regeneration in an immunocompetent rat osteochondral defect model. Cytotherapy 2016; 18(6): S13.
[85] Furuta T, Miyaki S, Ishitobi H, Ogura T, Kato Y, Kamei N, et al. Mesenchymal stem cell-derived exosomes promote fracture healing in a mouse model. Stem Cells Transl Med 2016; 5(12): 1620-30.
[86] Li H, Yang F, Wang Z, Fu Q, Liang A. MicroRNA-21 promotes osteogenic differentiation by targeting small mothers against decapentaplegic 7. Mol Med Rep 2015; 12(1): 1561-7.
[87] Meng Y-B, Li X, Li Z-Y, Zhao J, Yuan X-B, Ren Y, et al. microRNA-21 promotes osteogenic differentiation of mesenchymal stem cells by the PI3K/β-catenin pathway. J Orthop Res 2015; 33(7): 957-64.
[88] Sun Y, Xu L, Huang S, Hou Y, Liu Y, Chan K-M, et al. mir-21 overexpressing mesenchymal stem cells accelerate fracture healing in a rat closed femur fracture model. Biomed Res Int 2015; 2015: 412327.
[89] Zhang S, Chu WC, Lai RC, Lim SK, Hui JHP, Toh WS. Exosomes derived from human embryonic mesenchymal stem cells promote osteochondral regeneration. Osteoarthr Cartil 2016; 24(12): 2135-40.
[90] Qi X, Zhang J, Yuan H, Xu Z, Li Q, Niu X, et al. Exosomes secreted by human-induced pluripotent stem cell-derived mesenchymal stem cells repair critical-sized bone defects through enhanced angiogenesis and osteogenesis in osteoporotic

rats. Int J Biol Sci 2016; 12(7): 836-49.
[91] Nakamura Y, Miyaki S, Ishitobi H, Matsuyama S, Nakasa T, Kamei N, et al. Mesenchymal-stem-cell-derived exosomes accelerate skeletal muscle regeneration. FEBS Lett 2015; 589(11): 1257-65.
[92] Wang X, Zhang X, Ren X-P, Chen J, Liu H, Yang J, et al. MicroRNA-494 targeting both proapoptotic and antiapoptotic proteins protects against ischemia/reperfusion-induced cardiac injury. Circulation 2010; 122 (13): 1308-18.
[93] Ferreira E, Porter RM. Harnessing extracellular vesicles to direct endochondral repair of large bone defects. Bone Joint Res 2018; 7(4): 263-73.
[94] Lee DE, Ayoub N, Agrawal DK. Mesenchymal stem cells and cutaneous wound healing: novel methods to increase cell delivery and therapeutic efficacy. Stem Cell Res Ther 2016; 7(1): 37.
[95] Shabbir A, Cox A, Rodriguez-Menocal L, Salgado M, Van Badiavas E. Mesenchymal stem cell exosomes induce proliferation and migration of normal and chronic wound fibroblasts, and enhance angiogenesis in vitro. Stem Cells Dev 2015; 24(14): 1635-47.
[96] Zhang J, Guan J, Niu X, Hu G, Guo S, Li Q, et al. Exosomes released from human induced pluripotent stem cells-derived MSCs facilitate cutaneous wound healing by promoting collagen synthesis and angiogenesis. J Transl Med 2015; 13: 49.
[97] Fang S, Xu C, Zhang Y, Xue C, Yang C, Bi H, et al. Umbilical cord-derived mesenchymal stem cell-derived exosomal MicroRNAs suppress myofibroblast differentiation by inhibiting the transforming growth factor-β/SMAD2 pathway during wound healing. Stem Cells Transl Med 2016; 5(10): 1425-39.
[98] Liang X, Zhang L, Wang S, Han Q, Zhao RC. Exosomes secreted by mesenchymal stem cells promote endothelial cell angiogenesis by transferring miR-125a. J Cell Sci 2016; 129(11): 2182.
[99] Zhang B, Wu X, Zhang X, Sun Y, Yan Y, Shi H, et al. Human umbilical cord mesenchymal stem cell exosomes enhance angiogenesis through the Wnt4/β-catenin pathway. Stem Cells Transl Med 2015; 4(5): 513-22.
[100] Pu C-M, Liu C-W, Liang C-J, Yen Y-H, Chen S-H, Jiang-Shieh Y-F, et al. Adipose-derived stem cells protect skin flaps against ischemia/reperfusion injury via IL-6 expression. J Invest Dermatol 2017; 137(6): 1353-62.
[101] Rhim T, Lee DY, Lee M. Drug delivery systems for the treatment of ischemic stroke. Pharm Res 2013; 30(10): 2429-44.
[102] Thompson BJ, Ronaldson PT. Chapter six — Drug delivery to the ischemic brain. In: Davis TP, editor. Advances in pharmacology. Academic Press; 2014. p. 165-202. [Internet]. Available from: http://www.sciencedirect.com/science/article/pii/S1054358914000143.
[103] Tian T, Zhang H-X, He C-P, Fan S, Zhu Y-L, Qi C, et al. Surface functionalized exosomes as targeted drug delivery vehicles for cerebral ischemia therapy. Biomaterials 2018; 150: 137-49.
[104] Alvarez-Erviti L, Seow Y, Yin H, Betts C, Lakhal S, Wood MJA. Delivery of siRNA to the mouse brain by systemic injection of targeted exosomes. Nat Biotechnol 2011; 29: 341.
[105] Ohno S, Takanashi M, Sudo K, Ueda S, Ishikawa A, Matsuyama N, et al. Systemically injected exosomes targeted to EGFR deliver antitumor microRNA to breast cancer cells. Mol Ther 2013; 21(1): 185-91.
[106] Fuhrmann G, Serio A, Mazo M, Nair R, Stevens MM. Active loading into extracellular vesicles significantly improves the cellular uptake and photodynamic effect of porphyrins. In: 3rd Symposium on Innovative Polymers Control Delivery SIPCD 2014; 205.2015. p. 35-44.
[107] Luan X, Sansanaphongpricha K, Myers I, Chen H, Yuan H, Sun D. Engineering exosomes as refined biological nanoplatforms for drug delivery. Acta Pharmacol Sin 2017; 38(6): 754-63.
[108] Sun D, Zhuang X, Xiang X, Liu Y, Zhang S, Liu C, et al. A novel nanoparticle drug delivery system: the anti-inflammatory activity of curcumin is enhanced when encapsulated in exosomes. Mol Ther 2010; 18(9): 1606-14.
[109] Haney MJ, Klyachko NL, Zhao Y, Gupta R, Plotnikova EG, He Z, et al. Exosomes as drug delivery vehicles for Parkinson's disease therapy. J Control Release 2015; 207: 18-30.
[110] Didiot M-C, Hall LM, Coles AH, Haraszti RA, Godinho BM, Chase K, et al. Exosome-mediated delivery of hydrophobically modified siRNA for huntingtin mRNA silencing. Mol Ther 2016; 24(10): 1836-47.
[111] Wahlgren J, De L, Karlson T, Brisslert M, Vaziri Sani F, Telemo E, Sunnerhagen P, et al. Plasma exosomes can deliver exogenous short interfering RNA to monocytes and lymphocytes. Nucleic Acids Res 2012; 40(17): e130.
[112] Shtam TA, Kovalev RA, Varfolomeeva EY, Makarov EM, Kil YV, Filatov MV. Exosomes are natural carriers of exogenous siRNA to human cells in vitro. Cell Commun Signal 2013; 11: 88.
[113] Kooijmans SAA, Stremersch S, Braeckmans K, de Smedt SC, Hendrix A, Wood MJA, et al. Electroporation-induced siRNA precipitation obscures the efficiency of siRNA loading into extracellular vesicles. J Control Release 2013; 172 (1): 229-38.
[114] Momen-Heravi F, Bala S, Bukong T, Szabo G. Exosome-mediated delivery of functionally active miRNA-155 inhibitor to macrophages. Nanomedicine Nanotechnol Biol Med 2014; 10(7): 1517-27.
[115] Tian Y, Li S, Song J, Ji T, Zhu M, Anderson GJ, et al. A doxorubicin delivery platform using engineered natural membrane vesicle exosomes for targeted tumor therapy. Biomaterials 2014; 35(7): 2383-90.
[116] Johnsen KB, Gudbergsson JM, Skov MN, Christiansen G, Gurevich L, Moos T, et al. Evaluation of electroporation-induced adverse effects on adipose-derived stem cell exosomes. Cytotechnology 2016; 68(5): 2125-38.
[117] Kim MS, Haney MJ, Zhao Y, Mahajan V, Deygen I, Klyachko NL, et al. Development of exosome-encapsulated paclitaxel to overcome MDR in cancer cells. Nanomedicine Nanotechnol Biol Med 2016; 12(3): 655-64.
[118] Sato YT, Umezaki K, Sawada S, Mukai S, Sasaki Y, Harada N, et al. Engineering hybrid exosomes by membrane fusion with liposomes. Sci Rep 2016; 6: 21933.
[119] Jamur MC, Oliver C. Permeabilization of cell membranes. In: Oliver C, Jamur MC, editors. Immunocytochemical methods and protocols. Totowa, NJ: Humana Press; 2010. p. 63-6. [Internet]. Available from https://doi.org/10.1007/978-1-59745-324-0_9.

[120] Batrakova EV, Kim MS. Using exosomes, naturally-equipped nanocarriers, for drug delivery. J Control Release 2015; 219: 396-405.
[121] Pascucci L, Coccè V, Bonomi A, Ami D, Ceccarelli P, Ciusani E, et al. Paclitaxel is incorporated by mesenchymal stromal cells and released in exosomes that inhibit in vitro tumor growth: a new approach for drug delivery. J Control Release 2014; 192: 262-70.
[122] Lv L-H, Wan Y-L, Lin Y, Zhang W, Yang M, Li G-L, et al. Anticancer drugs cause release of exosomes with heat shock proteins from human hepatocellular carcinoma cells that elicit effective natural killer cell antitumor responses in vitro. J Biol Chem 2012; 287(19): 15874-85.
[123] Jang SC, Kim OY, Yoon CM, Choi D-S, Roh T-Y, Park J, et al. Bioinspired exosome-mimetic nanovesicles for targeted delivery of chemotherapeutics to malignant tumors. ACS Nano 2013; 7(9): 7698-710.
[124] Lee J, Kim J, Jeong M, Lee H, Goh U, Kim H, et al. Liposome-based engineering of cells to package hydrophobic compounds in membrane vesicles for tumor penetration. Nano Lett 2015; 15(5): 2938-44.
[125] Banizs AB, Huang T, Dryden K, Berr SS, Stone JR, Nakamoto RK, et al. In vitro evaluation of endothelial exosomes as carriers for small interfering ribonucleic acid delivery. Int J Nanomedicine 2014; 9: 4223-30.
[126] Zhang Y, Li L, Yu J, Zhu D, Zhang Y, Li X, et al. Microvesicle-mediated delivery of transforming growth factor β1 siRNA for the suppression of tumor growth in mice. Biomaterials 2014; 35(14): 4390-400.
[127] Liu Y, Li D, Liu Z, Zhou Y, Chu D, Li X, et al. Targeted exosome-mediated delivery of opioid receptor Mu siRNA for the treatment of morphine relapse. Sci Rep 2015; 5: 17543.
[128] Katakowski M, Buller B, Zheng X, Lu Y, Rogers T, Osobamiro O, et al. Exosomes from marrow stromal cells expressing miR-146b inhibit glioma growth. Cancer Lett 2013; 335(1): 201-4.
[129] Munoz JL, Bliss SA, Greco SJ, Ramkissoon SH, Ligon KL, Rameshwar P. Delivery of functional anti-miR-9 by mesenchymal stem cell-derived exosomes to glioblastoma multiforme cells conferred chemosensitivity. Mol Ther Nucleic Acids 2013; 2(10): e126.
[130] Fonsato V, Collino F, Herrera MB, Cavallari C, Deregibus MC, Cisterna B, et al. Human liver stem cell-derived microvesicles inhibit hepatoma growth in SCID mice by delivering antitumor microRNAs. Stem Cells 2012; 30(9): 1985-98.
[131] Lee S-T, Im W, Ban J-J, Lee M, Jung K-H, Lee SK, et al. Exosome-based delivery of miR-124 in a Huntington's disease model. J Mov Disord 2017; 10(1): 45-52.
[132] Yang J, Zhang X, Chen X, Wang L, Yang G. Exosome mediated delivery of miR-124 promotes neurogenesis after ischemia. Mol Ther Nucleic Acids 2017; 7: 278-87.
[133] Gu J, Zhang H, Ji B, Jiang H, Zhao T, Jiang R, et al. Vesicle miR-195 derived from endothelial cells inhibits expression of serotonin transporter in vessel smooth muscle cells. Sci Rep 2017; 7: 43546.
[134] Zhang Y, Yu M, Dai M, Chen C, Tang Q, Jing W, et al. miR-450a-5p within rat adipose tissue exosome-like vesicles promotes adipogenic differentiation by targeting WISP2. J Cell Sci 2017; 130(6): 1158.
[135] Gu D, Zou X, Ju G, Zhang G, Bao E, Zhu Y. Mesenchymal stromal cells derived extracellular vesicles ameliorate acute renal ischemia reperfusion injury by inhibition of mitochondrial fission through miR-30. Stem Cells Int 2016; 2016: 2093940.
[136] Zhang H, Bai M, Deng T, Liu R, Wang X, Qu Y, et al. Cell-derived microvesicles mediate the delivery of miR-29a/c to suppress angiogenesis in gastric carcinoma. Cancer Lett 2016; 375(2): 331-9.
[137] Yang J, Zhou C-Z, Zhu R, Fan H, Liu X-X, Duan X-Y, et al. miR-200b-containing microvesicles attenuate experimental colitis associated intestinal fibrosis by inhibiting epithelial-mesenchymal transition. J Gastroenterol Hepatol 2017; 32(12): 1966-74.
[138] Waldenström A, Gennebäck N, Hellman U, Ronquist G. Cardiomyocyte microvesicles contain DNA/RNA and convey biological messages to target cells. PLoS ONE 2012; 7(4): e34653.
[139] Lamichhane TN, Raiker RS, Jay SM. Exogenous DNA loading into extracellular vesicles via electroporation is size-dependent and enables limited gene delivery. Mol Pharm 2015; 12(10): 3650-7.
[140] García-Romero N, Carrión-Navarro J, Esteban-Rubio S, Lázaro-Ibáñez E, Peris-Celda M, Alonso MM, et al. DNA sequences within glioma-derived extracellular vesicles can cross the intact blood-brain barrier and be detected in peripheral blood of patients. Oncotarget 2016; 8(1): 1416-28.
[141] Cambier L, de Couto G, Ibrahim A, Echavez AK, Valle J, Liu W, et al. Y RNA fragment in extracellular vesicles confers cardioprotection via modulation of IL-10 expression and secretion. EMBO Mol Med 2017; 9(3): 337-52.
[142] Yokoi A, Yoshioka Y, Yamamoto Y, Ishikawa M, Ikeda S, Kato T, et al. Malignant extracellular vesicles carrying MMP1 mRNA facilitate peritoneal dissemination in ovarian cancer. Nat Commun 2017; 8: 14470.
[143] Mizrak A, Bolukbasi MF, Ozdener GB, Brenner GJ, Madlener S, Erkan EP, et al. Genetically engineered microvesicles carrying suicide mRNA/protein inhibit schwannoma tumor growth. Mol Ther 2013; 21(1): 101-8.
[144] Sugars KL, Rubinsztein DC. Transcriptional abnormalities in Huntington disease. Trends Genet 2003; 19(5): 233-8.
[145] Cai J, Han Y, Ren H, Chen C, He D, Zhou L, et al. Extracellular vesicle-mediated transfer of donor genomic DNA to recipient cells is a novel mechanism for genetic influence between cells. J Mol Cell Biol 2013; 5(4): 227-38.
[146] Théry C, Duban L, Segura E, Véron P, Lantz O, Amigorena S. Indirect activation of naïve CD4+ T cells by dendritic cell-derived exosomes. Nat Immunol 2002; 3: 1156.
[147] Hsu D-H, Paz P, Villaflor G, Rivas A, Mehta-Damani A, Angevin E, et al. Exosomes as a tumor vaccine: enhancing potency through direct loading of antigenic peptides. J Immunother 2003; 26(5): 440-50. [Internet]. Available from: https://journals.lww.com/immunotherapy-journal/Fulltext/2003/09000/Exosomes_as_a_Tumor_Vaccine_Enhancing_Potency.7.aspx.
[148] Morse MA, Garst J, Osada T, Khan S, Hobeika A, Clay TM, et al. A phase I study of dexosome immunotherapy in patients with advanced non-small cell lung cancer. J Transl Med 2005; 3(1): 9.
[149] Dai S, Wei D, Wu Z, Zhou X, Wei X, Huang H, et al. Phase I clinical trial of autologous ascites-derived exosomes

combined with GM-CSF for colorectal cancer. Mol Ther 2008; 16(4): 782-90.
[150] Besse B, Charrier M, Lapierre V, Dansin E, Lantz O, Planchard D, et al. Dendritic cellderived exosomes as maintenance immunotherapy after first line chemotherapy in NSCLC. Oncoimmunology 2015; 5(4): e1071008.
[151] Nooshabadi VT, Mardpour S, Yousefi-Ahmadipour A, Allahverdi A, Izadpanah M, Daneshimehr F, et al. The extracellular vesicles-derived from mesenchymal stromal cells: a new therapeutic option in regenerative medicine. J Cell Biochem 2018; 119(10): 8048-73.
[152] Park JS, Suryaprakash S, Lao Y-H, Leong KW. Engineering mesenchymal stem cells for regenerative medicine and drug delivery. Methods 2015; 84: 3-16.
[153] Schäfer R, Spohn G, Baer PC. Mesenchymal stem/stromal cells in regenerative medicine: can preconditioning strategies improve therapeutic efficacy? Transfus Med Hemother 2016; 43(4): 256-67.
[154] Shyam H, Singh SK, Kant R, Saxena SK. Mesenchymal stem cells in regenerative medicine: a new paradigm for degenerative bone diseases. Regen Med 2017; 12(2): 111-4.
[155] Kusuma GD, Carthew J, Lim R, Frith JE. Effect of the microenvironment on mesenchymal stem cell paracrine signaling: opportunities to engineer the therapeutic effect. Stem Cells Dev 2017; 26(9): 617-31.
[156] Park WS, Ahn SY, Sung SI, Ahn J-Y, Chang YS. Strategies to enhance paracrine potency of transplanted mesenchymal stem cells in intractable neonatal disorders. Pediatr Res 2017; 83: 214.
[157] Katsuda T, Kosaka N, Takeshita F, Ochiya T. The therapeutic potential of mesenchymal stem cell-derived extracellular vesicles. Proteomics 2013; 13(10-11): 1637-53.
[158] Zhuang X, Xiang X, Grizzle W, Sun D, Zhang S, Axtell RC, et al. Treatment of brain inflammatory diseases by delivering exosome encapsulated anti-inflammatory drugs from the nasal region to the brain. Mol Ther 2011; 19(10): 1769-79.
[159] Amzallag N, Passer BJ, Allanic D, Segura E, Théry C, Goud B, et al. TSAP6 facilitates the secretion of translationally controlled tumor protein/histamine-releasing factor via a nonclassical pathway. J Biol Chem 2004; 279(44): 46104-12.
[160] Alonso R, Rodríguez MC, Pindado J, Merino E, Mérida I, Izquierdo M. Diacylglycerol kinase α regulates the secretion of lethal exosomes bearing Fas ligand during activationinduced cell death of T lymphocytes. J Biol Chem 2005; 280(31): 28439-50.
[161] Islam A, Shen X, Hiroi T, Moss J, Vaughan M, Levine SJ. The brefeldin A-inhibited guanine nucleotide-exchange protein, BIG2, regulates the constitutive release of TNFR1 exosomelike vesicles. J Biol Chem 2007; 282(13): 9591-9.
[162] Parolini I, Federici C, Raggi C, Lugini L, Palleschi S, De Milito A, et al. Microenvironmental pH is a key factor for exosome traffic in tumor cells. J Biol Chem 2009; 284(49): 34211-22.
[163] Greening DW, Xu R, Ji H, Tauro BJ, Simpson RJ. A protocol for exosome isolation and characterization: evaluation of ultracentrifugation, density-gradient separation, and immunoaffinity capture methods. In: Posch A, editor. Proteomic profiling: methods and protocols. New York, NY: Springer New York; 2015. p. 179-209. [Internet]. Available from: https://doi.org/10.1007/978-1-4939-2550-6_15.
[164] Helwa I, Cai J, Drewry MD, Zimmerman A, Dinkins MB, Khaled ML, et al. A comparative study of serum exosome isolation using differential ultracentrifugation and three commercial reagents. PLoS ONE 2017; 12(1): e0170628.
[165] Sunkara V, Woo H-K, Cho Y-K. Emerging techniques in the isolation and characterization of extracellular vesicles and their roles in cancer diagnostics and prognostics. Analyst 2016; 141(2): 371-81.
[166] Muller L, Hong C-S, Stolz DB, Watkins SC, Whiteside TL. Isolation of biologically-active exosomes from human plasma. J Immunol Methods 2014; 411: 55-65.
[167] Soares Martins T, Catita J, Martins Rosa I, A B Da Cruz E Silva O, Henriques AG. Exosome isolation from distinct biofluids using precipitation and column-based approaches. PLoS ONE 2018; 13(6): e0198820.
[168] Aiastui A. Should cell culture platforms move towards EV therapy requirements? Front Immunol 2015; 6: 8.

第20章

外泌体作为药物在各种临床情况下的可能性
The potential of exosomes as theragnostics in various clinical situations

Ju-Seop Kang

Department of Pharmacology & Clinical Pharmacology Lab, College of Medicine, Hanyang University, Seoul, Ripublic of Korea

一、外泌体作为疾病的生物标志物和感染的治疗或疫苗候选物

外泌体是一些由真核细胞释放进入循环系统的细胞内膜基小囊泡。这些所谓的 EV 在细胞间通信中具有重要功能,健康受试者和各种疾病患者体液中的外泌体显示出不同的蛋白质和其他的细胞内容物,如 mRNA 和 microRNA,这些都可以作为潜在的诊断标志物进行测量[1-3]。肿瘤来源外泌体富含的 miRNA 可作为肿瘤标志物[4-6]。例如,多形性胶质母细胞瘤患者血清 EV 中的 RNA 含量与健康受试者存在明显差异[7,8],显示出其作为生物标志物的诊断潜力。

多形性胶质母细胞瘤患者体循环外泌体中的 EGFRvⅢ mRNA 水平升高,所以可将其作为该疾病的诊断生物标志物[9],起到液体活检的作用,从而避免从大脑中取出组织样本来检测 EGFRvⅢ 蛋白。外泌体膜上的 EGFR 也被检测出可能作为肺癌的诊断生物标志物[10]。蛋白多糖-磷脂酰肌醇聚糖-1(glypican-1,GP1)阳性外泌体具有很高的特异性和敏感性,通过血清检测,可以将胰腺癌患者、健康人群和良性胰腺疾病患者区分开来[11]。GP1 阳性外泌体的水平与肿瘤患者术前和术后的疗效和生存率相关,提示这也是一种有价值的胰腺癌预后标志物。在小鼠中,GP1 阳性外泌体在检测胰腺腹腔病变方面是可靠的,即使 MRI 结果为阴性。来源于前列腺腺泡细胞的血浆外泌体被研究作为诊断前列腺癌的新生物标志物[12]。外泌体的蛋白质组学分析显示了该病的潜在生物标志物[13]。肝细胞癌肝移植术后复发患者的血清外泌体中 miRNA 生物标志物水平升高[14]。

外泌体也被评估为多种器官非肿瘤疾病的生物标志物,包括 CNS[15]、肝脏[16]、肾脏[17]、肺[18]和动脉[19]。在 CNS 中,细胞外积聚异常加工的 tau 蛋白导致了 tau 介导的神经病理[20]。tau 蛋白似乎可以通过外泌体扩散,在 M1C 细胞神经母细胞蛋白瘤模型中,CSF 中 AD 早期的生物标志物 AT270 磷酸化 tau 蛋白增加。由于 CSF 外泌体部分相对于 CSF 总 tau 蛋白选择性丰度较高,轻度至中度散发性 AD 患者 CSF 中 AT270 磷酸化 tau 蛋白水平升高。AD 发作时,CSF 磷酸化 tau 蛋白水平的增加与 CSF 中外泌体相关部分的增加有关。在另一项研究中,神经源性血清外泌体中自噬溶酶体蛋白(组织蛋白酶 D、溶酶体相关膜蛋

白1和泛素化蛋白)的水平将临床前AD患者与匹配对照和额颞叶痴呆患者区分开来[21]。神经退行性疾病相关的CSF、血液外泌体中改变的microRNA谱可能是早期诊断AD和PD的新生物标志物[22],而且外泌体可以传递siRNA,这也为AD的治疗提供了可能性[23,24]。血清外泌体的蛋白质组学分析表明,与健康受试者相比,PD患者存在丰富的蛋白质[25]。

就肺部疾病而言,相比健康受试者,从哮喘患者支气管肺泡灌洗液中分离的外泌体显示出不同的miRNA谱[18]。哮喘相关的关键细胞,如肥大细胞、嗜酸性粒细胞、DC、T细胞和支气管上皮细胞释放的外泌体反过来又能激活或抑制其他哮喘相关细胞,进一步刺激过敏反应[26,27]。DC衍生外泌体(DC-derived exosome,Dex)的表面有可刺激过敏原特异性Th2细胞的协同刺激分子[28,29]。哮喘患者的嗜酸性粒细胞来源外泌体数量增加,在调节哮喘中有重要作用[30,31]。严重哮喘患者的外泌体miRNA含量与健康受试者相比有显著差异[32]。这些失调的miRNA与气道完整性相关的通路以及某些临床特征,如嗜酸性粒细胞计数或FEV1相关[33]。在另一项研究中,重症哮喘患者的外泌体miRNA表达谱与TGF-β和ErbB信号通路及黏着斑相关[34]。

外泌体还可作为过敏性疾病的疫苗[35]。从小鼠支气管肺泡灌洗液中分离的外泌体可诱导小鼠对橄榄花粉变应原的过敏反应产生耐受和保护[31]。

血清外泌体中miR-192水平的升高可以预测急性心肌梗死后心力衰竭的发展[36]。最后,尿外泌体已用作肾、泌尿生殖系统和全身疾病诊断生物标志物的起始材料[17,37]。

尽管许多研究表明EV生物标志与多种疾病相关,但个别的研究结果显示出不一致的趋势,可能可以用EV纯化方法上的差异来解释这种矛盾[38]。对于一个给定的应用,必须检查该方法的敏感性和特异性,包括明确设置的质量控制措施。外泌体也是弓形虫病、白喉、结核病和非典型严重急性呼吸综合征(severe acute respiratory syndrome,SARS)等传染病的疫苗优先候选对象。有报道称,健康小鼠口服带有刚地弓形虫抗原(*Toxoplasma gondii* antigen,T-Ag)的DC后产生免疫,可产生保护作用来抵抗弓形虫毒株,但是很难获得足够数量的DC用于接种[39-41]。小鼠骨髓来源的DC与完整的白喉毒素(diphtheria toxin,DT)释放的外泌体在体外刺激后,注射到小鼠体内,显示出特异性的IgG2b和IgG2a应答[42]。结核分枝杆菌感染能刺激巨噬细胞释放外泌体,而且含有结核分枝杆菌肽-MHC-Ⅱ复合物的外泌体可诱导抗菌性T细胞应答[43,44]。外泌体作为疫苗接种材料在SARS相关冠状病毒(coronavirus,CoV)中也进行了研究,CoV是一种能引起致命非典型肺部疾病的感染。Kuate等[35]发现,带有SARS-CoV spike S蛋白的外泌体产生的中和抗体滴度,可以通过SARS-S外泌体疫苗启动,然后用目前应用的腺病毒载体疫苗进行增强,从而进一步加强中和抗体滴度[35]。

激发有效、普遍的细胞毒性T淋巴细胞(cytotoxic T lymphocyte,CTL)免疫反应对包括病毒感染在内的各种疾病具有治疗潜力。例如,诱导抗埃博拉病毒(Ebola virus,EboV)特异性CTL免疫在治疗和预防环境中都有好处[45]。事实上,在急性EboV感染的幸存者已经发现了病毒特异性CTL的刺激[46],而病毒特异性CTL免疫在包括猕猴在内的一些非人类灵长类动物的保护中发挥了关键作用[47]。此外,将感染小鼠的含有小鼠适应EboV的

CD8$^+$ T淋巴细胞输注到幼稚受体小鼠体内,可保护小鼠免受 EboV 感染[48]。强大的 CTL 相关免疫反应对甲型流感病毒[49]和 HCV 感染[50]也有相关的治疗效果。Anticoli 等[45]提出了一种基于外泌体的疫苗平台,用于设计体内含有人乳头瘤病毒(human papilloma virus,HPV)E7 蛋白的外泌体。该方法涉及肌内注射 HPV-E7 编码的 DNA 载体,该载体在外泌体锚定 Nef 突变蛋白(Nef^{mut})C 端融合。HIV-1 Nef^{mut}是一种 27 kDa 的蛋白[51],与细胞膜上的 raft 微域连接[52]。Nef^{mut}缺少一些通常由野生型 Nef 引起的抗细胞作用,包括 CD4 下调、HIV-1 感染性增强、PAK-2 刺激和 MHC I 类下调,并且发现在外泌体中其水平很高[53,54]。在这种比对中,≈11-kDa E7 蛋白产生了强而有效的抗原特异性 CTL 免疫。为了确定该技术的普遍应用,我们对各种来源、大小的病毒产物包括 EboV、西尼罗病毒 NS3 和 HCV NS3 进行了免疫原性研究。与 Nef^{mut}融合后,所有抗原都比较稳定,与 Nef^{mut}相比都能在一定程度上转移到外泌体中。将表达各种融合产物的 DNA 载体注射到小鼠体内,产生一种明显可检测到的抗原特异性 CD8$^+$ T 细胞应答,其细胞毒性足以杀死装载肽或表达抗原的同基因细胞[45]。

DC 是抗原提呈能力最强且唯一能够刺激幼稚 T 细胞产生适应性免疫反应的 APC[55]。事实上,我们可以将肿瘤免疫监测定义为 T 细胞有效杀死肿瘤细胞的一个逐步结果阶段。具体来说,DC 捕获和处理肿瘤新抗原是第一阶段,这一过程依赖于分子信号,如促炎细胞因子、共刺激配体、死亡肿瘤细胞来源分子和肠道微生物组产物[56]。因此,基于 DC 的有效肿瘤疫苗的研究已经有一段时间了,也出现了一些积极的结果,如 Sipuleucel-T 免疫疗法用于去势抵抗性前列腺癌[57]。然而,基于 DC 的肿瘤疫苗的多样化应用显示出一些主要的局限性[58,59]。图 20-1 描述了基于 DC 的免疫治疗策略。基于 Dex 的肿瘤疫苗最近已成为一种可能克服其中一些障碍的替代方法。首先,Dex 分子成分易于分析,因此可以对验证参数进行严格定义[60]。其次,肽-MHC II 类配合物中 Dex 成分更为丰富,产量更高[58,60]。再次,Dex 与 DC 相比,可耐受较长时间的冷冻贮藏,可达 6 个月[58]。除这些优点之外,免疫抑制肿瘤微环境通常会抑制 DC 对抗原提呈和 T 细胞的刺激,但这不会影响外泌体[61,62]。最后,外泌体与使用活细胞相关的大多数风险(如产生免疫功能障碍或微血管闭塞)都无关[63]。肿瘤肽脉冲 Dex 在体内产生 CTL 启动,肿瘤生长抑制和肿瘤缓解。的确,单次皮内注射一周后引起了显著的肿瘤生长抑制,60 天后 40%～60% 的动物肿瘤消失[62]。此外,这些无细胞免疫治疗疫苗比直接注射可存活的 DC 疫苗更有效,后者只有 20% 的小鼠在 60 天后脱离了肿瘤。这些差异可能说明外泌体对肿瘤微环境的免疫调节作用具有抵抗力,而免疫调节作用可阻断 DC 抗原提呈的能力[62]。在过去的十年中,已经进行了几项成功的临床试验,评估基于 Dex 的肿瘤疫苗在 NSCLC 癌(non-small cell lung cancer,NSCLC)[64]和转移性黑色素瘤[65]患者中的可行性、安全性和有效性,总体而言结果是有希望的。在这两项试验中,患者接受了四剂含有多种不同 MHC II 类肽的自体 Dex 疫苗。疫苗生产被证明是可行的,而且这种疗法的耐受性很好,只有轻微的 1～2 级不良反应[64,65]。最近的一项 II 期临床试验评估了晚期 NSCLC 癌患者一线化疗后用 IFN-γ-Dex 作为维持免疫治疗的效果[66]。这项研究表明 IFN-乙酰胆碱凝胶生产的可行性和安全性,26 例患者中只有 1 例出现 3 级肝毒性。根据实体肿瘤疗效评价标准,该试验在临床结果中没有显示任何客观的肿瘤疗效。然而,研究表明,无进展生存期最长的患者在 Dex 治疗后 NK 细胞功能有显著改善,说明外泌体可刺激晚期 NSCLC 患者抗肿瘤免疫的 NK 细胞臂[66]。

肿瘤来源的外泌体也可作为抗原递送系统,能够阻断 $CD4^+$ 和 $CD8^+$ T 细胞依赖模式下的肿瘤进展[67]。正因为如此,基于肿瘤来源外泌体的细胞游离疫苗是临床应用的另一种可能性。然而,肿瘤来源的外泌体分离不方便,制备效率低,从患者体外培养的肿瘤细胞中获得的产量低[68]。然而,黑色素瘤患者的恶性积液中富含外泌体,它可将肿瘤抗原传递给 DC,进而刺激肿瘤特异性 CTL 在体外产生有效的抗肿瘤反应[69]。一项Ⅰ期临床试验检测了从晚期 CRC 患者腹水中提取的外泌体作为免疫治疗的效果,结果表明,与单独使用肿瘤外泌体相比,肿瘤外泌体与 GM-CSF 联合使用可更有效地诱导全身抗肿瘤免疫和 CTL 应答。仅使用肿瘤外泌体治疗的患者未表现出治疗效果,而在使用腹水来源的外泌体联合 GM-CSF 治疗的组中,观察到 1 名病情稳定的患者和 1 名临床略有反应的患者[68]。尽管到目前为止进行了许多尝试,作为一种新的肿瘤控制方法——基于 Dex 的免疫疗法仍然非常令人鼓舞。外泌体是免疫反应的熟练介质,其免疫刺激特性(通过供体 DC)的管理技术简单,加上相对于全细胞应用的优势,证实了它们的治疗前景[60]。

这一节特别有意思的是,外泌体可以通过建立免疫抑制微环境来促进肿瘤的生长和侵袭,也可以通过诱导抗原提呈和 $CD4^{+[70]}$、$CD8^{+[69]}$ T 细胞来刺激肿瘤细胞的破坏,或者通过天然免疫系统的组成部分,如 NK 细胞,来作为肿瘤免疫监视的试剂。

二、胞外囊泡作为药物传递系统

成功的纳米载体最重要的特征是有良好的体内行为。作为给药系统,EV 的发展需要了解其给药后的体内动力学。然而,对 EV 的细胞外行为、细胞摄取途径和亚细胞途径的了解仍不清楚。我们发现了各种细胞释放的 EV,并且这些囊泡在血液循环和生物液中相对稳定。这一现象表明,在生物系统中,EV 的清除速度要比人工合成的纳米载体慢得多。然而,不同的体内药代动力学研究表明,当 EV 注入循环后,会被迅速清除。B16 黑色素瘤细胞和脾细胞的 EV 静脉给药后会被迅速清除,如小鼠静脉给药后半衰期很短,只有大约 2 分钟[72,73]。尿外泌体中胎球蛋白-A 水平升高与急性尿路损伤相关[74]。

外泌体和微囊泡参与身体多种过程,装载了集中的遗传和蛋白质组信息,因此被认为在细胞间通信中起着重要作用。分泌小泡能以不同的方式传递信息。首先,它们可以通过表面表达的配体刺激受体靶细胞。例如,已经证实来源于 DC 的抗原提呈外泌体可在体内诱导 T 细胞介导的免疫应答[75]。此外,外泌体的配体受体信号也可以在其他调控过程中发挥作用,如血管生成[76]、止血[77]、肿瘤进展[78]和转移[79]。其次,分泌的 EV 可通过与靶细胞的质膜融合将表面受体从一个细胞转移到另一个细胞[80,81]。通过这种机制,HIV 将 CD4 受体从受感染细胞转移到完整的细胞中来增加易感性[82]。EV 具有许多优点,如高输送能力、固有靶向性和低免疫原性,所以可以让它成为从小分子到大分子核酸和蛋白质的有效生物传递系统[83](表 20-1)。

表 20-1　EV 用于治疗性给药的利弊[1,24,68,83-87]

优　点	缺　点
—纳米级囊泡在体液中的生物相容性和稳定性 —天然的低免疫原性 —对抗免疫系统的隐形能力 —可减少目标以外影响的固有目标特性 —引导治疗物质越过生物屏障的能力,尤其是 BBB —能够装载特定的小分子,如 miRNA 和药物 —能够使膜与靶细胞直接融合的独特成分,能有效地吸收细胞 —临床试验安全 —固有毒性低	—分泌和吸收机制,成分和生物学功能还不清楚 —对目标细胞的影响未知 —缺乏高效、稳产的分离技术 —规模化生产困难——没有最佳的净化方法;大规模生产成本高且具有挑战性 —缺乏不破坏 EV 完整性的有效装载方法 —体内研究数据较少,体内跟踪需要进一步研究 —治疗性给药缺乏临床研究 —具有异质成分的囊泡具有免疫原性

尽管基于 EV 的各种递送方法在不断发展,但主要问题是缺乏标准化、高效、合理的 EV 提取方法。当考虑到细 EV 的重复性、产量、纯度和功能特性时,需要对分离方法进行验证。此外,存储时间也没有经过标准程序验证,需要对基于 EV 产品进行仔细评估[88]。图 20-1 是各种基于外泌体制剂方法的总体示意图[89]。

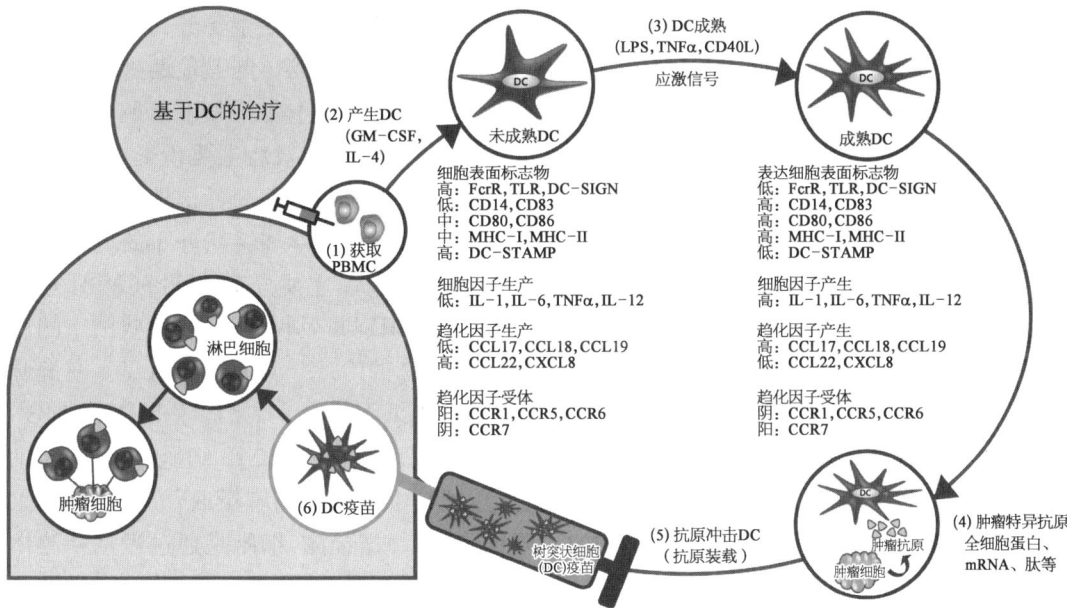

图 20-1　转化医学和临床医学中基于外泌体的各种诊断和治疗方法的总体示意图

此外,在 EV 上装载治疗药物的效率仍存在不足。在不降低膜完整性的前提下,相对紧密有序的双层脂质阻碍了药物有效地进入 EV。这种损伤可能会改变 EV 的免疫导向特性,并使其暴露在单核吞噬细胞系统下[89]。因此,理想的装载方法不仅要具有较高的装载效率,而且要保持 EV 的结构完整性和治疗学的功能完整性[83]。

人们对于基于纳米技术的各种 DDS 的应用越来越感兴趣,如脂质体、聚合物纳米颗粒、树枝状大分子和磁性纳米颗粒[90]。这些输送介质可以用于运送各种类型的物质,包括化疗药物、抗炎药和miRNA[91,92]。这些DDS的纳米直径有助于通过血液和淋巴系统进行有效的药物载量[93]。此外,我们对EV的体内药代动力学行为也有了进一步的认识,如循环半衰期、体内组织分布、细胞摄取和细胞生命等。这一认识对于阐明外泌体的生物学功能和外泌体治疗学的实际应用具有重要意义。明确外泌体药代动力学的第一步,包括体内组织分布的评估,也就是所谓的外泌体的生物分布。本文介绍了几种小分子亲脂性荧光染料标记方法,将其用于体内示踪。虽然体内分析的可靠性会因外泌体释放的游离染液而降低,但依然是一种有效评估外泌体在组织中定位作用的方法[94,95]。PKH67是一种亲脂性荧光染料,用来标记高转移性B16F10小鼠黑色素瘤细胞衍生的外泌体,这些外泌体积聚在肺、骨髓、脾脏和肝脏中,增强了肺的内皮通透性,促进了肿瘤向肺的转移[96]。除荧光染料外,亲油性近红外染料,如1,1′-双十八烷基-3,3,3′,3′-四甲基吲哚二碳菁高氯酸盐(DiD)和1,1′-双十八烷基四甲基吲哚三碳菁碘(DiR)已广泛用于外源性外泌体的成像。正常小鼠静脉给药后,标记的MSC外泌体均匀分布于脾脏和肝脏[94]。另一方面,在小鼠急性肾损伤模型中,这些外泌体在静脉内注射后积聚在肾脏以及脾脏和肝脏中。这一发现可以解释静脉注射MSC来源的外泌体是如何刺激SCID小鼠从顺铂诱导的急性肾损伤中恢复[97]。在对B16F10小鼠黑色素瘤细胞、C2C12小鼠成肌细胞、骨髓源性DC、人胚肾细胞HEK293T等不同细胞的DiR标记外泌体的体内行为研究中,外泌体在静脉给药后主要分布于肝、脾、肺和胃肠道。在这些外泌体中,B16F10小鼠黑色素瘤细胞来源的外泌体与其他两种小鼠细胞来源的外泌体相比,主要聚集在肺部,而DC外泌体和C2C12外泌体在脾脏和肝脏中积聚最多。HEK293T外泌体静脉注射后主要积聚在肝脏,腹腔或皮下注射后主要积聚在肝脏、胰腺和胃肠道[98]。与荧光染料或化学发光蛋白标记相比,用放射性示踪剂标记外泌体具有更高的灵敏度和稳定性,是一种更适合于定量评估外泌体药代动力学和组织分布的方法。例如,经标记的PC3外泌体在静脉注射后迅速从血液循环中消失,主要分布于肝脏(每24小时的注射剂量为12%[ID]/g)[99]。由于多种类型细胞都会识别并吸收外泌体,这些细胞的鉴定对于进一步探索外泌体的生物学特性和完善基于外泌体的治疗学具有重要意义。在静脉给药后,来源于小鼠DC的外泌体被脾脏和肝脏中的巨噬细胞摄取[90];来源于MDA-MB-231乳腺肿瘤细胞的外泌体被肺和脑中的巨噬细胞吸收;来源于C2C12细胞、NIH3T3细胞、MAEC细胞和RAW264.7细胞的外泌体主要被肝脏中的巨噬细胞摄取[100]。这些结果表明,巨噬细胞是主动吸收外源性外泌体的主要细胞[101]。据预测,细胞是通过识别外泌体膜上的表面分子而将其吸收。许多研究对于一些可能有助于外泌体的体内药代动力学的分子进行了分析。体外研究证明,外泌体膜上的碳水化合物参与了外泌体的细胞摄取过程[102]。转移到肺(MDA-MB-231和4175)或肝(BxPC-3和HPAF-Ⅱ)的肿瘤细胞外泌体分别集中于肺和肝脏。外泌体的蛋白质组学分析表明,整合素α6β4和αVβ5具有高表达。从整合素β4敲减的4175细胞中收集到的外泌体在肺中累积数量减少。这些结果表明,整合素在外泌体的药代动力学和组织分布中起着关键作用[101]。表达iRGD肽的未成熟转基因DC细胞的外泌体在αv整合素阳性肿瘤组织中呈选择性分布[103]。

除了依赖于细胞内传递的小RNA分子来实现其内在功能,EV还被应用于递送化疗药物,用于提高其疗效和减少不良反应。某项研究使用外泌体来输送姜黄素来治疗炎症性疾病[104],利用外泌体与姜黄素形成复合物来增强姜黄素的抗癌活性[105]。在小鼠乳腺肿瘤模型中,与化疗药物阿霉素相比,静脉注射整合素靶向 DC 源性 EV 可显著抑制肿瘤生长。此外,将阿霉素装载到 EV 中对心脏损伤较小,这是其最重要的剂量限制不良反应[103]。与脂质体阿霉素相比,外泌体阿霉素的优势在于外泌体膜蛋白的自然定向及其与靶细胞质膜受体相互作用[106,107]。此外,与游离紫杉醇相比,外泌体包裹紫杉醇在控制 Lewis 肺癌转移瘤生长时更为有效,并在各种化疗药物治疗耐药肿瘤方面具有很大潜力[108]。与游离顺铂相比,反复腹腔注射载顺铂的 EV 可提高卵巢癌荷瘤小鼠的长期存活率,静脉注射阿霉素负载的 EV 可延缓已形成的皮下肝癌生长[109]。重要的是,给药后总是能够观察到这些外泌体包被的药物并没有对肝肾功能产生不良影响。

遗憾的是,大蛋白通过 BBB 受到严重限制。事实上,因为无法越过 BBB,98%可能治疗各种 CNS 疾病的强效药物都没有在临床上应用[110]。为了克服这一困难,人们开发了各种纳米药物制剂[111,112]。PD 被认为与脑炎症、小胶质细胞活化和分泌性神经毒性活动(包括 ROS)有关[113,114]。PD 患者的脑组织样本显示,氧化还原酶、过氧化氢酶、超氧化物歧化酶和其他抗氧化剂的水平降低[115-117],表明这些患者对氧化应激和神经退化的抵抗力受损。在这些分子中,过氧化氢酶是最有效的天然抗氧化剂之一,它通过催化反应清除 100 万个自由基。因此,成功地将过氧化氢酶送入大脑可能是治疗 PD 的一个重要方式[84]。EV 被认为是治疗 PD 的治疗载体。外泌体在体外很容易被神经元细胞吸收,经鼻给药后在 PD 小鼠脑内检测到大量的外泌体。与游离过氧化氢酶相比,负载过氧化氢酶的外泌体(catalase-loaded exosomes,ExoCAT)能更有效地抑制小胶质细胞的活化,保护神经元免受活性氧的侵害[84]。因此,ExoCAT 是一种更适用于治疗炎症和退行性疾病(如 PD)的方法[84,118]。尽管这些只是初步报道,但结果表明,外泌体有望成为治疗多种疾病的药物传递系统。

来源于人脂肪组织源性 MSC 的外泌体被认为对 AD 有治疗价值[119]。外泌体可作为携带活性肾胰岛素残基溶酶(neprilysin,NEP)的载体在体内使用,NEP 是使 Aβ 在大脑中降解最重要的酶。在体外培养神经母细胞瘤株 N2A 时,MSC 来源的外泌体也能降低细胞内和细胞外的 Aβ 水平。因此,从 Aβ 的降解能力角度出发,人脂肪组织来源的 MSC 外泌体被认为是一种潜在的 AD 治疗方法。近期研究表明,多能 MSC 在脑卒中后的神经血管重建和神经功能恢复方面具有广阔前景。已有研究表明,MSC 来源外泌体对脑卒中有神经保护作用,部分原因是在脑卒中过程中和脑卒中后改变了外泌体的 miRNA 图谱[120]。

当我们思考与目前多种纳米颗粒传递系统相关的问题时,外泌体作为"自然传递系统"的模拟体,是上述生物分子传递的一种潜在选择。由于其体积小且来源于宿主细胞,可避免被巨噬细胞吞噬或降解,能在体内长期循环。这些运输工具有一个优点,它们能够穿过 BBB 到达 CNS[121]。由于对外泌体的性质及其在整体健康与疾病的病理生理学中的作用认识不足,使得长期安全性和治疗效果的预测变得复杂且困难。当外泌体在体内运输时,人们需要通过了解运输型治疗药物的装载方式,理解其生物命运及其对靶器官的影响[122]。目前,对于高纯度的外泌体分离还没有明确最佳的提纯技术[123]。目前的分离方法产生的外泌体数量较少,而且大规模生产用于临床研究,后续的药物批准昂贵且复杂[38]。未来的临床应用很可能需要外泌体的混合设计[124],当与治疗药物结合时,可能会表现出不良反应。尽管人们已经了解广义外泌体生物学,外泌体包含异质成分且有可能基于供体细胞的性质表现出免疫原性(刺激或抑制)效应。外泌体为各种合成生物分子的传递提供了广阔前景,是细胞治疗的一个新领域。作为药物传递系统,外泌体呈现出一个主要优势是:肝脏中的外泌体没有聚集、归巢现象或首过效应。具有长期安全性、充分表征的外泌体在细胞之间以及通过难以穿过的膜屏障,如 BBB 递送核酸和治疗分子将具有重大的实际意义。然而,在这些药物传递系统成为现实治疗方法之前,包括免疫反应在内的成分和过程需要澄清[122]。显而易见,肿瘤细胞源性外泌体具有独特性质,可能会被用来开发一种比合成药物载体更好的外泌体给药系统。然而,在基于外泌体的药物递送系统应用于临床之前,必须克服一些限制和障碍。重要的问题仍然需要自体解决,或者是非免疫原性外泌体工厂。因此,需要制订一种产生治疗应用型囊泡的策略,包括建立产生细胞类型、制备囊泡纳米粒的物理方法、提高 EV 产量和规模、EV 效果的衡量方法以及 EV 启发的生物工程人工囊泡。最近,一些研究人员研发了一种制备外泌体模拟囊泡的方法,该方法可以克服天然外泌体的局限性,如载药效率低和外泌体产量低[125]。这些载有化疗药物的纳米囊泡(直径为 100~200 nm)通过连续挤压使其经过孔径减小的过滤器分解细胞而产生[126]。这进一步表明,这些具有外泌体模拟特性的纳米囊泡可以作为 RNAi 转移到细胞质[127]。然而,外泌体膜中高水平的胆固醇、神经节苷脂和鞘磷脂导致其双层结构比它们的母体细胞更为坚硬[128],这表明它们与脂质颗粒的融合需要苛刻的条件[129],如积极的冻融过程[130]。为了避免这种情况,Yang 等设计了一种模拟病毒的融合性外泌体平台,将整合的血管口炎病毒 G 蛋白(一种病毒融合蛋白)导入靶细胞膜[131]。有趣的是,通过将来自修饰细胞的外泌体与插入肽、抗体或聚乙二醇的脂质体融合,外泌体修饰变得容易。

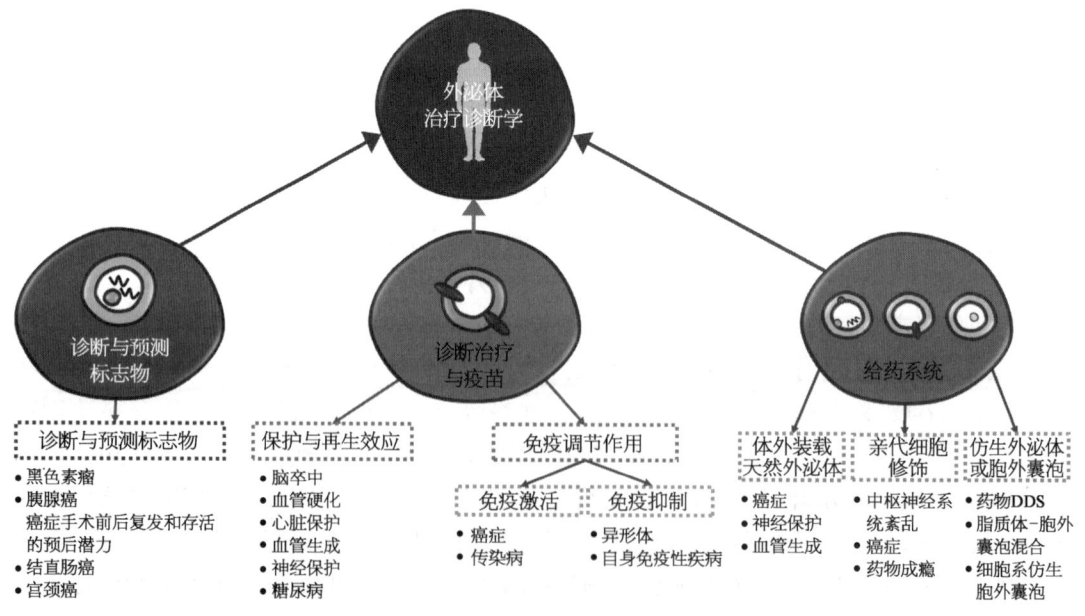

图 20-2 转化医学和临床医学中基于外泌体的诊断和治疗方法的各种策略示意图

尽管目前在治疗肿瘤和其他疑难杂症方面仍存在许多挑战，但外泌体，包括外泌体模拟纳米囊泡在内，被认为是有效的诊断生物标志物和有前景的治疗工具。此外，随着化学、物理、细胞和基因工程技术的发展，许多现有的外泌体修饰方法有望应用于各种临床情况(图20-2)。

（田思嫚 译，董江涛 审校）

参考文献

[1] Clayton A, Harris CL, Court J, et al. Antigen-presenting cell exosomes are protected from complement-mediated lysis by expression of CD55 and CD59. Eur J Immunol 2003; 33(2): 522-31.

[2] Pant S, Hilton H, Burczynski ME. The multifaceted exosome: Biogenesis, role in normal and aberrant cellular function, and frontiers for pharmacological and biomarker opportunities. Biochem Pharmacol 2012; 83(11): 1484-94.

[3] Revenfeld ALS, Bæk R, Nielsen MH, et al. Diagnostic and prognostic potential of extracellular vesicles in peripheral blood. Clin Ther 2014; 36(6): 830-46.

[4] Kumar D, Gupta D, Shankar S, et al. Biomolecular characterization of exosomes released from cancer stem cells: possible implications for biomarker and treatment of cancer. Oncotarget 2015; 6(5): 3280.

[5] Mishra PJ. Non-coding RNAs as clinical biomarkers for cancer diagnosis and prognosis. Expert Rev Mol Diagn 2014; 14(8): 917-9.

[6] Schwarzenbach H. The clinical relevance of circulating, exosomal miRNAs as biomarkers for cancer. Expert Rev Mol Diagn 2015; 15(9): 1159-69.

[7] Noerholm M, Balaj L, Limperg T, et al. RNA expression patterns in serum microvesicles from patients with glioblastoma multiforme and controls. BMC Cancer 2012; 12(1): 22.

[8] Taylor DD, Gercel-Taylor C. MicroRNA signatures of tumor-derived exosomes as diagnostic biomarkers of ovarian cancer. Gynecol Oncol 2008; 110(1): 13-21.

[9] Skog J, Würdinger T, Van Rijn S, et al. Glioblastoma microvesicles transport RNA and proteins that promote tumour growth and provide diagnostic biomarkers. Nat Cell Biol 2008; 10(12): 1470.

[10] Yamashita T, Kamada H, Kanasaki S, et al. Epidermal growth factor receptor localized to exosome membranes as a possible biomarker for lung cancer diagnosis. Pharmazie 2013; 68(12): 969-73.

[11] Melo SA, Luecke LB, Kahlert C, et al. Glypican-1 identifies cancer exosomes and detects early pancreatic cancer. Nature 2015; 523(7559): 177.

[12] Tavoosidana G, Ronquist G, Darmanis S, et al. Multiple recognition assay reveals prostasomes as promising plasma biomarkers for prostate cancer. Proc Natl Acad Sci U S A 2011; 108(21): 8809-14.

[13] Duijvesz D, Burnum-Johnson KE, Gritsenko MA, et al. Proteomic profiling of exosomes leads to the identification of novel biomarkers for prostate cancer. PLoS One 2013; 8(12): e82589.

[14] Sugimachi K, Matsumura T, Hirata H, et al. Identification of a bona fide microRNA biomarker in serum exosomes that predicts hepatocellular carcinoma recurrence after liver transplantation. Br J Cancer 2015; 112(3): 532.

[15] Kawikova I, Askenase PW. Diagnostic and therapeutic potentials of exosomes in CNS diseases. Brain Res 2015; 1617: 63-71.

[16] Masyuk AI, Masyuk TV, LaRusso NF. Exosomes in the pathogenesis, diagnostics and therapeutics of liver diseases. J Hepatol 2013; 59(3): 621-5.

[17] Spanu S, van Roeyen CR, Denecke B, et al. Urinary exosomes: a novel means to non-invasively assess changes in renal gene and protein expression. PLoS ONE 2014; 9(10): e109631.

[18] Levänen B, Bhakta NR, Paredes PT, et al. Altered microRNA profiles in bronchoalveolar lavage fluid exosomes in asthmatic patients. J Allergy Clin Immunol 2013; 131(3): 894-903. e898.

[19] Hoefer IE, Steffens S, Ala-Korpela M, et al. Novel methodologies for biomarker discovery in atherosclerosis. Eur Heart J 2015; 36(39): 2635-42.

[20] Saman S, Kim W, Raya M, et al. Exosome-associated tau is secreted in tauopathy models and is selectively phosphorylated in cerebrospinal fluid in early Alzheimer disease. J Biol Chem 2012; 287(6): 3842-9.

[21] Goetzl EJ, Boxer A, Schwartz JB, et al. Altered lysosomal proteins in neural-derived plasma exosomes in preclinical Alzheimer disease. Neurology 2015; 85(1): 40-7.

[22] Gui Y, Liu H, Zhang L, et al. Altered microRNA profiles in cerebrospinal fluid exosome in Parkinson disease and Alzheimer disease. Oncotarget 2015; 6(35): 37043-53.

[23] Cheng L, Doecke JD, Sharples RA, et al. Prognostic serum miRNA biomarkers associated with Alzheimer's disease shows concordance with neuropsychological and neuroimaging assessment. Mol Psychiatry 2014; 20: 1188.

[24] van den Boorn JG, Schlee M, Coch C, et al. SiRNA delivery with exosome nanoparticles. Nat Biotechnol 2011; 29(4): 325.

[25] Tomlinson PR, Zheng Y, Fischer R, et al. Identification of distinct circulating exosomes in Parkinson's disease. Ann Clin Transl Neurol 2015; 2(4): 353-61.

[26] Fujita Y, Yoshioka Y, Ito S, et al. Intercellular communication by extracellular vesicles and their microRNAs in asthma. Clin Ther 2014; 36(6): 873-81.

[27] van den Berge M, Tasena H. Role of microRNAs and exosomes in asthma. Curr Opin Pulm Med 2019; 25(1): 87-93.

[28] Admyre C, Grunewald J, Thyberg J, et al. Exosomes with major histocompatibility complex class II and co-stimulatory molecules are present in human BAL fluid. Eur Respir J 2003; 22(4): 578-83.

[29] Admyre C, Telemo E, Almqvist N, et al. Exosomes - nanovesicles with possible roles in allergic inflammation. Allergy 2008; 63(4): 404-8.

[30] Mazzeo C, Cañas JA, Zafra MP, et al. Exosome secretion by eosinophils: a possible role in asthma pathogenesis. J Allergy Clin Immunol 2015; 135(6): 1603-13.

[31] Prado N, Marazuela EG, Segura E, et al. Exosomes from bronchoalveolar fluid of tolerized mice prevent allergic reaction. J Immunol 2008; 181(2): 1519-25.
[32] Mortaz E, Alipoor SD, Varahram M, et al. Exosomes in severe asthma: update in their roles and potential in therapy. Biomed Res Int 2018; 2018: 2862187. 1-10.
[33] Francisco-Garcia A, Martinez-Nunez RT, Rupani H, et al. LSC abstract-altered small RNA cargo in severe asthma exosomes. Eur Respir J 2016; 48: 101.
[34] Suzuki M, Konno S, Makita H, et al. Altered circulating exosomal RNA profiles detected by next-generation sequencing in patients with severe asthma. Eur Respir Soc 2016; 48(S60): PA3410.
[35] Kuate S, Cinatl J, Doerr HW, et al. Exosomal vaccines containing the S protein of the SARS coronavirus induce high levels of neutralizing antibodies. Virology 2007; 362(1): 26-37.
[36] Matsumoto S, Sakata Y, Nakatani D, et al. Circulating p53-responsive microRNAs are predictive indicators of heart failure after acute myocardial infarction. Circ Res 2013; 113(3): 322-6.
[37] Huebner AR, Somparn P, Benjachat T, et al. Exosomes in urine biomarker discovery urine proteomics in kidney disease biomarker discovery. Springer; 2015; 43-58.
[38] Taylor DD, Shah S. Methods of isolating extracellular vesicles impact down-stream analyses of their cargoes. Methods 2015; 87: 3-10.
[39] Aline F, Bout D, Amigorena S, et al. Toxoplasma gondii antigen-pulsed-dendritic cell-derived exosomes induce a protective immune response against T. gondii infection. Infect Immun 2004; 72(7): 4127-37.
[40] Beauvillain C, Juste MO, Dion S, et al. Exosomes are an effective vaccine against congenital toxoplasmosis in mice. Vaccine 2009; 27(11): 1750-7.
[41] Beauvillain C, Ruiz S, Guiton R, et al. A vaccine based on exosomes secreted by a dendritic cell line confers protection against T. gondii infection in syngeneic and allogeneic mice. Microbes Infect 2007; 9(14-15): 1614-22.
[42] Colino J, Snapper CM. Exosomes from bone marrow dendritic cells pulsed with diphtheria toxoid preferentially induce type 1 antigen-specific IgG responses in naive recipients in the absence of free antigen. J Immunol 2006; 177(6): 3757-62.
[43] Ramachandra L, Qu Y, Wang Y, et al. Mycobacterium tuberculosis synergizes with ATP to induce release of microvesicles and exosomes containing major histocompatibility complex class Ⅱ molecules capable of antigen presentation. Infect Immun 2010; 78(12): 5116-25.
[44] Singh PP, LeMaire C, Tan JC, et al. Exosomes released from M. tuberculosis infected cells can suppress IFN-γ mediated activation of naïve macrophages. PLoS ONE 2011; 6(4): e18564.
[45] Anticoli S, Manfredi F, Chiozzini C, et al. An exosome-based vaccine platform imparts cytotoxic T lymphocyte immunity against viral antigens. Biotechnol J 2018; 13(4): 1700443.
[46] McElroy AK, Akondy RS, Davis CW, et al. Human Ebola virus infection results in substantial immune activation. Proc Natl Acad Sci U S A 2015; 112(15): 4719-24.
[47] Sullivan NJ, Hensley L, Asiedu C, et al. CD8+ cellular immunity mediates rAd5 vaccine protection against Ebola virus infection of nonhuman primates. Nat Med 2011; 17(9): 1128.
[48] Bradfute SB, Warfield KL, Bavari S. Functional CD8+ T cell responses in lethal Ebola virus infection. J Immunol 2008; 180(6): 4058-66.
[49] Fontana JM, Christos PJ, Michelini Z, et al. Mucosal immunization with integrase-defective lentiviral vectors protects against influenza virus challenge in mice. PLoS ONE 2014; 9(5): e97270.
[50] Liang TJ. Current progress in development of hepatitis C virus vaccines. Nat Med 2013; 19(7): 869.
[51] Pereira EA, daSilva LL. HIV-1 Nef: taking control of protein trafficking. Traffic 2016; 17(9): 976-96.
[52] Lenassi M, Cagney G, Liao M, et al. HIV Nef is secreted in exosomes and triggers apoptosis in bystander CD4+ T cells. Traffic 2010; 11(1): 110-22.
[53] D'Aloja P, Santarcangelo AC, Arold S, et al. Genetic and functional analysis of the human immunodeficiency virus (HIV) type 1-inhibiting F12-HIVnef allele. J Gen Virol 2001; 82(11): 2735-45.
[54] Lattanzi L, Federico M. A strategy of antigen incorporation into exosomes: comparing crosspresentation levels of antigens delivered by engineered exosomes and by lentiviral virus-kike particles. Vaccine 2012; 30(50): 7229-37.
[55] Théry C, Amigorena S. The cell biology of antigen presentation in dendritic cells. Curr Opin Immunol 2001; 13(1): 45-51.
[56] Chen DS, Mellman I. Oncology meets immunology: the cancer-immunity cycle. Immunity 2013; 39(1): 1-10.
[57] Kantoff PW, Higano CS, Shore ND, et al. Sipuleucel-T immunotherapy for castration-resistant prostate cancer. N Engl J Med 2010; 363(5): 411-22.
[58] Andre F, Escudier B, Angevin E, et al. Exosomes for cancer immunotherapy. Ann Oncol 2004; 15(Suppl. 4): iv141-4.
[59] Pitt JM, Charrier M, Viaud S, et al. Dendritic cell-derived exosomes as immunotherapies in the fight against cancer. J Immunol 2014; 193(3): 1006-11.
[60] Pitt JM, André F, Amigorena S, et al. Dendritic cell-derived exosomes for cancer therapy. J Clin Invest 2016; 126(4): 1224-32.
[61] Gabrilovich DI, Ciernik IF, Carbone DP. Dendritic cells in antitumor immune responses: I. Defective antigen presentation in tumor-bearing hosts. Cell Immunol 1996; 170(1): 101-10.
[62] Zitvogel L, Regnault A, Lozier A, et al. Eradication of established murine tumors using a novel cell-free vaccine: dendritic cell derived exosomes. Nat Med 1998; 4(5): 594.
[63] Zhang B, Yin Y, Lai RC, et al. Immunotherapeutic potential of extracellular vesicles. Front Immunol 2014; 5: 518.
[64] Morse MA, Garst J, Osada T, et al. A phase I study of dexosome immunotherapy in patients with advanced non-small cell lung cancer. J Transl Med 2005; 3(1): 9.
[65] Escudier B, Dorval T, Chaput N, et al. Vaccination of metastatic melanoma patients with autologous dendritic cell (DC) derived-exosomes: results of thefirst phase I clinical trial. J Transl Med 2005; 3(1): 10.
[66] Besse B, Charrier M, Lapierre V, et al. Dendritic cell-derived exosomes as maintenance immunotherapy after first line

chemotherapy in NSCLC. Oncoimmunology 2016; 5(4): e1071008.
[67] Wolfers J, Lozier A, Raposo G, et al. Tumor-derived exosomes are a source of shared tumor rejection antigens for CTL cross-priming. Nat Med 2001; 7(3): 297.
[68] Dai S, Wei D, Wu Z, et al. Phase I clinical trial of autologous ascites-derived exosomes combined with GM-CSF for colorectal cancer. Mol Ther 2008; 16(4): 782-90.
[69] Andre F, Schartz NE, Movassagh M, et al. Malignant effusions and immunogenic tumourderived exosomes. Lancet 2002; 360(9329): 295-305.
[70] Raposo G, Nijman HW, Stoorvogel W, et al. B lymphocytes secrete antigen-presenting vesicles. J Exp Med 1996; 183 (3): 1161-72.
[71] Viaud S, Terme M, Flament C, et al. Dendritic cell-derived exosomes promote natural killer cell activation and proliferation: a role for NKG2D ligands and IL-15Rα. PLoS ONE 2009; 4(3): e4942.
[72] Saunderson SC, Dunn AC, Crocker PR, et al. CD169 mediates the capture of exosomes in spleen and lymph node. Blood 2014; 123(2): 208-16.
[73] Takahashi Y, Nishikawa M, Shinotsuka H, et al. Visualization and in vivo tracking of the exosomes of murine melanoma B16-BL6 cells in mice after intravenous injection. J Biotechnol 2013; 165(2): 77-84.
[74] Zhou H, Pisitkun T, Aponte A, et al. Exosomal Fetuin-A identified by proteomics: a novel urinary biomarker for detecting acute kidney injury. Kidney Int 2006; 70(10): 1847-57.
[75] Théry C, Duban L, Segura E, et al. Indirect activation of naïve CD4+ T cells by dendritic cell-derived exosomes. Nat Immunol 2002; 3(12): 1156.
[76] Martinez MC, Andriantsitohaina R. Microparticles in angiogenesis: therapeutic potential. Circ Res 2011; 109(1): 110-9.
[77] Aharon A, Brenner B. Microparticles, thrombosis and cancer. Best Pract Res Clin Haematol 2009; 22(1): 61-9.
[78] Cho JA, Park H, Lim EH, et al. Exosomes from ovarian cancer cells induce adipose tissuederived mesenchymal stem cells to acquire the physical and functional characteristics of tumor-supporting myofibroblasts. Gynecol Oncol 2011; 123 (2): 379-86.
[79] Xu J, Lamouille S, Derynck R. TGF-β-induced epithelial to mesenchymal transition. Cell Res 2009; 19(2): 156.
[80] Al-Nedawi K, Meehan B, Kerbel RS, et al. Endothelial expression of autocrine VEGF upon the uptake of tumor-derived microvesicles containing oncogenic EGFR. Proc Natl Acad Sci U S A 2009; 106(10): 3794-9.
[81] Baj-Krzyworzeka M, Majka M, Pratico D, et al. Platelet-derived microparticles stimulate proliferation, survival, adhesion, and chemotaxis of hematopoietic cells. Exp Hematol 2002; 30(5): 450-9.
[82] Ratajczak J, Wysoczynski M, Hayek F, et al. Membrane-derived microvesicles: important and underappreciated mediators of cell-to-cell communication. Leukemia 2006; 20(9): 1487.
[83] Lu M, Xing H, Yang Z, et al. Recent advances on extracellular vesicles in therapeutic delivery: challenges, solutions, and opportunities. Eur J Pharm Biopharm 2017; 119: 381-95.
[84] Haney MJ, Klyachko NL, Zhao Y, et al. Exosomes as drug delivery vehicles for Parkinson's disease therapy. J Control Release 2015; 207: 18-30.
[85] Klumperman J, Raposo G. The complex ultrastructure of the endolysosomal system. Cold Spring Harb Perspect Biol 2014; 6(10): a016857.
[86] Rufino-Ramos D, Albuquerque PR, Carmona V, et al. Extracellular vesicles: novel promising delivery systems for therapy of brain diseases. J Control Release 2017; 262: 247-58.
[87] Viaud S, Ploix S, Lapierre V, et al. Updated technology to produce highly immunogenic dendritic cell-derived exosomes of clinical grade: a critical role of interferon-γ. J Immunother 2011; 34(1): 65-75.
[88] Lener T, Gimona M, Aigner L, et al. Applying extracellular vesicles based therapeutics in clinical trials - an ISEV position paper. J Extracell Vesicles 2015; 4(1): 30087.
[89] Batrakova EV, Kim MS. Development and regulation of exosome-based therapy products. Wiley Interdiscip Rev Nanomed Nanobiotechnol 2016; 8(5): 744-57.
[90] Kim OY, Lee JW, Gho YS. Extracellular vesicle mimetics: novel alternatives to extracellular vesicle-based theranostics, drug delivery, and vaccines. Semin Cell Dev Biol 2017; 67: 74-82.
[91] De Jong WH, Borm PJ. Drug delivery and nanoparticles: applications and hazards. Int J Nanomedicine 2008; 3 (2): 133.
[92] Wilczewska AZ, Niemirowicz K, Markiewicz KH, et al. Nanoparticles as drug delivery systems. Pharmacol Rep 2012; 64(5): 1020-37.
[93] Sercombe L, Veerati T, Moheimani F, et al. Advances and challenges of liposome assisted drug delivery. Front Pharmacol 2015; 6: 286.
[94] Grange C, Tapparo M, Bruno S, et al. Biodistribution of mesenchymal stem cell-derived extracellular vesicles in a model of acute kidney injury monitored by optical imaging. Int J Mol Med 2014; 33(5): 1055-63.
[95] Kotmakçı M, Çıntaş VB. Extracellular vesicles as natural nanosized delivery systems for small-molecule drugs and genetic material: steps towards the future nanomedicines. J Pharm Pharm Sci 2015; 18(3): 396-413.
[96] Peinado H, Alečkovi M, Lavotshkin S, et al. Melanoma exosomes educate bone marrow progenitor cells toward a pro-metastatic phenotype through MET. Nat Med 2012; 18(6): 883-91.
[97] Bruno S, Grange C, Collino F, et al. Microvesicles derived from mesenchymal stem cells enhance survival in a lethal model of acute kidney injury. PLoS One 2012; 7(3): e33115.
[98] Wiklander OP, Nordin JZ, O'Loughlin A, et al. Extracellular vesicle in vivo biodistribution is determined by cell source, route of administration and targeting. J Extracell Vesicles 2015; 4(1): 26316.
[99] Smyth TJ. Exploration of the drug delivery potential of tumor-derived exosomes. (Doctor of Philosophy). University of Colorado at Denver, Anschutz Medical Campus; 2014. Pharmaceutical Sciences Program.
[100] Charoenviriyakul C, Takahashi Y, Morishita M, et al. Cell type-specific and common characteristics of exosomes derived from mouse cell lines: yield, physicochemical properties, and pharmacokinetics. Eur J Pharm Sci 2017; 96: 316-22.

[101] Morishita M, Takahashi Y, Nishikawa M, et al. Pharmacokinetics of exosomes — an important factor for elucidating the biological roles of exosomes and for the development of exosome-based therapeutics. J Pharm Sci 2017; 106(9): 2265-9.
[102] Hao S, Bai O, Li F, et al. Mature dendritic cells pulsed with exosomes stimulate efficient cytotoxic T-lymphocyte responses and antitumour immunity. Immunology 2007; 120(1): 90-102.
[103] Tian Y, Li S, Song J, et al. A doxorubicin delivery platform using engineered natural membrane vesicle exosomes for targeted tumor therapy. Biomaterials 2014; 35(7): 2383-90.
[104] Sun D, Zhuang X, Xiang X, et al. A novel nanoparticle drug delivery system: the anti-inflammatory activity of curcumin is enhanced when encapsulated in exosomes. Mol Ther 2010; 18(9): 1606-14.
[105] Dhillon N, Aggarwal BB, Newman RA, et al. Phase II trial of curcumin in patients with advanced pancreatic cancer. Clin Cancer Res 2008; 14(14): 4491-9.
[106] Adlakha YK, Saini N. Brain microRNAs and insights into biological functions and therapeutic potential of brain enriched miRNA-128. Mol Cancer 2014; 13(1): 33.
[107] Xitong D, Xiaorong Z. Targeted therapeutic delivery using engineered exosomes and its applications in cardiovascular diseases. Gene 2016; 575(2): 377-84.
[108] Kim MS, Haney MJ, Zhao Y, et al. Development of exosome-encapsulated paclitaxel to overcome MDR in cancer cells. Nanomedicine 2016; 12(3): 655-64.
[109] Tang K, Zhang Y, Zhang H, et al. Delivery of chemotherapeutic drugs in tumour cell-derived microparticles. Nat Commun 2012; 3: 1282.
[110] Pardridge WM. Drug transport across the blood-brain barrier. J Cereb Blood Flow Metab 2012; 32(11): 1959-72.
[111] Kabanov AV, Batrakova EV. Polymer nanomaterials. In: Neuroimmune Pharmacology. Springer; 2008. p. 691-707.
[112] Silva GA. Nanotechnology applications and approaches for neuroregeneration and drug delivery to the central nervous system. Ann N Y Acad Sci 2010; 1199(1): 221-30.
[113] Ebadi M, Srinivasan SK, Baxi MD. Oxidative stress and antioxidant therapy in Parkinson's disease. Prog Neurobiol 1996; 48(1): 1-19.
[114] McGeer P, Itagaki S, Boyes B, et al. Reactive microglia are positive for HLA-DR in the substantia nigra of Parkinson's and Alzheimer's disease brains. Neurology 1988; 38(8): 1285.
[115] Abraham S, Soundararajan C, Vivekanandhan S, et al. Erythrocyte antioxidant enzymes in Parkinson's disease. Indian J Med Res 2005; 121(2): 111-5.
[116] Ambani LM, Van Woert MH, Murphy S. Brain peroxidase and catalase in Parkinson disease. Arch Neurol 1975; 32(2): 114-8.
[117] Riederer P, Sofic E, Rausch WD, et al. Transition metals, ferritin, glutathione, and ascorbic acid in parkinsonian brains. J Neurochem 1989; 52(2): 515-20.
[118] Kim SH, Bianco N, Menon R, et al. Exosomes derived from genetically modified DC expressing FasL are anti-inflammatory and immunosuppressive. Mol Ther 2006; 13(2): 289-300.
[119] Katsuda T, Oki K, Ochiya T. Potential application of extracellular vesicles of human adipose tissue-derived mesenchymal stem cells in Alzheimer's disease therapeutics. In: Stem cell renewal and cell-cell communication. Springer; 2014. p. 171-81.
[120] Li Y, Cheng Q, Hu G, et al. Extracellular vesicles in mesenchymal stromal cells: a novel therapeutic strategy for stroke. Exp Ther Med 2018; 15(5): 4067-79.
[121] Tran T-H, Mattheolabakis G, Aldawsari H, et al. Exosomes as nanocarriers for immunotherapy of cancer and inflammatory diseases. Clin Immunol 2015; 160(1): 46-58.
[122] Ha D, Yang N, Nadithe V. Exosomes as therapeutic drug carriers and delivery vehicles across biological membranes: current perspectives and future challenges. Acta Pharm Sin B 2016; 6(4): 287-96.
[123] Petersen KE, Manangon E, Hood JL, et al. A review of exosome separation techniques and characterization of B16-F10 mouse melanoma exosomes with AF4-UV-MALS-DLS-TEM. Anal Bioanal Chem 2014; 406(30): 7855-66.
[124] Rana S, Bajaj A, Mout R, et al. Monolayer coated gold nanoparticles for delivery applications. Adv Drug Deliv Rev 2012; 64(2): 200-16.
[125] He C, Zheng S, Luo Y, et al. Exosome theranostics: biology and translational medicine. Theranostics 2018; 8(1): 237-55.
[126] Jang SC, Kim OY, Yoon CM, et al. Bioinspired exosome-mimetic nanovesicles for targeted delivery of chemotherapeutics to malignant tumors. ACS Nano 2013; 7(9): 7698-710.
[127] Lunavat TR, Jang SC, Nilsson L, et al. RNAi delivery by exosome-mimetic nanovesicles — implications for targeting c-Myc in cancer. Biomaterials 2016; 102: 231-8.
[128] Parolini I, Federici C, Raggi C, et al. Microenvironmental pH is a key factor for exosome traffic in tumor cells. J Biol Chem 2009; 284(49): 34211-22.
[129] Armstrong JP, Holme MN, Stevens MM. Re-engineering extracellular vesicles as smart nanoscale therapeutics. ACS Nano 2017; 11(1): 69-83.
[130] Sato YT, Umezaki K, Sawada S, et al. Engineering hybrid exosomes by membrane fusion with liposomes. Sci Rep 2016; 6: 21933.
[131] Yang Y, Hong Y, Nam GH, et al. Virus-mimetic fusogenic exosomes for direct delivery of integral membrane proteins to target cell membranes. Adv Mater 2017; 29(13): 1605604.

第 21 章

外泌体、芽球、泛生和达尔文
Exosomes, gemmules, pangenesis and Darwin

Denis Noble

Department of Physiology, Anatomy & Genetics, University of Oxford, Oxford, United Kingdom

一、概述

本章采用历史笔记的形式,首先对最近发现的外泌体及其重要性与 Charles Darwin 在其著作和信件中表达的一些观点强烈一致的原因做出解释。之后,本章节将解释为什么这些观点会在 1882 年 Charles Darwin 去世后至 20 世纪上半叶新达尔文主义现代综合理论的形成过程中被刻意从标准进化生物学中删除。最后,将评论当前进化生物学的趋势,这些趋势可以被视为是回到了 Darwin 更微妙的多机制观点的现代形式。通过简要回顾现代研究可以发现,通过精子进行隔代遗传的机制是存在且有效的。

二、达尔文主义观点

如果 Charles Darwin 还活着,他会如何看待外泌体的发现及其重要性? 他会怎么评价这本书? 要回答这些问题,我们需要了解 Darwin 作为科学家和思想家的性格,以及他对自己理论的怀疑时是如何应对的。

(一) 物种起源

Darwin 是一个谨慎而迟钝的思想家。1859 年,他出版了其开创性著作《物种起源》(*The Origin of Species*)[1]。由于 Alfred Russel Wallace 一直在紧追,他在马来群岛的工作中得到了支持同样观点的重要信息,这使得 Darwin 匆忙完成了这本书。1831 年至 1836 年,自 Darwin 乘坐小猎犬号进行著名的航行以来已经过去了三十年,在这期间,他允许自己对于自然选择进化理论的想法在得到发表前缓慢成熟,即使如此,他依然不确定是否完全达到了他的目标。

《物种起源》完成后,Darwin 在给地质学家 Charles Lyell 的信中写道:

> 我认为我是一个非常迟钝的思想家,你或许会很惊讶,我花了那么多年去看清楚一些问题是什么,哪些问题必须被解答——例如,性状分化原则的必要性、中间品种在连续区域内的逐步灭绝、不育单次杂交和不育杂种的双重问题等。

由于本书的仓促出版,Darwin 直到第三版才完全认可他前辈的理论,其中甚至包括他的祖父 Erasmus Darwin。因此 Charles Darwin 知道,他绝不是第一个提出物种转化理论的人(当时进化论被称为物种转化理论)。在第三版(1861 年)中,他提到了至少 30 位他所承认的前辈,其中也包括 Aristotle。在第四版(1866 年)中,这个名单已增加到了 38 个,其中最著名的是 Jean-Baptiste Lamarck,Darwin 在提及他的时候写道:

"这是位当之无愧的博物学家……他坚持主张包括人类在内的所有物种都是由其他物种进化而来的。"

他有充分的理由赞扬 Lamarck。早在半个世纪前,Lamarck 在 1809 年出版的《动物哲学》(*Zoologie Philosophique*)[2](正好比 Darwin 的《物种起源》早 50 年)一书中阐述了支持物种转化理论的理由,因此他不得不像 Darwin 一样,在科学界同行的严厉批评中进行自我辩护。Darwin 在辩护中得到了号称"Darwin 的牛头犬"Thomas Henry Huxley 的极大帮助。当 Darwin 本人在乡下的家中默默工作时,Huxley 则完全扮演了达尔文主义代言人的角色。然而,Lamarck 本人却不得不在充斥着智慧与挑战的巴黎文化中,独自与 Georges Cuvier 等强大的对手舌战。Cuvier 曾写过一篇讣告辞,全面地诋毁了 Lamarck 的名誉。这篇致辞是在 Lamarck 贫民殡葬上宣读的,它像丧钟一样回荡在时间的长河中。这是一篇高度偏颇的文章。Cuvier 提出了一种神创论,即在全球灾难发生后,新物种会被单独创造出来。他强烈反对 Lamarck 相较于他更为激进的进化论观点(从一个物种到另一个物种的渐进进化)。

Darwin 的谨慎在他 1876 年写给探险家和自然历史学家 Moritz Wagner 的一封信中也得以展现:

在我看来,我所犯的最大错误是没有考虑到除自然选择以外的独立环境因素,如食物、气候等条件的直接作用。

值得注意的是,这封信写得比《物种起源》第四版的序言晚。因为他的怀疑似乎随着时间而逐渐增加。另外,他在信中所指的并非是自然选择,而是各种环境因素的直接作用。新达尔文主义过分强调了,并将一切结果都归因于自然选择,这是非常不寻常的。这是将达尔文主义视为新达尔文主义的错误原因之一,但绝不是唯一的原因。

人们通常认为,Lamarck 和 Darwin 虽然都赞成物种的渐进演化,但他们对于进化过程的问题的看法是截然不同的。其中的分歧主要体现在两方面。一方面,Lamarck 的理论通常被描述为"生命之梯",即复杂程度不断递增的单一连续;而 Darwin 的理论则被描述为"生命之树",表达了进化是从一个共同的起源辐射出多个分支的分化过程(图 21-1)。另一方面,Lamarck 支持的获

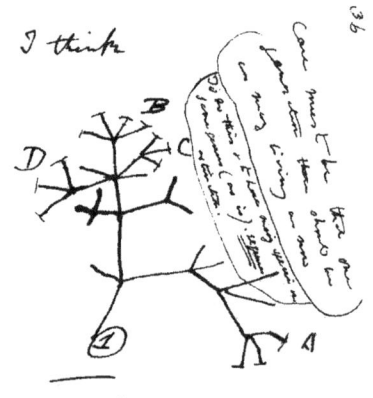

图 21-1　Darwin 生命进化树的第一个草图。摘自 Darwin 1837 年"B"笔记本

得性遗传成就了他的盛名（或恶名），而 Darwin 则以他的自然选择理论而闻名，但是在新达尔文主义看来，获得性遗传在自然选择的过程中是不必要的。

（二）生命之树

历史资料消除了人们对于拉马克主义和达尔文主义差异的误解。

首先，让我们思考一下是谁发明了生命之梯和生命之树。1809 年，当 Lamarck 发表他的著作《动物哲学》时，他就描述了生命之梯的想法，生命演化的进程通过一种被他称之为"le Pouvoir de la Vie"的趋势向上移动，以增加复杂性。因这句话被翻译为"生命的力量"，Lamarck 被误解为是一个支持"生命力"观点的活力论者。然而事实并非如此，法国遗传学及历史学家 André Pichot 在 Flammarion 出版社于 1994 年重印版本中的序言里写道：

> Lamarck 声明：有生命的物体和无生命的物体之间存在着根本的区别，这可能会使人们认为 Lamarck 是一个活力论者。但他不是。相反，他的生物学观点是对当时提出主流理论 Bichat 的生理活力论的机械回应，后者当时是主导理论（译自 Pichot 的法语记录）。

但更重要的是，在这本书的结尾，在一个不太为人所知的附录中，Lamarck 完全改变了他的想法。在对蠕虫的研究中，他无情地得出一个结论：所谓的"内部蠕虫"（如绦虫）和"外部蠕虫"（如蚯蚓）不可能同时存在于单一的生命阶梯内。当他意识到这一点时，许多其他的真相也随之出现。结果如图 21 - 2 所示：在 1809 年科学理论的框架中，Lamarck 在一定程

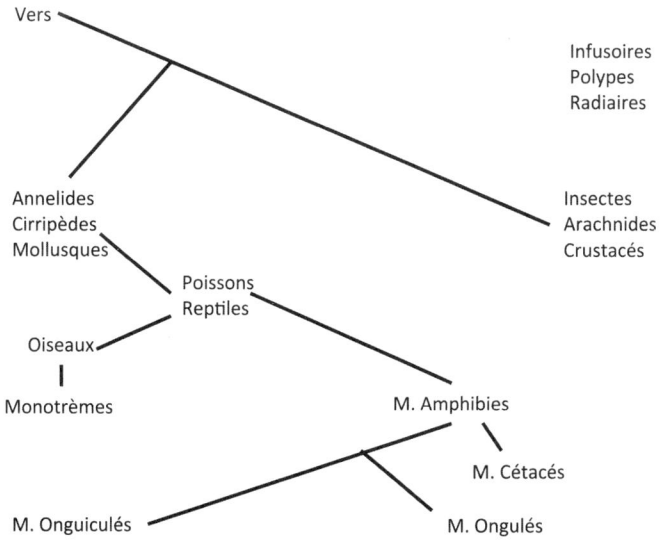

图 21 - 2　Lamarck 的生命之树。摘自《动物哲学》附录，1809 年

度上构建了一棵绝对清晰的生命之树。这个发现比 Darwin 1837 年的笔记本早 28 年，Darwin 不可能在 Lamarck 的书中知道这个图。

Lamarck 不仅在 1809 年的书中改变了他的理论，还在 1815 年[4]和 1820 年[5]出版的两本书中明确地重复了生命的分支树理论。因此，1809 年的附录并不仅仅是一时的心血来潮。

Stephen J Gould 在回顾 Lamarck 这一方面的研究时写道：

> 我们如何看待他（Lamarck）愿意逐渐承认自己的逻辑错误，以及他愿意构建一个全新的、相反的解释，而不是仅仅把他视作是一种英雄行为，这是值得我们钦佩的事情，这也是认为 Lamarck 是生物学历史上最杰出的智者之一的理由[6]。

在生命之树理论上，Lamarck 无疑早于 Darwin。现在让我们转向另一个广泛假设的差异。

（三）获得性状的遗传

为什么 Darwin 在给 Moritz Wagner 的信中（参见上文）说道：他（Darwin）没有"足够重视环境因素的直接作用，如食物、气候等，这些是独立于自然选择之外的"。如果环境因素不是获得性遗传的决定因素之一，那么它在"独立于自然选择"的条件下将会产生什么样的影响呢？我们确实在《物种起源》中找到了证据。Ernst Mayr 在哈佛大学 1964 年再版的《物种起源》的前言中写道：

> 奇怪的是，很少有进化论者注意到，除了自然选择，Darwin 同样承认用进废退是一种重要的进化机制。在这一点上，他有着非常清晰的证据。例如，在第 137 页中，鼹鼠和其他穴居哺乳动物的眼睛变小"可能是由于不用而逐渐变小，但也可能是自然选择的结果"。他在洞穴动物的例子中谈到失去眼睛时"我把这一性状的退化完全归因于废弃"（第 137 页）。在第 455 页，他明确说道："性状的退化或者器官选择性的退化会发生在生命周期的任意阶段……"在他的理论中，用进废退是十分重要的，其重要性则体现在《物种起源》一书中这个词的高频引用。我在第 11 页、第 43 页、第 134 页、第 135 页、第 136 页、第 137 页、第 447 页、第 454 页、第 455 页、第 472 页、第 479 页和第 480 页找到参考文献[7]。

正如 Lamarck 在其 1809 年的著作《生命之树》中提到的那样，我们可以猜想这是否只是 Darwin 理论中的一个过渡阶段。虽然许多进化生物学家都这么认为，但这种猜测是完全错误的。Darwin 在他 1859 年的书中提到了用进废退不仅仅是一种机制。事实上，他已经将其发展为一种理论，并且可以解释它是如何发生的。

Darwin 看到的问题是，我们并不清楚这一过程是如何在拥有单独生殖系统的多细胞生物中发生的。如果体细胞的变化是适应环境的结果，那么生殖细胞是无法改变的，除非这种新的性状可以通过某种方式影响到它们。例如，眼睛这样的感觉器官作为体细胞的一部分，它对于环境适应性的改变如何影响到遥远的生殖器官中的精子或卵细胞？必须有某种物质将信息传递给生殖细胞，从而遗传给下一代。为了解决这个问题，Darwin 发明了芽球的概念，他认为这些小颗粒（大概是通过血液流动）可以携带相关的遗传信息。Darwin 在 1868 年的著作《饲养动植物的变异》*The Uariation of Animals and Plants under Domestication*[8] 中提出了被称为泛生论的芽球理论。

在这本关于外泌体的书里，读者不必深入研究什么是 Darwin 的芽球。

我想我们可以回答本章开头提出的问题了：如果 Darwin 看到他的理论以这种方式反映在现代的理论探索中，他肯定会激动不已。当然，发现外泌体本身并不能证明它们是按照 Darwin 设想的方式出现的。

三、新达尔文主义（现代综合）观点

Darwin 的工作是在没有遗传学理论的情况下完成的。Mendel 在豌豆杂交遗传学上的工作直到 19 世纪晚期才被重新重视，当时也完成了第一个获得性状遗传的实验。

（一）获得性状遗传的早期实验

1890 年，August Weismann 第一次做了这个实验[9]。他决定不把动物，尤其是它们的胚胎放置在不同的环境中，而是通过手术方式干预。这一做法至关重要。

实验内容包括切断老鼠的尾巴，然后观察这是否对后代产生影响。答案无疑是否定的。这项工作是新达尔文主义的基石，所以它是否确切地回答了相关问题是至关重要的。正如 Lamarck 自己所表述的拉马克主义的旧观点所说，这是一种奇怪的不恰当的验证方法。其观点是，拉马克遗传可能发生在生物体与环境之间的功能性相互作用中，通过对生物体结构和功能的使用和废弃，而依靠外科手术所获得的非功能性结果是不能遗传的。

此外，Darwin 一定已经知道，这种遗传并非会受到动物饲养者的影响。无论繁殖了多少代，出于审美原因对狗进行断尾并不会导致后代的尾巴发育不良。用一种更现代的方式来说，生殖是否独立于环境因素的影响。如果要用断尾实验或任何其他实验来回答这个问题，主要是出于改变环境使无尾成为一种优势性状来考虑的。除了为什么手术导致的变化应该遗传这个显而易见的问题，即使是一个标准的拉马克学者也会注意到，除手术之外，环境因素并没有什么不同。此外，实验也不会考虑有利于无尾的环境因素。

20 世纪 50 年代，Conrad Waddington 研究环境对胚胎的影响，为此类实验指明了一条更为成功的道路。他在 1957 年出版的经典著作《基因策略》（*The Strategy of the Genes*）[10] 中所做的实验表明，将胚胎暴露在用于测试的环境，经过十几代左右的时间，获得的性状就可以被整合到基因组中。

然而，断尾实验让 Weismann 和其他人清楚了拉马克主义是不成立的。随后，将生殖细胞从体细胞中分离出来的 Weismann 成了新达尔文主义向现代综合理论发展的基石。直接引用 Weismann 的话：

> 在我看来,这(遗传物质)只能是生殖细胞的物质,这种物质把它的遗传倾向一代又一代地传递下去,起初不变,而且总是不受个体在生命周期中逆境的影响。如果这些观点是正确的,我们有关于通过行为(用进废退)改变物种性状的所有观点,如 Lamarck 提出的,并在某些情况下被 Darwin 接受的,都完全崩溃了。
>
> (1883 年关于遗传的讲座)

这表明,Weismann 充分意识到 Darwin 将后天获得性状的遗传作为进化理论的一部分是错误的。

至少可以说,这样一位杰出的、广受赞誉的科学家应该推翻这个不恰当的稻草人论证。更奇怪的是,这么多其他杰出的科学家竟然把它作为一个主要进化理论的基础。今天,没有哪一项重要的已发表的科学能够基于如此脆弱和不恰当的证据。为什么 Weismann 和他的继任者们要这么做?

在 Weismann 的实验中,部分答案基于一个鲜为人知的事实:他完全承认,他的实验只是否认了由于手术导致的残疾的遗传。他做这些实验是因为他知道"拉马克学说"认为这种残疾是可以遗传的。激进的拉马克学派已经建立起了稻草人理论,例如,他们声称,在几代人中反复进行割礼手术,可能会导致婴儿出生时没有包皮。他很清楚实验的局限性,也知道他们不成熟的实验是对一种类似的不成熟和不正确的理论的反应。

这个谜题的答案是,Weismann 已经确定他的另一个假设,即变异具有随机性是正确的。在 1883 年的同一场演讲中(在他的断尾实验之前),他拒绝接受后天获得性状遗传的观点,并对 Darwin 在《物种起源》中用进废退的例子提出了另一种解释。但是,对 Darwin 的例子有其他解释并不能证明他所说的这些解释是正确的。据我所知,Weismann 所做的断尾实验是唯一的直接实验。

(二)突变的随机性

人们还认为,Weismann 早在 1889 年就在他关于遗传的论文[11]中提出了这样一个观点,即生殖细胞的变化基本上是随机的,这与魏斯曼屏障一样,成了一种教条。因此,他对现代综合理论的两个主要假设负有责任,并经常被认为是在 20 世纪 30 年代和 20 世纪 40 年代,将 Darwin 与现代综合理论联系起来的最重要的进化生物学思想家。在 1982 年出版的权威著作《生物学思想的发展》(*The Growth of Biological Thought*[12])的作者 Ernst Mayr,将他描述为"有史以来最伟大的生物学家之一"。

(三)魏斯曼屏障现在被纳为"分子生物学的中心法则"了吗?

我们现在知道魏斯曼屏障不是绝对的,它存在许多其他的漏洞,例如,对于母系和父系的影响是如何跨代传播的[13]。现在一个重要的问题是,外泌体能够在多大限度上参与这种传播。因此,经过进化生物学家多年来的研究,我们已经知道基于种系绝对隔离的理论是不正确的。

那么,为什么新达尔文主义在 20 世纪后半叶,这些影响被发现时没有被抛弃呢?毕竟,将新达尔文主义与 Darwin 自己的理论区别开来的主要原因是排除了后天获得性状的遗传性。这正是二者差异的本质所在,也得到了 Alfred Russel Wallace 的支持,他和 Weismann 一样,在这个问题上采取了强硬立场。

Darwin 于 1882 年去世,正好在 Weismann 在 1883 年发表影响深远的演讲的前一年,所以这个问题在 Darwin 的一生中从未被讨论过。

细胞屏障是可渗透的这一认识导致了屏障概念的微妙转变。一些新达尔文主义理论家不再为所谓的"魏斯曼屏障"的绝对性质进行辩护,而是提出它已经成为分子生物学的中心法则,即核苷酸序列可以指定氨基酸序列,但氨基酸序列的变化不能用来确定核苷酸序列的变化。

魏斯曼屏障"正是中心法则"的观点现在广为流传,它甚至出现在维基百科关于中心法则的简单条目上:"中心法则是魏斯曼屏障的现代版本。"[b]

维基百科主页上的声明则更为谨慎:"这(魏斯曼屏障)并没有预测到中心法则,但确实预测了其以基因为中心的生命观,尽管是在非分子术语中。"维基百科上这一简要但极具误导性的声明反复出现在一个为小学生设计的网站上。[c]

这种错误是不幸的。生殖细胞和基因组之间存在根本性的区别。细胞包含的不仅仅是它的基因组。在地球上的大多数生命中,它都是完整的有机体。此外,可以证明细胞其余部分的信息含量与基因组[14]的信息含量相匹配。那么,中心法则即魏斯曼屏障的想法是如何产生的呢?

(四)改变基因的定义

这种发展可以用基因定义的转变来解释。1909 年,当 Johannsen 首次引入这个词时,它被定义为一种可遗传的表型特征[15]。这也是孟德尔学说的基本概念。因此,他们关于基因的定义应该适用于所有拥有生殖细胞的生物。Johannsen 解释说,这种基因可能是生物体中拥有遗传特性的任何东西(ein etwas)。如果他知道这些,RNA、DNA 和组蛋白上的表观遗传标记,以及使复制和遗传成为可能的细胞结构,都应该被包括在内。这显然不是现代分子生物学对基因的定义,后者仅限于形成蛋白质模板的 DNA 序列[16,17]。

这种定义上的重大转变在现代综合理论形成时还不为人所知。当时人们甚至不知道 DNA 是遗传物质,因此,定义上的转变对那些制订现代综合理论的人来说无关紧要也就不足为奇了。例如,在群体遗传学的数学理论方面取得的巨大进展[18]非常适合将基因定义为表型特征。事实上,对于遗传学在社会科学中的大多数应用,如经济学和社会学,保留表型的定义是重要的,甚至是必要的。

但是,回到基因的定义上来,表型和基因型定义之间的差异对于新达尔文主义的不同版本有着巨大的影响,如自私基因理论,它是建立在区分复制子(被认为是 DNA)和载体(表型)的基础上的[19]。

新达尔文主义的自私基因版本有两个致命的缺陷。首先,从生理学的角度来看,它的结果是不可预测的。问题是,自私基因理论的核心定义并不独立于该理论的唯一实验结果,即定义为 DNA 序列的基因是否实际上是自私的,例如,它们在基因库中的频率是否增加了[20]。其次，DNA不能被看作是一个与细胞分离的复制子[16]。细胞的功能，尤其是它的生理功能，是使DNA得以忠实复制的原因。

这一缺陷导致了中心法则发展的下一个错误，因为细胞才是复制的载体，而并非DNA。这是核心的问题，所以我现在将解释中心法则是如何错误发展的。

当中心法则首次被提出时，Watson和Crick承认他们受Schrödinger的著作《生命是什么？》(What is Life?)所启发[21]。在那本书中，Schrödinger做了两个预测，一个非常成功，另一个则显然是错误的[22]（第176～181页）。

正确的预测是，他所称之为非周期性的晶体其实就是遗传物质。如果把一种聚合物看成一种晶体，这就是对DNA的一种很好的描述。

错误的预测是分子的行为就像一个确定的晶体。这一观点直接导致了对中心法则的误解，认为复制的准确性和决定性的品质仅仅是因为DNA。

如果比较子细胞和亲本细胞的DNA，会发现在一个完整的基因组中，复制错误率不到一个碱基对。错误率大约只有十亿分之一个碱基对，这是非常精确的。但是，现在假设我们可以在复制后立即比较DNA序列，将发现大约有万分之一的错误率，这在一个30亿碱基对的基因组中意味着数百万的错误。没有任何真核细胞能在这样的误差率下存活。因此Schrödinger关于分子本身的行为就像一个确定晶体的观点是错误的。晶体结构的生长方式是对的，但这对DNA来说却是一种错误的比喻，这不是它生长和复制的方式。就其本身而言，这种方式将会留下数以百万计的错误。

它只在一个完整的细胞中精确地复制，这种复制包含了所有使细胞存活的客观功能。细胞通过一个非常复杂的三阶段过程来实现DNA的精确复制，在这个过程中，数以百万计的错误被检测和纠正。著名的基因组"不朽"实际上是整个细胞的功能，而不仅仅是基因组的功能。

此外，纠错过程由细胞控制，而不是由基因组本身控制，这一事实导致基因组不仅仅是一个"现成"的数据库。改变纠错的效率，允许插入和删除，使生物能够执行James Shapiro所说的自然基因工程[23-25]。

四、新趋势观点

关于新达尔文主义是否需要微调、扩展，或者可能完全放弃，现在有相当多的争论。在我回答这个问题之前，我想承认一个事实：新达尔文主义的现代综合理论非常有用。如果没有现代综合理论作为一个框架，整个数学生物学领域，如群体遗传学，可能不会在20世纪蓬勃发展。

但是，我也认为在新达尔文主义现代综合体的问题上已经达到了一个分水岭。正如我在其他地方详细论证的那样[22]，对Weismann和Wallace提出的原始理论有太多的实验性突破。如果我们使用一个不同的框架来发展一个更具包容性的理论，进化生物学将会进展得更快，如图21-3和图21-4所示。图21-3显示了扩展的进化合成EES(Pigliucci and Mueller[26])。

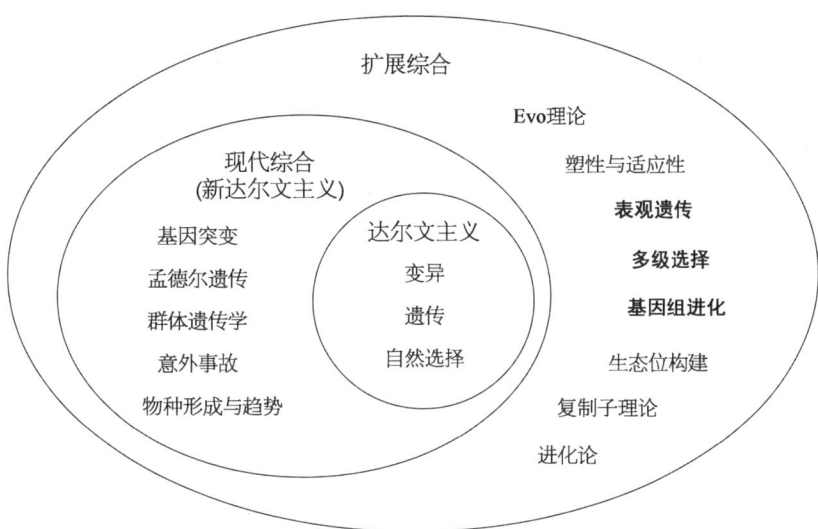

图 21-3 进化合成的扩展。每一个扩展都包含了以前的所有内容。基于 Pigliucci and Mueller[26]

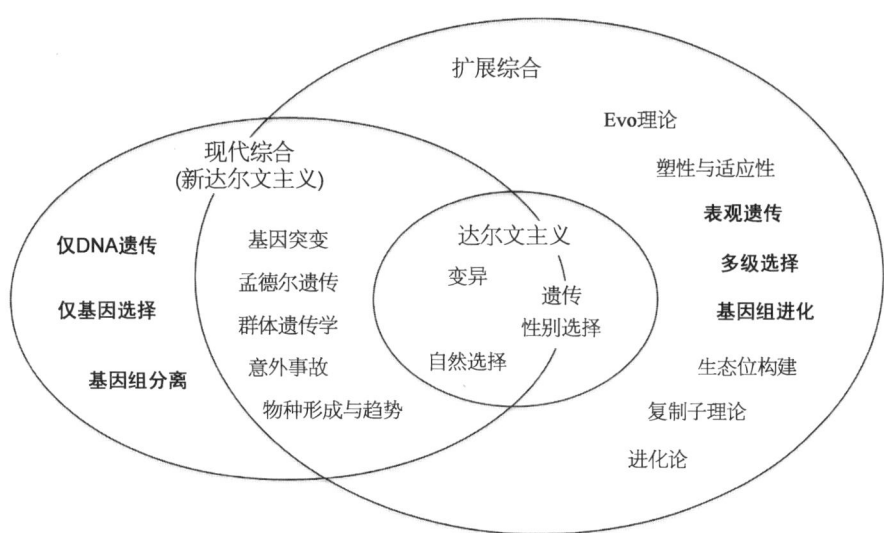

图 21-4 综合进化合成。Darwin 主义不再完全包含在新 Darwin 主义中,而是包含在综合之中。来自 Noble 2017[27]

我认为图 21-4 更好地代表了本章的结论,其中有几个重要的区别。首先,它代表了 Darwin 遗传观里包含了获得性状的遗传,而新达尔文主义排除了这一点。因此,Darwin 的遗传概念在一定程度上被排除在新达尔文主义现代综合理论之外,他的性别选择理论也是如此[28]。其次,它代表了扩展综合(在图 21-3 和图 21-4 中以粗体突出)的特征,这超出了 Weismann 和 Wallace 所定义的新达尔文主义的范围。该理论的特征被排除在相应的黑体字项目中。最左边的突出显示的项目与最右边的突出显示的项目对应,性别选择也包括两种达尔文主义的综合[29]。

如图 21-4 所示,集成综合作为达尔文思想的延伸比作为新达尔文主义的延伸更自然。我相信,实验事实的一个关键领域将使我们能够更准确地决定一个更具包容性的理论是外泌体研究,即本书的重点。这个领域正处于现代生物学基础问题的前沿,这就是为什么这本书会引起广泛关注的原因。因此,在结束这一章时,我将简要回顾一下关于外泌体和精子细胞传递 DNA 和 miRNA 的现代工作。

五、外泌体和 miRNA 跨代作用的现代研究

外泌体可能的作用之所以引起人们的极大兴趣,是因为任何外泌体 RNA、DNA、蛋白质转录因子等的传递都是通过生殖细胞越过魏斯曼屏障[30]。此外,这种分子模式的传递将至少在一定程度上代表外泌体来源细胞的基因组调控状态。Smith 和 Spadafora 在 2005 年回顾了这一领域,并总结道:

> 精子在几乎所有物种的转基因过程中都起着重要作用。SMGT(精子介导的基因转移)的潜在机制最好被看作是一种反转录转位介导的过程。由于精子细胞是外生遗传信息的载体,毫无疑问,它们有可能在各种物种的个体中引起遗传和表型的改变,值得进一步方法学研究,以优化其在生物技术中的应用[31]。

Spadafora 最近的一篇评论进一步证实了这一结论:

> 表观遗传学越来越被认为是一个潜在的促进进化的因素。基于看起来是不相关的结果,在这里我提出,含有 RNA 的纳米囊泡,主要是微小的调控 RNA,自体细胞组织往血液中释放,穿过魏斯曼屏障,到达附睾,最终被精子吸收。此后,这些信息在受精时传递给卵母细胞[32]。

Lavitrano 等[33]已经证明 SMGT 可以用于生产转基因猪,从而有可能发展出适合于人体器官移植的多基因转基因动物。类似的方法已经在小鼠[34]中得到了证明。在人类中,精液外泌体中 RNA 的表达谱可作为男性不育机制的标志[35,36]。

Valadi 等[37]已经证明,由外泌体传递的 miRNA 在不同物种之间转移时可以发挥功能,他们发现在将小鼠外泌体 RNA 转移到人类肥大细胞后,在受体细胞中发现了新的小鼠蛋白质,表明转移的外泌体 mRNA 在进入另一个细胞后可以被翻译。

这是一个迅速发展的领域。我们可能还没有听过 Darwin 的"芽球"理论,而 Lamarck 的理论也没有消失。

致谢

这一章的部分引用了我最近的一些出版物,这些出版物包括在参考文献中。

(关洁莹　译,朱颖婷　审校)

参考文献

[1] Darwin C. On the origin of species by means of natural selection, or the preservation of favoured races in the struggle for life. London: John Murray; 1859.
[2] Lamarck J-B. Philosophie zoologique, original edition of 1809 with introduction by Andre Pichot. Paris: Flammarion; 1994.
[3] Pichot A. Introduction. In: Philosophie zoologique. Paris: Flammarion; 1994.
[4] Lamarck, J-B., Histoire naturelle des animaux sans vertebres. 1815-1822, Paris: Verdiere.
[5] Lamarck J-B. Système analytique des connaissances positives de l'homme. Paris: Flammarion; 1820.
[6] Gould SJ. A tree grows in Paris: Lamarck's division of worms and revision of nature. In: The lying stones of Marrakech. Harmony Books; 2000.
[7] Mayr E. Introduction. In: On the origin of species. Cambridge, MA: Harvard; 1964. p. xxv-xxvi.
[8] Darwin C. The variation of animals and plants under domestication. London: John Murray; 1868.
[9] Weismann A. The germ-plasm: a theory of heredity. New York: Charles Scribner's Sons; 1893.
[10] Waddington CH. The strategy of the genes. London: Allen and Unwin; 1957.
[11] Weismann A. Essays upon heredity and kindred biological problems. Oxford University Press; 1889.
[12] Mayr E. The growth of biological thought. Cambridge, Mass: Harvard; 1982.
[13] Hanson M, Skinner M. Developmental origins of epigenetic transgenerational inheritance. Environ Epigenet 2016; https://doi.org/10.1093/eep/dvw002.
[14] Noble D. Differential and integral views of genetics in computational systems biology. Interface Focus 2011; 1: 7-15.
[15] Johannsen W. Elemente der Exakten Erblichkeitslehre. Jena: Gustav Fischer; 1909.
[16] Noble D. Central dogma or central debate? Physiology 2018; 33: 246-9. https://doi.org/10.1152/physiol.00017.2018.
[17] Kohl P, et al. Systems biology: an approach. Clin Pharmacol Ther 2010; 88: 25-33.
[18] Fisher RA. The genetical theory of natural selection. Oxford: Oxford University Press; 1930.
[19] Dawkins R. The selfish gene. vol.2006. Oxford: OUP; 1976.
[20] Noble D. Neo-Darwinism, the modern synthesis, and selfish genes: are they of use in physiology? J Physiol 2011; 589: 1007-15.
[21] Schrödinger E. What is life? Cambridge: Cambridge University Press; 1944.
[22] Noble D. Dance to the tune of life. In: Biological relativity. Cambridge: Cambridge University Press; 2016.
[23] Shapiro JA. Revisiting the central dogma in the 21st century. Ann N Y Acad Sci 2009; 1178: 6-28.
[24] Shapiro JA. Evolution: a view from the 21st century. Upper Saddle River, NJ: Pearson Education Inc.; 2011.
[25] Shapiro JA. Biological action in read-write genome evolution. Interface Focus 2017; 7. https://doi.org/10.1098/rsfs.2016.0115.
[26] Pigliucci M, Müller GB. Evolution — the extended synthesis. Cambridge, MA: MIT Press; 2010.
[27] Noble D. Evolution viewed from physics, physiology and medicine. Interface Focus 2017; 7. https://doi.org/10.1098/rsfs.2016.0159.
[28] Darwin C. The descent of man, and selection in relation to sex. London: John Murray; 1871.
[29] Noble R, Noble D. Harnessing stochasticity. How organisms make choices. Chaos 2018; 28. https://doi.org/10.1063/1.5039668.
[30] Smythies J, Edelstein L, Ramachandran V. Molecular mechanisms for the inheritance of acquired characteristics — exosomes, microRNA shuttling, fear and stress: Lamarck resurrected? Front Genet 2014; 5: 133.
[31] Smith K, Spadafora C. Sperm-mediated gene transfer: applications and implications. Bioessays 2005; 27: 551-62.
[32] Spadafora C. The "evolutionary field" hypothesis. Non-Mendelian transgenerational inheritance mediates diversification and evolution. Prog Biophys Mol Biol 2018; 134: 27-37.
[33] Lavitrano M, et al. Sperm-mediated gene transfer. Reprod Fertil Dev 2006; 18: 19-23.
[34] Lavitrano M, et al. Sperm cells as vectors for introducing foreign DNA into eggs: genetic transformation of mice. Cell 1989; 57: 717-23.
[35] Abu-Halima M, et al. Altered micro-ribonucleic acid expression profiles of extracellular microvesicles in the seminal plasma of patients with oligoasthenozoospermia. Fertil Steril 2016; 106: 1061-9.
[36] Barcelo M, et al. Exosomal microRNAs in seminal plasma are markers of the origin of azoospermia and can predict the presence of sperm in testicular tissue. Hum Reprod 2018; 33: 1087-98.
[37] Valadi H, et al. Exosome-mediated transfer of mRNAs and microRNA is a novel mechanism of genetic exchange between cells. Nat Cell Biol 2007; 9: 654-9.